Manual of Obstetrics and Gynecology for the Postgraduates

(Previously known as Master Pass in Obstetrics and Gynaecology)

Special Features

- Information provided, format of presentation and the method of learning, are consistent with the current system of education and evaluation
- Case-based rather than disease-based approach has been made. This is for the integration of knowledge with the clinical issues of diagnosis, investigations and management
- Unmatched content with complete coverage of the latest results from clinical trials
- Simple answers even for complex questions
- Discussion with the most advanced treatment modalities
- Adequate references at the end of each chapter for further study and clarification
- A number of relevant clinical images, drawings, illustrations, tables and summary lists, for easy understanding and reproducibility
- Targeted answers to more than 4,500 clinical questions
- Answers with explanations—more than 900 SBA and MCQs covering both the Obstetrics and Gynecology
- Wide coverage of 84 topics, with exciting new approach
- Model questions and answers with explanations for University Examination as well as MRCOG, MRCPI and MICOG Examinations
- Most trusted resource in Obstetrics and Gynecology.

Other Books by Author

- DC Dutta's Textbook of Obstetrics (8th Edition), Edited by Dr Konar
- DC Dutta's Textbook of Gynecology (7th Edition), Edited by Dr Konar
- Bedside Clinics and Viva-Voce in Obstetrics and Gynecology (4th Edition)
- A Guide to Clinical Obstetrics and Gynecology (4th Edition)
- Emergencies in Manipulative and Operative Obstetrics (4th Edition)
- Medical Disorders in Pregnancy—An Update (4th Edition)

Manual of Obstetrics and Gynecology for the Postgraduates

(Previously known as Master Pass in Obstetrics and Gynaecology)

Second Edition

Hiralal Konar (Hons; Gold Medalist)
MBBS (Cal), MD (PGI), DNB (India)
MNAMS, FACS (USA), FRCOG (London)
Chairman, Indian College of Obstetricians and Gynecologists (2013)
Professor, Department of Obstetrics and Gynecology
Calcutta National Medical College and Hospital, Kolkata, West Bengal, India

One-time Professor and Head, Department of Obstetrics and Gynecology
Midnapore Medical College and Hospital, West Bengal University of Health Sciences, Kolkata, India

Rotation Registrar in Obstetrics, Gynecology and Oncology
Northern and Yorkshire Region, Newcastle-upon-Tyne, UK
Examiner of MBBS, DGO, MD and PhD of different Indian Universities and National Board of Examination, New Delhi, India and other International Colleges (MRCPI) and Universities

Foreword
BN Chakravorty

JAYPEE *The Health Sciences Publisher*
New Delhi | London | Philadelphia | Panama

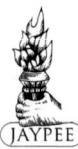 **Jaypee Brothers Medical Publishers (P) Ltd**

Headquarters

Jaypee Brothers Medical Publishers (P) Ltd.
4838/24, Ansari Road, Daryaganj
New Delhi 110 002, India
Phone: +91-11-43574357
Fax: +91-11-43574314
Email: jaypee@jaypeebrothers.com

Overseas Offices

J.P. Medical Ltd.
83, Victoria Street, London
SW1H 0HW (UK)
Phone: +44-20 3170 8910
Fax: +44-(0)20 3008 6180
Email: info@jpmedpub.com

Jaypee-Highlights Medical Publishers Inc.
City of Knowledge, Bld. 237, Clayton
Panama City, Panama
Phone: +1 507-301-0496
Fax: +1 507-301-0499
Email: cservice@jphmedical.com

JP Medical Inc.
325 Chestnut Street, Ste 412
Philadelphia, PA 19106
Phone: +1-267-519-9789
Email: support@jpmedus.com

Jaypee Brothers Medical Publishers (P) Ltd.
17/1-B, Babar Road, Block-B, Shaymali
Mohammadpur, Dhaka-1207, Bangladesh
Mobile: +08801912003485
Email: jaypeedhaka@gmail.com

Jaypee Brothers Medical Publishers (P) Ltd.
Bhotahity, Kathmandu, Nepal
Phone: +977-9741283608
Email: kathmandu@jaypeebrothers.com

Website: www.jaypeebrothers.com
Website: www.jaypeedigital.com

© 2017, Mrs Madhusri Konar

The views and opinions expressed in this book are solely those of the original contributor(s)/author(s) and do not necessarily represent those of editor(s) of the book.

All rights reserved. No part of this publication may be reproduced, stored or transmitted in any form or by any means, electronic, mechanical, photocopying, recording or otherwise, without the prior permission in writing of the publishers.

All brand names and product names used in this book are trade names, service marks, trademarks or registered trademarks of their respective owners. The publisher is not associated with any product or vendor mentioned in this book.

Medical knowledge and practice change constantly. This book is designed to provide accurate, authoritative information about the subject matter in question. However, readers are advised to check the most current information available on procedures included and check information from the manufacturer of each product to be administered, to verify the recommended dose, formula, method and duration of administration, adverse effects and contraindications. It is the responsibility of the practitioner to take all appropriate safety precautions. Neither the publisher nor the author(s)/editor(s) assume any liability for any injury and/or damage to persons or property arising from or related to use of material in this book.

This book is sold on the understanding that the publisher is not engaged in providing professional medical services. If such advice or services are required, the services of a competent medical professional should be sought.

Every effort has been made where necessary to contact holders of copyright to obtain permission to reproduce copyright material. If any have been inadvertently overlooked, the publisher will be pleased to make the necessary arrangements at the first opportunity.

Inquiries for bulk sales may be solicited at: jaypee@jaypeebrothers.com

Manual of Obstetrics and Gynecology for the Postgraduates

First Edition: **2013**
Second Edition: **2017**

ISBN: 978-93-86056-28-3

Printed at: Samrat Offset Pvt. Ltd.

Dedicated

to

*those who strive relentlessly
to develop quality care
for
women's health*

Foreword

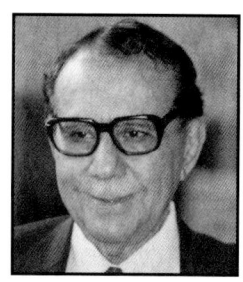

There are many objectives with which a book in medical discipline is written or compiled. The first and foremost is to propagate contemporary and currently available new information and discoveries in the topic on which a chapter has been written. The second objective is to suggest some new ideas or concepts, based on which further improvement in our knowledge about pathogenesis, diagnosis and management can be achieved. The last and most important objective is to outline the materials in each chapter in such a manner which is easily understandable and reproducible even by a new entrant in medical discipline.

The first two objectives will help those who are already in profession or proactive for quite sometime and the last one will benefit immensely the fresh candidates who are aspiring for medical graduation or if they are already graduates, to acquire higher postgraduate diplomas or degrees. It gives me immense pleasure to write about **Manual of Obstetrics and Gynecology for the Postgraduates**. Examination system all over the world is under constant refinement. Progressive advancement in technology and science, virtually has changed every area of obstetrics and gynecology substantially. Simultaneously the examination system has changed to produce quality medical graduates and specialists in the discipline.

The earlier pattern of essay questions and long clinical case, have been proved unreliable methods of assessing candidates' knowledge, clinical as well as communication skills. Essay questions have been replaced by more reliable methods like—Short Review Questions, Multiple Choice Questions (MCQs), Single Best Answer (SBA) and Extended Matching Questions (EMQs). Clinical skills are assessed by Objective Structured Clinical Examinations (OSCEs).

Manual of Obstetrics and Gynecology for the Postgraduates is primarily aimed to help a candidate to qualify and to pass the examination for obtaining the postgraduate degree. This book is designed to provide new format of testing knowledge and clinical skills. This book, to my knowledge, is the first of its kind to have all the component of new assessment system.

I am proud to say that Professor Hiralal Konar, is one of my brilliant students. He has proved his excellency through dedication in the profession and also in the largest national organization of the country, The Federation of Obstetric and Gynaecological Societies of India (FOGSI) and as the Chairman of Indian College of Obstetricians and Gynaecologists (ICOG). He is well known for his two other books that are widely read in India as well as abroad, DC Dutta's Textbook of Obstetrics and DC Dutta's Textbook of Gynecology.

I believe, this book would be of immense help to the students, residents and all the specialists in this discipline of Obstetrics and Gynecology.

I congratulate him and wish his endeavor a huge success.

Professor (Dr) BN Chakravorty
MO, FRCOG, DSc
Director, Institute of Reproductive Medicine
HB-36/A/3, Sector – III
Salt Lake City
Kolkata 700106

Preface to the Second Edition

Manual of Obstetrics and Gynecology for the Postgraduates is designed to provide a synoptic review of management issues covering the key areas in obstetrics and gynecology. The textbook with its classic presentation provides knowledge that has no alternative. But failure of clinical application of the same, makes a difference in examination performance. This book is focussed to polish examination performance to improve the chance of passing the theory, clinical as well as the table viva-voce part of the examination.

Case-based rather than disease-based discussions have been made to provide the updated and evidence-based information to the candidate.

This book addresses the new format of examination system currently pursued all over the world. Extensive discussions have been made with Objective Structured Clinical Examinations (OSCEs), Single Best Answer (SBA), Multiple Choice Questions (MCQs) and Extended Matching Questions (EMQs). Model questions with answers in all the above-mentioned areas have been provided and these are of distinct values. This book aims to help candidates to test and assess their knowledge and to find out the areas of weakness.

The current examination system explores the candidates' analytical power rather than simple factual recall. ***Manual of Obstetrics and Gynecology for the Postgraduates*** helps appropriate application of textbook knowledge in respect of an individual clinical scenario.

Commonly discussed topics are selected. A broad range of themes have been incorporated in different sections (84 chapters) of this book with graded difficulty. I am ever grateful to my teacher Professor (Dr) BN Chakravorty for his contribution of the topic 'Infertility and Assisted Reproductive Technology (ART)' (Section 5) in this book. History in medicine and eponyms have been presented (Section 12). I personally feel, one should know about the ideals, whose footsteps we follow while working in the discipline.

While writing this book, I have deviated from the traditional approach of a textbook, with expectation that core knowledge to be covered by a textbook. Attempts have been made to incorporate much of the available evidences upon which our practice in obstetrics and gynecology should base.

Manual of Obstetrics and Gynecology for the Postgraduates is intended to help medical students, residents aspiring as well appearing for the postgraduate examinations MS, MD, DGO (University), DNB, FNB, Fellowship Exit Examination (National Board), RCPI, MICOG, MRCOG (membership examination of international colleges), American Board (USMLE), specialized nurses (BSc, MSc), midwives as well as specialists in the discipline of obstetrics and gynecology.

I do hope this comprehensive book will be of immense educational resource to the readers.

I do welcome the views of students/teachers for their suggestions, comments through our website: www.hiralalkonar.com.

Hiralal Konar

Preface to the First Edition

'Master Pass' is designed to provide comprehensive review of management issues covering the key areas in Obstetrics and Gynaecology. Textbook knowledge has got no alternative. But failure of clinical application of the same, makes the examination performance poor. 'Master Pass' focuses polishing examination performances to improve the chance of passing the theory, clinical, as well as the table viva-voce part of the examination.

Case-based and topic-based discussions have been made to provide the updated and evidence-based information to the candidate.

'Master Pass' addresses the new format of examination system currently persued all over the world. Extensive discussions have been made with Objective Structured Clinical Examinations (OSCEs), Multiple Choice Questions (MCQs), Extended Matching Questions (EMQs) and Short Answer Questions (SAQs). Model approach with questions and answers in all the above-mentioned areas have been made and these are of distinct value. This book aims to help the candidate to test and assess their knowledge and to find out the areas of weakness.

The current examination system explores the candidates' analytical power rather than simple factual recall. 'Master Pass' helps appropriate application of textbook knowledge in respect of an individual clinical scenario.

Commonly discussed topics are selected. A broad range of themes have been incorporated in different sections (total 6) of this book with graded difficulty. I am so grateful to my teacher Prof BN Chakravorty for his contribution of the topic 'Infertility' (Section III) in the book.

History in medicine and eponyms have been presented (Section VI). I personally feel, one should know the characters in whose steps we follow while working in the discipline.

While writing 'Master Pass', I have moved away from the traditional approach of a textbook, with expectation that core knowledge to be covered by a textbook. Attempts have been made to incorporate much of the available evidences upon which our practice in Obstetrics and Gynaecology should base.

Master Pass is intended to help medical students, residents aspiring for, as well appearing the master examination [MS, MD, DGO (University), DNB, FNB, Fellowship Exit Examination (National Board)], MICOG, MRCOG, specialized nurses (BSc, MSc), midwives as well as specialists in the discipline of Obstetrics and Gynaecology.

I do hope this comprehensive book will be of immense educational resource to the readers.

I do welcome the views of the students/teachers for their suggestions, comments through our website: www.hiralalkonar.com.

This book is dedicated to all who work relentlessly in Obstetrics and Gynaecology to develop quality care for women's health.

Hiralal Konar

Acknowledgments

I have consulted many of my esteemed colleagues in the country and abroad, a multitude of eminent authors, many current evidence-based studies, guidelines and recommendations particularly RCOG, London; ACOG; WHO; RANZCOG; SOGC. I do sincerely acknowledge my legacy to all of them including the related authors and publishers.

I am deeply indebted to my esteemed teachers Professor KM Gun, MO, FRCOG, FRCS, FACS; Professor BN Chakravorty, MO, FRCOG, DSc, Director, Institute of Reproductive Medicine (IRM), Kolkata; Prof DC Dutta, MO (Late), author of Textbook of Obstetrics and Textbook of Gynecology. I sincerely acknowledge the following teachers across the country and abroad for their valuable feedback to enrich our books. Their comments, suggestions have helped to shape this new edition. I hope, I have listed all those who have contributed and apologize if any names have been missed inadvertently.

Professor Sabaratnam Arulkumaran, St George's, University of London, President FIGO (Past); Paul Fogarty, Senior Vice President, RCOG, London; Mr Michael O'Connel, Royal College of Physicians, Dublin; Mr. Tony Hollingworth, Queen Mary, University of London; Professor PS Chakraborty, IPGMER, Kolkata; Professor P Mukherjee, Kolkata Medical College; Professor C Das, NRSMCH; Professor A Biswas, CNMC, Kolkata; Professor Habibullah, Professor P Desari, JIPMER, Puducherry; Professor A Pedicaile, CMC Vellore; Professor A Kriplani, Professor KK Ray, AIIMS, New Delhi; Professor V Das, KGMU, Lucknow; Professor RL Singh, RIMS, Imphal; Professor Ng Indra Kumar, Imphal; Professor Santa Singh, NEGRIMS, Shillong; Professor R Chauhan NSCB, Jabalpur; Prof V Das, PGIMER, Chandigarh; Professor (Mrs) L Das, Professor PC Mahapatra, Professor Maya Padhi, Professor S Kanungo, SCBMC, Cuttack; Professor NR Agarwal, Professor LK Pandey, Banaras Hindu University, Banaras; Professor Ava Rani Sinha, Patna; Professor Hemali Sinha, AIIMS. Patna; Professor A Bhaniwad, JSS MCH, Mysore; Professor A Huria GMCH, Chandigarh; Professor RShrivastava BRDMCH, Gorakhpur; Professor S Murthy Davangare, Karnataka; Professor K Pandey, GSVMMC, Kanpur; Professor S Minhans, IGMC, Shimla, Himachal Pradesh; Professor R Bulusu, MVJMCH, Bengaluru; Professor Jayanthi, Kempegowda Medical College, Bengaluru; Professor S Rani, Thanjavur MCH, Tamil Nadu. Professor Hemant Deshpande, Professor Himadri Bal, Pune; Professor R Ahmed, Dibrugarh; Professor A Goswami, Guwahati; Professor S Dutta, NBMCH, Siliguri; Professor M Sarkar MMCH, Malda; Professor J Mukherjee, NBMCH, Siliguri; Professor BK Kanungo, Gangtok; Professor M Pradhan, Tripura; Professor DK Bhowmik, JNMCH, Maharashtra; Professor Renu Rohatgi, Patna; Professor Gita B Banerjee, Bankura; Professor Farhana Dewan, Professor Kohinoor Begum, Dhaka; Professor Rokeya Begum, Chittagong; Professor Rowshan Ara Begum, Professor Sabera Khatun, Dhaka; Professor S Nurjahan Bhuiyan, Chittagong; Professor Jyoti Bindal, GRMC, Gwalior; Professor Seema Hakim, AMU, Aligarh; Professor RP Wadhwa, GMC, Mewat, Haryana; Professor Beena Bhatnagar, NIMS, Jaipur; Professor Manpreet Kaur, DMC, Ludhiana; Professor MG Hiremath, Hubli; Professor MB Bellad, Belgium; Professor Ajith, Kannur; Professor Malik Goonewardene, University of Ruhuna, Sri Lanka; Professor HR Seneviratne, Colombo, Sri Lanka; Professor Jyandip Nath, Guwahati; Professor Murali Pai, KMC, Manipal; Professor Nilesh Dalal, MGMC, Indore; Professor Sudesh Agarwal, SPMC, Bikaner; Professor Pushpa Dahiya, Rohtak, PIMS; Professor Sumangala, GMC, Calicut; Professor Mary Daniel, PIMS, Puducherry; Professor

Sasikala, SMVMCH, Puducherry; Professor Atiya Sayed, AIMS, J&K; Professor N Chaudhury, HIMS, Dehradun; Professor Shehnaz Taing, GMC, Srinagar; Professor Abha Singh, LHMC, Delhi; Professor S Nanda, PGI, Rohtak; Professor N Chutani, SMC and Professor SS Gulati, SMC, Greater Noida; Professor Raksha Arora, SMC, Ghaziabad; Professor Jaya Chaturvedi, AIIMS, Rishikesh; Professor Abha Singh, JNMCH, Raipur; Professor Rehana Nazam, TMU, Moradabad; Professor Bharati Misra, MKCG, Brahmapur; Professor Neelam Pradhan, Professor Meeta Singh, Tribhuvan University and Teaching Hospital (TU and TH), Kathmandu; Professor S Mishra, VMC, Nepal; Professor Sujatha Sharma, GMC, Amritsar; Professor Madhu Nagpal, SGRDMC, Amritsar; Professor Promila Jindal; PIMS, Jalandhar.

I would like to extend my thanks to many of the readers including the residents and students, who have contacted me with suggestions and seeking clarifications through e-mails. Their inputs have been valuable and are much appreciated. I wish I could mention their names individually.

I am extremely grateful to Mrs Madhusri Konar, MA, BEd for all her insightful secretarial accomplishment in support of the book. I thank Dr Dorothy Dessa for her assistance throughout. I sincerely thank Md Jakir Hossain, MSc, BEd for his diligent and expert work to accomplish the entire Second Edition of this book.

I sincerely thank Shri JP Vij (Group Chairman), Mr Ankit Vij (Group President), Ms Chetna Malhotra Vohra (Associate Director–Content Strategy), Mr PS Ghuman (AGM Production), Jaypee Brothers Medical Publishers (P) Ltd and production staff to maintain the commitment for this book.

Contents

Section 1: Obstetrics

1. **Objective Structured Clinical Examination in Obstetrics** 3
   - Case 1: Severe Pre-eclampsia *3*
   - Case 2: Counseling *6*
   - Case 3: Ectopic Pregnancy *7*
   - Case 4: Abruptio Placentae; Placenta Previa *10*
   - Case 5: Unstable Lie *12*
   - Case 6: Nonprogress of Labor *13*
   - Case 7: Cardiotocography-I *15*
   - Case 8: Cardiotocography-II *18*
   - Case 9: Management of Labor (Partograph-I) *20*
   - Case 10: Management of Labor (Partograph-II) *22*
   - Case 11: Primary Postpartum Hemorrhage *25*
   - Case 12: Secondary Postpartum Hemorrhage *27*
   - Case 13: Surgical Management of Postpartum Hemorrhage (PPH) *29*
   - Case 14: Pregnancy and Labor in a Woman with Prior Cesarean Delivery *36*
   - Case 15: Puerperal Pyrexia *37*
   - Case 16: Multiple Pregnancy *38*
   - Case 17: Neural Tube Defects *40*
   - Case 18: Anencephaly *41*
   - Case 19: Hydrocephalus *43*
   - Case 20: Cystic Hygroma *44*
2. **Self-Assessment in Obstetrics** 46

Section 2: Gynecology

3. **Objective Structured Clinical Examination (OSCE) in Gynecology** 107
   - Case 1: Polycystic Ovarian Syndrome (PCOS) *107*
   - Case 2: Endometriosis *110*
   - Case 3: Primary Amenorrhea *115*
   - Case 4: Secondary Amenorrhea *118*
   - Case 5: Pelvic Pain *119*
   - Case 6: Infertility *120*
   - Case 7: Hematocolpos *123*
   - Case 8: Infertility *124*

Case 9: Hydatidiform Mole   126
Case 10: Endometriosis   129
Case 11: Cervical Fibroid   130
Case 12: Carcinoma Cervix   131
Case 13: Carcinoma Endometrium   135
Case 14: Carcinoma of the Ovary   138
Case 15: Carcinoma Cervix   141
Case 16: Menopause and Hormone Replacement Therapy (HRT)   144
Case 17: Carcinoma Cervix   146
Case 18: Hysterectomy and Oophorectomy   148
Case 19: Postmenopausal Bleeding   149
Case 20: Inherited Cancers and the Management   152

4. **Self-Assessment in Gynecology** 154

Section 3: Obstetric Discussion

5. **Preterm Birth and Management Issues** 225
6. **Gestational Diabetes Mellitus** 230
7. **Obesity in Pregnancy** 237
8. **Monochorionic Twin Pregnancy** 242
9. **Prenatal Screening for Fetal Abnormalities** 250
10. **Severe Pre-eclampsia and Eclampsia** 258
11. **HELLP Syndrome** 263
12. **Cesarean Section** 266
13. **Placenta Previa, Placenta Previa Accreta and Vasa Previa** 271
14. **Perimortem Cesarean Section** 276
15. **Puerperal Sepsis** 279
16. **Maternal Near Miss** 285
17. **Cesarean Delivery on Maternal Request** 289
18. **Classification of Evidence Levels and Grades of Recommendations** 294

Section 4: Gynecology Discussion

19. **Recurrent Miscarriage (First and Second Trimesters)** 299
20. **Tubal Ectopic Pregnancy** 307
21. **Cervical Insufficiency (Incompetence)** 310
22. **Heavy Menstrual Bleeding** 314
23. **Urinary Incontinence** 319

24. Polycystic Ovary Syndrome 323
25. Male and Female Sterilization 327
26. Gestational Trophoblastic Disease 334
27. Carcinoma of the Endometrium (Early Stage Diseases) 339
28. Pregnancy of Unknown Location 343
29. Abnormal Uterine Bleeding 348
30. Endoscopy in Gynecology (Laparoscopic Surgery) 352
31. Robotic Surgery in Gynecology 355

Section 5: Infertility and Assisted Reproductive Technology (ART)

32. Current Concept in Physiology of Ovulation 361
33. Infertility Evaluation and Management 367
34. Female Infertility 370
35. Male Infertility 383
36. Assisted Reproductive Technology (ART) 388
37. Management Strategies for Low Responder Woman 396
38. Third Party Reproduction 400

Section 6: Maternal Medicine (Short Obstetric Reviews)

39. Obstetric Case Presentation 405
40. Anemia in Pregnancy 407
41. Hemoglobinopathy 411
42. Sickle Cell Disease in Pregnancy 414
43. Thyroid Dysfunction in Pregnancy 418
44. Heart Disease in Pregnancy 425
45. Gestational Age and Cesarean Delivery 429
46. Place of Thromboprophylaxis during Pregnancy 432
47. External Cephalic Version 434
48. Diminished Fetal Movements 436
49. Transfusion in Obstetrics 441
50. Obstetric Cholestasis 445
51. Diabetic Nephropathy 446
52. Renal Transplant 448
53. Non Hemorrhagic Shock in Obstetrics 450

Section 7: Short Reviews in Gynecology

54. **Place of Prophylactic Salpingectomy or Salpingo-oophorectomy in Current Gynecologic Practice** 463
55. **Endometrial Carcinoma** 466
56. **Bariatric Surgery in Gynecology and Obstetrics** 469
57. **Fertility Conserving Options for Women with Gynecologic Malignancies** 473
58. **Fertility Conserving Options for Women with Cervical Cancer** 476
59. **Fertility Conserving Options for Women with Endometrial Cancer** 478
60. **Advances in Contraception** 480
61. **Interventional Radiology in Obstetrics and Gynecology** 487
62. **Surgical Site Infection** 489
63. **Abnormal Uterine Bleeding: Investigations and Management Issues** 491
64. **Subfertility and Pelvic Endometriosis** 497
65. **Medical Methods of Termination of Pregnancy** 499

Section 8: Intrapartum Electronic Fetal Monitoring

66. **Fetal Response in Labor** 503
67. **Fetal Heart Rate Patterns** 505
68. **Fetal ECG** 509
69. **Management of Nonreassuring Fetal Status (NRFS)** 511

Section 9: Perinatal Medicine

70. **Immunization during Pregnancy and Breastfeeding** 517
71. **Noninvasive Prenatal Testing for Fetal Chromosomal Abnormality** 521
72. **Congenital Perinatal and Neonatal Infections** 525
73. **Congenital HIV Infection and AIDS** 527
74. **Varicella Zoster Virus (Chickenpox) Infection** 530
75. **Rubella in Pregnancy** 532
76. **Cytomegalovirus Infection in Pregnancy** 534
77. **Viral Hepatitis in Pregnancy** 536
78. **Listeriosis in Pregnancy** 540
79. **Toxoplasmosis in Pregnancy** 542
80. **Group B Streptococci Infection in Pregnancy** 545

Section 10: MRCOG Examination

81. **PART I MRCOG Examination** 549
82. **PART II MRCOG Examination** 574

Section 11: MRCOG (EMQs)

83. **Extended Matching Questions (EMQs)** 585

Section 12: In Whose Footsteps We Follow

84. **History in Obstetrics and Gynecology** 597

Index 603

Abbreviations

AACE	American Association of Clinical Endocrinology	BPP	Biophysical Profile
AC	Abdominal Circumference	BPV	Bioprosthetic Heart Valves
ACA	Anticardiolipin Antibodies	BSO	Bilateral Salpingo-oophorectomy
ACE	Angiotensin Converting Enzyme	BTB	Breakthrough Bleeding
ACHOIS	Australian Carbohydrate Intolerance Study	CBAVD	Congenital Bilateral Absence of Vas Deferens
ACOG	American College of Obstetricians and Gynecologists	CC	Clomiphene Citrate
		CDC	Centers for Disease Control and Prevention
ACS	Acute Chest Syndrome	CDMR	Cesarean Delivery on Maternal Request
ACTH	Adrenocorticotropic Hormone	CECT	Contrast-enhanced Computed Tomography
ADA	American Diabetes Association		
AEDF	Absent End-diastolic Flow	CEMACH	Confidential Enquiry into Maternal and Child Health
AEDs	Antiepileptic Drugs		
AFASS	Affordable, Feasible, Accessible, Sustainable and Safe	cff-DNA	Cell-free Fetal DNA
		CFTR	Cystic Fibrosis Transmembrane Regulator
AFC	Antral Follicle Count	CGH	Comparative Genomic Hybridization
AFE	Amniotic Fluid Embolism	CIN	Cervical Intraepithelial
AFP	Alpha-fetoprotein	CIS	Carcinoma *in situ*
AFS	American Fertility Society	CMV	Cytomegalovirus
AIDS	Acquired Immune Deficiency Syndrome	CNS	Central Nervous System
		CO	Combined Obesity
ALT	Alanine Transaminase	COCs	Combine Oral Contraceptives
AMH	Anti-Müllerian Hormone	COS	Controlled Ovarian Stimulation
APA	Antiphospholipid Antibody	COX	Cycloxygenase
APAS	Antiphospholipid Antibody Syndrome	CPD	Cephalopelvic Disproportion
		CPR	Cardiopulmonary Resuscitation
API	Association of Physicians of India	CPR	Cumulative Pregnancy Rate
ARM	Artificial Rupture of the Membranes	CPT	Complete Perineal Tear
ART	Assisted Reproductive Technology	CRH	Corticotropin-releasing Hormone
ASRM	American Society for Reproductive Medicine	CRS	Congenital Rubella Syndrome
		CS	Cesarean Section
AST	Aspartate Transaminase	CSF	Cerebrospinal Fluid
ASTEC	A Study in the Treatment of Endometrial Cancer	CT	Computed Tomography
		CTG	Cardiotocography
ATA	American Thyroid Association	CTPA	Computed Tomographic Pulmonary Angiography
BBT	Basal Body Temperature	CVD	Cardiovascular Disease
BMD	Bone Mineral Density	CVS	Chorionic Villus Sampling
BMI	Body Mass Index	CZ	Carbimazole
BP	Blood Pressure	D&C	Dilatation and Curettage
BPAD	Bipolar Affective Disorder	DF	Dominant Follicle
BPD	Biparietal Diameter	DFMC	Daily Fetal Movement Count
BPM	Beats per Minute	DHEAS	Dehydroepiandosterone Sulphate

DIC	Disseminated Intravascular Coagulation	HC	Head Circumference
DIPSI	Diabetes in Pregnancy Society of India	hCG	Human Chorionic Gonadotropin
		HCV	Hepatitis C Virus
DMPA	Depot Medroxyprogesterone Acetate	HDFN	Hemolytic Disease of the Fetus and Newborn
DPG	Diphosphoglycerate	HDL	High Density Lipoprotein
DTIC	Distal Tubal Intraepithelial Carcinoma	HDR	High Dose Radiation
		HDU	High Dependency Unit
DVT	Deep Vein Thrombosis	HFEA	Human Fertilization and Embryology Authority
E	Eclampsia	HELLP	Hemolysis, Elevated Liver Enzymes, Low Platelet count
E2	Estradiol		
EC	Endometrial Curettage	hGH	Human Growth Hormone
ECG	Electrocardiogram	HGSOC	High-grade Serous Ovarian Cancer
ECV	External Cephalic Version	HIV	Human Immunodeficiency Virus
EGF	Epidermal Growth Factor	HLA	Human Leukocyte Antigen
EOCs	Epithelial Ovarian Cancers	HMB	Heavy Menstrual Bleeding
EPAU	Early Pregnancy Assessment Unit	HMG	Human Menopausal Gonadotropin
ESHRE	European Society of Human Reproduction and Embryology	HPL	Human Placental Lactogen
		HPV	Human Papilloma Virus
		HRT	Hormone Replacement Therapy
		HWY	Hundred Woman Years (Pregnancy)
FBC	Full Blood Count		
FDP	Fibrinogen Degradation Products	IADPSG	International Association of Diabetes and Pregnancy Study Groups
FET	Frozen Embryo Transfer		
FFP	Fresh Frozen Plasma	IAP	Intrapartum Antibiotic Prophylaxis
FGR	Fetal Growth Restriction	ICD	International Statistical Classification of Disease
FIGO	International Federation of Gynaecology and Obstetrics		
		ICSI	Intracytoplasmic Sperm Injection
FISH	Fluorescence *in situ* Hybridization	ICU	Intensive Care Unit
FL	Femur Length	IDDM	Insulin-dependent Diabetes Mellitus
FOGSI	Federation of Obstetricians and Gynaecologists of India	IFA	Immunofluorescence Assay
		IGF	Insulin-like Growth Factor
FSH	Follicle Stimulating Hormone	IPV	Inactivated Polio Vaccine
FVS	Fetal Varicella Syndrome	ITP	Idiopathic Thrombocytopenic Purpura
GBS	Group B Streptococci		
GDM	Gestational Diabetes Mellitus	ITS	Indian Thyroid Society
GIFT	Gamete Intrafallopian Transfer	ITU	Intensive Therapy Unit
GIT	Gastrointestinal Tract	IUCD	Intrauterine Contraceptive Device
GnRH	Gonadotropin Releasing Hormone	IUD	Intrauterine Device
GO	Generalized Obesity	IUFD	Intrauterine Fetal Demise
GSI	Genuine Stress Incontinence	IUGR	Intrauterine Growth Restriction
GTD	Gestational Trophoblastic Disease	IUI	Intrauterine Insemination
GTN	Gestational Trophoblastic Neoplasia	IVC	Inferior Vena Cava
		IVF-ET	*In vitro* Fertilization and Embryo Transfer
HAART	Highly Active Antiretroviral Therapy		
HAPO	Hyperglycemia and Adverse Pregnancy Outcome	IVH	Intraventricular Hemorrhage
		IVIG	Intravenous Immunoglobulin
HAV	Hepatitis A Virus	LAC	Lupus Anticoagulant
HbF	Fetal Hemoglobin	LARVT	Laparoscopic Assisted Radical Vaginal Trachelectomy
HBV	Hepatitis B Virus		

LAVH	Laparoscopic Assisted Vaginal Hysterectomy	**MTX**	Methotrexate
LBC	Liquid-based Cytology	**MVA**	Manual Vacuum Aspiration
LDH	Lactate Dehydrogenase	**MVP**	Maximum Vertical Pocket
LDL	Low Density Lipoprotein	**NEC**	Necrotizing Enterocolitis
LFT	Liver Function Test	**NICE**	National Institute for Health and Clinical Excellence
LGSOC	Low-grade Serous Ovarian Cancer	**NICHD**	National Institute of Child Health and Human Development
LH	Luteinizing Hormone	**NICU**	Neonatal Intensive Care Unit
LLETZ	Large Loop Excision of the Transformation Zone	**NIPT**	Noninvasive Prenatal Testing
LMP	Last Menstrual Period	**NSAIDs**	Nonsteroidal Antiinflammatory Drugs
LMWH	Low Molecular Weight Heparin	**NTD**	Neural Tube Defects
LNG-IUD	Levonorgestrel-intrauterine Device	**OA**	Occiput Anterior
LNG-IUS	Levonorgestrel-intrauterine System	**OAB**	Overactive Bladder
LOA	Left Occiput Anterior	**OAT**	Oligoasthenoteratozoospermia
LOD	Laparoscopic Ovarian Drilling	**OGTT**	Oral Glucose Tolerance Test
LOS	Laparoscopic Ovarian Surgery	**OHSS**	Ovarian Hyperstimulation Syndrome
LPD	Luteal Phase Defect	**OP**	Occiput Posterior
LSCS	Lower Segment Cesarean Section	**OSCE**	Objective Structured Clinical Examination
LUF	Luteinized Unruptured Follicle	**OTA**	Oligoasthenoteratozoospermia
LVSI	Lymphovascular Space Involvement	**PAPP-A**	Pregnancy Associated Plasma Protein-A
MAHA	Microangiopathic Hemolytic Anemia	**PCOS**	Polycystic Ovarian Syndrome
MAP	Mean Arterial Pressure	**PCR**	Polymerase Chain Reaction
MC	Monochorionic	**PDA**	Patent Ductus Arteriosus
MCA	Middle Cerebral Artery	**PE**	Pulmonary Embolism
MCA-PSV	Middle Cerebral Artery Peak Systolic Velocity	**PESA**	Percutaneous Epididymal Sperm Aspiration
MCDA	Monochorionic Diamniotic	**PET**	Positron Emission Tomography
MCTP	Monochorionic Twin Pregnancy	**PGD**	Prenatal Genetic Diagnosis
MDTA	Multidisciplinary Team Approach	**PID**	Pelvic Inflammatory Disease
MEA	Microwave Endometrial Ablation	**PMB**	Postmenopausal Bleeding
MFR	Monthly Fecundity Rate	**PMS**	Premenstrual Syndrome
MgSO$_4$	Magnesium Sulfate	**POD**	Pouch of Douglas
MHV	Mechanical Heart Valves	**POF**	Premature Ovarian Failure
MMK	Marshall-Marchetti-Krantz	**POP**	Pelvic Organ Prolapse
MMR	Maternal Mortality Rate	**POP**	Progestin only Pill
MNM	Maternal Near Miss	**PORTEC**	Postoperative Radiation Therapy in Endometrial Cancer
MOM	Multiple of the Median	**PPA**	Primary Peritoneal Adenocarcinoma
MPGS	Massively Parallel Genomic Sequencing	**PPIUCD**	Postpartum Intrauterine Contraceptive Devices
MRg FUS	MR-guided Focused Ultrasound	**PRBCs**	Packed Red Blood Cells
MRI	Magnetic Resonance Imaging	**PRES**	Posterior Reversible Encephalopathy Syndrome
MRSA	Methicillin-resistant *Staphylococcus Aureus*	**PROM**	Premature Rupture of Membranes
MSAFP	Maternal Serum Alpha-fetoprotein	**PSOC**	Papillary Serous Ovarian Cancer
MTCT	Mother-to-child Transmission		
MTHFR	Methylenetetrahydrofolate Reductase		
MTP	Medical Termination of Pregnancy		

PSP1	Pregnancy Specific Protein 1	**TIC**	Tubal Intraepithelial Carcinoma
PSTT	Placental Site Trophoblastic Tumor	**TLH**	Total Laparoscopic Hysterectomy
PTD	Postpartum Thyroid Dysfunction	**TNFs**	Tumor Necrosis Factors
PT	Prothrombin Time	**TOT**	Transobturator Tape
PTT	Partial Thromboplastin Time	**TPO**	Thyroid Peroxidase
PTU	Propylthiouracil	**TPOAbs**	Thyroid Anti-TPO Antibodies
PUL	Pregnancy of Unknown Location	**TRAP**	Twin Reverse Arterial Perfusion
PVD	Peripheral Vascular Disease	**TRH**	Thyrotropin Releasing Hormone
RALH	Robotic Assisted Laparoscopic Hysterectomy	**TSHRAbs**	Thyrotropin Receptor Autoantibodies
RCOG	Royal College of Obstetrics and Gynecology	**TTN**	Transient Tachypnea of the Newborn
RCTs	Randomized Controlled Trials	**TTTS**	Twin-twin Transfusion Syndrome
RDS	Respiratory Distress Syndrome	**TVS**	Transvaginal Sonography
RFM	Reduced Fetal Movements	**TVT**	Tension-free Vaginal Tape
RMI	Risk of Malignancy Index	**TZ**	Transformation Zone
ROMA	Risk of Ovarian Malignancy Algorithm	**UAE**	Uterine Artery Embolization
		UE3	Unconjugated Estriol
RVT	Radical Vaginal Trachelectomy	**UFH**	Unfractionated Heparin
SAMM	Severe Acute Maternal Morbidity	**UI**	Urinary Incontinence
SCD	Sickle Cell Disease	**USG**	Ultrasonography
SCJ	Squamocolumnar Junction	**UTI**	Urinary Tract Infections
SGA	Small for Gestational Age	**VaIN**	Vaginal Intraepithelial Neoplasia
SHBG	Sex Hormone Binding Globulin	**VBAC**	Vaginal Birth After Cesarean
SI	Shock Index	**VBAC-TOL**	Vaginal Birth After Cesarean-Trial of Labor
SIL	Squamous Intraepithelial Lesion		
SIS	Saline Infusion Sonography	**VCB**	Vaginal Cuff Brachytherapy
SLE	Systemic Lupus Erythematosus	**VEGF**	Vascular Endothelial Growth Factor
SSI	Surgical Site Infections	**VIA**	Visual Inspection using Acetic Acid
STIs	Sexually Transmitted Infections	**VKA**	Vitamin K Antagonist
SUI	Stress Urinary Incontinence	**VTE**	Venous Thromboembolism
SUZI	Subzonal Insemination	**VVF**	Vesicovaginal Fistula
TAH	Total Abdominal Hysterectomy	**VZIG**	Varicella Zoster Immunoglobulin
TBEA	Thermal Balloon Endometrial Ablation	**VZV**	Varicella Zoster Virus
TCRE	Transcervical Resection of Endometrium	**WHO**	World Health Organization
		WLTC	Women with Life-threatening Condition
TEC	Thromboembolic Complications		

SECTION 1

Obstetrics

Section Outline

Ch. 1. Objective Structured Clinical Examination in Obstetrics
- Case 1: Severe Pre-eclampsia
- Case 2: Counseling
- Case 3: Ectopic Pregnancy
- Case 4: Abruptio Placentae; Placenta Previa
- Case 5: Unstable Lie
- Case 6: Nonprogress of Labor
- Case 7: Cardiotocography-I
- Case 8: Cardiotocography-II
- Case 9: Management of Labor (Partograph-I)
- Case 10: Management of Labor (Partograph-II)
- Case 11: Primary Postpartum Hemorrhage
- Case 12: Secondary Postpartum Hemorrhage
- Case 13: Surgical Management of Postpartum Hemorrhage (PPH)
- Case 14: Pregnancy and Labor in a Woman with Prior Cesarean Delivery
- Case 15: Puerperal Pyrexia
- Case 16: Multiple Pregnancy
- Case 17: Neural Tube Defects
- Case 18: Anencephaly
- Case 19: Hydrocephalus
- Case 20: Cystic Hygroma

Ch. 2. Self-Assessment in Obstetrics

SECTION 1

Obstetrics

Section Outline

Ch. 1. Objective Structured Clinical Examination in Obstetrics
- Case 1: Severe Pre-eclampsia
- Case 2: Counseling
- Case 3: Ectopic Pregnancy
- Case 4: Abruptio Placentae; Placenta Previa
- Case 5: Unstable Lie
- Case 6: Nonprogress of Labor
- Case 7: Cardiotocography-I
- Case 8: Cardiotocography-II
- Case 9: Management of Labor (Partograph-I)
- Case 10: Management of Labor (Partograph-II)
- Case 11: Primary Postpartum Hemorrhage
- Case 12: Secondary Postpartum Hemorrhage
- Case 13: Surgical Management of Postpartum Hemorrhage (PPH)
- Case 14: Pregnancy and Labor in a Woman with Prior Cesarean Delivery
- Case 15: Puerperal Pyrexia
- Case 16: Multiple Pregnancy
- Case 17: Neural Tube Defects
- Case 18: Anencephaly
- Case 19: Hydrocephalus
- Case 20: Cystic Hygroma

Ch. 2. Self-Assessment in Obstetrics

1 Objective Structured Clinical Examination in Obstetrics

CASE 1: SEVERE PRE-ECLAMPSIA

Case Summary

Mrs CR in her first pregnancy was admitted with the diagnosis of severe pre-eclampsia. Complete hemogram revealed Hb of 9.8 g/dL, which was 11.6 g/dL 1 week ago. LFT revealed AST = 150 IU/L, ALT = 200 IU/L, alkaline phosphatase = 180 IU/L and LDH = 1,000 IU/L. Platelet count was 85,000/mL.

Q. What is the probable diagnosis?

Ans. Hemolysis, Elevated Liver enzymes, Low Platelet count (HELLP) syndrome.

Q. How do you diagnose it?

Ans. Presence of hemolysis, elevated liver enzymes and low platelet count in a patient with severe pre-eclampsia.

Q. What do you understand by severe pre-eclampsia?

Ans. Severe pre-eclampsia includes:
- BP > 160 mm Hg systolic or > 110 mm Hg diastolic
- Proteinuria > 5 g/24 hours
- Onset of acute renal failure
- Oliguria: Urine < 500 mL/24 hours
- Pulmonary edema
- HELLP syndrome
- Thrombocytopenia (< 100,000/µL)
- Symptoms due to end organ involvement—headache, epigastric pain, visual disturbances
- Fetal growth restriction.

Q. What is the diagnostic criteria for HELLP syndrome?

Ans. The diagnostic criteria include:
- Hemolysis
- AST > 70 IU/L
- Platelets < 100,000/mm^3
- LDH > 600 IU/L
- ALT > 70 IU/L
- Serum bilirubin > 1.2 mg/dL
- Abnormal peripheral blood smear (schistocytes).

Q. What other investigations should be done for her?
Ans. Other investigations should be done are—coagulation profile, serum uric acid, creatinine, urine analysis and ophthalmoscopy.

Q. What is the risk of eclampsia in HELLP syndrome when compared to severe pre-eclampsia?
Ans. Eclampsia is more common in HELLP syndrome in comparison to severe pre-eclampsia.

Q. What would be the appropriate management of the case?
Ans. Patient should be managed in a tertiary care center:
- **To stabilize maternal condition**
    - Antihypertensive therapy—hydralazine 5 mg IV bolus to be followed by infusion (25 mg in 200 mL normal saline) at the rate of 2.5 mg/hour to be doubled every 30 minutes till the diastolic BP is < 110 mm Hg. Labetalol IV (200 mg in 200 mL of normal saline) at the rate of 20 mg/hour can also be used as an alternative.
    - Antiseizure prophylaxis with $MgSO_4$ (IM or IV regimen).
    - CT or USG of abdomen if subcapsular hematoma of liver is suspected.
    - To correct coagulopathy if any: Fresh (relatively) whole blood transfusion, platelet transfusion if count is < 10,000 mm³.
- **To evaluate fetal wellbeing**
    - Nonstress test
    - Biophysical profile
    - Doppler flow study of umbilical artery.
- **Termination of pregnancy (delivery)**
    - Pregnancy > 34 weeks → corticosteroid therapy → delivery
    - Pregnancy < 34 weeks →

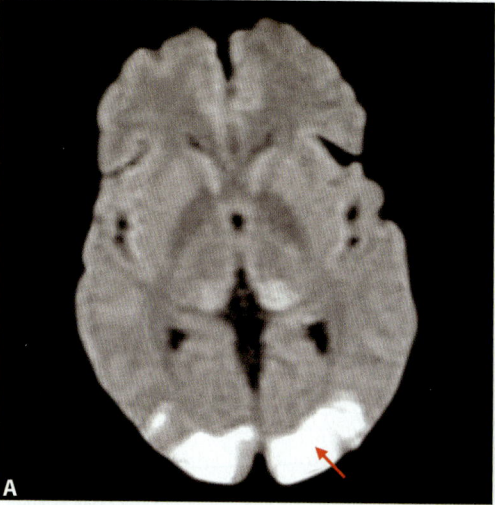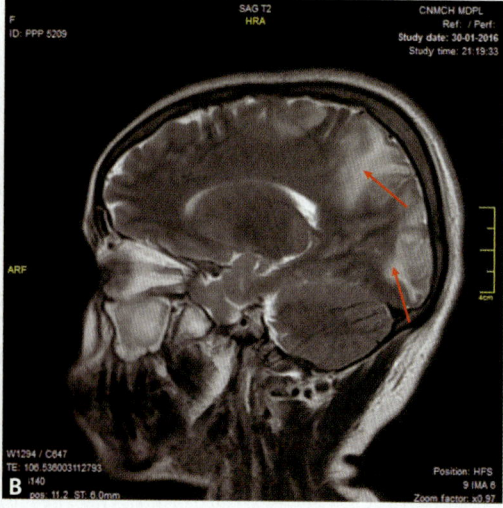

Figs 1.1A and B: MRI of the brain axial and sagittal views showing posterior reversible encephalopathy syndrome (PRES) in a patient with eclampsia. Massive areas of the occipital and parietal lobes show infarction and vasogenic edema. T2 flair lesions are seen (*see* arrows)

Q. What is posterior reversible encephalopathy syndrome (PRES)?

Ans. Cerebral changes in severe pre-eclampsia and eclampsia have been demonstrated with many neurodiagnostic tests including MRI, cerebral Doppler velocimetry and cerebral angiography (Figs 1.1A and B). Cerebral pathology in eclampsia is mainly due to **loss of cerebral autoregulation**. Important findings on MRI are:
- Hypodense areas of diffuse white matter
- Loss of normal cortical sulci
- Cerebral infarction (low attenuation)
- Edema of the occipital lobe
- Cerebral hemorrhage (high density area)
- Acute hydrocephalus.

Posterior reversible encephalopathy syndrome is similar to hypertensive encephalopathy. It is due to reversible cerebral vasoconstriction. Such lesions may also be seen in frontal lobes, temporal lobes, basal ganglia and thalamus. Occipital lobe edema may cause blindness, although reversible lesions due to cerebral infarctions may show persistent pathology.

CASE 2: COUNSELING

Case Summary

Mrs AK, 26-year-old, married for 1 year is planning to have a baby. She has come to you for counseling about pre-eclampsia. She came to know about the problems of high blood pressure and convulsions during pregnancy, while she was reading the 'Women's Health' magazine.

Q. What are the predisposing factors for pre-eclampsia?
Ans.
- Young and elderly primigravidae
- Positive family history (genetic)
- Pregnancy complications—multiple pregnancy, diabetes
- New paternity
- Many others (genetic and immunological).

Q. Can you predict pre-eclampsia?
Ans. There are many screening methods. Doppler study (Fig. 1.2) to detect 'notch' in the early diastole wave especially in the uterine arteries, at 24 weeks of gestation can predict the possible development of pre-eclampsia. Other tests like **Roll over test** and **Angiotensin infusion test** have been tried. Unfortunately, positive predictive value of all these tests is poor.

Q. Can you prevent pre-eclampsia?
Ans. Pre-eclampsia is not a totally preventable disease. Use of low-dose aspirin, calcium, antioxidants (vitamins C and E) have been tried in the high-risk groups to reduce the onset of severe disease.

Q. Can you predict and prevent eclampsia?
Ans. Eclampsia may present in atypical ways though in majority it is preceded by severe pre-eclampsia. So, effective management of pre-eclampsia is the only way to prevent eclampsia.

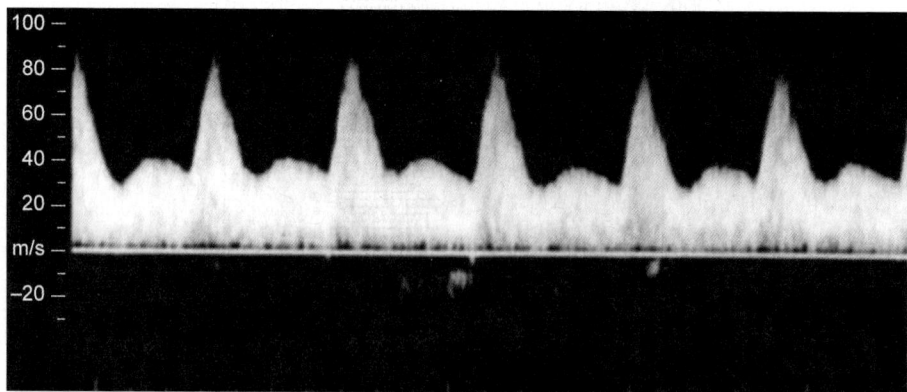

Fig. 1.2: Flow velocity waveform (Doppler velocimetry) of the uterine artery at 26 weeks of gestation. This shows early diastole 'notch'. Presence of this notch and elevated resistive index (RI) or pulsatility index (PI) at advanced weeks of gestation indicate high uterine vascular resistance and reduced placental blood flow. This is thought to be due to failure of trophoblastic invasion of the spiral arteries

CASE 3: ECTOPIC PREGNANCY

Case Summary

Mrs NS, 26-year-old nurse, $P_{1+0+1+1}$ was seen in the outpatient clinic for the lower abdominal pain and irregular vaginal bleeding. It is nearly 6 weeks that she had her last menstrual period (LMP). On clinical examination, she was hemodynamically stable and there was some discomfort on pelvic examination (Fig. 1.3).

Q. What are the most likely diagnoses?
Ans. Complications (bleeding) of early pregnancy—threatened or incomplete miscarriage (*See* Konar & Dutta's Bedside Clinics and Viva-voce in Obstetrics and Gynecology, p. 99) and ectopic pregnancy.

Q. What investigations you will recommend?
Ans. Urine for hCG and pelvic ultrasonography [transvaginal scan (TVS)].
Investigation report
Urine hCG = positive; serum β-hCG = 1,850 IU/L; pelvic ultrasonography—Uterus: NS; cavity: empty. Mass in the right adnexae; no fluid in the pouch of Douglas (POD), left tube and ovary—not visualized (Fig. 1.3).

Q. What would be your next step of management?
Ans. Diagnostic laparoscopy—double puncture procedure.
On laparoscopy—pathology revealed as shown in Figure 1.4.

Q. What is your diagnosis?
Ans. Unruptured tubal ectopic pregnancy.

Q. Mention some predisposing factors of this pathology?
Ans. Pelvic inflammatory disease, previous induced abortion, tubal surgery (tubal sterilization or reversal of sterilization), *in vitro* fertilization and embryo transfer.

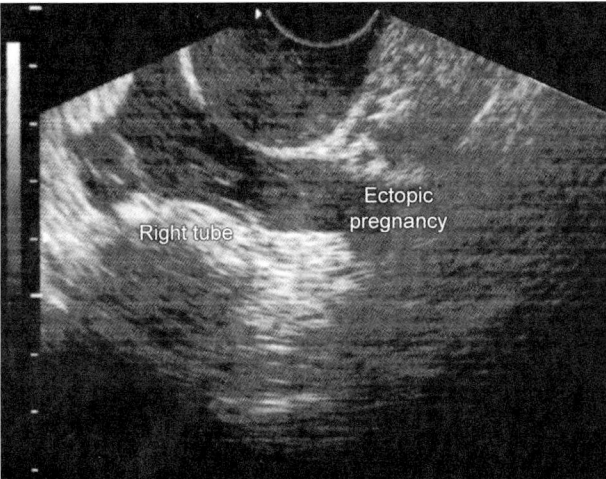

Fig. 1.3: Sonogram showing ectopic pregnancy
Courtesy: Dr (Mrs) S Ghosh and Prof BN Chakravorty, IRM, Kolkata

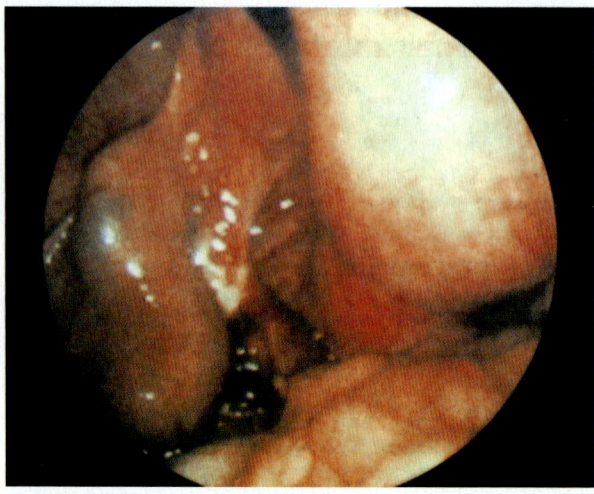

Fig. 1.4: Laparoscopic view of tubal ectopic pregnancy (unruptured)

Q. What is the value of serum β-hCG and serum progesterone to predict the diagnosis?

Ans. Serum β-hCG > 2000 IU/L with empty uterine cavity on TVS suggests ectopic pregnancy. Serum progesterone > 25 ng/mL suggests viable intrauterine pregnancy.

Q. What would be the appropriate management for her?

Ans. Conservative management for unruptured tubal ectopic pregnancy.

Procedure may be either medical or surgical:
- **Medical:** Systemic methotrexate (MTX) or direct local into the sac with agents, like MTX, PGF2α or potassium chloride.
- **Surgical:** Salpingostomy or salpingotomy (Fig. 1.5).

Q. Are all the cases suitable for medical management?

Ans. No. Contraindications are: (i) Tubal diameter > 4 cm; (ii) presence of fetal cardiac activity; (iii) presence of intraperitoneal bleeding or tubal rupture.

Q. Does she need any follow-up following the initial treatment?

Ans. She should be followed up with estimation of serum β-hCG weekly till the values are normal. **But level of serum β-hCG remained plateau on the 10th day of treatment.**

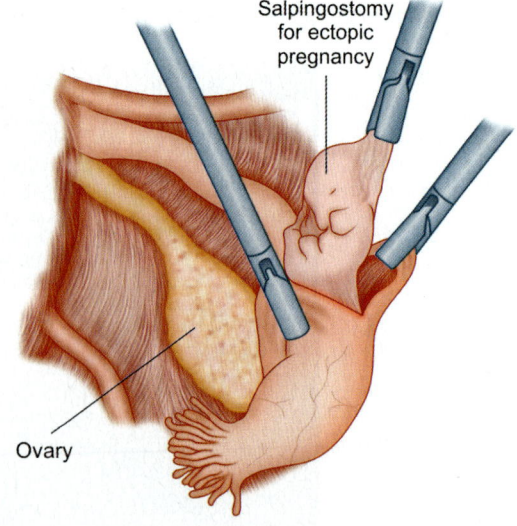

Fig. 1.5: Laparoscopic surgery for tubal ectopic pregnancy

Q. *What would you do for her?*
Ans. She should be treated with systemic chemotherapy (MTX 50 mg/m^2) IM single dose. After the completion of treatment, she wants to know from you the following questions.

Q. *What is the risk of recurrence of tubal ectopic pregnancy?*
Ans. About 10–15%.

Q. *What precautionary measures she may take to minimize the risk?*
Ans. To avoid the use of intrauterine device (IUD) contraceptive and progestin only pills.

Q. *How best you can reassure her?*
Ans. She is advised to report whenever she misses her period. Serum β-hCG and pelvic ultrasonography should be done to confirm the diagnosis as well as to detect the site of pregnancy.

CASE 4: ABRUPTIO PLACENTAE; PLACENTA PREVIA

Case Summary

Mrs CX, 27-year-old, $P_{1+0+0+1}$, at 37 weeks of gestation was admitted in emergency with the complaints of abdominal pain and vaginal bleeding. On examination, she looked pale, BP 140/96 mm Hg. Uterus was found tender.

Q. What is the most likely diagnosis?
Ans. Abruptio placentae.

Q. What other signs she may have?
Ans. Difficulty in palpating the fetal parts, difficulty in auscultating the fetal heart sound (FHS), height of the fundus—more than the period of amenorrhea and presence of uterine tenderness.

Q. What are the common causes of the problem?
Ans. The exact cause is obscure. The observed associations are:
- Pre-eclampsia
- Sudden uterine decompression (following delivery of the first baby of twins)
- Circumvallate placenta (Fig. 1.6)
- Trauma
- Folic acid deficiency
- Smoking, cocaine abuse and thrombophilias.

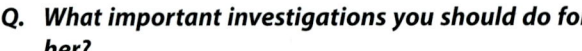

Fig. 1.6: Stillbirth following placental abruption in a case with circumvallate placenta

Q. What important investigations you should do for her?
Ans. Blood for Hb%, hematocrit, platelets, coagulation profile, ABO and Rh grouping and cardiotocography.

Q. What definitive management you would do for her?
Ans. Resuscitation and termination of pregnancy. Patient may go into labor spontaneously. Otherwise labor may be induced by ARM ± oxytocin.

Q. What are the indications of cesarean section in such a condition?
Ans.
- Evidences of fetal distress
- Where amniotomy could not be done as the cervix is unfavorable
- Nonprogress of labor even with amniotomy ± oxytocin
- Associated obstetric complications (breech).

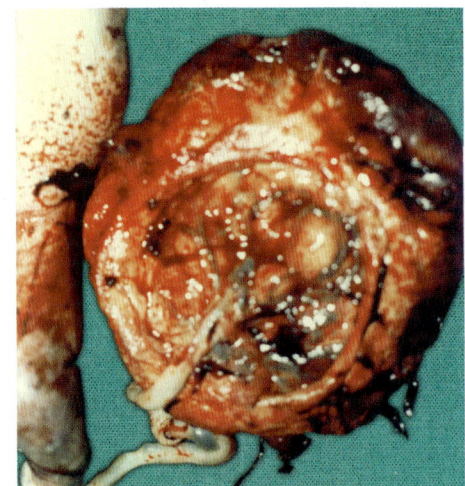

Fig. 1.7: Circumvallate placenta with abruption

Q. How do you explain the indeterminate bleeding?
Ans. The diagnosis of unclassified bleeding is made after exclusion of placental and local causes. Rupture of vasa previa (*See* Dutta's Textbook of Obstetrics, 8th Edition, p. 301), marginal sinus, circumvallate placenta (Fig. 1.7) or marked decidual reaction on endocervix may be the possible cause.

Q. How do you manage a case of vasa previa?
Ans. Color Doppler (TVS) is helpful for antenatal diagnosis. Bleeding cases with vasa previa need delivery by category-I cesarean section. Antenatal corticosteroids should be given in a case with preterm delivery. Management depends on gestational age, severity and the recurrence of bleeding. Pregnancy ≥ 37 weeks → delivery. Expectant management is done in selected cases only (*See* Dutta's Textbook of Obstetrics, 8th Edition, p. 301). Neonatal blood transfusion may be needed.

Q. What is the relationship between previous cesarean section and incidence of placenta previa?
Ans. Women with a previous cesarean delivery have an increased risk of abnormal placental location (placenta previa). In addition, these women have an increased risk of morbid adherent placenta (placenta accreta, increta or percreta). Risk of placenta accreta with placenta previa without any uterine scar is about 3%. However, this risk increases in cases with prior cesarean delivery (scarred uterus). **The overall risk of placenta accreta with placenta previa with prior cesarean delivery is 11%, 40% and 60% after the first, second and third cesarean delivery respectively.** Morbidly adherent placenta leads to significant hemorrhage during cesarean section (CS). This may lead to cesarean hysterectomy. **Hence, in such a case, operation should be done by an experienced person and blood or blood products should be made available.**

CASE 5: UNSTABLE LIE

Case Summary

Mrs CD is seen in the antenatal clinic at 38 weeks of gestation of her second pregnancy. Single fetus with oblique lie was observed. Antenatal card record revealed that her last visit in the clinic was a week ago and baby was in transverse lie.

Q. What is the diagnosis?
Ans. Unstable lie.

Q. What should be the appropriate investigations for her?
Ans. Ultrasonography to detect any cause for unstable lie specially placenta previa.

Q. What are the important complications of this problem?
Ans. Prelabor rupture of the membranes and cord prolapse.

Q. What would be the appropriate approach for management?
Ans. Admission in the hospital and close monitoring.
   If no cause is detected, lie may become stable. In that case she may go into spontaneous labor or may be induced (stabilizing induction). Otherwise, she should be delivered by CS.

Q. What advise she should be given when she is admitted in the ward?
Ans. To maintain kick-chart (*See* Dutta's Textbook of Obstetrics, 8th Edition, p. 121). In case the membrane ruptures (leakage of liquor), she should inform the on duty nurse and should not take anything orally until examined by her doctor.

CASE 6: NONPROGRESS OF LABOR

Case Summary

Mrs AD, 26-year-old primigravida, is admitted in labor at 39 weeks of pregnancy. Cervix was 3 cm dilated and membranes were intact. She was having 2–3 contractions at every 10 minutes and each contraction lasting for 10–20 seconds. Fetal heart sound on auscultation was 146 beats/min and were regular. Three hours later, repeat examination revealed that cervix was till 3 cm.

Q. What is the diagnosis?
Ans. Nonprogress of labor.

Q. What do you mean by nonprogress of labor?
Ans. When the rate of cervical dilatation is less than 1 cm/hour and the descent of the presenting part is less than 1 cm/hour, the condition is known as ***slow progress of labor***. But when there is no change in terms of cervical dilatation and descent of the presenting part over a period of at least 2 hours, the condition is known as ***nonprogress of labor***.

Q. What are the reasons for nonprogress of labor?
Ans. The underlying etiologies are often not clearly determined. Weak or abnormal uterine contractions, deflexion of the fetal head, cephalopelvic disproportion, malposition, inadequate or lack of labor analgesia, maternal dehydration are often associated with nonprogress of labor.

Q. What would be the next appropriate step to rectify the abnormality?
Ans.
- Maternal rehydration
- Artificial rupture of the membranes (ARM)
- To reassess the woman once again.

Q. What would be the next step of management if the situation is not improved?
Ans. Once cephalopelvic disproportion has been excluded, labor process may be augmented with escalating dose of oxytocin infusion.
After 4 hours of regular and strong contractions, she was found fully dilated. Head was at +3 (perineum). Sagittal suture was in the anteroposterior diameter of the pelvis. She was found completely exhausted and was unable to push down (bear down).

Q. What would be your next step of management?
Ans.
- To continue oxytocin infusion
- To give her adequate analgesia
- To expedite the delivery by outlet forceps.

Q. What are the abnormalities of the active phase of labor?
Ans.
- Protracted active phase
- Arrest of active phase.

Q. What do you understand by protracted and arrest of active phase and how do you manage them?
Ans.
- Protraction of labor (WHO, 1994) is defined when the cervical dilatation is less than 1 cm/hour for a minimum of 4 hours during the active phase of labor.
- Arrest of labor in the active phase is defined when there is no dilatation of the cervix for 2 hours or more.

Management: Protraction and arrest disorders during the active phase of labor may be due to poor or incoordinate uterine contractions, malposition, malpresentations or due to cephalopelvic disproportion (CPD).

Management is initiated according to its cause. Expectant management with support, and amniotomy with or without oxytocin augmentation may be effective.

Cases with CPD need to be delivered by CS.

CASE 7: CARDIOTOCOGRAPHY-I

Case Summary

Mrs SC, 27-year-old school teacher, presents in her first pregnancy at 38 weeks of gestation with diminished fetal movements. The cardiotocography was done and is shown in the Figures 1.8 to 1.10.

Q. What is the baseline FHR?
Ans. 150 beat per minute (bpm).

Q. What is the baseline variability?
Ans. 10–20 bpm.

Q. Is there any sinusoidal pattern?
Ans. Nil.

Q. How many accelerations are there in the trace?
Ans. Six within the period of 20 minutes.

Q. Is there any deceleration?
Ans. Nil.

Q. What about the nonstress test?
Ans. Fetal movements are evidenced by black blocks in the graph. Simultaneously with the fetal movements there is acceleration of the FHR. So, the nonstress test is normal (reassuring pattern).

Q. What are the criteria of a normal (reactive) trace?
Ans.
- Baseline FHR between 120 bpm and 160 bpm (RCOG, NICE: 100–160 bpm)
- Baseline variability between 10 bpm and 25 bpm
- Two accelerations in 20 minutes observation
- No deceleration.

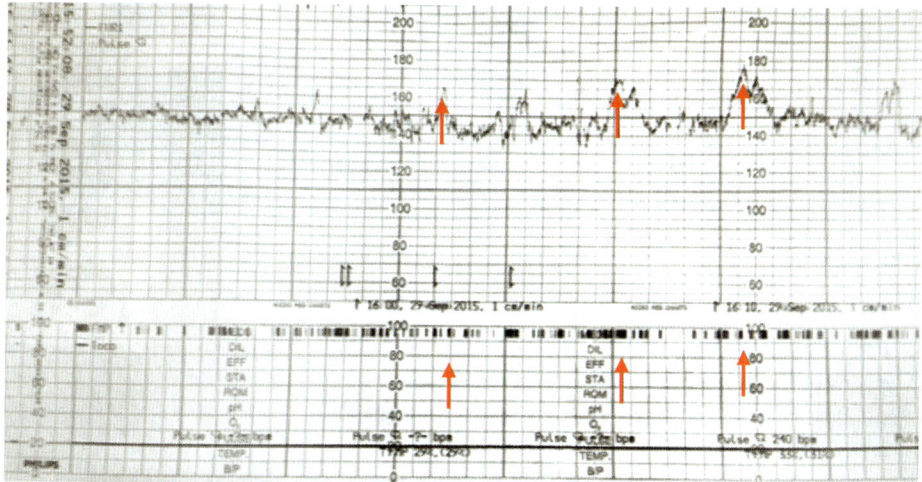

Fig. 1.8: Cardiotocograph showing reactive nonstress test indicated by fetal movements (blocks) with cardiac accelerations (*see* arrows)

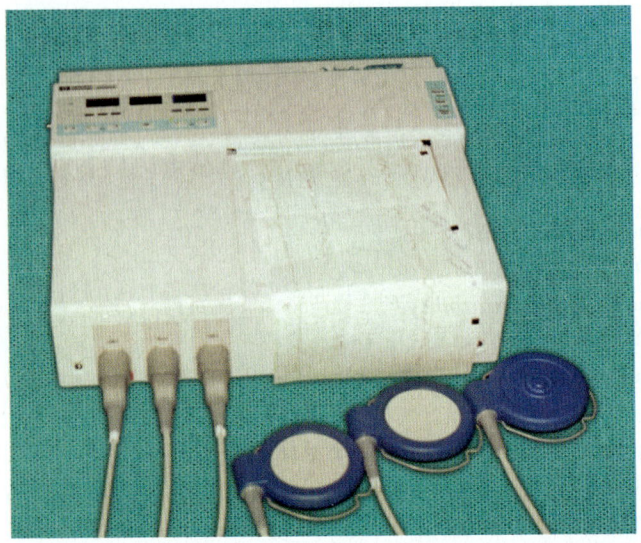

Fig. 1.9: Fetal monitor with the abdominal transducers

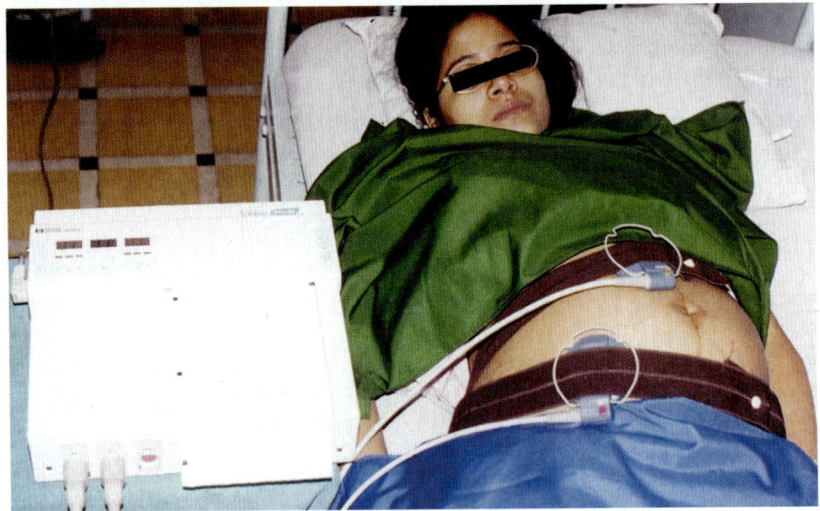

Fig. 1.10: Cardiotocography is in progress

Q. When a trace pattern is called abnormal?

Ans. Pathological trace
- Baseline heart rate < 100 bpm or > 160 bpm
- Baseline variability < 5 bpm for 90 minutes or more
- No acceleration in 40 minutes
- Repetitive early or variable deceleration
- Repetitive late deceleration
- Sinusoidal pattern.

Q. How the CTG traces are categorized?
Ans. Categorization of CTG traces are: According to **RCOG and NICE** the categories are: (a) Normal, (b) suspicious, (c) pathological. Four features are considered for categorization of a CTG trace: **These are: (a) Baseline FHR, (b) variability, (c) decelerations and (d) accelerations.**
- **Normal:** All the four features are reassuring.
- **Suspicious:** One non-reassuring and the rest are reassuring.
- **Pathological:** Two or more features are non-reassuring.
  According to NICHD (2008) and ACOG (2009)
- Interpretation (*See* Dutta's Textbook of Obstetrics, 8th Edition, p. 694).
  - **Category I:** Normal (based on all the four parameters, mentioned above).
  - **Category II:** Indeterminate (all tracings not in the category of I or III).
  - **Category III:** Abnormal (besides others, sinusoidal pattern is considered as abnormal).

Q. Name some common causes of fetal bradycardia and tachycardia?
Ans. Fetal bradycardia
- Fetal distress
- Acidosis
- Fetal heart conduction defect
- Drugs to mother (pethidine, methyldopa)

Fetal tachycardia
- Drugs to mother (β-adrenergic agents)
- Infection (mother or fetus)
- Anemia (maternal or fetal)
- Fetal distress.

Q. What about the tocograph in the trace?
Ans. The tocograph showed absence of uterine contractions.

Q. What are the indications of continuous electronic fetal monitoring during labor?
Ans. Where there is increased risk of intrapartum fetal hypoxia. Conditions are as follows:
- Intrauterine growth restriction (IUGR)
- Meconium stained amniotic fluid
- Maternal hypertension or diabetes
- Malposition (OP) or presentation (breech)
- Previous CS.

18 Manual of Obstetrics and Gynecology for the Postgraduates

CASE 8: CARDIOTOCOGRAPHY-II

Case Summary

Mrs ZC, 26-year-old housewife, $P_{0+0+0+0}$, was admitted at 35.4 weeks of gestation because she was epileptic and the baby was small for gestation. A 30 minutes cardiotocography (CTG) was done when she complained of diminished fetal movements. The CTG trace is shown in the Figure 1.11.

Q. What abnormalities are shown in the trace?
Ans. Baseline fetal heart rate was 140 bpm with unprovoked repeated decelerations lasting for more than 3 minutes.

Q. What would be the next plan of management?
Ans. Patient should be admitted for continuous monitoring and for biophysical scoring. *Further CTG showed the trace as shown in the Figure 1.12.*

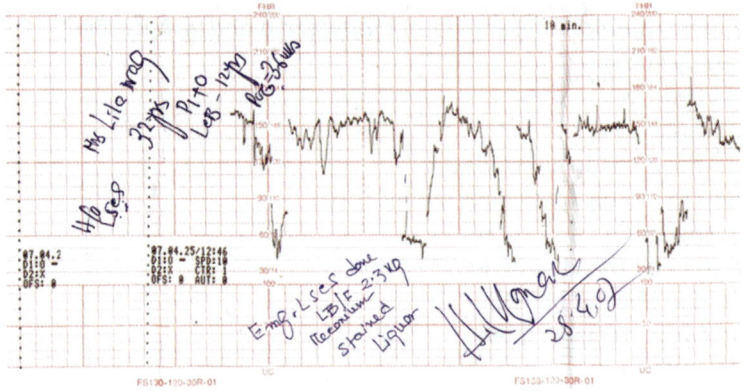

Fig. 1.11: Abnormal nonstress test showing repeated decelerations > 40 bpm and lasting > 3 minutes

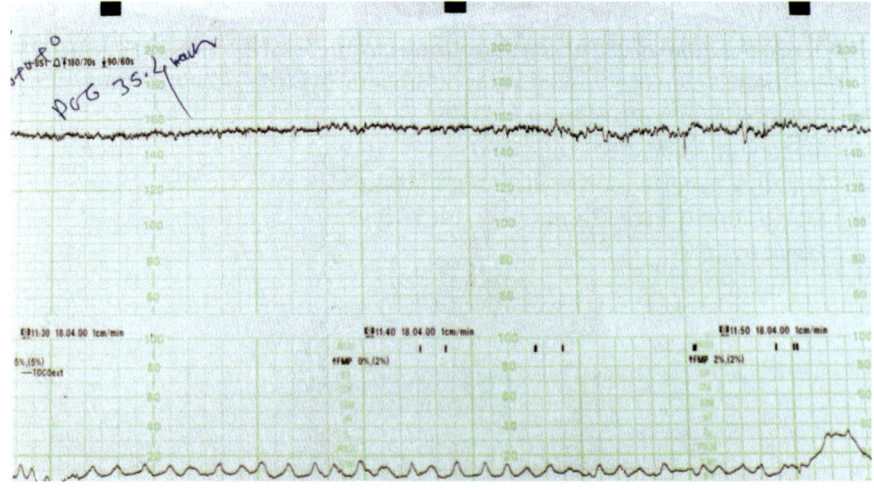

Fig. 1.12: Cardiotocogram showing sinusoidal pattern

Q. What abnormalities are shown in the trace (Fig. 1.12)? This trace pattern remained persistent on two more occasions.

Ans. *Sinusoidal pattern*
Fetal baseline heart rate is 155 bpm
Baseline variability is < 5 bpm
Acceleration: Nil.

Q. What would be your advice?

Ans. To organize delivery.
On examination, cervix was found unfavorable. She was delivered by lower segment cesarean section (LSCS). The baby on examination revealed as shown in Figure 1.13. The baby weighted 1.2 kg.

Q. What are the complications for the baby?

Ans.
- Presence of other congenital malformations
- Feeding problem
- Speech problem
- Delayed dentition
- Repeated chest infection due to regurgitation.

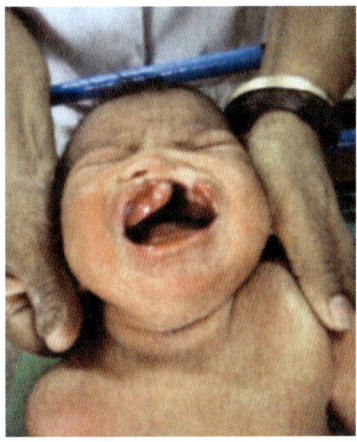

Fig. 1.13: Neonate with IUGR showing cleft lip and palate

CASE 9: MANAGEMENT OF LABOR (PARTOGRAPH-I)

Case Summary

Mrs LT, 23-year-old, was admitted with labor pain following a term pregnancy. Her partograph is shown in the Figure 1.14.

Q. What was the cervical dilatation at the time of admission at 3 am?
Ans. Cervix was only 1 cm dilated.

Q. At what time she entered into the active phase of labor?
Ans. At 11 am (8 hours after admission) cervix was 4 cm dilated.

Q. At what time she became fully dilated?
Ans. At 2 pm (11 hours since admission) cervix was 10 cm (fully) dilated.

Q. What was the duration of the latent phase of labor?
Ans. 8 hours (3 am to 11 am).

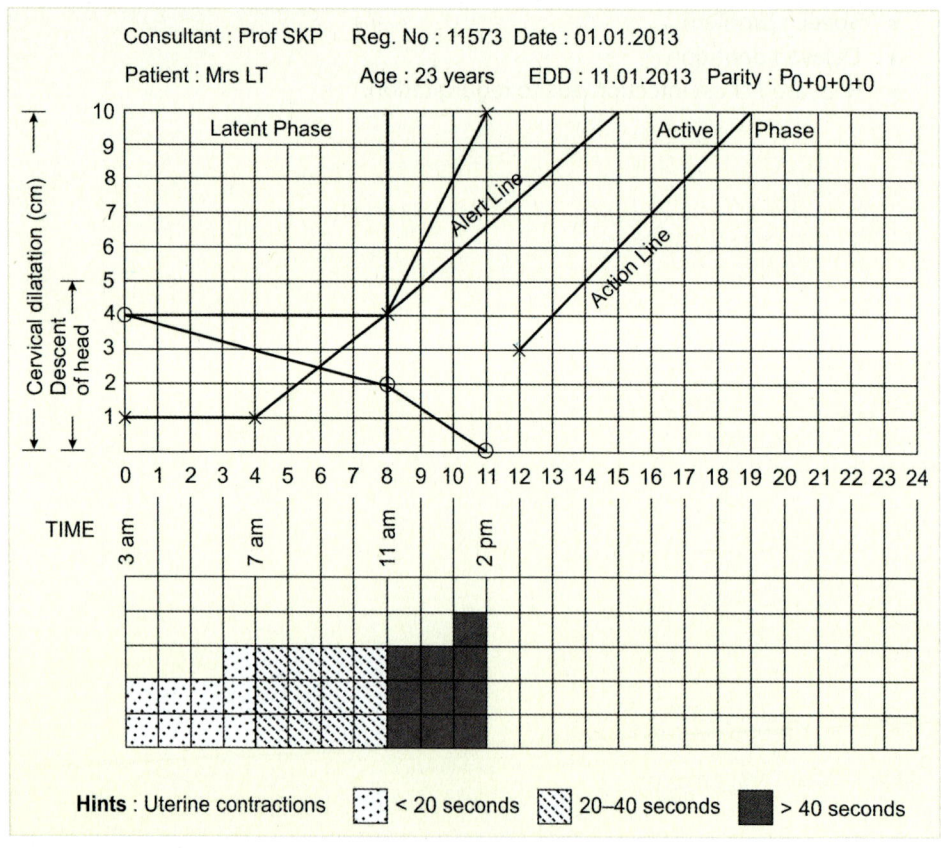

Fig. 1.14: Partograph representing graphically the important observations in labor[1]

Q. *What was the duration of the active phase of labor?*
Ans. 3 hours (11 am to 2 pm).

Q. *How were the uterine contractions for the first 3 hours and the last 1 hour of labor since admission?*
Ans. For the first 3 hours, uterine contraction were 2 per 10 minutes and each lasted for less than 20 seconds. For the last 1 hour, the frequency of uterine contractions were 4 per 10 minutes and each lasted more than 40 seconds.

CASE 10: MANAGEMENT OF LABOR (PARTOGRAPH-II)

Case Summary

Mrs CZ was $G_2 P_{1+0+0+1}$, admitted with labor pain following a term pregnancy. Her partograph is shown in the Figure 1.15.

Q. What was the total duration of labor?
Ans. The total duration of labor was 8 hours.

Q. What was the situation of the head at the time of admission?
Ans. Head was five-fifths above the pelvic brim at 6 am at the time of admission.

Q. At what time the head was engaged?
Ans. 4 hours following admission (at 10 am) head was found engaged (two-fifths were felt above the brim).

Q. What was the FHR and maternal blood pressure when she entered the active phase of labor?
Ans. Fetal heart rate was 140 bpm; BP was 120/80 mm Hg.

Q. What was the color of the liquor?
Ans. Clear (as donated by 'C').

Q. When was the cervix fully dilated?
Ans. 8 hours following admission (at 2 pm) cervix was fully dilated.

Q. In a labor process, when is the latent phase prolonged?
Ans. When the duration is more than 8 hours, it is called prolonged latent phase.

Q. What should be the appropriate management for the prolonged latent phase of labor?[3]
Ans. To make the cervix favorable by using prostaglandin E2 gel, if required. This is followed by amniotomy [artificial rupture of the membranes (AROM)] and oxytocin infusion.

Q. Where should be the plotting of cervical dilatation in normal labor?
Ans. In a normal labor, the plotting of cervical dilatation should either on the alert line or to the left of it.

Q. What is your impression when cervical dilatation plotting crosses the alert time?
Ans. The labor is going to be prolonged.

Q. What steps you should take when the cervical dilatation has crossed the alert line and has reached the action line?
Ans. To reassess the situation as regard the maternal health, uterine contractions, FHR, position of the presenting part, pelvic adequacy and color of the liquor. Depending on these, decision is made either for termination of labor or for augmentation of labor.

Q. What do you mean by augmentation of labor?
Ans. Amniotomy is done if the membranes are intact. Oxytocin infusion is started in an escalating drop rate at an interval of 30 minutes. It is adjusted against uterine contractions. Ideally,

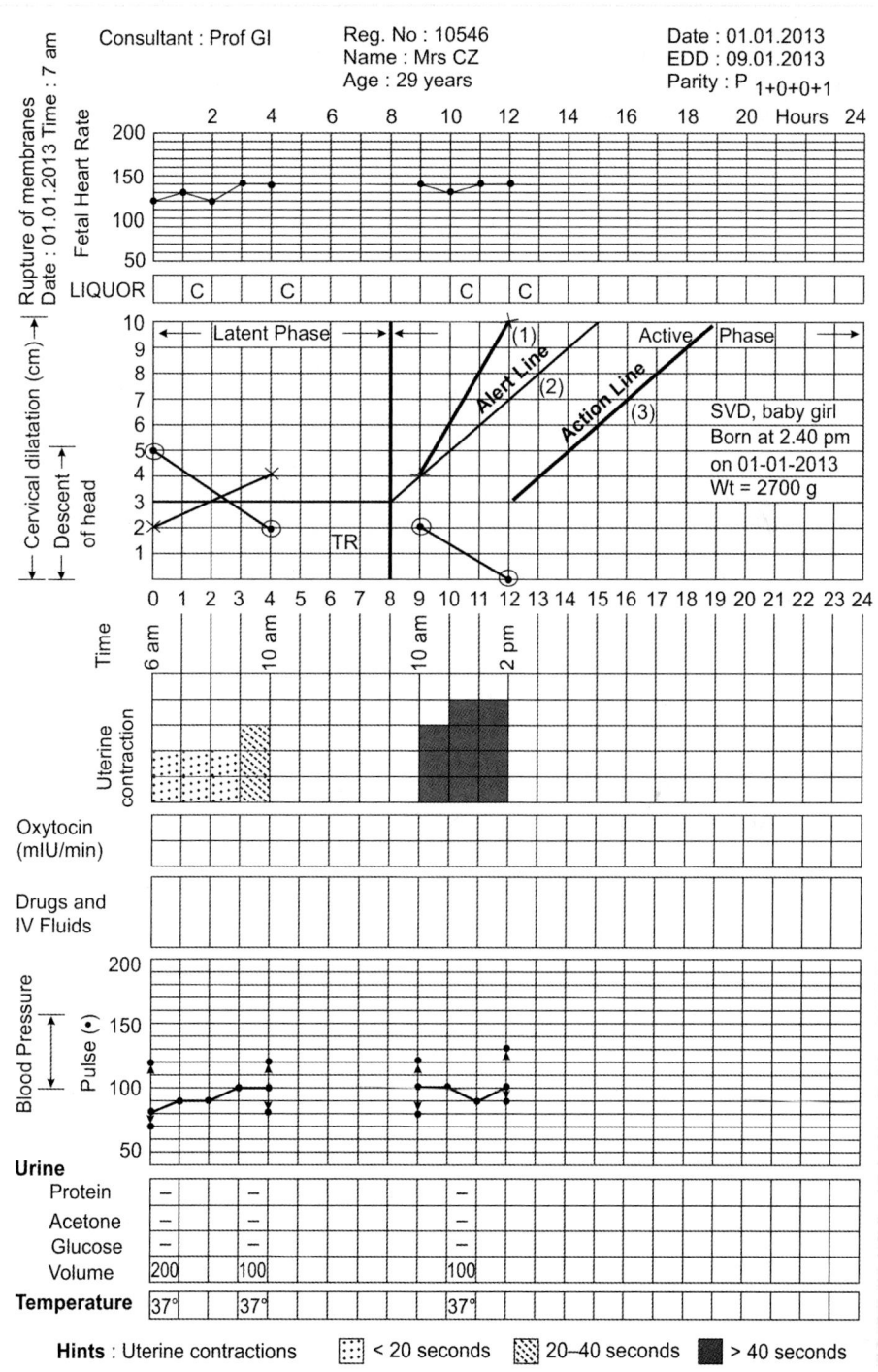

Fig. 1.15: Partograph representing graphically the important observations for labor[2]

3–4 contractions in 10 minutes time and each lasting for 40 seconds are optimum. Infusion once started, should be maintained at that rate throughout the second and third stage of labor.

Other aspects of management are:
- Maternal hydration must be adequately maintained
- Pain relief during labor must be adequate
- Labor should be reassessed at an frequent interval for fetal and maternal wellbeing
- Labor is terminated, if there is no satisfactory progress by another 4 hours time.

References

1. **World Health Organisation.** Preventing prolonged labor: A practical guide. The partograph. Unpublished document WHO/FHE/MSM/93.8/9/10/11. Geneva. World Health Organisation, 1993.
2. **World Health Organisation.** Maternal Health and Safe Motherhood Programme. World Health Organisation partograph in management of labor. Lancet. 1994;343(8910):1399-1404.
3. **World Health Organisation (WHO).** Care in normal birth: A practical guide WHO/FRH/MSM/96.4. Geneva, 1996.

CASE 11: PRIMARY POSTPARTUM HEMORRHAGE

Case Summary

Mrs AR has been delivered vaginally. She started bleeding severely following delivery of the placenta. Placenta was found complete on examination.

Q. What is this condition called?
Ans. Primary postpartum hemorrhage (PPH).

Q. What management you would do immediately?[1]
Ans. To commence IV infusion with crystalloid (Ringer's solution). To send blood for ABO grouping, Rh typing and cross matching, continuous catheterization and to call for help of the obstetric registrar.

Q. What are the possible causes of this problem?
Ans. Causes are divided by 'four Ts':
  1. Tone (atonicity)
  2. Trauma (genital tract)
  3. Tissue (retained products of conception)
  4. Thrombin (coagulopathy).

Q. What are the different medical management of this problem?[1]
Ans.
- Airway to maintain
- Crystalloid infusion
- Foley catheterization
- IV access (14 gauge cannula × 2)
- Blood transfusion as early as possible
- To massage the uterus.
- To give oxytocin IV by infusion (10 units in 500 mL N saline, 40 drops/minute)
- Injection methergin 0.2 mg IV or injection 15-methyl $PGF2\alpha$ 250 mg IM or misoprostol (PGE_1) 1,000 µg rectum depending on the response.

Q. What are the different surgical management of this problem?
Ans.
- Exploration of the uterus under general anesthesia
- To repair any injury to the cervix, vagina or perineum
- Uterine tamponade:
  - Tight intrauterine packing (in low resource settings before transfer of patient)
  - Bimanual compression
  - Balloon tamponade using different types of hydrostatic balloon catheter (Foley catheter, Bakri balloon, Sengstaken–Blakemore tube, inflated with 200–500 mL of saline) has been found effective. This can avoid hysterectomy in 78% cases. Mechanism of action is similar to tight intrauterine packing.
- Uterine brace suture (Fig. 1.16) B-Lynch or its modifications are done by oversewing the uterus
- Uterine devascularization procedure:
  - Ligation of uterine and ovarian vessels
  - Ligation of internal iliac arteries
  - Angiographic embolization of hypogastric artery by gelfoam.
- Hysterectomy (rarely).

Once bleeding is controlled, patient is observed in ICU or in high-dependence unit.

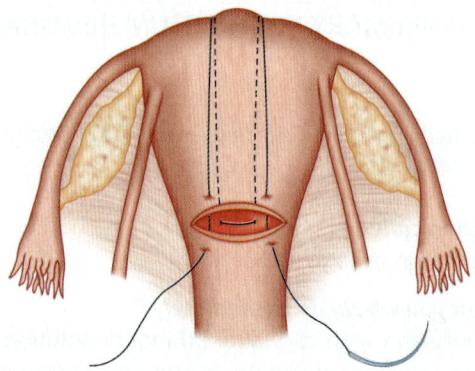

Fig. 1.16: B-Lynch (1997) uterine brace suture. In *modified brace suture*, the uterine cavity is not opened. A chromic catgut (no. 2) suture is passed from anterior to posterior surface of the uterus and is tied tightly over the fundus. Similarly, it is done on the other side. This acts by compression effect

Q. How optimal management of PPH could be organized?
Ans. Training of all birth attendants in the management of PPH should be organized (rehearsal).

Q. What other important issues to be considered in the management of PPH?
Ans. Accurate documentation of all events from delivery, medical and surgical management, soft involvement in respect of time must be done. It minimizes the risk of litigation.

Reference

1. RCOG. Prevention of postpartum hemorrhage; Green Top Guidelines No. 35: 2009.

CASE 12: SECONDARY POSTPARTUM HEMORRHAGE

Case Summary

Mrs CD had her vaginal delivery 12 days back. She had slight vaginal bleeding since then but for last 2 days she is bleeding heavily.

Q. What is this abnormal bleeding called?
Ans. Secondary postpartum hemorrhage (PPH).

Q. What is the immediate management?
Ans. She is admitted in the hospital, IV infusion is started with Ringer's solution. Blood is sent for grouping and cross matching.

Q. What are the possible causes?
Ans. Endometritis, retained products of conception, blood clots or infection.

Q. What investigations would you organize for her?
Ans. Blood for Hb%, TLC, DLC, high vaginal swab and midstream urine for culture and sensitivity, ultrasonography (including Doppler study) of the uterus.

Q. What would be the management?
Ans. Antibiotics (combination of ampicillin, gentamicin and metronidazole), blood transfusion and may need evacuation of the uterus under general anesthesia, if retained products are there. **This antibiotic therapy does not prevent breastfeeding**.

Q. What are the other causes for such secondary PPH?
Ans. There may be few rare but important causes of secondary PPH. These are post-traumatic uterine artery pseudoaneurysm and arteriovenous fistula formation. Uterine arteriovenous malformations may be acquired or congenital in origin.

Q. What is the usual presentation of a case with secondary PPH due to uterine vascular malformations?
Ans.
- Such women have the history of previous obstetric operation (CS) or any gynecologic surgery
- Woman presents with sudden onset of fresh vaginal bleeding
- Recurrent admissions with postpartum hemorrhage
- Bleeding: The uterine bleeding is usually heavy and often intractable and not controlled by uterotonic agents
- Failure to respond with uterine evacuation.

Q. How the diagnosis of such case of uterine arteriovenous malformations could be made?
Ans.
- Clinical presentation of such cases are very characteristic
- Ultrasonography with the use of color Doppler is an important diagnostic tool
- Pelvic angiography is considered as the gold standard investigation in the diagnosis of vascular malformations
- Color Doppler will demonstrate the blood flow within the lesion and a 'to and fro' phenomenon. The 'to and fro' sign differentiates the pseudoaneurysm from other pelvic lesions (hematoma or abscess).

Q. What is the possible etiology of such arteriovenous malformations?

Ans. It may be congenital. In obstetrics CS is commonly found to be associated with the formation of vascular abnormalities. However, pseudoaneurysm has been reported following spontaneous vaginal delivery. Gynecological surgery may also result in pseudoaneurysm formation.

Q. How this condition of arteriovenous malformations could be prevented?

Ans. Congenital arteriovenous malformations cannot be prevented. Therefore, early diagnosis is helpful. Iatrogenic vascular malformations could be prevented by doing CS carefully and avoiding extension of uterine incision. The suture is to be placed beyond the apex of extension. These measures may help to avoid the formation of pseudoaneurysm of the uterine artery.

Q. How the condition of secondary PPH due to arteriovenous pseudoaneurysm formation is managed?

Ans. Natural healing process may seal the injured artery and the condition maybe self-limiting. Uterine artery embolization (UAE) has been successful in the management of PPH. Uterine artery embolization is a minimally invasive procedure and is performed under local anesthesia. The UAE can preserve the uterus and, hence, the fertility potential of the woman.

Q. How the procedure of uterine artery embolization is done?

Ans. It is performed via percutaneous femoral artery catheterization (see Figs 61.1A and B). Angiography helps to identify the anatomy and possible source of hemorrhage. Gelatin sponge is commonly used as it reduces perfusion pressure and stops hemorrhage. It also allows eventual recanalization of the vessels.

Q. What are the complications of UAE?

Ans. Infection, endometritis, neurologic damage may occur. Bladder necrosis and ovarian failure have been reported. The effect of UAE on future fertility is still unknown.

CASE 13: SURGICAL MANAGEMENT OF POSTPARTUM HEMORRHAGE (PPH)

Surgical procedures for the control of PPH in order to preserve the uterus, are many. Whereas, the decision to perform hysterectomy in such a situation is rather easy, compared to preservation of the uterus. Different surgical measures including bilateral ligation of the internal iliac (hypogastric) artery could be done.

One is definitely profited, when successful in preserving the uterus, if not, inevitably the patient succumbs to death. Time and the decision to perform the type of surgery are the important factors. As such, the factors: expertize of surgery, environment (resources available) and patient's condition, are all to be assessed prior to contemplating surgery and the specific type. Time does not permit one to try all the different types of conservative surgeries one after the especially in a case with atonic PPH.

Golden hour of PPH management is **the initial one hour** of standard management (*See* Manual of Obstetrics and Gynecology for the Postgraduates, p. 25) with resuscitation of the woman to maintain her vitals. It is observed that chance of survival of the woman decreases unless she is effectively resuscitated in the golden first one hour.

Q. How the vital parameters of the woman can indicate severity of the situation?

Ans. It is commonly expressed as the **rule of 30** when she has lost 30% of her blood volume and in a state of moderate shock. It is manifested with the following features:
- Drop of systolic BP by 30 mm Hg
- Rise in pulse rate by 30 bpm
- Rise in respiratory rate more than 30 breaths per minute
- Drop of hemoglobin or hematocrit by 30%
- Urine output less than 30 mL/hour.

Shock Index (SI) is considered to correlate better for obstetric hemorrhage rather than any other parameter when assessed alone. SI is calculated, dividing the heart rate by systolic blood pressure. The normal value lies between 0.5 and 0.7. SI: 0.9–1.1 suggests significant hemorrhage.

Q. What are the different surgical methods to control PPH?

Ans. *Several methods are used, depending upon the type of hemorrhage.*
- ***Traumatic PPH*** needs repair of genital tract injuries (perineum, vagina and cervix). Such a procedure may has to be done under general anesthesia.
- ***Atonic PPH*** is managed surgically when all conventional medical measures have failed.

    Surgical measures for atonic PPH are:
    - Balloon tamponade (*See* Manual of Obstetrics and Gynecology for the Postgraduates, p. 25)
    - Uterine compression sutures (different types *See* Manual of Obstetrics and Gynecology for the Postgraduates, p. 30)
    - Stepwise uterine devascularization
    - Angiographic selective arterial embolization (*See* Manual of Obstetrics and Gynecology for the Postgraduates, Ch 61)
    - Hysterectomy as the last resort.

Q. What is tamponade test?

Ans. When firm bimanual compression of the uterus, in a case with atonic PPH is effective in controlling hemorrhage, it is accepted as the positive tamponade test. This suggests that some balloon tamponade or brace suture could be effective.

Uterine compression sutures have been used for atonic postpartum hemorrhage. Several techniques have been used. These are: B-Lynch suture, Hayman vertical suture, Pereira transverse and vertical sutures and also multiple square sutures. Thick absorbable suture (chromic catgut no. 2) are passed both anteriorly and posteriorly on the external surface of the uterus. They are tied firmly so that adequate uterine compression occurs. It is effective in 50–75% of cases.

Stepwise Uterine Devascularization

The different vessels that are stepwise ligated:
- **Uterine artery ligation** (unilateral/bilateral) (*see* below)
- Uterine artery embolization (UAE)
- **Utero-ovarian vessels ligation:** This is done by ligating the uterine branch of the ovarian artery at the point of anastomosis with the uterine artery (Fig. 1.17). Compared to the ligation at the infundibulopelvic ligament, this procedure allows the blood supply to the tube and ovary. This is the preferred method and is done in addition to uterine artery ligation (unilateral/bilateral)
- **Hypogastric artery ligation** (unilateral/bilateral).

Uterine Artery Ligation (O'Leary-1966) (Fig. 1.17)

- It may be done before performing ligation of internal iliac artery. During pregnancy maximum blood supply (90%) to the pregnant uterus is made by the uterine arteries.
- This surgical procedure is simple, safe, easy to perform and effective.
- The uterine artery is ligated at the junction of upper and lower uterine segment. The suture passes through the myometrium (2 cm deep).
- Bilateral ligation of uterine and utero-ovarian vessels may also be done.

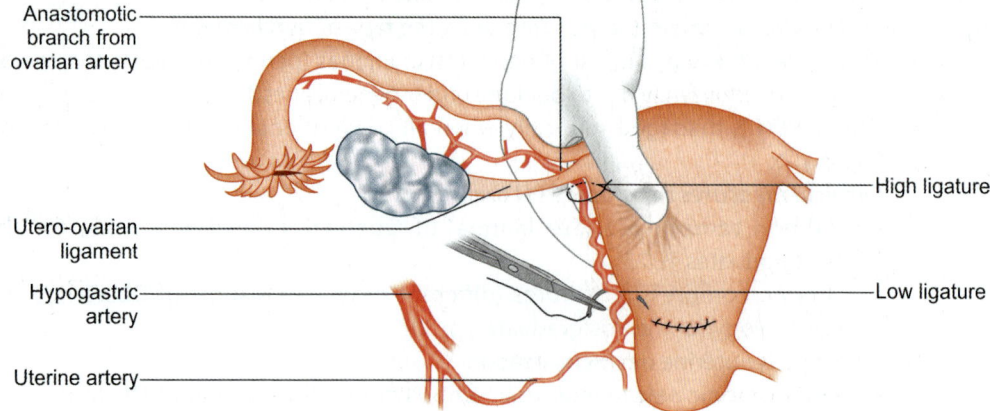

Fig. 1.17: Ligation of the uterine artery and the utero-ovarian vessels

- Bilateral ligation of uterine arteries is effective in 85% cases of PPH.
- As it is done at a higher level, injuries to the ureters are avoided.

Hypogastric Artery Ligation

Q. What is the rationale of hypogastric artery ligation in obstetrics?

Ans. In cases with acute obstetric hemorrhage, at times, identification of specific bleeding vessels technically is impossible. It may be due reasons like tissue friability leading to oozing from different sites or retraction of the bleeding vessels. As a life saving measure, prompt decision has to be made, often desperately, to ligate the anterior division of the internal iliac artery (hypogastric artery) to control the hemorrhage.

Pelvic collateral circulation: Collateral circulation in the female pelvis is extensive. It restores circulation in no time following bilateral hypogastric artery ligation. Bilateral hypogastric artery ligation was first performed by Howard Kelly (1893), to control pelvic hemorrhage. Successful pregnancy has been observed following bilateral ligation of hypogastric arteries, where the uterus was preserved. The main arterial groups having collateral circulation with the hypogastric artery are:

- Branches from the aorta
- Branches from the external iliac artery
- Branches from the femoral artery.

The pathways of collateral circulation has been demonstrated by the aortogram (*See* Manual of Obstetrics and Gynecology for the Postgraduates, p. 218, Fig. 4.1).

Ligation of internal iliac artery and development of collateral circulation

Systemic artery		Internal iliac artery
1. Lumbar (aorta) ⟶	with ⟵	Iliolumbar
2. Middle sacral (aorta) ⟶	with ⟵	Lateral sacral
3. Superior rectal (inferior mesenteric) ⟶	with ⟵	Middle rectal
4. Ovarian (aorta) ⟶	with ⟵	Uterine
5. Inferior epigastric (external iliac) ⟶	with ⟵	Obturator
6. Lateral circumflex femoral (femoral) ⟶	with ⟵	Inferior gluteal
7. Medial circumflex femoral (femoral) ⟶	with ⟵	Inferior gluteal
8. Deep circumflex iliac (external iliac) ⟶	with ⟵	Superior gluteal

Indications of Internal Iliac (Hypogastric) Artery Ligation

- Broad ligament hematoma following
  - Rupture of the uterus
  - Extension of uterine incision during LSCS
  - Cervical tear
- When bleeding cannot be controlled by hemostatic sutures.
- Unilateral hypogastric ligation is effective.
- Atonic PPH: When all conventional measures have failed
- Morbid adherent placenta with uncontrolled bleeding
- Secondary PPH from uterine scar (cesarean), when hemostasis cannot be effectively achieved due to friable tissues.

Hemodynamic Alterations Following Ligation of Internal Iliac Artery
After ligation, pulsation virtually ceases, in arteries distal to ligation.

Side of ligation	Pulse pressure	Mean Pressure	Blood flow
Opposite	14	10	–
Same	77	22	49
Bilateral	85	24	48

Approach: In obstetrics ***transabdominal infraumbilical route*** is always preferred. In cases with unilateral broad ligament hematoma, it is not wise to proceed through extraperitoneal route.
Advantages of transabdominal route approach:
- It is convenient to perform the hypogastric artery ligation unilaterally or even bilaterally
- Ligation of utero-ovarian vessels is possible whenever required
- Hysterectomy could be done when decided
- Operations could be facilitated either by eventrating the uterus or pushing the uterus to the opposite side.

Complications of the operations:
- Injury to the internal iliac and external iliac veins
- Injury to the ureter
- Ischemia of the central pelvic area followed by tissue necrosis (rare).

Limitations: Poor result in some cases may be due to its delay in performance.
This mainly due to:
- Patient already is in irreversible hemorrhagic shock
- Coagulation failure started already.

Failures: Even after ligation of hypogastric arteries bleeding fails to stop.
The reasons are:
- Simultaneous venous bleeding
- Dislodgement of clots as the blood pressure rises
- Presence of large aberrant arterial branches that supply blood to the pelvis
- Severe necrosis following infection destroys the vessels.

Q. What is the mechanism of hemostasis following ligation of internal iliac artery?

Ans.
- There is reduction of pulse pressure in the vessels distal to the tie. This reduction of pulse pressure is to the extent of 85%.
  - This procedure converts arterial pressure system to that of venous circulation. This mechanism helps hemostasis with the formation of a stable clot.
  - It is successful in about 50% of cases (ACOG).

Techniques of Ligation (Figs 1.18A and B)
- Adequate exposure of the operating field is essential
- Ligation of the internal iliac artery is done at 4–5 cm distal to its origin. This usually saves the branches of the posterior division
- It is done carefully to avoid injuries to the internal iliac vein.

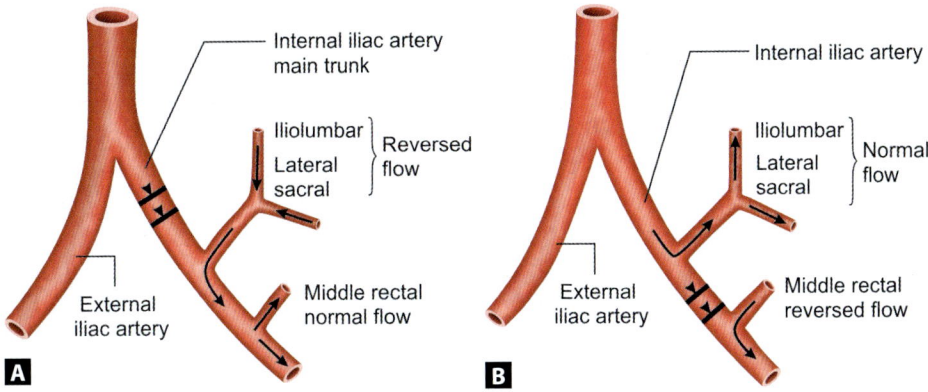

Figs 1.18A and B: Ligation of the internal iliac artery. **A.** Above the origin of the posterior division (main trunk), **B.** Below the origin of the posterior division (anterior division)

Steps of Internal Iliac (Hypogastric) Artery Ligation (Fig. 1.19)

- Common iliac artery and its bifurcation up to the external and internal iliac arteries are visualized through the peritoneum. These vessels are then palpated also.
- The posterior peritoneum is opened on the lateral side of the common iliac artery near its bifurcation and is extended down for 4–6 cm. The incision is made lateral to the ureter. The hypogastric artery is posterior and medial to the external iliac artery. Internal iliac vein lies posterior and slightly lateral to the artery (Fig. 1.20A).
- Posterior division has to be clearly identified.

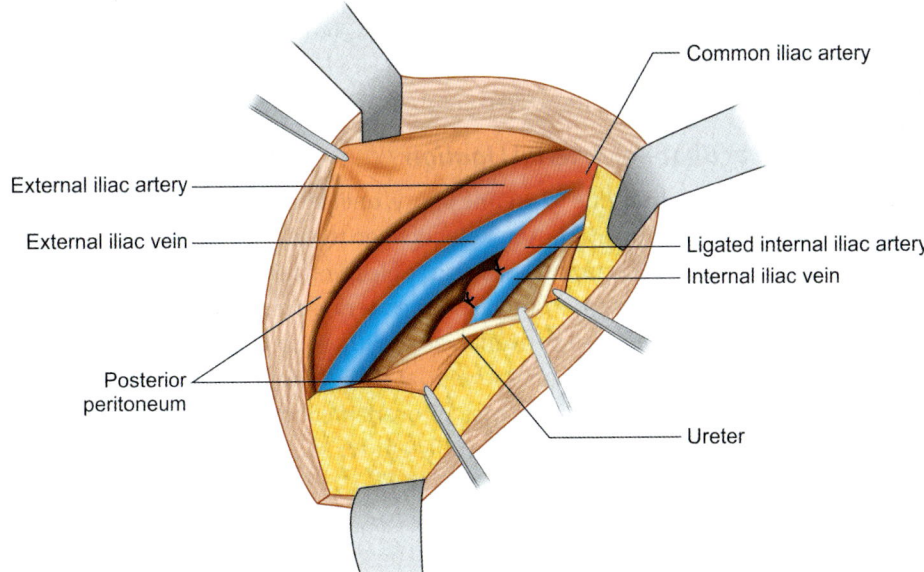

Fig. 1.19: Ligation of the internal iliac artery at two sites. The artery is not transected (*See* Manual of Obstetrics and Gynecology for the Postgraduates, p. 218).

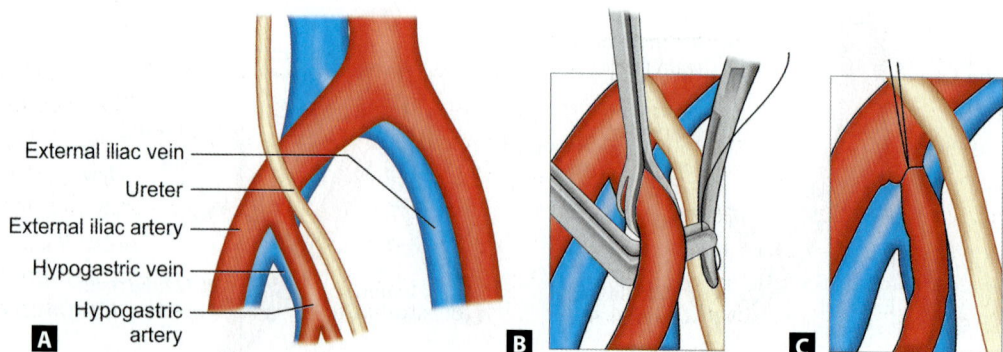

Figs 1.20A to C: A. Anatomy of the pelvic vessels and the ureter, **B.** Dissection of the hypogastric artery and passage of silk thread with a right angle forceps, **C.** Ligation of the hypogastric artery close the origin

- The areolar tissue that joins the posterior wall of the internal iliac artery to the anterior wall of the vein is carefully separated by blunt dissection.
- A Babcock clamp is placed on the hypogastric artery and is elevated from the anterior surface of internal iliac vein.
- A right angle clamp (Fig. 1.20B) or an aneurysm needle is passed below the artery from lateral to the medial, while the Babcock clamp elevates the artery.
- Silk suture no. 1 is used to tie. To avoid recanalization, it should be tied twice (Figs 1.19 and 1.20C).
- It is important to check the pulsation of the branches of the external iliac artery before and after the procedure.
- Not to transect the artery in between the ties. There may be chance of retraction and bleeding from the ends.
- The peritoneum is closed with interrupted catgut sutures.

Place of Unilateral or Bilateral Arterial Ligation

- In broad ligament hematoma due to uterine injury, unilateral ligation on the affected side is done. However, because of great anastomosis between these two vessels, the procedure may have to be employed on the opposite side also, if bleeding fails to control.
- But when the bleeding is of uterine origin and the uterine preservation is required, bilateral ligation of the hypogastric as well as ovarian arteries have to be done. In emergency, if the ovarian artery cannot be isolated from the vein, at the infundibulopelvic ligament, both are to be ligated. In such cases, there is chance of ovarian congestion with polycystic ovarian changes. However, collateral circulation is sufficient for subsequent ovarian function to be reasonably normal.

Maintenance of Reproductive Function

Provided the patient has a normal reproductive genital tract, menstruation resumes as in other cases. Even when bilateral ligation of ovarian arteries are done along with bilateral ligation of the internal iliac artery, future obstetric outcome has not been found to be adversely affected.

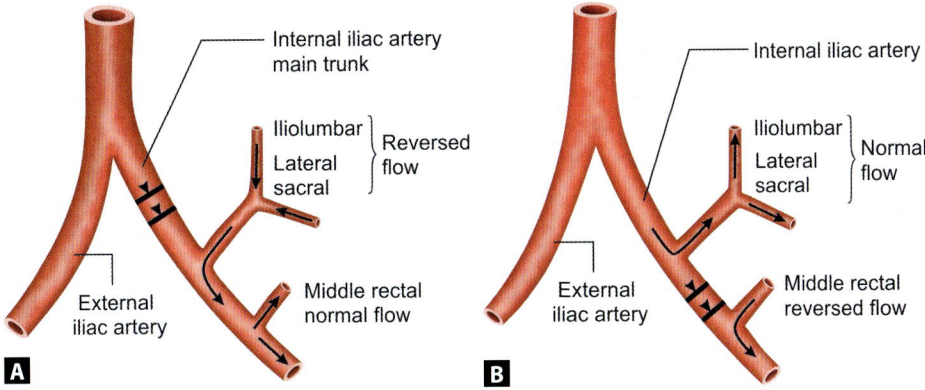

Figs 1.18A and B: Ligation of the internal iliac artery. **A.** Above the origin of the posterior division (main trunk), **B.** Below the origin of the posterior division (anterior division)

Steps of Internal Iliac (Hypogastric) Artery Ligation (Fig. 1.19)

- Common iliac artery and its bifurcation up to the external and internal iliac arteries are visualized through the peritoneum. These vessels are then palpated also.
- The posterior peritoneum is opened on the lateral side of the common iliac artery near its bifurcation and is extended down for 4–6 cm. The incision is made lateral to the ureter. The hypogastric artery is posterior and medial to the external iliac artery. Internal iliac vein lies posterior and slightly lateral to the artery (Fig. 1.20A).
- Posterior division has to be clearly identified.

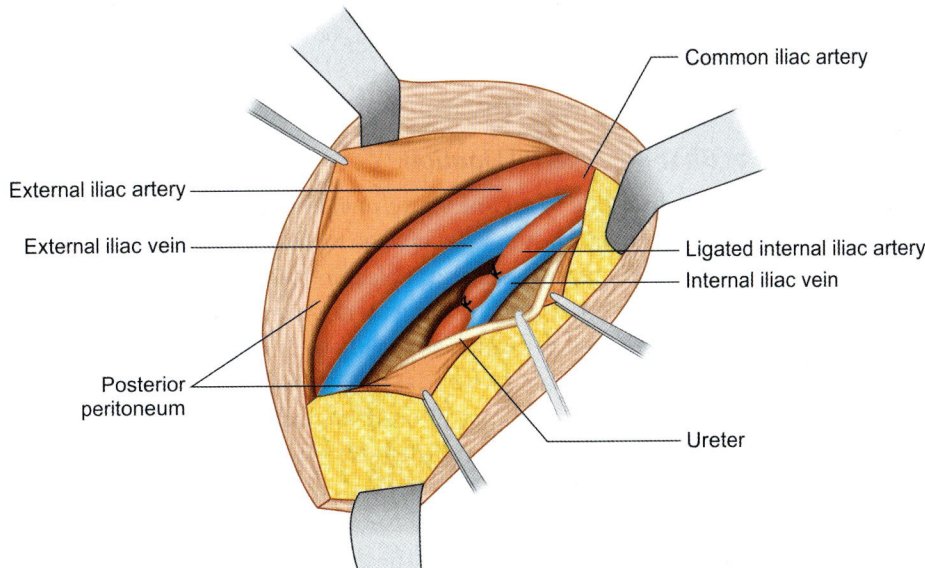

Fig. 1.19: Ligation of the internal iliac artery at two sites. The artery is not transected (*See* Manual of Obstetrics and Gynecology for the Postgraduates, p. 218).

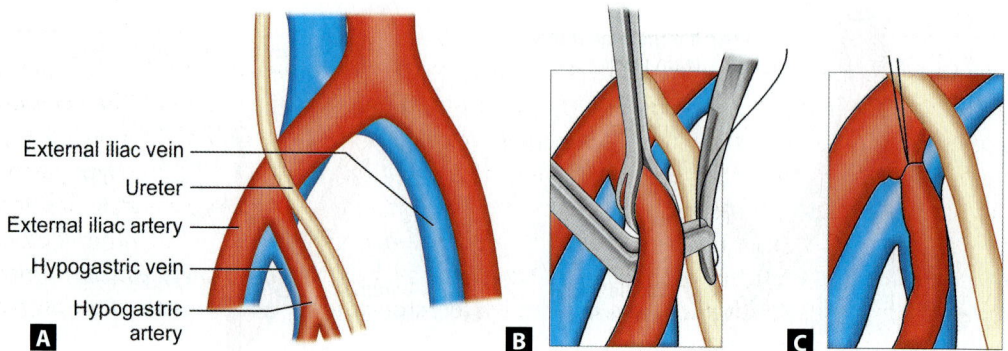

Figs 1.20A to C: A. Anatomy of the pelvic vessels and the ureter, **B.** Dissection of the hypogastric artery and passage of silk thread with a right angle forceps, **C.** Ligation of the hypogastric artery close the origin

- The areolar tissue that joins the posterior wall of the internal iliac artery to the anterior wall of the vein is carefully separated by blunt dissection.
- A Babcock clamp is placed on the hypogastric artery and is elevated from the anterior surface of internal iliac vein.
- A right angle clamp (Fig. 1.20B) or an aneurysm needle is passed below the artery from lateral to the medial, while the Babcock clamp elevates the artery.
- Silk suture no. 1 is used to tie. To avoid recanalization, it should be tied twice (Figs 1.19 and 1.20C).
- It is important to check the pulsation of the branches of the external iliac artery before and after the procedure.
- Not to transect the artery in between the ties. There may be chance of retraction and bleeding from the ends.
- The peritoneum is closed with interrupted catgut sutures.

Place of Unilateral or Bilateral Arterial Ligation

- In broad ligament hematoma due to uterine injury, unilateral ligation on the affected side is done. However, because of great anastomosis between these two vessels, the procedure may have to be employed on the opposite side also, if bleeding fails to control.
- But when the bleeding is of uterine origin and the uterine preservation is required, bilateral ligation of the hypogastric as well as ovarian arteries have to be done. In emergency, if the ovarian artery cannot be isolated from the vein, at the infundibulopelvic ligament, both are to be ligated. In such cases, there is chance of ovarian congestion with polycystic ovarian changes. However, collateral circulation is sufficient for subsequent ovarian function to be reasonably normal.

Maintenance of Reproductive Function

Provided the patient has a normal reproductive genital tract, menstruation resumes as in other cases. Even when bilateral ligation of ovarian arteries are done along with bilateral ligation of the internal iliac artery, future obstetric outcome has not been found to be adversely affected.

CONCLUSION

Hypogastric ligation either unilateral or bilateral in obstetrics is a life-saving procedure. It requires lot of surgical skill and also courage, so as to perform it in a desperately ill patient. The decision to perform it following hysterectomy for uterine trauma is rather easy and well-formulated. But attempted preservation of the uterus hopefully at the cost of ligation of both the hypogastric and ovarian arteries requires lot of expertize, courage and thoughts. One is definitely profited with it if successful, but if it is not, inevitably leads to patient's death. As such, other factors like—personal expertize, environment and the patient's condition are all to be assessed prior contemplating conservative surgery vis-à-vis hysterectomy, especially in a case with atonic postpartum hemorrhage.

CASE 14: PREGNANCY AND LABOR IN A WOMAN WITH PRIOR CESAREAN DELIVERY

Case Summary

A woman in her second pregnancy was admitted in the labor ward at 39 weeks of gestation. She had the history of cesarean delivery in her first pregnancy. Labor was progressing satisfactorily, until about 4 hours later, she complained unusual pain in the suprapubic region and it was associated with vaginal bleeding. She was found to have tachycardia and hypotension. Cardiotocography revealed irregularities of the fetal heart rate.

Q. What would be the possible diagnosis?
Ans. Scar dehiscence or scar rupture of uterus. (*See* Manual of Obstetrics and Gynecology for the Postgraduates, p. 266, Fig. 12.1).

Q. What is the immediate management?
Ans. Resuscitation of the patient with IV infusion (crystalloid), blood sample for grouping and cross matching and to organize urgent laparotomy.

Q. What would be the actual management?
Ans. This will depend on the extent and type of rupture. Delivery of the baby is done first. If it is just a scar dehiscence then repair of the uterus is done following delivery. If it is extensive then it may need subtotal hysterectomy. But in such a patient it is unlikely.

Q. What additional steps you may consider in this case?
Ans. To consider bilateral tubectomy when repair of the scar is done. However, it depends on adequate counseling with the couple and with informed consent before she would be taken to the operation theater.

Q. How are you going to deliver her in next pregnancy?
Ans. By elective cesarean section (CS) after 38 completed weeks of gestation.

Q. Had there been a classical scar on the uterus, when is it more likely to rupture?
Ans. During pregnancy, rupture occurs commonly in the third trimester.

Q. Is there any place of induction and/or augmentation of labor in a woman who is undergoing vaginal birth after cesarean (VBAC)?
Ans. There is an increased risk of uterine rupture in women planned for VBAC when they were induced with prostaglandins (ACOG). However, oxytocin can be used judiciously for induction of labor. Oxytocin can be used to augment labor when labor has started spontaneously. Labor monitoring should be close for assessment of uterine contractions and scar tenderness. Continuous electronic fetal heart rate monitoring should be used. These are important for women undergoing VBAC when oxytocin is given either for induction or augmentation.

Q. After a VBAC, should the uterine scar be explored as a routine?
Ans. There is no benefit from transcervical exploration of the uterine scar following VBAC as a routine. If there is no bleeding per vaginam and the uterus is well retracted, there is no need of exploration. Asymptomatic scar dehiscence, even if present, needs no treatment. Such dehiscence generally heal well. However, presence of excessive vaginal bleeding, maternal tachycardia and hypotension need prompt assessment to exclude scar rupture.

Q. Is there any place of epidural analgesia to a woman who is undergoing VBAC-TOL?
Ans. Vaginal birth after cesarean delivery (VBAC) trial of labor is not a contraindication for the use of epidural analgesia. Epidural analgesia does not mask the signs and symptoms of uterine rupture.

CASE 15: PUERPERAL PYREXIA

Case Summary

A 26-year-old woman developed temperature (39°C) on the 4th day of her puerperium following spontaneous vaginal delivery at the end of a term pregnancy.

Q. What could be the possible reasons?
Ans.
- Infection of the episiotomy wound
- Breast infection
- Urinary tract infection
- Respiratory tract infection or deep vein thrombosis.

Q. Enumerate few important symptoms and signs for the patient.
Ans.
- Offensive vaginal discharge and perineal pain
- Engorged breasts with pain and tenderness
- Dysuria and frequency of micturition
- Cough, chest pain and crepitations
- Swollen legs with pain and tenderness.

Q. Organize few important investigations for her.
Ans. It will depend on the clinical examination findings. Common investigations are:
- Wound swab for culture and sensitivity
- Midstream urine for culture and sensitivity
- Chest X-ray
- Ultrasound scan with Doppler flow study of the calf veins.

Q. She faced difficulty in breastfeeding her baby. How are you going to help her?
Ans. Correct position of the mother, frequent feeding and correct attachment of the baby with the breast can improve the outcome. For any other difficulties, a trained nurse may be helpful.

CASE 16: MULTIPLE PREGNANCY

Q. What important measures in the management of multiple pregnancy may improve the perinatal outcome?

Ans.
- Early diagnosis with sonography
- Diagnosis of chorionicity and zygocity within 14 weeks
- Selective fetal reduction (*See* Dutta's Textbook of Obstetrics, 8th Edition, p. 245)
- Early detection of fetal congenital malformation
- Frequent antenatal visit at every 2–3 weeks from 32 weeks of gestation onwards
- Diet with additional calories (+300 Kcal/day)
- Extra rest at home and early cessation of work
- Increased supplementation of iron (100–200 mg/day), folic acid, calcium and vitamins
- Counseling the woman about the risks of preterm labor and preterm babies
- Fetal growth monitoring by serial ultrasound (every 2–3 weeks interval) examinations. Early detection of intrauterine growth restriction (IUGR)
- Hospitalization and management of any complications like preterm labor, pre-eclampsia, polyhydramnios, single fetal death and twin-twin transfusion syndrome
- Delivery in an equipped center with facilities of neonatal intensive care unit (NICU).

Q. What happens when one twin dies in uterus?

Ans.
- When death occurs in the **first trimester** → the dead fetus is completely absorbed.
- **Death beyond the first trimester** → the dead fetus may persist as a small, dried and flattened mass known as **fetus papyraceus**.

    The risk to the surviving fetus is when the death of one fetus occurs in the second or third trimester. The risk to the surviving fetus depends upon the following factors—(i) time of death (first trimester or beyond), (ii) chorionicity and zygocity of twins and (iii) time interval between the death of one twin to the delivery of the surviving twin. Monochorionic twins are at increased risks.

Q. How is the diagnosis of twin-twin transfusion syndrome (TTTS) made?

Ans. *The diagnosis of TTTS is made on ultrasound criteria*. These are as mentioned below:
- Monochorionic placenta
- Same sex gender
- Oligohydramnios with maximum vertical pocket (MVP) less than 2 cm in one sac and polyhydramnios (MVP ≥ 8 cm) in other sac
- Discordant growth and bladder appearance—severe TTTS
- Hemodynamic and cardiac compromise—severe TTTS.

Q. Discuss the pathophysiology involved in TTTS?

Ans. In TTTS, blood is transfused from the donor twin to its recipient. Donor becomes anemic, growth restricted, hypovolemic, pale and oliguric whereas the recipient becomes polycythemic, hypervolemic, plethoric and polyuric. The recipient suffers from the problem of cardiac failure due to circulatory overload. There is difference in the amniotic fluid between the two sacs. Donor twin suffers from oligohydramnios whereas the recipient develops polyhydramnios. Due to oligohydramnios in the donor twin sac, the fetus fails to move (stuck twin). The polyhydramnios and oligohydramnios complex ('poly-oli' syndrome) results in IUGR, pulmonary hypoplasia of one (donor) twin and cardiac failure and PROM in the other (recipient) twin.

In TTTS, there is unidirectional flow through arteriovenous anastomoses. This unidirectional flow leads to an imbalance in blood volumes and hemodynamics. Deoxygenated blood from the donor is pumped into the recipient.

In the donor twin ischemia may be due to hypotension, anemia or due to both. The recipient twin also suffers from ischemia due to episodes of hypotension. Neurological damage in multiple pregnancy is due to ischemic necrosis.

Cerebral pathology is due to cavitary lesions following ischemia. Cerebral palsy, microcephaly or multicystic encephalomalacia are the common cerebral lesions.

Q. Why is selective fetal reduction in multiple gestation done?
Ans. Maternal and perinatal complications are more in pregnancy complicated by quadruplets or greater number of fetuses. Pregnancy outcome is improved significantly by reducing the number of fetuses in early pregnancy. It is safe in multichorionic multifetal pregnancy. Selective fetal reduction is usually done at 10–13 weeks of pregnancy. Intracardiac injection of potassium chloride is usually done **under ultrasound guidance**.

FETAL CONGENITAL MALFORMATIONS

CASE 17: NEURAL TUBE DEFECTS

Case Summary

A 32-year-old, unbooked woman was admitted at 36+ weeks of gestation in labor. She delivered without any delay. The baby looked like as shown in Figure 1.21.

Q. What is most likely the diagnosis?
Ans. Open neural tube defects—encephalocele with spina bifida.

Q. How the prenatal diagnosis could have been made?
Ans. By fetal anatomy scan with ultrasound.

Q. Which biochemical test is helpful to make the diagnosis?
Ans. Estimation of maternal serum alpha fetoprotein (MSAFP) at 15–18 weeks of gestation. The level is elevated (> 2.5 MOM) in such a case (*See* Manual of Obstetrics and Gynecology for the Postgraduates, p. 255).

Q. Who are the mothers that have the high-risk for this abnormality?
Ans.
- Women over 35 years of age
- Family history or previous birth of neural tube defects
- History of recurrent miscarriage
- Epileptic mother with anticonvulsants (sodium valproate)
- Diabetic mother
- Obesity (BMI > 35 kg/m^2)
- Use of folic acid antagonists (methotrexate)
- Women with malabsorption syndrome.

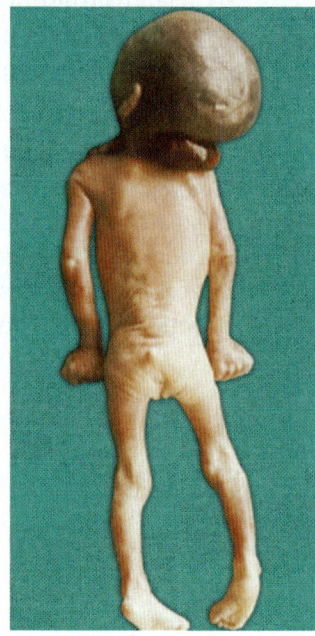

Fig. 1.21: Encephalocele with spina bifida

Q. What is the risk of recurrence and how could this be prevented?
Ans. Recurrence risk after one child is 4%.

Pregnancy counseling is essential. Folic acid supplementation (4 mg daily) at the beginning of 1 month before conception to about 12 weeks of pregnancy is recommended.

CASE 18: ANENCEPHALY

Case Summary

A 28-year-old, unbooked woman, $P_{1+0+1+1'}$ was admitted in labor at 36 weeks of gestation. She delivered without delay. The baby looked like as shown in Figure 1.22.

Q. What is the diagnosis?
Ans. Anencephaly—defect of the neural tube.

Q. What are the possible pregnancy complications with this abnormality?
Ans. Hydramnios (70%), malpresentation (breech), tendency of postmaturity, failure of induction and shoulder dystocia.

Q. How the prenatal diagnosis could be made?
Ans.
- Sonography
- Elevated maternal serum alpha fetoprotein (MSAFP) estimation at 15–18 weeks of gestation.

Q. What is the risk of future pregnancy?
Ans. Recurrence rate after one affected child is 4%.

Q. How the recurrence of this abnormality could be prevented?
Ans. Prepregnancy counseling is important. Folic acid supplementation (4 mg daily) at the beginning of 1 month before conception to about 12 weeks of pregnancy.

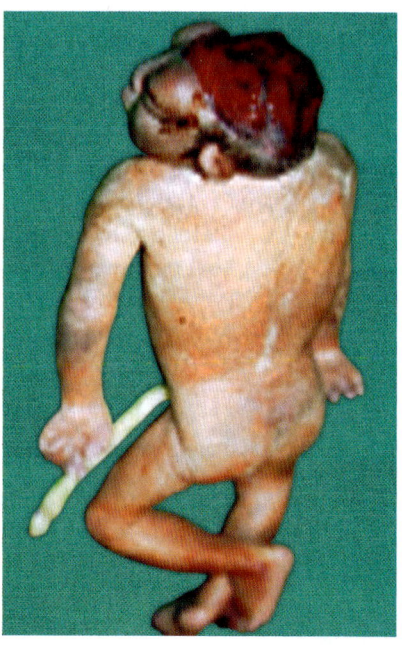

Fig. 1.22: Anencephaly, absence of cranial vault (calvarium) and telencephalon

Q. Who are the high-risk women for neural tube defects?
Ans. It is not possible to identify all the high-risk women. But in general the high-risk women are:
- Woman with a previous pregnancy affected with neural tube defect (NTD)
- Maternal diabetes mellitus
- Maternal drug intake (valproic acid, carbamazepine)
- Woman with her husband or close relative who has an NTD.

Q. Why folic acid supplementation is recommended before conception?
Ans. Randomized controlled trials have shown that women who had a previous child with a NTD, intake of high dose of folic acid (4 mg/day) decreased the risk by 70%. Centers for Disease Control and Prevention (CDC) recommends that women who had one previous NTD affected pregnancy should be supplemented with 4 mg of folic acid per day. Therapy should begin at least 4 weeks before conception and to be continued through the first trimester.

Women with no history of NTD affected pregnancy should take 400 μg (0.4 mg) of folic acid similar to that of the high-risk women.

Q. What are neural tube defects?
Ans. These are a severe form of birth anomalies. These are due to lack of closure of the neural tube at either upper or lower end in the 3rd to 4th week after conception (D26 to D28 postconception).

Q. Is there any other benefits of taking folic acid prepregnancy?
Ans. The other benefits of prepregnancy folic acid supplementation are:
- Prevention of NTDs
- Reduction in the risk of other problems like:
    - Congenital heart defects
    - Orofacial defects
    - Cleft lip and cleft palate
    - Low-birth-weight babies
    - Preterm births
    - Autism.

Q. Is there any adverse effects of intake of folic acid?
Ans. Folic acid supplementation of 400 mcg (0.4 mg)/day can be taken for years. No adverse effects have been observed.

Q. What should be the dose of supplementation of folic acid for high-risk women?
Ans. Folic acid 400 mcg (0.4 mg)/day is recommended. It should be started at least 4 weeks before the conception and to be continued throughout the first trimester.

CASE 19: HYDROCEPHALUS

Case Summary

A 30-year-old, unbooked woman, $P_{1+0+1+1}$, was admitted at term pregnancy. She was delivered by lower segment cesarean section (LSCS) because of tenderness of the scar of previous CS. Baby looked like as shown in Figure 1.23.

Q. What is the abnormality?

Ans. Hydrocephalus.

Q. What are the pregnancy complications with this abnormality?

Ans. Undiagnosed cases when left uncared for, labor will become prolonged and obstructed. Rupture of uterus may occur. Fetal outcome is extremely poor.

Q. How could it be diagnosed prenatally?

Ans. By ultrasonography: Dilated lateral ventricles and thinning out of cortex (Fig. 1.24). Clinical examination during labor — gaping of suture lines and tense fontanelles.

Q. How could the baby be delivered vaginally where there is no other contraindication?

Ans. In labor when the cervix is 3–4 cm dilated, decompression of the head (**cephalic presentation**) is done by sharp pointed scissors or a perforator.

In **breech presentation,** during assisted vaginal breech delivery to deliver the after coming head, laminectomy at the cervical region is done to open up the spinal canal to drain cerebrospinal fluid (CSF) and for decompression.

Abdominal decompression (cephalocentesis) with a large bore lumbar puncture needle may also be done.

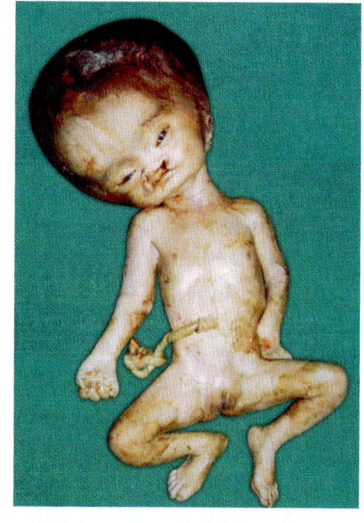

Fig. 1.23: Hydrocephalus

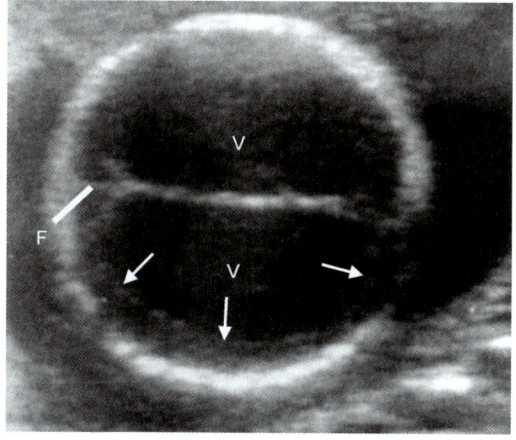

Fig. 1.24: Ultrasonography showing marked ventricular enlargement (F. flax) with thinning of the cortex (V)

Q. What is the risk of future pregnancy?

Ans. Risk of recurrence in subsequent pregnancy is about 5%.

CASE 20: CYSTIC HYGROMA

Case Summary

Mrs PK in her first pregnancy had a prenatal diagnosis and opted for pregnancy termination at 18 weeks of gestation. The fetus is seen in the photograph (Fig. 1.25).

Q. What is the abnormality?
Ans. Huge cystic hygroma.

Q. What are the common causes of the abnormality?
Ans. Turner's syndrome (45XO).
Trisomy 18; trisomy 21; triploidy.

Q. How is it diagnosed prenatally?
Ans. By ultrasonography (Figs 1.26 and 1.27).
Important markers are:
- Nuchal thickness > 3 mm (subcutaneous edema at the level of the neck due to dilatation of the lymphatic capillaries) (Fig. 1.26) is associated with chromosomal abnormalities like 45X, trisomies (13, 18, 21), triploidy and aneuploidy
- Hydrops—trisomy (13, 18, 21), 45XO
- Short femur—trisomy 21
- Banana sign (banana configuration of the cerebellum)—dysplastic cerebellum
- Lemon sign (frontal concave scalloping)—Figure 1.27 (*see* arrow)
- Banana sign and lemon sign are observed in cases with open spina bifida.

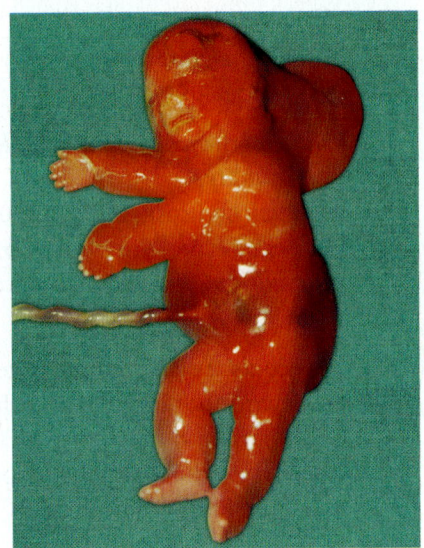

Fig. 1.25: Cystic hygroma (fetus with Turner's syndrome)

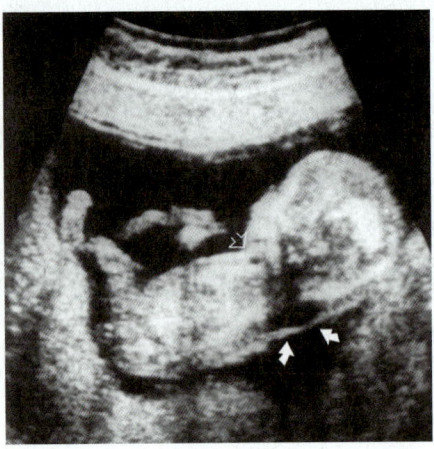

Fig. 1.26: Ultrasonography of the fetus showing thickened nuchal translucency (*see* arrows)

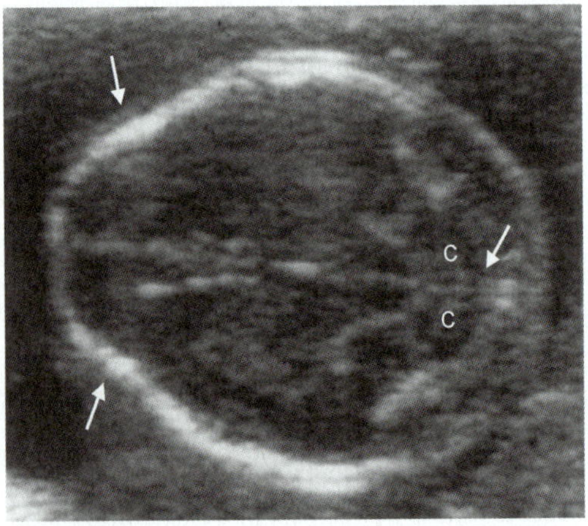

Fig. 1.27: Ultrasonography showing lemon sign and banana sign (*see* arrows)

Q. What are the high-risk factors for such an abnormality?
Ans.
- History of recurrent miscarriage
- Previous birth of a chromosomally abnormal fetus
- Previous child mentally retarded
- Family history of chromosomal abnormality
- Parental chromosomal abnormality (translocation).

Q. Who are the high-risk women to have an infant with chromosomal abnormality?
Ans.
- Maternal age ≥ 35 years
- Previous baby with NTD
- Previous baby with chromosomal abnormality
- Family history of NTD
- Abnormal maternal serum screening tests
- Abnormal fetus on ultrasound
- Chromosomal abnormality in either parent (aneuploidy, balanced translocation).

Q. What different investigations are performed to detect fetal, genetic, chromosomal and structural abnormalities?
Ans. Screening and diagnostic procedures for early detection of fetal (i) genetic, (ii) chromosomal and (iii) structural abnormalities are as below:

Tests for Prenatal Diagnosis (See Manual of Obstetrics and Gynecology for the Postgraduates for the references in the table below)

Screening tests	Diagnostic tests
- Maternal serum alpha fetoprotein (MSAFP) (p. 255) - Triple test (combined test): ↓ MSAFP, ↓ unconjugated estriol (uE3) and ↑ hCG (p. 255) - Quadruple test: ↓ MSAFP, ↓ uE3, ↑ hCG, ↑ inhibin - Integrated test (p. 255) - Integrated serum test (p. 255) - High-resolution ultrasonography - 3D or 4D ultrasound with increased resolution (p. 252)	- Chorionic villus biopsy (p. 198) - Amniocentesis (p. 68) - Cordocentesis (p. 95, 521) - Fetoscopy - Fetal cell isolation from maternal blood - Genetic analysis from isolated fetal nucleated red blood cells or trophoblast cells (free fetal DNA) (p. 521) - Peri-implantation genetic diagnosis (p. 391)

Q. What is the current recommendation for prenatal genetic diagnosis?
Ans. All pregnant women should be offered screening for Down's syndrome (RCOG clinical guideline 2007), with a test which provides detection rate above 75% and a false-positive rate of less than 3%. These tests should be age standardized and based on a cut off value of 1 in 250 or greater.

Q. What is the detection rate of first trimester screening for trisomies 13, 18 and 21?
Ans. Different parameters considered are maternal age, fetal nuchal translucency thickness (NT), FHR, serum β-hCG and PAPP-A. Combined parameters when used, can detect about 90% of cases of trisomy 21 and 95% cases of trisomies 18 and 13. False-positive rate is about 5%. Currently, screening for fetal aneuploidies based on the analysis of cell free fetal DNA (cffDNA) from maternal plasma has been introduced (See Manual of Obstetrics and Gynecology for the Postgraduates, p. 521). Evidence suggests that analysis of cffDNA in maternal blood can detect about 99% of cases of trisomy 21, 97% cases of trisomy 18 and 92% of trisomy 13. The false-positive rates (FPRs) were 0.08%, 0.15% and 0.2% respectively. However, testing of cffDNA is expensive at the moment.

2

Self-Assessment in Obstetrics

SINGLE BEST ANSWER (SBA) AND MULTIPLE CHOICE QUESTIONS (MCQs)

Q.1 The pelvis which has greater anteroposterior diameter at the inlet compared to that of transverse diameter is classified as:
- a. Gynecoid
- b. Android
- c. Anthropoid
- d. Platypelloid

Ans. c. *See Dutta's Textbook of Obstetrics, 8th Edition, p. 403.*

Q.2 Regarding germ cells:
- a. Following birth, there is mitotic division of the primary oocytes
- b. The final maturation of the oocytes occurs only before fertilization
- c. Ovulation occurs soon after formation of secondary oocytes
- d. Secondary oocytes completes the second meiotic division just before fertilization

Ans. c. At birth, there is no more mitotic division. Final maturation of the oocyte occurs after fertilization. Secondary oocyte completes the second meiotic division after fertilization (*See Dutta's Textbook of Gynecology, 7th Edition, p. 66*).

Q.3 Decidual space is obliterated by:
- a. 10th week
- b. 12th week
- c. 14th week
- d. 16th week

Ans. d. *See Dutta's Textbook of Obstetrics, 8th Edition, p. 28.*

Q.4 Tertiary villi are completed by:
- a. 17th day
- b. 19th day
- c. 21st day
- d. 23rd day

Ans. c. 21st day

Q.5 Regarding development, all the statements are correct except:
- a. Gonads are developed from mesoderm and endoderm
- b. Bartholin's glands are developed from endoderm
- c. Most of the genital tract is developed from the endoderm
- d. Urethra from endoderm

Ans. c. Most of the genital tract is developed from mesoderm.

Self-Assessment in Obstetrics

Q.6 Blood flow in the intervillous space per minute is approximately:
  a. 250 mL
  b. 300 mL
  c. 500 mL
  d. 700 mL
Ans. c. See Dutta's Textbook of Obstetrics, 8th Edition, p. 37.

Q.7 Regarding human chorionic gonadotropin (hCG) all are correct except:
  a. hCG is a glycoprotein
  b. Plasma half-life is 24 hours
  c. Site of origin is the syncytiotrophoblasts
  d. Maximum secretion is at 6–7 weeks
Ans. d. Maximum secretion is at 6–7 weeks (60–70 days).

Q.8 Thickness of the placental membrane at term approximately:
  a. 0.025 mm
  b. 0.002 mm
  c. 0.012 mm
  d. 0.02 mm
Ans. a. See Dutta's Textbook of Obstetrics, 8th Edition, p. 38.

Q.9 Deeper penetration of the villi is prevented by:
  a. Nitabuch's fibrinoid layer
  b. Trophosphere
  c. Mucopolysaccharides content of the decidua
  d. Enzyme in cytotrophoblast
Ans. a. Nitabuch's fibrinoid layer

Q.10 Fetal sex can be determined by examining the genitalia with ultrasonography (USG) at:
  a. 8th week
  b. 10th week
  c. 12th week
  d. 16th week
Ans. d. Fetal gender identification by USG is possible in the second trimester though third trimester is the appropriate time.

Q.11 The following changes occur in the vascular system of the newborn after birth:
  a. The proximal parts of the umbilical arteries become the lateral umbilical ligaments
  b. Anatomical closure of the ductus arteriosus occurs soon after birth
  c. Anatomical closure of the foramen ovale occurs with onset of respiration
  d. Ductus venosus becomes ligamentum venosum
Ans. d. The proximal parts of the umbilical arteries remain open as superior vesical arteries. Anatomical closure of the ductus arteriosus occurs at about 1–3 months. Anatomic closure of foramen ovale occurs at about 1 year.

Q.12 The following are related to delivery of head in normal labor except:
  a. During crowning, the biparietal diameter stretches the vulval outlet
  b. Successive parts of the fetal head to be born are face, brow and vertex
  c. Restitution occurs in the direction opposite to that of internal rotation
  d. Head is delivered with slow extension
Ans. b. The successive parts to be born are vertex, brow and face.

Q.13 During the active phase of labor, the effective dilatation of the cervix in primigravida should be at the rate of:
 a. 0.5 cm/hour
 b. 1 cm/hour
 c. 1.5 cm/hour
 d. 2 cm/hour
Ans. b. 1 cm/hour

Q.14 The following are related to a normal pelvis:
 a. Angle of inclination is 90°
 b. Sacrocotyloid diameter measures from the sacral promontory to the iliopubic eminence
 c. Waste space of Morris is about 2.5 cm
 d. Bispinous diameter is 8.5 cm
Ans. b; c. Waste space of Morris should not be more than 1 cm. a. = 55°; d. = 10.5 cm.

Q.15 The perineal injury can be prevented in normal labor by all except:
 a. To maintain flexion of the head
 b. Timely episiotomy as a routine
 c. Slow delivery of the head in between contractions
 d. Effective perineal guard
Ans. b. Episiotomy in selected cases only.

Q.16 Regarding hyperemesis gravidarum all are correct except:
 a. It is associated with weight loss of more than 5% of the body mass
 b. Glycosuria is commonly observed
 c. Thiamine supplementation is helpful
 d. Omeprazole may relieve the symptoms
Ans. b. Ketonuria is common; c. Thiamine prevents Wernicke's encephalopathy and pontine myelinolysis. Dextrose containing solutions should be avoided as they may precipitate Wernicke's encephalopathy and pontine myelinolysis; d. Proton pump inhibitor, omeprazole has been used successfully. Severe, intractable hyperemesis may need corticosteroids. (*See* Dutta's Textbook of Obstetrics, 8th Edition, p. 181).

Q.17 The following are the blood values following delivery:
 a. Immediately following delivery, there is increased blood volume
 b. Cardiac output remains as in prelabor value soon following delivery
 c. Fibrinogen level remains high up to 2nd week postpartum
 d. There is leukopenia
Ans. c. Immediately following delivery, there is slight decrease in blood volume and the cardiac output rises to about 60% above the prelabor values. There is leukocytosis.

Q.18 The following biochemical changes occur in hyperemesis gravidarum except:
 a. Fall in plasma sodium and potassium
 b. Fall in plasma chloride
 c. Fall in urinary ketone bodies
 d. Rise in blood urea and uric acid
Ans. c. *See* Dutta's Textbook of Obstetrics, 8th Edition, p. 182.

Q.19 Most common cause of first trimester miscarriage:
 a. Chromosomal abnormality of the fetus
 b. Endocrinal defect
 c. Antiphospholipid antibodies
 d. Immunological
Ans. a. *See* Dutta's Textbook of Obstetrics, 8th Edition, p. 187.

Self-Assessment in Obstetrics

Q.20 Most common known cause of midtrimester miscarriage:
a. Uterine malformation
b. Fibroid
c. Cervical incompetence
d. Chronic maternal illness

Ans. c. *See Dutta's Textbook of Obstetrics, 8th Edition, p. 187.*

Q.21 Pregnancy should be strongly discouraged in a woman who has:
a. Atrial septal defect
b. Patent ductus arteriosus
c. Eisenmenger syndrome
d. Rheumatic mitral stenosis

Ans. c. *See Dutta's Textbook of Obstetrics, 8th Edition, p. 187.*

Q.22 Elective time of cerclage operation for midtrimester recurrent abortion:
a. Around 8 weeks
b. Around 14 weeks
c. Around 20 weeks
d. Prepregnant state

Ans. b. *See Dutta's Textbook of Obstetrics, 8th Edition, p. 199.*

Q.23 The best method of evacuation of a missed abortion in uterus of more than 12 weeks:
a. Oxytocin infusion
b. Intramuscular prostaglandin (15 methyl PGF2α)
c. Prostaglandin E_1 vaginal (misoprostol) followed by evacuation of the uterus
d. Suction evacuation

Ans. c. Success rate is more than 90%. (*See Dutta's Textbook of Obstetrics, 8th Edition, p. 191*).

Q.24 Hydatidiform mole is principally a disease of:
a. Amnion
b. Chorion
c. Uterus
d. Decidua

Ans. b.

Q.25 Management of unruptured tubal ectopic pregnancy may be done by:
a. Expectantly in majority of the cases
b. Medically by Methotrexate in all cases
c. Laparoscopic conservative surgery is the gold standard
d. Salpingostomy, as it eliminates the risk of persistent ectopic pregnancy

Ans. c; a and b. Cases must be selected properly; d. Risk of persistence is 5–20%. (*See Dutta's Textbook of Obstetrics, 8th Edition, p. 216*).

Q.26 The advantages of hysterectomy in molar pregnancy are:
a. Chance of choriocarcinoma becomes nil
b. Follow-up is not required
c. Enlarged ovaries can be removed during operation
d. Chance of pulmonary embolization is minimal.

Ans. d. Chance of choriocarcinoma may be reduced significantly but cannot be to nil. Follow-up is mandatory and the lutein cyst should not be removed as a routine during surgery.

Q.27 The following are related to prophylactic chemotherapy in molar pregnancy:
a. It may be given in 'at risk' patients
b. Multiple agents are preferred
c. Malignant sequelae becomes nil
d. Follow-up is not required

Ans. a. Cytotoxic drugs are hazardous and often prove fatal. However, in high risk patient specially where facilities for follow-up are not available, prophylactic chemotherapy has got a place following evacuation of mole. (*See Dutta's Textbook of Obstetrics, 8th Edition, p. 228*).

Q.28 The most common type of monozygotic twins:
   a. Diamniotic-monochorionic
   b. Diamniotic-dichorionic
   c. Monoamniotic-monochorionic
   d. Monoamniotic-dichorionic

Ans. a. Types of placentations in twins are: Diamniotic-Dichorionic (Di-Di). Diamniotic-Monochorionic (Di-Mo) or Monoamniotic-Monochorionic (Mo-Mo). Dizygotic twins (80%) are always Di-Di. Monozygotic twins (20%) are Di-Mo in majority (13–14%), Di-Di in (6–7%) and Mo-Mo in only less than 1% of cases. (*See* Dutta's Textbook of Obstetrics, 8th Edition, p. 231, 240).

Q.29 Absolute proof of monozygosity is determined by:
   a. DNA finger printing
   b. Intervening membrane layers
   c. Sex of the babies
   d. Reciprocal skin grafting

Ans. a. *See* Dutta's Textbook of Obstetrics, 8th Edition, p. 235.

Q.30 Monozygotic twins are associated with all except:
   a. Twin transfusion syndrome
   b. Vanishing twin
   c. Different karyotype pattern
   d. Fetal anomalies

Ans. c. Fetal risks depend more on chorionicity than on zygosity.

Q.31 Gestational trophoblastic disease (GTD):
   a. Persistent trophoblastic tumor following H. mole is about 1%
   b. Placental site trophoblastic tumor is very responsive to chemotherapy
   c. Recurrence risk of GTD is 10%
   d. Risk of choriocarcinoma is about 2%

Ans. d; a. 15–20%; b. less responsive; c. about 1%.

Q.32 Concerning hemolysis, elevated liver enzyme levels, low platelet count (HELLP) syndrome:
   a. It is a manifestation of severe pre-eclampsia
   b. Platelet transfusions are often indicated
   c. Eclampsia is less likely to occur when compared to severe pre-eclampsia
   d. Use of dexamethasone improves the outcome

Ans. d. *See* Manual of Obstetrics and Gynecology for the Postgraduates, p. 265; a. HELLP syndrome complicates around 20% of all cases of severe pre-eclampsia; b. Platelet transfusions are not generally indicated unless the count is less than 40,000/mL; c. Eclampsia is more common in HELLP syndrome compared to pre-eclampsia.

Q.33 Best method of induction of labor in hydramnios:
   a. High rupture of the membranes
   b. Low rupture of the membranes
   c. Abdominal amniocentesis followed by stabilizing oxytocin drip
   d. Prostaglandins

Ans. c. It minimizes sudden decompression of the uterine cavity, placental abruption and incidence of cord prolapse. (*See* Dutta's Textbook of Obstetrics, 8th Edition, p. 215).

Q.34 Single umbilical artery is commonly associated with the following except:
   a. Babies born from diabetic mothers
   b. Congenitally malformed babies

c. More in twins
d. Is always associated with IUGR

Ans. d. *See* Dutta's Textbook of Obstetrics, 8th Edition, p. 254)

Q.35 About the recurrence all are true except:
a. Recurrence in HELLP syndrome is 5%
b. Recurrence of ectopic pregnancy is 10–15%
c. Recurrence in hydatidiform mole is 1–2%
d. Recurrence of abruptio placentae is 6–10%

Ans. a. It is about 20–25%.

Q.36 In twin pregnancy:
a. Fetal risks depend more on zygosity than on chorionicity
b. Chorionicity is best determined in the second trimester by USG
c. Presence of twin peak sign indicates dichorionicity
d. Monozygotic twins are always monochorionic

Ans. c; a. Fetal risk depend more on chorionicity than on zygosity; b. Accurate in the first trimester; d. about 80% of all twins are dichorionic. (*See* Dutta's Textbook of Obstetrics, 8th Edition, p. 237).

Q.37 The following are the criteria of gestational hypertension, except:
a. No underlying cause of hypertension
b. Unassociated with edema and/or proteinuria
c. Normalization of BP within 6 weeks, following delivery
d. Pregnancy outcome is often poor

Ans. d. Pregnancy outcome is usually similar or superior to that of normotensive pregnancy.

Q.38 The following are related to essential hypertension with pregnancy, except:
a. Family history is often present
b. Platelet count is markedly low
c. About 20% may be superimposed with pre-eclampsia
d. About 30% have permanent deterioration of hypertension following delivery

Ans. b.

Q.39 The best way to diagnose the degree of placenta previa:
a. Transvaginal sonography
b. Double set up examination
c. Observation during CS
d. Examination of placenta following delivery

Ans. a. *See* Dutta's Textbook of Obstetrics, 8th Edition, p. 286.

Q.40 The following statements are related to placenta previa, except:
a. Incidence of placenta previa is decreasing
b. Type III and IV constitute about one-third
c. Posterior placenta previa is easy to diagnose
d. The amount of blood loss is not related to the degree of placenta previa

Ans. c. It is difficult to diagnose even with USG. Incidence of placenta previa is related to high parity and it is decreasing due to small family norm.

52 Manual of Obstetrics and Gynecology for the Postgraduates

Q.41 Blood coagulopathy in abruptio placentae is mainly due to:
   a. Decreased synthesis of fibrinogen
   b. Consumption coagulopathy
   c. Enhanced fibrinolytic activity with raised FDP and D-dimer
   d. Increased activation of plasminogen

Ans. b. Consumption of fibrinogen intravascularly as well as retroplacentally. (*See* Dutta's Textbook of Obstetrics, 8th Edition, p. 296).

Q.42 The best way to tackle the blood coagulation disorders in abruptio placentae:
   a. Massive relatively fresh blood transfusion
   b. To administer antifibrinolytic substances
   c. To administer fibrinogen rich substances
   d. Heparin

Ans. a. Massive relatively fresh blood transfusion improves hypovolemic state, increases tissue perfusion and increases production of procoagulants either from the liver or reticuloendothelial cells. This is in addition to the supply of fibrinogen in fresh blood. (*See* Dutta's Textbook of Obstetrics, 8th Edition, p. 715).

Q.43 The incorrect statement in the management of couvelaire uterus is:
   a. It can be diagnosed only by laparotomy
   b. Most of the muscle dissociation occurs in the middle and outer muscle layers
   c. The myometrial hematoma more often interferes with uterine contraction
   d. Per se, it is not an indication for hysterectomy

Ans. c. Myometrial hematoma usually does not cause uterine atonicity. (*See* Dutta's Textbook of Obstetrics, 8th Edition, p. 296).

Q.44 The following tests are related to blood coagulation disorders in obstetrics except:
   a. Thrombocytopenia is a feature of fibrinolytic process and not of DIC
   b. In DIC, RBC will be 'helmet' shaped or fragmented but in fibrinolytic process, the cell morphology is normal
   c. Weiner clot observation test gives a rough estimate of total blood fibrinogen level
   d. Thrombocytopenia can be diagnosed from the peripheral smear

Ans. a. Thrombocytopenia is a feature of DIC and not of fibrinolytic process; c. If clotting time is < 6 minutes, fibrinogen level is > 150 mg%. (*See* Dutta's Textbook of Obstetrics, 8th Edition, p. 714).

Q.45 The physiological iron deficiency state during pregnancy is evidenced by the following except:
   a. Fall in hemoglobin concentration
   b. Fall in hematocrit value
   c. Low serum iron
   d. Low iron binding capacity

Ans. d. The serum iron binding capacity will be high. (*See* Dutta's Textbook of Obstetrics, 8th Edition, p. 306).

Q.46 The following statements are related to the therapy of iron deficiency anemia except:
   a. Oral iron can restore not only the serum iron but also the store iron
   b. Parenteral iron therapy markedly increases the reticulocytic count within 7–14 days
   c. Parenteral therapy is ideal during 30–36 weeks
   d. Blood transfusion may be useful in severe anemia beyond 36 weeks

Ans. a.

Q.47 Which of the following to be avoided in the treatment of thalassemia:
  a. Fresh (relatively) blood transfusion
  b. Folic acid
  c. Routine iron therapy
  d. Deferoxamine improves pregnancy outcome

Ans. c. There is usually no deficiency of iron and exogenous iron therapy may precipitate hemochromatosis.

Q.48 Safe and effective method of contraception in sickle cell anemia:
  a. Oral pill
  b. IUCD
  c. Barrier method
  d. Progestin (only contraceptives)

Ans. d. It can be use safely. It also reduces 'sickling'. (*See* Dutta's Textbook of Obstetrics, 8th Edition, p. 317).

Q.49 The statement that is not related to hemoglobinopathies is:
  a. Hemoglobinopathies are specific inherited disorders within the polypeptide chains of globin fraction
  b. Sickle cell disease is due to mutation causing substitution of valine for glutamic acid on the β chain
  c. β-thalassemia is confirmed when the level of HbA_2 ($α_2 δ_2$) is > 3.5% and HbF ($α_2 γ_2$) is > 2%
  d. α and β polypeptide chains are controlled by four genes

Ans. d. Two genes (chromosome 11) direct β chain and four genes (chromosome 16) direct α chain production.

Q.50 Patients with organic heart disease in pregnancy most commonly die during:
  a. 20–24 weeks of pregnancy
  b. First stage of labor
  c. Soon following delivery
  d. 2 weeks of postpartum

Ans. c. Due to congestive cardiac failure with increased cardiac load. (*See* Dutta's Textbook of Obstetrics, 8th Edition, p. 320).

Q.51 The best method of curtailing the second stage of labor in heart disease is by:
  a. Prophylactic forceps
  b. Ventouse
  c. Spontaneous delivery with episiotomy
  d. Cesarean section

Ans. b. Ventouse can be applied with the patient in dorsal postion. The lithotomy position during forceps delivery increases the venous return to the heart and may overload it. (*See* Dutta's Textbook of Obstetrics, 8th Edition, p. 322).

Q.52 Regarding cytomegalovirus (CMV) infection in pregnancy:
  a. Fetal organ damage occurs when infection is in the first trimester only
  b. Is associated with hepatosplenomegaly in infancy
  c. May be confirmed by culture of infant's nasal secretions
  d. CMV vaccine is protective

Ans. b and c. (*See* Dutta's Textbook of Obstetrics, 8th Edition, p. 349).

Q.53 The following are related to gestational diabetes, except:
  a. Fasting hyperglycemia (> 105 mg/dL) is associated with increased risk
  b. High risk for the development of type-2 diabetes in the postpartum period

c. Macrosomia is due to the proinsulin polypeptides (IGF–I and II)
d. Fetal anomalies are increased

Ans. d. It is only in overt diabetes. Fasting hyperglycemia is associated with increased risk of IUD and development of type-2 diabetes in the postpartum period.

Q.54 The following statements are related to diabetes with pregnancy except:
a. Good control of diabetes in prepregnant state reduces the incidence of congenital malformation of the fetus
b. The insulin requirement is diminished as pregnancy advances
c. There is increased risk of proliferative retinopathy and the need of laser photocoagulation
d. 'Unexplained' IUD may be due to fetal acidemia

Ans. b. The insulin requirement increases as pregnancy advances. (*See* Dutta's Textbook of Obstetrics, 8th Edition, p. 331).

Q.55 The following are related to red degeneration of fibroid except:
a. Usually occurs in a big fibroid
b. Usually occurs in second half of pregnancy
c. The color is due to hemolyzed red cells and hemoglobin
d. There is associated leukopenia

Ans. d. There is leukocytosis.

Q.56 Concerning preterm labor and tocolytics:
a. Indomethacin reduces the risk of neonatal mortality
b. β mimetics are associated with constriction of the fetal ductus arteriosus
c. Atosiban has been shown to prolong pregnancy for 7 days
d. β mimetics are associated with maternal pulmonary edema

Ans. c and d; a. It is associated with neonatal constriction of ductus arteriosus: Intraventricular hemorrhage, necrotizing enterocolitis and oligohydramnios. (*See* Dutta's Textbook of Obstetrics, 8th Edition, p. 584).

Q.57 Regarding anti-D prophylaxis in a RhD negative woman:
a. The use of anti-D has prevented all pregnant RhD negative women from developing anti-D antibodies
b. A 500 IU dose of anti-D is sufficient to cover a fetomaternal hemorrhage of 4 mL of red blood cells (125 IU/mL)
c. Antenatal prophylaxis of RhD negative women immunization during pregnancy will significantly reduce the sensitization
d. Kleihauer-Betke test is to note the number of maternal red bloods cells in fetal blood

Ans. b and c; a. Despite the use of anti-D IgG approximately 1% of the RhD negative women develop anti-D antibodies. (*See* Dutta's Textbook of Obstetrics, 8th Edition, p. 390).

Q.58 Which of the statements are almost noncontroversial in the management of a post cesarean pregnancy:
a. Once a CS, always a CS
b. Once a CS, a mandatory hospital delivery and individualization of the case
c. Following vaginal delivery, exploration of uterus is a must
d. Prophylactic forceps is a routine

Ans. b. *See* Dutta's Textbook of Obstetrics, 8th Edition, p. 383 and 384.

Self-Assessment in Obstetrics

Q.59 *The following statements are related to antibody formation against Rhesus-antigen except:*
   a. Detectable antibodies usually develop at 6 months following large volume of fetomaternal bleed
   b. 0.1 mL is considered as critical sensitising volume
   c. Antibody once formed remains throughout life
   d. Albumin agglutinin (IgG) is the first to appear and is not harmful to the fetus

Ans. d. IgM antibody is the first to appear and IgG crosses the placenta and is harmful to the fetus.

Q.60 *Ultimate cause of fetal death in hydrops fetalis is due to:*
   a. Chronic placental insufficiency
   b. Damage to the liver leading to hypoproteinemia and edema
   c. Cardiac failure
   d. Severe anemia and anoxia

Ans. c. See Dutta's Textbook of Obstetrics, 8th Edition, p. 571.

Q.61 *Anti-D gammaglobulin should be administered to all the Rh-negative mother following delivery except:*
   a. Baby is Rh-positive with direct Coombs' test negative
   b. Even when baby's Rh typing cannot be performed
   c. Associated ABO group incompatibility
   d. Baby is Rh-negative with absence of antibody

Ans. d.

Q.62 *The objectives of exchange transfusion in hemolytic disease of newborn with direct Coombs' test positive are all except:*
   a. To correct anemia by replacing sensitized red blood cells with Rh-negative cells
   b. To remove the circulatory antibodies
   c. To eliminate the circulatory bilirubin
   d. To alter the Rh-factor of the baby's blood

Ans. d. Rh-factor is not changed. (See Dutta's Textbook of Obstetrics, 8th Edition, p. 396).

Q.63 *The following statements are related to Rh-incompatibility:*
   a. Immunoprophylaxis against Rh-antigen by administration of 300 mg of anti-D gamma globulin following delivery is 100% protective
   b. Exchange transfusion to the baby is to alter temporarily the Rh-factor of the baby's blood
   c. The blood for exchange transfusion should be of group 'O' Rh-negative packed cells from unsensitized donors
   d. Detection of antibody (IgG) in mother is called direct Coombs' test

Ans. c; a. It is not cent percent guranated, ideally dose should be calculated by Kleihauer test; b. Not at all alter the Rh typing of the infant's blood; d. It is indirect Coombs' test.

Q.64 *The following are related to contracted pelvis:*
   a. The words contracted pelvis and cephalopelvic disproportion are interchangeable
   b. Engagement of the head clearly rules out contracted pelvis
   c. Radiopelvimetry is invaluable and can even replace clinical pelvimetry
   d. CT and MRI are accurate for the diagnosis

Ans. d. Contracted pelvis may be a cause of cephalopelvic disproportion (CPD) but CPD may occur even without contracted pelvis. Engagement of the head only rules out inlet contraction. Radiopelvimetry can be complementary to clinical pelvimetry but cannot replace it. (*See* Dutta's Textbook of Obstetrics, 8th Edition, p. 403).

Q.65 The correct statement related to contracted pelvis is:
   a. Trial of labor is conducted always in an institution
   b. Isolated outlet contraction is rare
   c. X-ray pelvimetry is less informative than clinical or MRI
   d. Muller-Munro Kerr is an abdominal method of pelvic assessment

Ans. d. Muller-Munro Kerr is an abdominovaginal method. (*See* Dutta's Textbook of Obstetrics, 8th Edition, p. 411).

Q.66 Regarding appendicitis in pregnancy:
   a. Incidence is less compared to nonpregnant state
   b. Predisposes to preterm labor
   c. Conservative management should be the choice
   d. Clinical features are very diagnostic

Ans. b. Incidence is same (1 in 2,000 pregnancies) as that of nonpregnant state. **Management is always surgical** and a **rate of 30% of normal appendices at laparotomy is justified**. Mortality is higher because of late diagnosis. Usual features of nausea, vomiting, leukocytosis in normal pregnancy, displacement of the position of the appendix by the gravid uterus and finally suspicion of other conditions (pyelonephritis, placental abruption) make the diagnosis often late. (*See* Dutta's Textbook of Obstetrics, 8th Edition, p. 354).

Q.67 Trial of labor is characterized by:
   a. Labor is usually induced
   b. Oxytocin stimulation should not be used
   c. Should not be initiated in nonengaged head
   d. Considered for cases with suspected cephalopelvic disproportion

Ans. d. Spontaneous onset of labor, oxytocin stimulation may be used.

Q.68 Diabetes in pregnancy with regard to labor and delivery:
   a. Maternal hyperglycemia predisposes to neonatal hypoglycemia
   b. Use of oxytocin is contraindicated
   c. Incidence of cesarean delivery is more than 50%
   d. The need of insulin is higher in breastfeeding woman

Ans. a and c; d. Insulin requirement falls in breastfeeding women. (*See* Dutta's Textbook of Obstetrics, 8th Edition, p. 333).

Q.69 The following are related to retraction ring (Bandl's ring) except:
   a. It is an end result of tonic uterine contraction and retraction
   b. It invariably follows obstructed labor
   c. It is always situated at the junction of upper and lower segment of the uterus
   d. It is stationary

Ans. d. It is not stationary. (*See* Dutta's Textbook of Obstetrics, 8th Edition, p. 420).

Self-Assessment in Obstetrics

Q.70 *The following names are related in the field of obstetrics and gynecology—point out the correct association:*
 a. Anatomical pelvic axis is named after Carus, a famous obstetrician
 b. Apgar name is related to an anesthetist. He innovated a scoring system to assess the cardiopulmonary status in the newborn
 c. Pincus in Japan was the first to introduce cyclic administration of progestogen preparation as contraception
 d. In a normal pelvis, waste space of Morris should not exceed 1 cm
Ans. d. Carus was an anatomist. Virginia Apgar was a lady anesthetist. Pincus in Puerto Rico introduced the cyclic hormone administration.

Q.71 *The following statements are related to occipitoposterior except:*
 a. Malrotation of occiput may cause occipitosacral arrest
 b. 10% cases are associated with anthropoid or android pelvis
 c. Incomplete forward rotation of occiput may cause deep transverse arrest
 d. Nonrotation of occiput may cause oblique posterior arrest
Ans. b. More than 50% cases are associated.

Q.72 *The following are related to face pubis delivery except:*
 a. Biparietal diameter (9.5 cm) stretches the perineum
 b. Suboccipito frontal diameter (10 cm) emerges out of the introitus
 c. Spontaneous delivery is common in anthropoid or gynecoid pelvis
 d. Head is born by flexion
Ans. b. Occipitofrontal diameter (11.5 cm) emerges out of the introitus.

Q.73 *Primary dysfunctional labor is due to all except:*
 a. Occipitoposterior position   b. Cephalopelvic disproportion
 c. Uterine dysfunction   d. Epidural analgesia
Ans. d. When the progress in the active phase of first stage is less than 1 cm/hour, is called primary dysfunctional labor. Epidural analgesia does not alter the progress of the first stage.

Q.74 *Time limit from the birth of the umbilicus up to delivery of the aftercoming head in breech should not exceed:*
 a. 1 minute   b. 2–3 minutes
 c. 5–7 minutes   d. 8–10 minutes
Ans. c. See Dutta's Textbook of Obstetrics, 8th Edition, p. 444.

Q.75 *Prolonged latent phase of labor:*
 a. Usually causes prolonged active phase
 b. It may be due to cephalopelvic disproportion
 c. It has no obstetric significance
 d. Normal duration of latent phase is 18 hours
Ans. b; c. It carries a high cesarean section rate.

Q.76 *The following are related to face presentation except:*
 a. The most common position is LMA
 b. Engaging diameter is submentobregmatic

c. The diameter distending the vulval outlet is mentovertical (14 cm)
d. During moulding, there is elongation of occipitofrontal diameter

Ans. c. The relevant diameter is submentovertical (11.5 cm) and not mentovertical. (*See* Dutta's Textbook of Obstetrics, 8th Edition, p. 450).

Q.77 The following statements related to prolonged labor are true except:
a. Prolonged labor is synonymous with inefficient uterine contraction
b. Combined duration of first and second stage is to be considered
c. CS may be justified even in prolonged second stage
d. Intervention is done when the cervicograph crosses the action line

Ans. a. Inefficient uterine contraction can be a cause of prolonged labor but prolonged labor may be due to other causes also. (*See* Dutta's Textbook of Obstetrics, 8th Edition, p. 463).

Q.78 Which of the following are not practised in the management of obstructed labor:
a. There is no place of wait and watch policy
b. Dehydration and ketoacidosis should be promptly corrected
c. Oxytocin has got a definite place in the management
d. Uterus should be explored as a routine, following delivery

Ans. c. Oxytocin has got no place in the management of obstructed labor. (*See* Dutta's Textbook of Obstetrics, 8th Edition, p. 468).

Q.79 Shoulder dystocia may occur in all except:
a. Big baby
b. Anencephaly
c. IUGR
d. Normal size baby

Ans. c. In about 50%, the weight of the baby is normal.

Q.80 The following are related to anencephaly except:
a. It is commonly associated with prematurity
b. Often associated with oligohydramnios
c. Increased association with female baby
d. Obstructed labor may occur

Ans. b. Increased association with polyhydramnios.

Q.81 The following statements are related to postpartum hemorrhage (PPH) except:
a. It is always a preventable condition
b. Atonicity of the uterus is the most common cause
c. Intravenous ergometrine with the delivery of the anterior shoulder is a prophylaxis
d. Blood loss during CS exceeds the quantitative definition of PPH

Ans. a. PPH is not always a preventable condition, although anticipation and early detection can minimize its severity. (*See* Dutta's Textbook of Obstetrics, 8th Edition, p. 475).

Q.82 Concerning HIV:
a. The prevalence of HIV infection in woman is rising
b. Majority of the cases in India are following blood transfusion
c. In majority, mother to child transmission (MTCT) occur antenatally
d. Vertical transmission to neonates is about 14–25%

Ans. a and d. Transmission from mother to child can occur at any stage of pregnancy, labor and puerperium (via breast milk), yet it is most common during vaginal delivery (labor). **Majority are following heterosexual transmission**. (*See* Dutta's Textbook of Obstetrics, 8th Edition, p. 350).

Q.83 The following statements are related to prophylaxis against rupture uterus except:
   a. Oxytocin should not be administered in obstructed labor
   b. During ECV, general anesthesia should be used
   c. Internal version should be done in shoulder presentation
   d. Failure of ventouse delivery should be completed by forceps.
Ans. a and b. Undue force should not be used during ECV. So general anesthesia should be avoided as it may mask the pain which is a warning signal.

Q.84 The following statements are related to surgical treatment of rupture uterus except:
   a. Hysterectomy is the surgery of choice unless there is sufficient reason to preserve the uterus
   b. There is hardly any place of repair in spontaneous rupture following obstructed labor
   c. Laparotomy should be done whenever there is any doubt of rupture
   d. Lower segment scar rupture must be tackled by subtotal hysterectomy
Ans. d. Repair with or without sterilization may be done. (*See* Dutta's Textbook of Obstetrics, 8th Edition, p. 498).

Q.85 Regarding manual vacuum aspiration (MVA):
   a. This procedure is done under general anesthesia
   b. The equipment should not be reused
   c. This method can be used up to a menstrual age of 12 weeks
   d. This procedure is more expensive than D and C
Ans. c. MVA is an outpatient or an office procedure. Paracervical block may be needed. b. The equipment can be reused provided that the syringe is kept clean and the cannulae are sterilized. d. It is cheaper than D and C. (*See* Dutta's Textbook of Obstetrics, 8th Edition, p. 646).

Q.86 The following are related to puerperal foot drop:
   a. It is usually unilateral
   b. Observed after the first 7 days of delivery
   c. It is due to stretching of the lumbosacral trunk or injury to peroneal nerve
   d. Surgical intervention is often needed
Ans. a and c. It is observed within a day or two following delivery. Conservative management is usually done.

Q.87 Immediate management of a preterm baby following birth are all, except:
   a. Delayed clamping of the cord
   b. Wrap the baby with a warm towel to maintain temperature at 37°C
   c. Adequate oxygenation with concentration not exceeding 35%
   d. Intramuscular administration of aqueous solution of vitamin K (1 mg)
Ans. a. The cord is to be clamped early in premature baby to prevent hypervolemia thus reducing cardiac load and hyperbilirubinemia.

Q.88 Concerning intrapartum care of a woman with HIV:
   a. Rupture of membranes > 4 hours during labor increases the risk of MTCT
   b. Presence of fetal distress during labor needs the use of fetal scalp electrode
   c. Fetal distress on cardiotocography suggests to perform fetal scalp blood sampling
   d. Cesarean section has high postoperative complications

Ans. a; b and c. These procedures should not be done, cesarean delivery may be an option in such a case; d. **No consensus as yet as regard the operative complications**. It does not appear to be high. (*See* Dutta's Textbook of Obstetrics, 8th Edition, p. 352).

Q.89 Concerning women with HIV:
  a. Infections like atypical tuberculosis may be associated
  b. Cervical screening should be done annually
  c. Treatment of infertility should be discouraged
  d. HIV viruses are DNA retroviruses

Ans. a and b; a. Secondary infections are common due to immune deficiency state; b. Due to increased risk of CIN and cervical cancer, annual screening is essential; c. Due to improvement in prognosis and as the risk of MTCT is so low, **HIV infection should not discourage a HIV positive woman to receive fertility treatment**. (*See* Dutta's Textbook of Obstetrics, 8th Edition, p. 351).

Q.90 As regard the treatment of HIV in pregnancy:
  a. Zidovudine monotherapy is the drug of choice
  b. Pregnant woman with HIV should receive antiretroviral therapy assessing the viral load and CD4$^+$ count
  c. Antiretroviral drug therapy is safe in pregnancy
  d. Each pregnancy worsens the prognosis of the disease

Ans. b. Combination therapy should be given (British HIV association); c. Experience as regard the safety of the drugs is limited specially to the fetus; d. Pregnancy per se has got no effect on the disease progression. (*See* Dutta's Textbook of Obstetrics, 8th Edition, p. 351).

Q.91 Indications of single agent chemotherapy following evacuation of hydatidiform mole are:
  a. A rise in hCG titre
  b. A plateau of hCG titre for 5–7 days
  c. Normalization of hCG by 6 weeks post evacuation
  d. Appearance of brain metastases

Ans. a. Single agent chemotherapy is indicated when the levels of hCG at remained elevated 8 weeks after evacuation; d. Combination chemotherapy is indicated when metastases are present.

Q.92 The oxytocin infusion is contraindicated in all except:
  a. Obstructed labor
  b. Trial of labor
  c. Hypovolemic state
  d. Cardiac disease

Ans. b.

Q.93 The following statements are related to prostaglandins:
  a. PGI$_2$ is a potent vasoconstrictor
  b. PGE$_2$ is at least 5 times more potent than PGF2α
  c. PGE$_2$ acts predominantly on the myometrium while PGF2α acts mainly on the cervix
  d. In the control of atonic PPH, PGE$_2$ is more effective than PGF2α

Ans. b. PGE$_2$ acts predominantly on the cervix while PGF2α acts mostly on the myometrium.

Q.94 Suppression of lactation may occur following the use of all except:
a. Oxytocin
b. Estrogen
c. Ergot derivatives
d. Bromocriptine

Ans. a. *See* Dutta's Textbook of Obstetrics, 8th Edition, p. 174.

Q.95 Regarding twin pregnancy and delivery:
a. Perinatal death is significantly more in the second twin born at term
b. Monoamniotic twins should be delivered by elective cesarean section
c. Cesarean delivery of the second twin following vaginal delivery of the first is about 8%
d. Overall incidence of cesarean section in twins is around 50%

Ans. a, b and d; c. It is around 3% (*RCOG* National Sentinal Cesarean Section Audit). (*See* Dutta's Textbook of Obstetrics, 8th Edition, p. 240).

Q.96 As regard the MTCT in HIV:
a. MTCT is nearly 60% for a HIV positive woman
b. When the maternal viral load is low, MTCT does not occur
c. Breastfeeding doubles the rate of HIV transmission
d. Proper interventions may reduce the transmission (MTCT) rate to 2%

Ans. c and d. Use of antiretrovirals, elective cesarean section delivery and avoidance of breastfeeding will reduce the transmission to less than 2%; b. Unfortunately, there is no level below which transmission is said to be nil. (*See* Dutta's Textbook of Obstetrics, 8th Edition, p. 351).

Q.97 Methods of ripening of cervix are all, except:
a. Oxytocin infusion
b. Misoprostol (PGE_1)—vaginally
c. Intravaginal prostaglandin (PGE_2) either pessary or gel
d. Prostaglandin F2α

Ans. d.

Q.98 The following are related to stripping of the membranes except:
a. It helps in ripening of the cervix
b. It is an effective method for induction of labor
c. It is done prior to rupture of the membranes
d. It reduces postmature pregnancies

Ans. b. Stripping of the membranes is not a useful method of induction. It is effective in ripening of the cervix. (*See* Dutta's Textbook of Obstetrics, 8th Edition, p. 598).

Q.99 Time of insertion of IUD are all except:
a. 2–3 days after the menses
b. During menses
c. Any time during lactation amenorrhea
d. One week following first trimester MTP

Ans. d. Soon following the procedure. (*See* Dutta's Textbook of Obstetrics, 8th Edition, p. 616).

Q.100 As regard LNG–IUD:
a. Hormone contained is levonorgestimate
b. Risk of menorrhagia is same as with other IUDs
c. Serum progesterone is raised
d. Improves dysmenorrhea and premenstrual tension syndrome

Ans. d.

Q.101 Estrogen is added to the 'oral pill' preparation for all the following functions except:
   a. Better cycle control
   b. To prevent breakthrough bleeding
   c. Inhibiting FSH rise thereby preventing ovulation
   d. To potentiate the action of progestogen in producing changes in the cervical mucus
Ans. c. Estrogen and progestogen synergistically act on the hypothalamus to prevent LH surge and ovulation. (*See* Dutta's Textbook of Obstetrics, 8th Edition, p. 622).

Q.102 Conventional 'pill' (21 tab) should be taken usually in the following manner except:
   a. To start from 5th day of every cycle and to continue for 3 weeks
   b. To start from day 1 of a cycle and then three weeks on and 1 week off regime
   c. It can be taken as long as she desires for spacing of birth with periodic check-up
   d. Active liver disease is a contraindication
Ans. a. From day 1 of the cycle.

Q.103 Regarding contraception during lactation all are correct except:
   a. Combined oral pills affect lactation adversely
   b. Minipill is an alternative
   c. Lactation suppresses ovulation
   d. After 6 weeks following childbirth, combined pills may be started in lactating mothers
Ans. d. After 6 months following childbirth pills may be started in lactating mothers. (*See* Dutta's Textbook of Obstetrics, 8th Edition, p. 177).

Q.104 The best method of contraception in a newly married healthy couple (wife aged 25, husband aged 32):
   a. Condom
   b. IUD
   c. Rhythm method
   d. Oral pill
Ans. d. *See* Dutta's Textbook of Obstetrics, 8th Edition, p. 622, 637.

Q.105 The following statements are related to oral pill used in apparently healthy women:
   a. Ovulation returns within 3 months following stoppage of pills
   b. It may produce infertility
   c. Pregnancy immediately following its withdrawal may have some adverse effect on the fetus
   d. Long-term user may have premature menopause
Ans. a.

Q.106 Beneficial effects of 'pill users' are all except:
   a. Reduced ovarian malignancy
   b. Improvement of endometriosis
   c. Decreased menstural loss
   d. Reduced cervical malignancy
Ans. d. Pill user should have regular cytology screening. (*See* Dutta's Textbook of Obstetrics, 8th Edition, p. 627).

Q.107 The progesterone in the combined pill produces the following side effects except:
   a. Hypomenorrhea
   b. Acne
   c. Weight gain
   d. Increased libido
Ans. d. Libido is decreased.

Q.108 **The estrogen in the combined pill produces the following side effects except:**
   a. Nausea, vomiting and headache
   b. Rise in total cholesterol
   c. Hypertension
   d. Insulin resistance and hyperglycemia
Ans. d. This is due to progestogen effects. (*See* Dutta's Textbook of Obstetrics, 8th Edition, p. 625).

Q.109 **Following statements are related to postpill amenorrhea except:**
   a. It is observed in about 1% of cases
   b. It is pituitary in origin
   c. It may be associated with galactorrhea
   d. Investigations are same as in secondary amenorrhea
Ans. b. It is observed in less than 1% of cases and of hypothalamic in origin.

Q.110 **The following statements are related to the endocrinal status in 'pill users' except:**
   a. Gonadotropin level remains low as found in early proliferative phase
   b. Ovarian function remains quiescent
   c. Endometrium shows stromal edema, and decidual reaction
   d. Estrogen decreases the hepatic synthesis of fibrinogen and factor VII, X
Ans. d. Estrogen increases their synthesis. (*See* Dutta's Textbook of Obstetrics, 8th Edition, p. 627).

Q.111 **The following statements are related to injectable steroids (Depo-provera) except:**
   a. It inhibits ovulation
   b. It can be used safely during lactation
   c. Menorrhagia is a known side effect
   d. Protective against endometrial cancer
Ans. c. It reduces menorrhagia as the endometrium is atrophic. (*See* Dutta's Textbook of Obstetrics, 8th Edition, p. 628).

Q.112 **In ideal contraceptive prescription—match the following:**
   a. Newly married couple   1. IUD
   b. Parous women for spacing   2. Minipill
   c. Elderly woman   3. Combined oral pills
   d. To stop future pregnancy   4. Sterilization/CuT 380A
Ans. a = 3; b = 1; c = 2; d = 4.

Q.113 **Regarding chickenpox in pregnancy:**
   a. The incubation period is 7–10 days
   b. Maternal infection after 20 weeks may cause fetal varicella syndrome (FVS)
   c. Oral Acyclovir within 24 hours of rash can reduce the severity of symptoms
   d. Varicella zoster immunoglobulin (VZIG) within 24 hours of contact can prevent FVS
Ans. c; a. Incubation period is 10–20 days; b. Maternal infection before 20 weeks only can cause FVS in 1–2% of cases; c. Oral Acyclovir should be given after 20 weeks of gestation only; d. There is no evidence that VZIG can prevent FVS. (*See* Dutta's Textbook of Obstetrics, 8th Edition, p. 349).

Q.114 **Folic acid deficiency is manifested by:**
   a. Hypersegmentation of neutrophils
   b. Angular stomatitis
   c. Microcytes
   d. Anemia
Ans. a and d.

Q.115 The following statements are related to vasectomy operation except:
  a. Following the operation, the person is not sterile immediately
  b. The sperm are absorbed although the semen is passed during intercourse
  c. In the interim period, condom should be used
  d. Pregnancy rate following reversal of vasectomy is about 90%

Ans. d. Pregnancy rate is low (50%).

Q.116 As regard episiotomy:
  a. It should be done just prior to crowning
  b. Timed episiotomy can prevent stress urinary incontinence
  c. It protects the newborn from intracranial hemorrhage
  d. In forceps delivery, it is often performed after the blades are applied

Ans. a; d. There is no evidence to support the views expressed in b and c. Therefore routine episiotomy in primigravida is not recommended.

Q.117 The following statements are related to forceps operation except:
  a. It is associated with more maternal trauma than ventouse
  b. All outlet forceps are low forceps but not all low forceps are outlet forceps operations
  c. Failed vaginal delivery with forceps is high compared to ventouse
  d. Types of forceps operation depends on the station of the head

Ans. c. Failure of ventouse delivery is more compared to forceps.

Q.118 The following statements are related to forceps delivery:
  a. Prophylactic forceps can be applied when the conditions of low mid-forceps delivery are fulfilled
  b. Trial forceps as applied in operation theater in cases of outlet contraction
  c. Failed forceps means failure of descent of the head even with forcible traction
  d. Kielland's forceps are for rotation and correction of asynclitism

Ans. d. Prophylactic forceps is a low forceps operation. Trial forceps is related to midpelvic contraction. Failed forceps includes not only traction failure but also failure in application of or in the locking of the blades.

Q.119 The following statements are related to symphysiotomy except:
  a. The operation should be done only when obstruction is anticipated
  b. Isolated outlet contraction is the ideal case
  c. FHS must be present
  d. Ventouse is preferable to forceps for extraction

Ans. a. Symphysiotomy is only done with established obstruction with presence of FHS and not in anticipated cases.

Q.120 The following vital statistics are expressed in relation to number of births as per FIGO:
  a. The maternal mortality ratio (MMR) is expressed as number of deaths per 100,000 total births
  b. Perinatal mortality rate (PMR) is expressed in terms of deaths per 1,000 live births
  c. Stillbirth rate is expressed in terms of deaths per 1,000 live births
  d. Neonatal death rate is expressed in terms of deaths per 1,000 live births

Ans. d. MMR is expressed per 100,000 live births. PMR is expressed per 1,000 total births. Stillbirth rate is expressed per 1,000 total births.

Q.121 *Among the important causes of maternal deaths in the developing countries—match the following:*
   a. Hemorrhage   1. 20%
   b. Hypertensive disorders   2. 13%
   c. Unsafe abortion   3. 12%
   d. Indirect causes   4. 25%

Ans. a = 4; b = 3; c = 2; d = 1. (WHO—1999).

Q.122 *The following are related to perinatal mortality:*
   a. The perinatal mortality rate includes stillbirths and first week neonatal deaths
   b. Babies dying due to lethal congenital abnormalities are excluded
   c. Anemia contributes significantly to the perinatal death
   d. Total number of live birth is used as a denominator

Ans. a; b. In corrected perinatal death it is excluded. c. Low birth weight is a significant cause. d. It is the number of total births.

Q.123 *The most common cause of perinatal death in India:*
   a. Prematurity   b. Asphyxia
   c. Intracranial hemorrhage d. Congenital malformation

Ans. a.

Q.124 *Regarding HIV in women:*
   a. Presence of sexually transmitted infections (STIs) increase the infectivity of HIV
   b. HIV positive women on antiretroviral therapy should be discouraged from pregnancy
   c. Progesterone pill is recommended as a contraception to avoid transmission
   d. Risk of transmission by needle prick during surgery is about 0.3%

Ans. a and d; b. Women with HIV should be counseled about the different interventions that may reduce MTCT. a. Presence of other STIs makes HIV more infectious. (*See* Dutta's Textbook of Obstetrics, 8th Edition, p. 350, 351).

Q.125 *The following statements related to continuous fetal monitoring are true except:*
   a. Beat-to-beat variation is not a reliable index of the intrauterine fetal status
   b. Late deceleration is suggestive of chronic placental insufficiency
   c. Variable deceleration is due to cord compression
   d. Early deceleration is due to head compression

Ans. a. Beat-to-beat variation is the most reliable index of intrauterine fetal status.

Q.126 *Regarding epilepsy in pregnancy:*
   a. Seizure frequency decreases in majority
   b. Monotherapy is preferred than polydrug therapy
   c. No increase in incidence of epilepsy in offspring
   d. Breastfeeding is contraindicated

Ans. b; a. Either remains unchanged or increases in some. c. The risk increases by five-fold. d. Not contraindicated but drug dosage needs readjustment. (*See* Dutta's Textbook of Obstetrics, 8th Edition, p. 338).

Q.127 *Better births initiative (WHO) recommends the following:*
   a. Routine acceleration of labor
   b. Routine amniotomy (ARM)

c. No routine suctioning of neonates who have not been exposed to meconium
d. Women in labor must be restricted to bed as a routine

Ans. c. There is no evidence of any benefit for routine interventions like routine enemas, amniotomy, acceleration of labor, episiotomy, restriction to bed for all women and routine suctioning to all neonates. These interventions are therefore to be avoided as a routine practice.

Q.128 Concerning active phase of labor:
a. Starts when the cervix is 6 cm dilated
b. Cervix dilates at the rate of 1 cm/hour
c. Epidural analgesia slows the progress
d. Oxytocin should not be used

Ans. b; a. When cervix is 3 cm dilated. d. Oxytocin may be needed.

Q.129 Hemodynamic changes in pregnancy are all except:
a. Increase in cardiac output
b. Increase in heart rate
c. Reduction in vascular resistance
d. Increase in mean arterial pressure (MAP)

Ans. d. Mean arterial pressure falls in first trimester and reaching a nadir by midpregnancy. Thereafter MAP increases slowly to reach the nonpregnant level at term pregnancy. (*See* Dutta's Textbook of Obstetrics, 8th Edition, p. 60).

Q.130 The following statements are related to retained placenta except:
a. The retained placenta is more often than not due to uterine atonicity
b. Simple adherent is more common than morbid adherent
c. Focal adherent is more common than complete adherent
d. Hysterectomy is the treatment of choice

Ans. d. It is indicated in selected cases. (*See* Dutta's Textbook of Obstetrics, 8th Edition, p. 418).

Q.131 The following statements are related to PPH except:
a. CS is one of the common causes of PPH
b. PPH with atonic uterus almost always rules out traumatic bleeding
c. HELLP syndrome and Sheehan syndrome are related to PPH
d. In precipitate labor, the uterus becomes hypotonic to cause PPH

Ans. b. Even with atonic uterus, traumatic bleeding may coexist.

Q.132 The most important factor in hemostasis following placental separation:
a. Uterine contraction
b. Uterine retraction
c. Thrombosis
d. Myotamponade

Ans. b.

Q.133 Concerning levonorgestrel intrauterine system (LNG-IUS):
a. Daily release of 20 mg/day of levonorgestrel is effective in preventing endometrial proliferation
b. Ectopic pregnancy rate is similar to copper bearing IUCDs
c. Around 75% of women continue to ovulate with LNG-IUS *in situ*
d. Uterine fibroids are absolute contraindication

Ans. a and c. *See* Dutta's Textbook of Obstetrics, 8th Edition, p. 615.

Q.134 Concerning chickenpox in pregnancy:
a. Risk of FVS is about 1–2% when infection occurs within 20 weeks
b. VZIG should be given to the neonate after 2 weeks of birth
c. Following an exposure, the pregnant woman should have VZIG within 10 days
d. FVS is characterized by skin scarring

Ans. a; c and d; b. VZIG should be given to the neonate within 5 days of birth. (*See* Dutta's Textbook of Obstetrics, 8th Edition, p. 349).

Q.135 Regarding hemopoiesis in the fetus:
a. Red blood cells are predominantly nucleated until 37 weeks of gestation
b. Liver is the major site of hemopoiesis up to term
c. Serum folate level in the cord blood is almost same to that of the mother
d. Embryonic hemoglobins are Gower–1 ($\zeta_2 \varepsilon_2$), Gower–2 ($\alpha_2 \varepsilon_2$) and HbF ($\alpha_2 \gamma_2$)

Ans. d. After 12 weeks the red blood cells are all nonnucleated. By 10th week liver is the major site of hemopoiesis and thereafter hemopoiesis is taken over gradually by the bone marrow. Liver ceases its hemopoietic function by term pregnancy. In cord blood level of folic acid, ferritin and B_{12} are much higher than that of the mother. Embryonic (5–8 weeks) hemoglobins are $\zeta_2 \varepsilon_2$ – 42%, $\alpha_2 \varepsilon_2$ – 24% and $\alpha_2 \gamma_2$ – 34% (Fig. 2.1). (*See* Dutta's Textbook of Obstetrics, 8th Edition, p. 47).

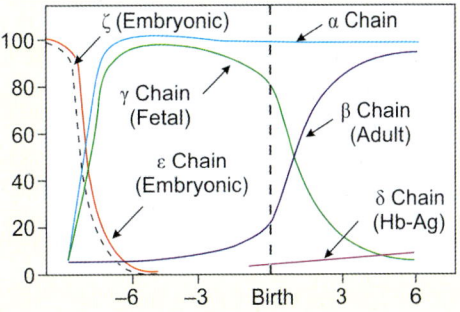

Fig. 2.1: Production of hemoglobin polypeptide chains in relation to gestational age

Q.136 Pick up the correct one in relation to PPH:
a. Atonic uterus always rules out traumatic bleeding
b. Contracted uterus clearly rules out atonic bleeding
c. Bleeding with contracted uterus in absence of genital tract injuries is a theoretical possibility
d. Intrauterine plugging has got no place in modern obstetrics

Ans. b. Intrauterine plugging has got a place in the management of PPH. Atonic uterus may be associated with traumatic bleeding. Bleeding with contracted uterus in absence of genital tract injuries may be due to blood coagulopathy specially following delivery in abruptio placentae.

Q.137 The following are related to placenta accreta except:
a. The most common cause is poor decidual formation with absence of Nitabuch's layer
b. The management is best achieved by hysterectomy unless there is sufficient reason to preserve the uterus
c. It is always associated with PPH
d. It may cause inversion of uterus

Ans. c.

Q.138 Regarding fetal monitoring by cardiotocography:
a. A sinusoidal FHR pattern is always associated with fetal hypoxia
b. Fetuses with congenital abnormalities always exhibit abnormal FHR patterns

c. Decelerations in the second stage is always pathological
d. Decreased baseline variability may be due to drugs
Ans. d. *See* Dutta's Textbook of Obstetrics, 8th Edition, p. 692.

Q.139 Regarding pregnancy and lupus anticoagulant:
a. Mortality is similar as in nonpregnant state
b. Coagulation time is reduced *in vitro*
c. Risk of deep vein thrombosis is high
d. May cause fetal congenital heart block

Ans. c and d. systemic lupus erythematosus (SLE) often flares up in pregnancy. Mortality is high in puerperium. Lupus anticoagulant prolongs clotting time *in vitro* but paradoxically produces thrombosis *in vivo*. Anti Ro (SS—A or anti SS—B) antibodies may cause fetal congenital heart block.

Q.140 Regarding prenatal diagnosis by early amniocentesis and CVS in the first trimester of pregnancy:
a. CVS has lower complications compared to midtrimester amniocentesis
b. CVS is a painful procedure
c. CVS can offer the karyotype result within few days compared to amniocentesis
d. CVS has lower complications compared to first trimester amniocentesis

Ans. c and d. Early first trimester amniocentesis has a complication rate higher than that of CVS. (*See* Dutta's Textbook of Obstetrics, 8th Edition, p. 129).

Q.141 In which fetal presentation, a vaginal delivery can be expected:
a. Face presentation when the chin lies direct to the sacrum
b. Brow presentation
c. Shoulder presentation
d. Face presentation when the chin lies under the symphysis pubis

Ans. d. *See* Dutta's Textbook of Obstetrics, 8th Edition, p. 452.

Q.142 Contraindications for VBAC-trial of labor in a subsequent pregnancy include:
a. When the first cesarean section was done for cephalopelvic disproportion (CPD)
b. Prior twice lower segment cesarean section
c. Prior cesarean section due to fetal distress
d. Nonavailability of X-ray pelvimetry

Ans. a and b. *See* Dutta's Textbook of Obstetrics, 8th Edition, p. 384.

Q.143 The risks of continuation of pregnancy in secondary abdominal pregnancy are all except:
a. Catastrophic hemorrhage
b. Fetal malformation
c. Increased perinatal loss
d. Increased incidence of pre-eclampsia

Ans. d. *See* Dutta's Textbook of Obstetrics, 8th Edition, p. 218.

Q.144 The term 'placental sign' denotes:
a. Alteration of fetal heart rate (FHR) on pressing the head into the pelvis
b. Spotting on the expected date of period in early months of pregnancy

    c. Permanent lengthening of the cord in third stage of labor
    d. Slight gush of bleeding in third stage of labor
- **Ans.** b. This is also called "Hartman's sign". (*See* Dutta's Textbook of Obstetrics, 8th Edition, p. 73).

Q.145 The following are always indications of CS except:
   a. Type IV placenta previa
   b. Abruptio placentae
   c. Stage 1B carcinoma cervix with pregnancy
   d. Active genital herpes at 38 weeks
- **Ans.** b.

Q.146 Iatrogenic causes of tubal pregnancy are all except
   a. Tubal plastic surgery
   b. Increased use of assisted reproductive technology (ART)
   c. Combined oral contraceptive (COC) pill
   d. Tubal sterilization operation
- **Ans.** c. COC is protective. (*See* Dutta's Textbook of Obstetrics, 8th Edition, p. 208).

Q.147 The Spiegelberg's criteria in the diagnosis of ovarian pregnancy are all except:
   a. Tube on the affected side must be intact
   b. The gestation sac must be in the position of the ovary
   c. The gestation sac is connected with infundibulopelvic ligament
   d. Ovarian tissue must be found on its wall on histological examination
- **Ans.** c. The gestation sac should be connected with ovarian ligament. (*See* Dutta's Textbook of Obstetrics, 8th Edition, p. 220).

Q.148 Indications of urgent delivery of the second baby in twin are all except:
   a. Abruptio placentae
   b. Cord prolapse of the second baby
   c. Inadvertent use of ergometrine IV with the delivery of the anterior shoulder of the first baby
   d. Breech presentation of the second baby
- **Ans.** d. *See* Dutta's Textbook of Obstetrics, 8th Edition, p. 242.

Q.149 Regarding cholestasis of pregnancy:
   a. Commonly seen in the mid-trimester
   b. Associated with postmaturity
   c. Associated with neonatal jaundice
   d. Marked geographical variation in incidence
- **Ans.** d; a. Common in third trimester. b. Preterm labor is common. (*See* Dutta's Textbook of Obstetrics, 8th Edition, p. 336).

Q.150 Indications of exchange transfusion in anemia with pregnancy are all except:
   a. Severe anemia with cardiac failure
   b. Cases of severe anemia requiring surgery
   c. Severe anemia with hematocrit less than 15%
   d. For correction of anemia in early pregnancy
- **Ans.** d.

Q.151 Causes of acute pain abdomen during first half of pregnancy are all except:
   a. Disturbed ectopic pregnancy
   b. Hydatidiform mole
   c. Acute hydramnios
   d. Multiple pregnancy
   Ans. d. See Dutta's Textbook of Obstetrics, 8th Edition, p. 355.

Q.152 As regard placental transfer—match the following:
   a. Oxygen   1. Pinocytosis
   b. Antibodies (IgG)   2. Active transfer
   c. Iron   3. Facilitated diffusion
   d. Glucose   4. Diffusion
   Ans. a = 4; b = 1; c = 2; d = 3.

Q.153 Sacrosciatic notch is most wide and shallow in:
   a. Gynecoid pelvis   b. Anthropoid pelvis
   c. Flat pelvis   d. Android pelvis
   Ans. b.

Q.154 The following are related to breech presentation except:
   a. Complete breech is common in multiparae
   b. Frank breech is the most common variety amongst incomplete breech
   c. Breech without associated complicating factor is called uncomplicated
   d. External cephalic version (ECV) should not be done beyond 38 weeks
   Ans. d. ECV may be done even in early labor.

Q.155 Salient features in diagnosis of anterior face presentation are all except:
   a. Vaginal examination may simulate as breech
   b. Cephalic eminence is to the side towards which the limbs lie
   c. Deep grove is there between the head and the back
   d. USG showing hyperextended head
   Ans. b. The cephalic eminence is to the side towards which the back lies.

Q.156 Rubella infection in pregnancy:
   a. Risk of the fetus is maximum in the third trimester
   b. IgM takes about 21 days to appear in the blood after infection
   c. Rubella immunization in pregnancy should be given
   d. Every pregnancy should be screened irrespective of earlier vaccination
   Ans. b and d. Fetal risk is maximum in the first trimester (10–50%). The virus is extremely teratogenic and each pregnancy should be screened to assess the immunity status.
   c. It is contraindicated during pregnancy and pregnancy should not occur after 3 months following immunization.

Q.157 The following are related to the management of acute obstetric inversion except:
   a. To replace the uterus urgently even without anesthesia before shock develops
   b. To replace the part inverted first
   c. If shock develops prior to replacement, resuscitation is to be done first
   d. Hydrostatic method is quite effective and less shock producing
   Ans. b. To replace the part which is inverted last. (See Dutta's Textbook of Obstetrics, 8th Edition, p. 488).

Self-Assessment in Obstetrics

Q.158 The following medical disorders often improve during pregnancy except:
- a. Asthma
- b. Iron deficiency anemia
- c. Depression
- d. Regional ileitis

Ans. b.

Q.159 Conditions which contraindicate breastfeeding are all except:
- a. Active pulmonary tuberculosis
- b. Puerperal psychosis
- c. Patient with hepatitis-B
- d. Galactosemia

Ans. c.

Q.160 The important functions of prostaglandins are all except:
- a. It helps in the process of ovulation
- b. It has got luteotrophic effect
- c. It has got ripening effect on the cervix
- d. It enhances myometrial contraction

Ans. b. It has luteolytic effect.

Q.161 Contraindications of epidural analgesia are all except:
- a. Kyphoscoliosis
- b. Patient having anticoagulant therapy
- c. Severe hemorrhage
- d. Pre-eclampsia

Ans. d. Epidural analgesia is advantageous in pre-eclampsia.

Q.162 Benefits of surgical induction (ARM) are all except:
- a. Lowers the blood pressure in pre-eclampsia
- b. Relieves the maternal distress in hydramnios
- c. Controls bleeding in placenta previa
- d. Reduces the need of cesarean section

Ans. c. Controls bleeding in abruptio placentae.

Q.163 The placenta of twins may be:
- a. Dichorionic and monoamniotic in dizygotic twins
- b. Dichorionic and monoamniotic in monozygotic twins
- c. Monochorionic and monoamniotic in dizygotic twins
- d. Dichorionic and diamniotic in monozygotic twins

Ans. d. *See* Dutta's Textbook of Obstetrics, 8th Edition, p. 236.

Q.164 The following statements are related to recent CPT:
- a. The common cause is extension of an episiotomy
- b. Perineal body is not affected but the anal sphincter is torn
- c. The operative steps are like those of old CPT repair
- d. End to end sphincter approximation (not overlapping) is done

Ans. a and d. There is total loss of perineal body along with anal sphincter in CPT. The operation is to be done without dissecting the flaps as done in old CPT repair.

Q.165 A 25-year-old lady has difficulty in voiding 6 hours postpartum. The most likely the cause is:
- a. Severe pre-eclampsia
- b. Excess oxytocin infusion during delivery

c. Epidural analgesia
d. Vulval hematoma

Ans. d. *See* Dutta's Textbook of Obstetrics, 8th Edition, p. 492.

Q.166 The following are the physical features of amniotic fluid:
a. The fluid is faintly acidic
b. Its specific gravity is about 1.016
c. Relatively hypertonic to the maternal serum at term
d. None of the above

Ans. d. The fluid is faintly alkaline. It has low specific gravity of 1.010 and is relatively hypotonic to maternal serum at term.

Q.167 The clinical entities arising out of the vestigeal structures of the umbilical cord following birth are all except:
a. Distal part of the vitelline duct may persist as Meckel's diverticulum
b. Parent allantois may communicate with the bladder producing leakage of urine through the umbilicus
c. Nonobliteration of the extraembryonic coelom may lead to congenital umbilical hernia or exomphalos
d. Right umbilical vein disappears by 4th month

Ans. a. Proximal part and not the distal part of the vitelline duct persists as the Meckel's diverticulum.

Q.168 The following are related to fetal erythropoiesis except:
a. In the embryonic phase, the erythropoiesis is first demonstrated in the primitive mesoderm
b. By 10th week, the liver becomes the major site
c. Near term, the bone marrow becomes the major site
d. At term, 75–80% of hemoglobin is fetal type (HbF)

Ans. a. Erythropoiesis is first demonstrated in the yolk sac.

Q.169 Lifespan of the fetal RBC approximately:
a. 60 days
b. 80 days
c. 100 days
d. 120 days

Ans. b.

Q.170 Gonadotrophic hormones are produced in the fetal pituitary as early as:
a. 10th week
b. 20th week
c. 30th week
d. None of the above

Ans. a.

Q.171 Regarding failure in medical termination of pregnancy (MTP) all are correct except:
a. It is more common than surgical termination
b. Failed surgical termination is common when it is done in less than 6 weeks of gestation
c. Routine visual inspection of the products of conception should be done
d. Histological confirmation of the product of conception is essential

Ans. d. The reported rate of failure following medical first trimester termination is 0.7% compared to that of surgical is 0.2%; b. early pregnancy (< 6 weeks) and those with congenital uterine anomalies, uterus acutely anteverted, or fibroids, have high risk of failure; d. Routine histological confirmation of the products of conception is not recommended. (*See* Dutta's Textbook of Obstetrics, 8th Edition, p. 202, 643).

Q.172 **The following statements are related to venous pressure during pregnancy except:**
  a. Antecubital venous pressure is raised
  b. Femoral venous pressure is markedly increased in later months of pregnancy
  c. Distensibility of the veins is increased due to progesterone
  d. There is stagnation of blood in the venous system specially below the uterus
Ans. a. It is unaffected.

Q.173 **Regarding postpartum hemorrhage:**
  a. It is reduced by active management of third stage of labor
  b. Is usually due to genital tract injury
  c. Is more common in women with previous history of PPH
  d. Less common in multiparous women
Ans. a and c; b. Uterine atony is the most common cause (90%). Multiparity and history of PPH are known causes. (*See* Dutta's Textbook of Obstetrics, 8th Edition, p. 474).

Q.174 **Glucose tolerance test during pregnancy reveals the following findings except:**
  a. Slightly high level of fasting blood sugar
  b. There is hyperinsulinemia due to raised contra insulin factors
  c. Blood sugar level remains at a higher level than in the nonpregnant state after 2 hours
  d. Despite physiological blood sugar level, glucose may be excreted in the urine
Ans. a. The fasting blood sugar level remains slightly at a lower level than in the nonpregnant state due to fetal consumption.

Q.175 **The following are related to uterine souffle except:**
  a. It is a soft blowing systolic murmur heard on the sides of pregnant uterus
  b. The sound is synchronous with the maternal pulse
  c. It is due to increased blood flow through the placental site
  d. It can be heard even in a big fibroid
Ans. c. It is due to increase in blood flow through the dilated uterine vessels.

Q.176 **The following are related to funic souffle except:**
  a. It is soft blowing murmur synchronous with the fetal heart sounds
  b. It is due to rush of blood through the intervillous space
  c. It is heard in about 15% cases
  d. When present is diagnostic of pregnancy
Ans. b. It is due to rush of blood through the compressed umbilical arteries.

Q.177 **The following statements are related to hemolytic disease of the newborn except:**
  a. Rh-incompatibility is more common than ABO blood group incompatibility
  b. The first ABO blood group incompatible baby may be affected
  c. Affection of future babies due to ABO blood group incompatibility is unlikely
  d. Once Rh-affected baby is born, all future children will be affected unless they are Rh-negative
Ans. a. ABO blood group incompatibility is more common.

Q.178 The following are evidences of iron deficiency in a pregnant woman except:
   a. A progressive decline in serum iron
   b. A progressive increase in serum ferritin
   c. An increase in total iron binding capacity
   d. Microcytosis and hypochromia in peripheral blood film
Ans. b. There is progressive decrease in serum ferritin.

Q.179 The following are related to the use of heparin during pregnancy except:
   a. Low molecular weight heparin (fragmin) crosses the placental barrier
   b. With a cofactor antithrombin III, it has powerful antithrombin action
   c. Its effect can be neutralized by slow protamine IV
   d. Heparin therapy is monitored by partial thromboplastin time (PTT) estimation
Ans. a. It does not cross the placental barrier.

Q.180 Regarding sickle cell (HbSS) disease in pregnancy:
   a. Risks of pulmonary disease is increased
   b. Epidural anesthesia is contraindicated
   c. Fluids are restricted in labor to avoid cardiac overload
   d. Oral pill is suitable for contraception
Ans. a. Sickle cell hemoglobinopathy is an inherited disorder. It may be HbAS (trait) or HbSS (disease).

Q.181 Fetal bradycardia observed during external cephalic version in breech presentation at 36 weeks should be tackled by:
   a. Stop the procedure and repeat it after 30 minutes
   b. To bring back the podalic pole into the lower pole of the uterus and monitor the fetus
   c. To complete the version quickly
   d. Deliver the fetus by immediate cesarean section
Ans. b.

Q.182 The common maternal side effects following isoxsuprine therapy to arrest preterm labor are all, except:
   a. Tachycardia
   b. Hypokalemia
   c. Hypertension
   d. Hyperglycemia
Ans. c. It causes hypotension.

Q.183 The most accurate method for diagnosis of preterm rupture of the membranes (PROM):
   a. Nitrazine test
   b. Amniotic fluid crystallization (ferning)
   c. Testing the pH of vaginal fluid
   d. Detecting clear fluid passing from the cervical canal
Ans. d. Amniotic fluid pH is 7.0–7.5; a. Nitrazine paper test for pH > 6.6, suggests rupture of membranes. But it has false-positive result also (blood).

Q.184 Congenital heart disease is most likely in the newborn of mothers suffering from all except:
   a. Systemic lupus erythematosus
   b. Rheumatoid arthritis
   c. Diabetes in pregnancy
   d. Congenital heart disease of the mother
Ans. b.

Self-Assessment in Obstetrics

Q.185 *Contraindications in the use of beta adrenergic therapy in arresting preterm labor are all except:*
  a. Cervical dilatation > 3 cm
  b. Regular uterine contractions with or without pain
  c. Chorioamnionitis
  d. Pregnancy beyond 34 weeks
Ans. b.

Q.186 *The following are related to plasma volume in pregnancy:*
  a. The peak increase is at about 34 weeks
  b. The increase is more in primi than multipara
  c. The increase is more in multiple pregnancy than in singleton one
  d. The increase in more in pre-eclampsia
Ans. c. The peak value is at 30–32 weeks. The increase is more in multipara and in multiple pregnancy.

Q.187 *The best biochemical marker of pre-eclampsia:*
  a. Uric acid
  b. Creatinine
  c. D-dimer
  d. NPN
Ans. a.

Q.188 *For prenatal diagnosis amniocentesis is performed at:*
  a. 10–12th week
  b. 14–16th week
  c. 18–20th week
  d. 20–24th week
Ans. b. However, in some centers, early amniocentesis is done at 10–12 weeks.

Q.189 *Regarding thrombocytopenia in pregnancy:*
  a. Gestational thrombocytopenia may be due to hemodilution
  b. Splenectomy is essential for immune thrombocytopenia (ITP)
  c. Severe pre-eclampsia causes neonatal thrombocytopenia
  d. Immunoglobulin therapy in ITP cannot improve the outcome
Ans. a; d. Immunoglobulin (IV) in high dose improves the maternal and fetal platelet counts in ITP. b. Splenectomy in pregnancy has a 10% mortality.

Q.190 *Regarding vomiting in pregnancy:*
  a. Hyperemesis gravidarum is commonly seen
  b. Steroid therapy may be needed in severe cases of hyperemesis
  c. *Helicobacter pylori* is the causative factor
  d. First pregnancy is generally not affected
Ans. b. Vomiting in pregnancy is common but not the hyperemesis. High level of human chorionic gonadotropin (hCG) is related, first pregnancy is commonly affected.

Q.191 *Definitive treatment of pre-eclampsia:*
  a. Prophylactic anticonvulsant therapy
  b. Diuretics
  c. Termination of pregnancy
  d. Antihypertensives
Ans. c. *See* Dutta's Textbook of Obstetrics, 8th Edition, p. 264.

Q.192 Spontaneous preterm labor is more common:
a. Amongst monozygotic twins
b. Amongst dizygotic twins
c. No correlation in twins
d. Twin transfusion syndrome

Ans. a. This is probably because of more association with hydramnios in monozygotic twins.

Q.193 The first evidence of recovery from eclampsia:
a. Subsidence of edema
b. Disappearance of proteinuria
c. Increase in urinary output
d. Normalization of BP

Ans. c.

Q.194 As regard to cardiac arrest during pregnancy:
a. Maintain circulation by chest compression: ventilation (mouth to mouth) = 5:1
b. Immediate tracheal intubation and ventilation with 100% O_2, if possible
c. Outcome is better compared to the nonpregnant state
d. Cesarean section (CS) is contraindicated

Ans. a and b. Outcome is less successful and has raised mortality rate. Cesarean section may be indicated for maternal and fetal survival. CS also avoids aortocaval compression which is an important cause.

Q.195 Hazards of furosemide therapy in pre-eclampsia are all except:
a. Maternal hypokalemia
b. Reduction of maternal plasma volume
c. Fetal hypernatremia
d. Fetal thrombocytopenia

Ans. c. It causes fetal hyponatremia.

Q.196 Regarding listeriosis in pregnancy:
a. Mode of transmission of infection is sexual
b. Is associated with meningoencephalitis of the newborn
c. May present with skin rash at birth
d. In labor liquor is meconium stained

Ans. b, c and d; a. Ingestion of contaminated food (cheese) is often the mode of infection.

Q.197 The following statements are related to hepatitis B virus (HBV):
a. HBV is teratogenic
b. Neonatal transmission is mainly transplacental
c. HBV vaccine is contraindicated during pregnancy
d. The carrier neonate may develop hepatocellular carcinoma

Ans. d. HBV is not teratogenic and transmission is mainly during delivery. HBV vaccine is not contraindicated during pregnancy. (*See* Dutta's Textbook of Obstetrics, 8th Edition, p. 336).

Q.198 Causes of nonimmune hydrops fetalis are all except:
a. Rh-isoimmunization
b. Chronic fetomaternal transfusion
c. Alpha thalassemia
d. Infection with cytomegalovirus

Ans. a. It is an immune variety. (*See* Dutta's Textbook of Obstetrics, 8th Edition, p. 571).

Q.199 *Early ultrasonic diagnosis is made for all these except:*
  a. Fetal sex at 16th week
  b. Renal tract abnormality at 16th–18th weeks
  c. Anencephaly at 12th week
  d. Hydrocephalus at 24th week

Ans. d. Hydrocephalus can be diagnosed as early as at 16th week.

Q.200 *Embedded IUD in the uterus with missing thread is best removed by:*
  a. Hook
  b. Artery forceps
  c. Uterine curettage
  d. Hysteroscopy

Ans. d. While all the other methods are commonly used with occasional failure, hysteroscopy offers a cent percent success rate.

Q.201 *The following are related to sonographic measurements of biparietal diameter:*
  a. The ultrasonically determined biparietal diameter is same as the external diameter of the head
  b. Biparietal diameter is measured from outside of the scalp on the near side to the outside of the skull on the far side
  c. The same is measured from outside the skull on the near side to the outside of the scalp on the far side
  d. It is measured at the level of cavum septum pellucidum

Ans. d. The correct procedure is to measure the distance from outside of the skull on the near side, to the inside of the skull on the far side of the parietal bone, at the level of thalami (*See* Dutta's Textbook of Obstetrics, 8th Edition, Fig. 41.3, p. 733).

Q.202 *The following are related with cervical incompetence except:*
  a. Typically causes painless midtrimester abortion
  b. Diameter of the internal os is > 1 cm by ultrasound
  c. Length of the cervical canal is < 2.5 cm on ultrasound
  d. Abdominal circlage is superior to Shirodkar's operation

Ans. d. Shirodkar's circlage (vaginal) is the first choice. Abdominal circlage is done when the cervix is too short or is lacerated.

Q.203 *Maternal smoking during pregnancy is associated with all except:*
  a. Increasing the level of carbon monoxide and carbon dioxide in blood
  b. Decreasing the blood oxygen tension
  c. Placenta previa and abruption
  d. Increased fetal congenital malformation

Ans. d.

Q.204 *Following are related to placental transfer and concentration level except:*
  a. Fetal glucose level is higher than the mother
  b. Neither parathormone nor calcitonin crosses the placenta
  c. Amino acid concentration is high in the fetus
  d. In cord blood, level of ferritin is high

Ans. a.

Q.205 The following are related to hCG except:
  a. It is a glycoprotein having a molecular weight approximately 30,000
  b. It helps in placental steroidogenesis
  c. It affects fetal sexual differentiation
  d. It helps in the differentiation of fetal zone in the adrenal glands
Ans. a. The molecular weight of hCG ranges between 36,000 and 40,000.

Q.206 The following are related to human placental lactogen (hPL) except:
  a. Its molecular weight is approximates by 22,000
  b. It is an insulin antagonist
  c. It has lipolytic and lactogenic effects
  d. The plasma level is raised in hydatidiform mole
Ans. d. The level is lowered in hydatidiform mole.

Q.207 Maternal serum alpha fetoprotein is raised in all except:
  a. Open neural tube defects   b. Trisomies
  c. Omphalocele   d. Renal agenesis
Ans. b.

Q.208 The following are related to placental transfer except:
  a. Maternal thyrotrophic hormone does not cross the placenta
  b. Thyroxin crosses the placenta freely to the fetus
  c. Chorionic thyrotropin passes mainly to maternal circulation
  d. Thyroid stimulating antibodies cross the placenta freely
Ans. b. Thyroid hormones cross the placenta to a very limited degree. (*See* Dutta's Textbook of Obstetrics, 8th Edition, p. 70).

Q.209 Regarding embryology:
  a. Interstitial implantation occurs commonly on the anterior wall of the fundus
  b. Implantation occurs in the morula stage
  c. Corpus luteum degenerates soon following implantation
  d. Implantation corresponds to 24th day of a regular menstrual cycle
Ans. a. Implantation occurs in blastocyst stage. Corpus luteum continues to grow and it reaches its maximum growth at 8th week. Implantation corresponds to about 20th day of a regular cycle. (*See* Dutta's Textbook of Obstetrics, 8th Edition, p. 25).

Q.210 Contraindications of the use of ventouse are:
  a. Premature baby   b. Hemorrhagic disease of the fetus
  c. Brow presentation   d. All of the above
Ans. d. There is chance of avulsion of the scalp and consequent hematoma formation. Chance of bleeding from the puncture site is more. In fetal distress, it is not suitable as the process takes longer and forceps is a better alternative. It is also not safe to apply in brow or face presentation.

Q.211 Regarding placental transfer of amino acids:
  a. Occurs even when fetal blood levels of amino aids are higher than maternal
  b. Is mediated by diffusion process
  c. It is independent of anoxia
  d. Endocytosis is a known process
Ans. a and d. *See* Dutta's Textbook of Obstetrics, 8th Edition, p. 40.

Q.199 Early ultrasonic diagnosis is made for all these except:
   a. Fetal sex at 16th week
   b. Renal tract abnormality at 16th–18th weeks
   c. Anencephaly at 12th week
   d. Hydrocephalus at 24th week

Ans. d. Hydrocephalus can be diagnosed as early as at 16th week.

Q.200 Embedded IUD in the uterus with missing thread is best removed by:
   a. Hook
   b. Artery forceps
   c. Uterine curettage
   d. Hysteroscopy

Ans. d. While all the other methods are commonly used with occasional failure, hysteroscopy offers a cent percent success rate.

Q.201 The following are related to sonographic measurements of biparietal diameter:
   a. The ultrasonically determined biparietal diameter is same as the external diameter of the head
   b. Biparietal diameter is measured from outside of the scalp on the near side to the outside of the skull on the far side
   c. The same is measured from outside the skull on the near side to the outside of the scalp on the far side
   d. It is measured at the level of cavum septum pellucidum

Ans. d. The correct procedure is to measure the distance from outside of the skull on the near side, to the inside of the skull on the far side of the parietal bone, at the level of thalami (*See* Dutta's Textbook of Obstetrics, 8th Edition, Fig. 41.3, p. 733).

Q.202 The following are related with cervical incompetence except:
   a. Typically causes painless midtrimester abortion
   b. Diameter of the internal os is > 1 cm by ultrasound
   c. Length of the cervical canal is < 2.5 cm on ultrasound
   d. Abdominal circlage is superior to Shirodkar's operation

Ans. d. Shirodkar's circlage (vaginal) is the first choice. Abdominal circlage is done when the cervix is too short or is lacerated.

Q.203 Maternal smoking during pregnancy is associated with all except:
   a. Increasing the level of carbon monoxide and carbon dioxide in blood
   b. Decreasing the blood oxygen tension
   c. Placenta previa and abruption
   d. Increased fetal congenital malformation

Ans. d.

Q.204 Following are related to placental transfer and concentration level except:
   a. Fetal glucose level is higher than the mother
   b. Neither parathormone nor calcitonin crosses the placenta
   c. Amino acid concentration is high in the fetus
   d. In cord blood, level of ferritin is high

Ans. a.

78 Manual of Obstetrics and Gynecology for the Postgraduates

Q.205 The following are related to hCG except:
   a. It is a glycoprotein having a molecular weight approximately 30,000
   b. It helps in placental steroidogenesis
   c. It affects fetal sexual differentiation
   d. It helps in the differentiation of fetal zone in the adrenal glands

Ans. a. The molecular weight of hCG ranges between 36,000 and 40,000.

Q.206 The following are related to human placental lactogen (hPL) except:
   a. Its molecular weight is approximates by 22,000
   b. It is an insulin antagonist
   c. It has lipolytic and lactogenic effects
   d. The plasma level is raised in hydatidiform mole

Ans. d. The level is lowered in hydatidiform mole.

Q.207 Maternal serum alpha fetoprotein is raised in all except:
   a. Open neural tube defects
   b. Trisomies
   c. Omphalocele
   d. Renal agenesis

Ans. b.

Q.208 The following are related to placental transfer except:
   a. Maternal thyrotrophic hormone does not cross the placenta
   b. Thyroxin crosses the placenta freely to the fetus
   c. Chorionic thyrotropin passes mainly to maternal circulation
   d. Thyroid stimulating antibodies cross the placenta freely

Ans. b. Thyroid hormones cross the placenta to a very limited degree. (*See* Dutta's Textbook of Obstetrics, 8th Edition, p. 70).

Q.209 Regarding embryology:
   a. Interstitial implantation occurs commonly on the anterior wall of the fundus
   b. Implantation occurs in the morula stage
   c. Corpus luteum degenerates soon following implantation
   d. Implantation corresponds to 24th day of a regular menstrual cycle

Ans. a. Implantation occurs in blastocyst stage. Corpus luteum continues to grow and it reaches its maximum growth at 8th week. Implantation corresponds to about 20th day of a regular cycle. (*See* Dutta's Textbook of Obstetrics, 8th Edition, p. 25).

Q.210 Contraindications of the use of ventouse are:
   a. Premature baby
   b. Hemorrhagic disease of the fetus
   c. Brow presentation
   d. All of the above

Ans. d. There is chance of avulsion of the scalp and consequent hematoma formation. Chance of bleeding from the puncture site is more. In fetal distress, it is not suitable as the process takes longer and forceps is a better alternative. It is also not safe to apply in brow or face presentation.

Q.211 Regarding placental transfer of amino acids:
   a. Occurs even when fetal blood levels of amino aids are higher than maternal
   b. Is mediated by diffusion process
   c. It is independent of anoxia
   d. Endocytosis is a known process

Ans. a and d. *See* Dutta's Textbook of Obstetrics, 8th Edition, p. 40.

Q.212 *The following are related to intervillous space:*
   a. Intervillous space embryologically consists of maternal and fetal components
   b. Blood in this space is of fetal origin
   c. It is lined internally on all sides by cytotrophoblasts
   d. Rohr stria at the bottom of this space is due to fibrin deposition

Ans. d; a. Intervillous space is absolutely fetal in origin—bounded in between the basal and chorionic plate. b. It contains paradoxically only the maternal blood. The maternal blood enters the space by piercing the basal plate and not the chorionic plate. (*See* Dutta's Textbook of Obstetrics, 8th Edition, p. 37).

Q.213 *The newborn of diabetic mothers can have the following special problems except:*
   a. Polycythemia   b. RDS
   c. Hypoglycemia   d. Anemia

Ans. d. Because of high insulin production, there is chance of hypoglycemia soon following birth. Because of relatively late development of lung surfactant and increased risk of acidosis, RDS is common.

Q.214 *The following are related to alpha-fetoprotein (AFP) except:*
   a. AFP is derived from fetal liver and yolk sac
   b. Peak levels of AFP in fetal blood are reached at the end of first trimester
   c. Maternal blood levels are higher in hydatidiform mole
   d. It is a glycoprotein

Ans. c.

Q.215 *The following are related to increased level of amniotic fluid AFP except:*
   a. Open neural tube defects   b. Omphalocele
   c. Hydrocephalus   d. Intestinal obstruction (fetal)

Ans. c.

Q.216 *The following are related to rise in the incidence of ectopic pregnancy except:*
   a. Increased STD   b. Reconstructive tubal surgery
   c. Assisted reproductive techniques d. Third generation IUDs

Ans. d. *See* Dutta's Textbook of Obstetrics, 8th Edition, p. 208.

Q.217 *Regarding malaria in pregnancy:*
   a. Once it is acquired, immunity is life long
   b. Organ damage is due to blockage of the capillaries
   c. Quinine should be avoided in the first trimester
   d. Hypoglycemia is common with P. vivax malaria

Ans. b. *See* Dutta's Textbook of Obstetrics, 8th Edition, p. 344.

Q.218 *HELLP syndrome related to severe pre-eclampsia includes the following except:*
   a. Hemolytic anemia   b. Elevated liver enzymes
   c. Leukopenia   d. Low platelet count

Ans. c. It consists of three features only.

Q.219 *The following chromosomal abnormalities are associated with fetal loss and live born except:*
   a. Autosomal trisomy is mostly associated with first trimester abortions
   b. Polyploidy is common in second trimester abortuses

c. Trisomy 18 is most common in stillbirths
d. Trisomy 21 is most common in live births

Ans. b. Polyploidy is rare in late pregnancies; instead autosomal trisomy and monosomy X are common.

Q.220 Regarding medical termination of pregnancy (MTP):
a. Misoprostol is an effective abortifacient only when used orally
b. Unsuccessful use of misoprostol for MTP may result in fetal malformation
c. Mifepristone is associated with the significant risk of fetal abnormality in the event of failed termination of pregnancy
d. Failed termination of pregnancy is overall 5% even when properly done

Ans. b and a. Misoprostol can be used for termination of pregnancy when used either orally or vaginally; b. Unsuccessful use of misoprostol as an abortifacient may result in abnormalities in the children born thereafter. Moebius syndrome (paralysis of facial muscles), ectopia vesice, limb defects and hydrocephalus have been reported. Continuation of pregnancy due to failure of MTP is around 1%. Mifepristone has not been reported to have significant risk of fetal malformations. (*See* Dutta's Textbook of Obstetrics, 8th Edition, p. 203, 204).

Q.221 As regard to the postmaturity syndrome all are correct except:
a. Stillbirth rate is increased by 6 fold from 37 weeks to 43 weeks
b. Fetal risks are: Meconium aspiration, intrapartum hypoxia and acidosis
c. Maternal risks are: Increased operative delivery and maternal morbidity
d. Elevated fetal cortisol level is the cause for prolonged pregnancy

Ans. d. Cortisol deficiency may contribute to prolonged pregnancy.

Q.222 Regarding use of combined oral contraceptives all are true except:
a. Risk of major congenital anomaly is high when taken in early pregnancy
b. Breast milk is affected adversely in quality and quantity when COC is taken during lactation
c. Breastfeeders may use DMPA or norplant safely
d. Return of ovulation usually occurs within 3 months of stoppage of pills

Ans. a. *See* Dutta's Textbook of Obstetrics, 8th Edition, p. 622.

Q.223 As regards to the deep transverse arrest all are correct except:
a. Head is deep into the pelvic cavity
b. Sagittal suture lies in the bispinous diameter
c. There is no progress at least for 1 hour following full dilatation of the cervix
d. Delivery should be done by immediate cesarean section

Ans. d. Mode of delivery should depend upon the cause. (*See* Dutta's Textbook of Obstetrics, 8th Edition, p. 431).

Q.224 As regard to deep vein thrombosis (DVT) and pulmonary embolism (PE) all are correct except:
a. High-risk factors are obesity, heart disease and presence of thrombophilia
b. Perfusion scan (ventilation/perfusion), blood gas study are important for diagnosis
c. Heparin IV is the drug of choice
d. Breastfeeding is contraindicated while on heparin

Ans. d. *See* Dutta's Textbook of Obstetrics, 8th Edition, p. 508, 510.

Self-Assessment in Obstetrics

Q.225 Active management of labor:
   a. Resident house surgeon must be actively involved
   b. Partogram is maintained to record the progress of labor
   c. Male person should not be present during the course of labor
   d. Any case can be considered for active management
Ans. b. Consultant obstetrician must be involved. Husband (partner) should be present. Not all cases are considered for active management.

Q.226 Regarding postpill amenorrhea:
   a. It is observed in about 5% of women after 6 months of pill use
   b. Spontaneous resumption of menstruation is rare
   c. It is more common in women who lose weight when using COC pill
   d. When it lasts longer than 6 months, investigations should be done
Ans. c and d; a. Postpill amenorrhea affects around 1% of women. b. Spontaneous resumption of menstruation is common. c. It is an observation though the exact mechanism is not known. d. It may signify the unmasking of underlying gynecological abnormalities such as PCOS, hyperprolactinemia or premature ovarian failure.

Q.227 Which one is not an indications for cesarean hysterectomy?
   a. Uncontrolled PPH due to atonic uterus
   b. Morbid adherent placenta
   c. Multiple fibroid uterus seen during CS
   d. Grossly infected uterus
Ans. c.

Q.228 As regard to epidural analgesia which one is incorrect:
   a. Bupivacaine 0.5% is commonly used
   b. Lumbar puncture is made between L_2 and L_3 space
   c. Postspinal headache is commonly due to infection
   d. Hypovolemia is a contraindication
Ans. c. Commonly due to cerebrospinal fluid (CSF) leakage. (*See* Dutta's Textbook of Obstetrics, 8th Edition, p. 590).

Q.229 Regarding partogram which one is incorrect:
   a. Records cervical dilatation and fetal head descent against time
   b. It reduces prolonged labor
   c. It reduces the rate of cesarean section
   d. Fetal monitoring with cardiotocography (CTG) is a must
Ans. d. *See* Dutta's Textbook of Obstetrics, 8th Edition, p. 605.

Q.230 Surgical management of atonic PPH includes all except:
   a. Bilateral ligation of internal iliac arteries
   b. Uterine brace suture
   c. Bilateral ligation of ovarian and uterine vessels
   d. Ligation of inferior vena cava
Ans. d. Inferior vena cava ligation is done in recurrent pulmonary embolism. b. (*See* Dutta's Textbook of Obstetrics, 8th Edition, p. 482, 511).

82 Manual of Obstetrics and Gynecology for the Postgraduates

Q.231 Regarding tuberculosis in pregnancy:
   a. Purified protein derivative (PPD) skin test of from swelling 5 mm is considered positive for a woman who is HIV positive (high-risk)
   b. The neonate should be isolated even if mother is under treatment
   c. Neonate should be given prophylactic isoniazid therapy for 3 months
   d. When mother is on isoniazid therapy neonate should be given isoniazid resistant Bacillus Calmette–Guérin (BCG) vaccination

Ans. a and c. According to Centers for Disease Control (1993) three drugs can make sputum sterile within 2 weeks. Isoniazid does not affect the immunogenecity of BCG. There is no contraindication of breastfeeding for a patient under treatment.

Q.232 As regard to the cervix carcinoma in pregnancy:
   a. Clinical diagnosis is always early compared to nonpregnant state
   b. Patient with microinvasive carcinoma may be followed up to term
   c. Stage for stage survival outcome is no different between pregnancy and nonpregnant state
   d. Radical surgery must not be done on the fetus *in situ*

Ans. b and c; a. Usually late. d. May be done with fetus *in situ* in early weeks.

Q.233 Heart disease in pregnancy:
   a. Rheumatic mitral stenosis is the most common heart disease
   b. Atrial septal defect is the most common congenital heart disease
   c. Elective cesarean section is preferred for coarctation of aorta
   d. Maternal mortality in primary pulmonary hypertension is about 10%

Ans. a, b and c; d. Mortality is as high as 50%. (*See* Dutta's Textbook of Obstetrics, 8th Edition, p. 319).

Q.234 Regarding megaloblastic anemia in pregnancy:
   a. Vitamin B_{12} deficiency in pregnancy is common
   b. Addisonian pernicious anemia is due to lack of intrinsic factor
   c. Daily requirement of folic acid is 5 mg
   d. The fetus also becomes anemic when mother suffers from anemia

Ans. b; a. It is rare, as the need of Vitamin B_{12} in pregnancy is 3 mg (300 mcg) which is supplied by any diet that contains animal products. c. Daily requirement is 4 mg (400 mcg). d. The fetus is never anemic, because of transplacental supply from mothers. (*See* Dutta's Textbook of Obstetrics, 8th Edition, p. 312).

Q.235 In pregnancy with chronic nephritis which one is incorrect:
   a. Pregnancy outcome mainly depends on the level of blood pressure (BP)
   b. Presently pregnancy outcome has improved when compared with the past pregnancy outcome
   c. Pregnancy outcome is poor when serum creatinine level is >250 mmol/L
   d. Superimposed pre-eclampsia worsens the pregnancy outcome

Ans. a. Outcome depends on the level of BP, proteinuria and serum creatinine.

Q.236 Diagnostic hematological picture in thalassemia:
   a. MCV is normal
   b. Serum ferritin reduced

c. HBA$_2$ ($\alpha_2\delta_2$) is raised
d. Serum iron binding capacity is raised

Ans. c. See Dutta's Textbook of Obstetrics, 8th Edition, p. 317.

Q.237 In monozygotic twin pregnancy all are correct except:
a. Complications are more compared to dizygotic twins
b. Risks of fetal anomalies are low
c. Twin-twin transfusion syndrome may occur
d. Twin peak sign may be observed

Ans. b.

Q.238 Regarding HIV infection—all are correct except:
a. In most Asian countries infection rates are less than 1%
b. Perinatal transmission is 14–25%
c. Triple chemotherapy is preferred as a first line defence
d. When CD4 + count is high and the HIV RNA is low, risk of disease progression is high

Ans. d. Viral load—HIV RNA is an important determinant for disease progression.

Q.239 Regarding HIV infection—all are correct except:
a. Worldwide infection rate in women is 25–30%
b. Male to female transmission is low compared to female to male transmission
c. The median time from infection to AIDS is about 10 years
d. Immunofluorescence assay (IFA) is a confirmatory test

Ans. b. See Dutta's Textbook of Obstetrics, 8th Edition, p. 350.

Q.240 All the definitions are accepted except:
a. Morula is a solid ball of cells formed by 16 or so blastomeres
b. A fluid filled space converts the morula to a blastocyst
c. Completed 7th week demarcates an embryo from a fetus
d. Blastomeres are the daughter cells derived from the blastocyst

Ans. d. Cells are derived from mitotic division of zygote. (See Dutta's Textbook of Obstetrics, 8th Edition, p. 24).

Q.241 Doppler studies for umbilical flow velocity:
a. Umbilical artery Doppler flow velocity waveform is helpful in the management of high-risk pregnancies
b. Normal pregnancy exhibits an increase in the systolic/diastolic (S/D) ratio with advancing gestational age
c. At term in a normal pregnancy, end-diastolic flow may be absent
d. It is not useful in the management of multiple gestations

Ans. a. See Dutta's Textbook of Obstetrics, 8th Edition, p. 123.

Q.242 Regarding thyrotoxicosis in pregnancy all are correct except:
a. Thyrotoxicosis may ameliorate due to production of blocking antibodies
b. Thyroid stimulating antibodies act like TSH
c. Breastfeeding is contraindicated in patients with antithyroid drugs
d. Neonatal thyrotoxicosis may occur due to transplacental passage of maternal thyroid stimulator antibodies

Ans. c. Ideally the neonatal thyroid function should be monitored and the drug dose should be kept low.

Q.243 Regarding endocrinology in pregnancy—all are correct except:
  a. Maternal pituitary gland is essential for continuation of pregnancy
  b. All pituitary hormones are secreted by the fetus before 17 weeks
  c. Fetal adrenal glands are larger in volume
  d. There is transplacental transfer of thyroxine
Ans. a. *See* Dutta's Textbook of Obstetrics, 8th Edition, p. 70.

Q.244 Important ultrasound markers and their association are as below except:
  a. Twin peak sign or lambda sign—dichorionic placenta
  b. Nuchal translucency > 3 mm—chromosomal abnormality
  c. Lemon sign—neural tube defects
  d. Omphalocele—prognostically better than gastroschisis
Ans. d. Prognosis of omphalocele is poor, it may be associated with multiple anomalies including chromosomal abnormality. (*See* Manual of Obstetrics and Gynecology for the Postgraduates, p. 44, 243).

Q.245 Regarding gestational age determination in the second trimester all are correct except:
  a. Most appropriate time is between 14 and 20 weeks
  b. Commonly used parameters are BPD, HC and AC
  c. Cavum septum pellucidi is the important intracranial landmark for measurements
  d. HC is measured at the level of BPD
Ans. b. Parameters are BPD, HC, AC and FL (femur length).

Q.246 Important USG observations and the correlations are all—match them appropriately:

a. Gestational sac		1.	9 weeks
b. Fetal cardiac activity		2.	7 weeks
c. Lower limb buds		3.	6 weeks
d. Spine		4.	5 weeks

Ans. a = 4; b = 3; c = 2; d = 1. (*See* Manual of Obstetrics and Gynecology for the Postgraduates, p. 429).

Q.247 Regarding ultrasonography in the first trimester of pregnancy all are correct except:
  a. CRL between 7 and 12 weeks of gestation is most accurate for dating
  b. Pseudogestational sac is central in location in the uterine cavity
  c. Double ring sign of chorion and decidua interface is present in true gestational sac
  d. Embryo is seen when gestational sac diameter is 12 mm
Ans. d. Embryo is seen when gestational sac diameters is more than 17 mm.

Q.248 Regarding fetal physiology—all are correct except:
  a. At term fetal hemoglobin ($\alpha_2\gamma_2$) is 70–80%
  b. IgM is predominantly of fetal origin
  c. Fetal breathing movements are first observed at 20 weeks
  d. Fetal thyroid starts functioning by the 11th week
Ans. c. Breathing movements are observed by 11th week (*See* Dutta's Textbook of Obstetrics, 8th Edition, p. 47).

Q.249 *As regard to lactation all are true except:*
 a. Lactation can suppress ovulation
 b. It is not inhibited by progesterone
 c. High estrogen level initiate lactation
 d. Bromocriptine suppress lactation
Ans. c; b. Mini pill can be used as contraception during lactation.

Q.250 *In neonatal resuscitation:*
 a. Apgar score at 1 minute is more valuable
 b. External cardiac massage is started when heart rate is 100 per minute
 c. Drugs (adrenalin and dopamine) are the immediate steps of management
 d. Maintenance of airway and circulation are the prime objectives
Ans. d. Long-term neurological sequele is related more to the 5 minute apgar score and it is of more value. Gentle external cardiac massage is started when the heart rate is < 60 per minute. Medications are rarely used during resuscitation.

Q.251 *Oxytocin:*
 a. It is a decapeptide
 b. Synthesized in the posterior lobe of pituitary gland
 c. Alcohol stimulates its release
 d. It has a half-life of 3–4 minutes
Ans. d. Oxytocin is a nonapeptide, alcohol inhibits its secretion, it is synthesized in the supraoptic and paraventricular nuclei of hypothalamus. (*See* Dutta's Textbook of Obstetrics, 8th Edition, p. 573).

Q.252 *The following are ultrasonographic markers for increased chromosomal abnormality except:*
 a. Nuchal translucency > 3 mm
 b. Short femur
 c. Rocker bottom feet
 d. Jejunal atresia
Ans. d. Duodenal atresia is associated with Down's syndrome.

Q.253 *Management of fetal distress in labor are all except:*
 a. Change maternal position
 b. Stop oxytocin if infusion is on
 c. Immediate cesarean section
 d. O_2 administration
Ans. c. It is not needed in all the cases.

Q.254 *Doppler ultrasonography in obstetrics:*
 a. Diastolic blood flow velocity normally decreases with advancing gestation
 b. Absent or reversed end-diastolic velocity (umbilical artery) indicates prompt delivery
 c. CTG is more sensitive than Doppler flow study
 d. Pulsatility index or resistance index is used to express the Doppler flow study
Ans. d; a. It increases. b. Not prompt delivery but intensive fetal surveillance is needed and delivery should be decided upon other **non-Doppler reasons.** c. It remains inconclusive.

Q.255 *Regarding the Doppler flow velocimetry:*
 a. The diastolic flow reduces as the vascular resistance decreases
 b. Middle cerebral artery blood flow is commonly studied

c. Abnormal venous waveform in inferior vena cava is pathological
d. Presence of 'notch' in uterine arteries at 24 weeks confirms development of IUGR and pre-eclampsia

Ans. c; a. Diastolic blood flow increases as the vascular resistance decreases. b. Umbilical artery. d. May predict but cannot confirm. (*See* Dutta's Textbook of Obstetrics, 8th Edition, p. 123).

Q.256 Regarding antenatal assessment of fetal wellbeing:
a. Clinical methods are poor for screening the high-risk cases
b. Biochemical methods are sensitive to detect the fetus at risk
c. Biophysical methods have significantly improved the perinatal outcome
d. No single method is optimum to detect a fetus at risk

Ans. d. Clinical methods can be used as screening tests. Biochemical methods are poor to detect a fetus at risk. Perinatal outcome is improved because of improved neonatal care. (*See* Dutta's Textbook of Obstetrics, 8th Edition, p. 119).

Q.257 Regarding ultrasonographic fetal biometry:
a. Abdominal circumference (AC) is the least sensitive parameter for detection of IUGR
b. In asymmetric IUGR, head circumference/abdominal circumference (HC/AC) is reduced
c. Serial biparietal diameter (BPD) is the only important measurement in IUGR
d. AC indirectly reflects fetal liver size and glycogen storage

Ans. d. Abdominal circumference is the most sensitive parameter. b. The HC/AC ratio is increased. AC is reduced as the stored liver glycogen is depleted. There is brain sparing effect to cause raised HC/AC. (*See* Dutta's Textbook of Obstetrics, 8th Edition, p. 535).

Q.258 Antenatal cardiotocography—according to FIGO:
a. Baseline FHR is 120–160 beat per minute (bpm)
b. Baseline variability is 5–15 bpm
c. Reactive CTG: It means two or more accelerations in 20 minutes
d. Recurrent variable decelerations are not pathological

Ans. c; a. 110–150 bpm; b. 10–25 bpm. (*See* Dutta's Textbook of Obstetrics, 8th Edition, p. 693).

Q.259 Side effects of oxytocin are all except:
a. Fetal distress
b. Hypernatremia
c. Amniotic fluid embolism
d. Uterine rupture

Ans. b. It may cause hypontremia.

Q.260 Regarding breech delivery—match the following:
a. Lovset's maneuver
b. Burn-Marshall method
c. Prague method
d. Groin traction

1. Aftercoming head delivery
2. Shoulder delivery
3. Occipitoposterior position of head
4. Delivery of the breech

Ans. a = 2; b = 1; c = 3; d = 4.

Q.261 Concerning erb's palsy in the neonate all are true except:
a. Caused by injury of C4, C5, C6 roots of the brachial plexus
b. Often needs surgical intervention for improvement

c. Hazard faced in shoulder dystocia
d. Characteristic position of the affected limb is 'waiter's tip'

Ans. b.

Q.262 Microcytic hypochromic anemia may be due to:
a. Folic acid deficiency
b. Vitamin B_{12} deficiency
c. Thalassemia
d. Acute blood loss

Ans. c. *See* Dutta's Textbook of Obstetrics, 8th Edition, p. 307.

Q.263 Induction of labor at term is associated with:
a. Increased cesarean section rate
b. Increased instrumental deliveries
c. Reduced perinatal mortality
d. Reduced neonatal seizure rate

Ans. c. Prospective randomized trial have shown no increase in the rate of cesarean section or instrumental delivery when induction is at 41st week. Neonatal seizures are also unaffected. (*See* Dutta's Textbook of Obstetrics, 8th Edition, p. 598).

Q.264 Decision for vaginal delivery after previous cesarean section:
a. Radiopelvimetry is important for pelvic assessment
b. Clinical pelvimetry in between pregnancy should be done
c. Partographic assessment during labor is more informative
d. Elective cesarean section is ideal following previous cesarean delivery

Ans. c; a. Less informative. b. Retrospective assessment is of little value. c. Chance of vaginal delivery is about 60% following one previous cesarean with nonrecurrent factors.

Q.265 Amnioinfusion in labor:
a. Reduces perinatal mortality
b. Increases maternal risk of infection
c. Reduces the risk of meconium aspiration
d. Does not reduce the risk of cord compression

Ans. c; d. Reduces the risk of cord compression and thereby reduces variable deceleration.

Q.266 Regarding flow velocimetry of umbilical artery:
a. Resistance index of 1.0 implies absent end-diastolic flow (AEDF)
b. AEDF is not associated with any risk of fetal structural or chromosomal abnormality
c. Higher the pulsatility index, greater is the placental vascular resistance
d. It correlates well with the spiral artery count

Ans. a; c and d. Umbilical artery waveforms correlate well with the spiral artery count. Waves of trophoblasts invasion (at 10–12 weeks and again at 12–16 weeks) in the spiral artery up to radial artery causes fall in the pulsatility index in normal pregnancy. There is funneling of the arteries which causes increase in the blood flow. Trophoblastic invasion is absent in pre-eclampsia. b. Absent or reversed end-diastolic flow carries increased risk of fetal structural (20%) and chromosomal (4%) abnormality.

Q.267 As regard to fetal circulation:
a. Umbilical vein carries deoxygenated blood from the fetus
b. Blood from right atrium (75%) enters the left atrium through foramen ovale

c. Ductus arteriosus diverts left ventricular blood into the descending aorta
d. Anatomical closure of foramen ovale occurs soon after birth

Ans. b. *See* Dutta's Textbook of Obstetrics, 8th Edition, p. 49.

Q.268 As regard shoulder dystocia:
a. Antenatal sonography can predict the diagnosis accurately
b. McRobert's position should be used promptly
c. Suprapubic pressure (Wood's maneuver) is of little value
d. Fundal pressure is effective and should be given

Ans. b; c. Suprapubic pressure is next step after step b; d. Fundal pressure should not be used as it causes high neonatal morbidity (neurological damage). (*See* Dutta's Textbook of Obstetrics, 8th Edition, p. 469).

Q.269 As regard to gestational diabetes:
a. Routine screening of all pregnant women is helpful
b. Obesity, unexplained polyhydramnios are risk factors
c. Congenital malformation is increased
d. Insulin is not required for the management

Ans. b; a. Selective screening based on risk factors is recommended, congenital malformation is not increased, insulin may be needed for glycemic control. (*See* Dutta's Textbook of Obstetrics, 8th Edition, p. 326).

Q.270 Endocrinology in pregnancy:
a. Human placental lactogen (hPL) is different from prolactin immunologically
b. There is no change in the thyroid gland as the level of TSH remains normal
c. There is progressive rise in plasma cortisol level
d. Parathyroid hormones cross the placenta

Ans. c. *See* Dutta's Textbook of Obstetrics, 8th Edition, p. 66.

Q.271 Pregnancy is contraindicated in the following cardiac conditions:
a. Severe pulmonary hypertension
b. Eisenmenger's syndrome
c. Left ventricular dysfunction with history of previous peripartum cardiomyopathy
d. Fallot's tetralogy (corrected)

Ans. a; b and c; d. After surgical correction, women tolerate pregnancy well.

Q.272 Features suggestive of IUGR are all except:
a. Reduced symphysiofundal height
b. Reduced end-diastolic flow on umbilical artery Doppler study
c. Poor weight gain during pregnancy
d. Amniotic fluid index is 15 cm

Ans. d.

Q.273 For ultrasound assessment of gestational age—match the following parameters:
a. 5 weeks post LMP   1. BPD measurement
b. 6 weeks post LMP   2. Yolk sac on transvaginal scan
c. 7 weeks post LMP   3. Cardiac motion on abdominal scan
d. 14–20 weeks post LMP   4. Gestational sac

Ans. a = 4; b = 2; c = 3; d = 1. (*See* Dutta's Textbook of Obstetrics, 8th Edition, p. 77).

Q.274 Intrahepatic cholestasis in pregnancy—all are true except:
 a. Second common cause of jaundice next to viral hepatitis
 b. May cause IUFD
 c. May recur in subsequent pregnancies (50–60%)
 d. Bilirubin level is usually > 5 mg/dL
Ans. d. Bilirubin level is usually < 5 mg/dL. (*See* Dutta's Textbook of Obstetrics, 8th Edition, p. 336).

Q.275 Following are true in imaging techniques during pregnancy except:
 a. Pelvimetry by computed tomography (CT) exposes the fetus to more radiation
 b. Radiopelvimetry is relatively safe compared to CT
 c. Pelvimetry by MRI is considered accurate and biologically safe
 d. *In utero* exposure up to 10 rad is permissible
Ans. c. In fetal, radiation exposure by different methods are (approximately): CT pelvimetry 0.2 rad, radiopelvimetry 0.5–1.1 rad depending upon how many views are taken. MRI uses either no or very minimum radiation. *In utero* exposure of less than 5 rad (0.05 Gy) have not been observed to cause congenital malformations or growth restriction.

Q.276 In hyperemesis gravidarum:
 a. Hypernatremia is common
 b. Thiamine deficiency can result in Wernicke's encephalopathy
 c. Pyrexia occurs
 d. Colicky abdominal pain is characteristic
Ans. b. *See* Dutta's Textbook of Obstetrics, 8th Edition, p. 183.

Q.277 Regarding medical disorders in pregnancy:
 a. Diabetes is associated more with postmaturity
 b. Insulin requirement falls with progress of pregnancy in diabetes
 c. Tocolysis with β-mimetics is contraindicated with heart disease
 d. Pulmonary edema is a complication following *P. vivax* infection
Ans. c; d. Pulmonary edema is common with *P. falciparum* infection.

Q.278 Current midwifery and obstetric practice is:
 a. All perineal tears must be sutured
 b. Dexon suture in episiotomy is more painful than catgut
 c. Dexon (polyglycolic acid) is completely absorbed by 60 days
 d. Third degree perineal tear is one when anal sphincter is involved
Ans. d; a It should be repaired only when it is large or is bleeding. b. Catgut suture causes more inflammation and is more painful. c. Absorbed by 120 days.

Q.279 Thrombophilias causing recurrent thromboembolism are due to deficiencies of all except:
 a. Antithrombin III
 b. Protein C
 c. Homocysteine
 d. Protein S
Ans. c. It is hyperhomocysteinemia, not the deficiency.

Q.280 Regarding breech presentation:
   a. It occurs in about 10% of all deliveries
   b. ECV is successful in about 60% of cases
   c. Version should ideally be performed under anesthesia
   d. Risk of entrapment of aftercoming head can be predicted with the use of **ultrasonography**

Ans. b; a. 3–4%. c. Undue force should not be used during ECV therefore anesthesia should not be used. d. It cannot be predicted always.

Q.281 Regarding increased glomerular filtration rate (GFR) in normal pregnancy all are correct except:
   a. Can lead to renal glycosuria
   b. Decreases maternal serum urea and creatinine concentration
   c. Can cause urinary tract infection
   d. Changes start in the late second trimester

Ans. d. Constituents like amino acids, folic acid, urea, creatinine are filtered by the kidney and their serum concentration fall. But the changes start in early first trimester. Renal glycosuria is the cause for urinary tract infection. (*See* Dutta's Textbook of Obstetrics, 8th Edition, p. 63).

Q.282 Regarding asymptomatic bacteriuria during pregnancy all are correct except:
   a. Bacterial count is over 10^5/mL
   b. Overall incidence is 5–10%
   c. It should be treated with appropriate antimicrobial agent
   d. Risk of progression to symptomatic state, if left untreated is rare

Ans. d. Risk is about 20–30%. (*See* Dutta's Textbook of Obstetrics, 8th Edition, p. 347).

Q.283 In normal pregnancy:
   a. O_2 carrying capacity of blood is raised by 15–20%
   b. A fall in hemoglobin concentration is due to anemia
   c. Dyspnea in later months is pathological
   d. Arteriovenous (A-V) oxygen difference increases

Ans. a; b. It is physiological due to hemodilution and not pathological due to anemia. c. In normal pregnancy it is physiological. d. Venous blood is slightly more saturated with O_2 and the A-V O_2 difference decreases.

Q.284 Preterm labor has been associated with all except:
   a. Infection with bacteroides and bacterial vaginosis
   b. Cytokines are mainly IL-6, TNF-α and leukotrienes
   c. Fetal fibronectin (FFN) in cervical discharge is detected
   d. Corticosteroid should be given to all the mothers

Ans. d. It is not needed if pregnancy is > 34 weeks. (*See* Dutta's Textbook of Obstetrics, 8th Edition, p. 365).

Q.285 Fetal affection by Rh antibody are all except:
   a. Nonimmune hydrops fetalis
   b. Icterus gravis neonatorum

Self-Assessment in Obstetrics 89

c. Congenital anemia of the newborn
d. Fetal death

Ans. a. *See* Dutta's Textbook of Obstetrics, 8th Edition, p. 388, 571.

Q.286 *Which of the following is not accepted in clinical obstetric practice:*
  a. First pregnancy at or above 30 years (FIGO>35 years) is called elderly primigravida
  b. Pregnant woman with previous four or more viable birth is called grand multipara
  c. Woman having three or more induced abortion is called recurrent abortion
  d. Uterine pregnancy coexisting with ectopic pregnancy is called heterotypic pregnancy

Ans. c. It should be spontaneous not induced.

Q.287 *Regarding the pelvis—match the following:*
  a. Android pelvis   1. Sacrocotyloid diameter of engagement
  b. Scoliotic pelvis   2. Narrow subpubic angle
  c. Anthropoid pelvis 3. Wide and shallow sacrosciatic notch
  d. Flat pelvis   4. Shortened oblique diameter

Ans. a = 2; b = 4; c = 3; d = 1. (*See* Dutta's Textbook of Obstetrics, 8th Edition, p. 403).

Q.288 *About occipitoposterior position all are true except:*
  a. The engaging diameter of the fetal head is suboccipitofrontal (10 cm) or occipitofrontal (11.5 cm)
  b. Complete anterior rotation of occiput occurs in majority (90%)
  c. It is the most common malpresentation
  d. Deflection of the fetal head favors this position

Ans. c. It is an abnormal position of the head. (*See* Dutta's Textbook of Obstetrics, 8th Edition, p. 426).

Q.289 *In relation to normal labor:*
  a. Bearing down efforts are exclusive of second stage
  b. In primigravida dilatation and effacement take place simultaneously
  c. Duration of latent phase in a primigravida is 18 hours
  d. Abdominal assessment of head by fifth formula (crichton) can reduce repeated vaginal examination

Ans. d.

Q.290 *About partographic management of labor:*
  a. Incidence of prolonged labor is reduced
  b. Alert line means to alert the anesthetist on duty
  c. Action line means immediate action by forceps or cesarean delivery
  d. Labor is expected to be completed by 12 hours

Ans. a and d. In cervicograph action line is drawn 4 hours (WHO–1994C) to the right and parallel to the alert line. Labor is considered abnormal when the cervical dilatation crosses the alert line and falls on zone 2 (*See* Manual of Obstetrics and Gynecology for the Postgraduates, Cases: 9 and 10, p. 20, 22) and intervention is required when it crosses the action line and falls on zone 3.

Q.291 *Diagnosis of unruptured tubal ectopic pregnancy can be made by:*
  a. Serum β-hCG level when titre is falling
  b. Transvaginal sonography showing empty uterine cavity

c. Combination of serum βhCG and transvaginal sonography
d. Careful history taking and examination in majority

Ans. c. See Dutta's Textbook of Obstetrics, 8th Edition, p. 216.

Q.292 The following are related to lactation:
a. An intact nerve supply is essential for the growth of mammary gland during pregnancy
b. Lactational amenorrhea depends on the frequency and duration of lactation
c. Presence of the infant or infant's cry can induce milk let down reflex
d. Bromocriptine is dopamine antagonist

Ans. b and c. Bromocriptine is dopamine agonist. (See Dutta's Textbook of Obstetrics, 8th Edition, p. 172).

Q.293 Hormonal changes in a lactating woman are:
a. Prolactin level is high
b. GnRH level is high
c. LH level is raised
d. Level of estrogen is high

Ans. a. Regarding b, c and d. levels are low. (See Dutta's Textbook of Obstetrics, 8th Edition, p. 66).

Q.294 The following statements are related to normal delivery:
a. Delivery in upright or traditional squatting position is beneficial
b. Enema should be a routine to accelerate the progress of labor
c. Sustained pushing (bearing down efforts) should be discouraged
d. Vaginal examination must be frequent to assess the progress of labor

Ans. a and c; b. Though enema is given traditionally, it has nothing to do with the labor progress. d. Vaginal examination is generally done at interval of 4 hours with the use of partograph. Usually 4 hours is the time interval between the alert line and action line. Reference : WHO (1994) The partograph : A managerial tool for the prevention of prolonged labor, Geneva: Maternal and child health unit.

Q.295 The following are the collateral pathways (demonstrated by aortogram) that develops following bilateral ligation of internal iliac arteries—match them appropriately:
a. Lumbar arteries
b. Superior rectal
c. Superficial and deep external
d. Inferior epigastric and medial circumflex femoral

1. Obturator artery
2. Internal pudendal artery
3. Middle and inferior rectal arteries pudendal
4. Iliolumbar artery

Ans. a = 4; b = 3; c = 2; d = 1. (See Dutta's Textbook of Gynecology, 7th Edition, p. 25).

Q.296 The important hemodynamic mechanism of hemostasis following ligation of internal iliac arteries:
a. Reducing the blood flow (50%) by ligation of vessels
b. Significant reduction (85%) in the pulse pressure
c. Effects are the same irrespective of the procedure (unilateral or bilateral)
d. Significant reduction (25%) of the mean arterial pressure

Ans. a, b and d. This helps to form stable clot to achieve effective hemostasis. Bilateral ligation should be done when the bleeding is of uterine origin. (See Manual of Obstetrics and Gynecology for the Postgraduates, p. 32).

Q.297 *Regarding injectable contraceptive steroids all are correct except:*
   a. DMPA (depot medroxyprogesterone acetate) injection is more reliable than combined oral pill
   b. Norplant is effective within 24 hours and lasts for 5 years
   c. DMPA and norplant both inhibit ovulation
   d. Menorrhagia is a known side effect for the both
Ans. d. Both DMPA and norplant control menorrhagia and improve anemia. (*See* Dutta's Textbook of Obstetrics, 8th Edition, p. 628).

Q.298 *Regarding levonorgestrel intrauterine system (LNG-IUS):*
   a. Increases the incidence of ectopic pregnancy than copper IUCD
   b. Specially useful in newly married woman
   c. Failure rate is lower than the copper IUCD
   d. Causes suppression of endometrium and improves menorrhagia
Ans. c and d. (*See* Dutta's Textbook of Obstetrics, 8th Edition, p. 615).

Q.299 *Regarding breakthrough bleeding (BTB) while using combined oral pills:*
   a. It has no clinical significance as regard to the efficacy of pills
   b. Usually observed after 6 months of use
   c. Patient should be advised to take higher dose estrogen pills immediately
   d. It is commonly due to subthreshold blood level of hormones
Ans. d; a. There are other causes of BTB which should be excluded before advising immediate change to higher dose pill. b. It is common during the first 3 months of use.

Q.300 *Increased incidence of venous thrombosis is associated with:*
   a. Use of progesterone only pill
   b. Factor V Leiden mutation
   c. Cases of thrombophilias
   d. Ovarian hyperstimulation syndrome
Ans. b; c and d.

Q.301 *Failure rate of contraceptive methods are as follows except:*
   a. DMPA—0–1 per HWY
   b. Norplant—0.1 per HWY
   c. LNG-IUS—0.02 per HWY
   d. Levonorgestrel (used as an emergency contraception)—3 per HWY
Ans. d. It is 0–1 per HWY on correct use. (*See* Dutta's Textbook of Obstetrics, 8th Edition, p. 611).

Q.302 *Regarding emergency contraception:*
   a. Yuzpe method taking of birth control pills within 5 days of unprotected sex
   b. IUCD must be used within 48 hours or earlier
   c. Risk of pregnancy following a single act of unprotected coitus (around ovulation) is 8%
   d. RU 486 must be used within 5 days
Ans. c; a. It should be taken as soon as possible after intercourse but not later than 72 hours. b. IUCD should be used within a maximum period of 5 days. d. Single dose (600 mg) must be taken within 27th day of the cycle.

Q.303 Regarding progestin only pill (POP):
a. It acts mainly by inhibiting ovulation
b. It is contraindicated in elderly women specially who smoke
c. It is taken with "3 weeks on and 1 week off" regime similar to combined pills
d. It is less reliable in obese women

Ans. d; a. It acts mainly on cervical mucous. b. It is indicated in such cases. c. It is taken continuously without any break.

Q.304 Regarding the drugs and teratogenecity—match them appropriately:
a. Alcohol   1. Nasal hypoplasia, stippled epiphyses
b. Isotretinoin   2. Hypocalvaria
c. Enalapril   3. Cleft palate, cardiac defect, hydrocephalus
d. Warfarin   4. Short palpebral fissures, hypoplastic filtrum

Ans. d; a = 4; b = 3; c = 2; d = 1. See Ref. Drug therapy in pregnancy (FDA-1980) (See Manual of Obstetrics and Gynecology for the Postgraduates, p. 261, 415; Dutta's Textbook of Obstetrics 8th Edition, p. 589).

Q.305 Regarding exposure of teratogens and gestational age all are true except:
a. Peri-implantation period has got all or none effects
b. Embryonic period has structural malformation effects
c. Fetal period is unaffected by teratogens
d. Effects within first 8 weeks is called embryopathy

Ans. c. Fetus is still vulnerable as brain growth continues throughout pregnancy.

Q.306 Regarding ultrasound screening for down's syndrome—all are correct except:
a. Nuchal translucency is the most sensitive marker
b. Congenital cardiac defect is observed in about 50% of cases
c. There is no need of further testing, when ultrasound scan is normal
d. In the first trimester ultrasound marker combined with biochemical marker increases the sensitivity

Ans. c. Only about 30% cases of down's syndrome have structural malformation.

Q.307 Screening for Down's syndrome:
a. Sensitivity of quadruple test (AFP + hCG + uE3 + Inhibin A) is 90%
b. Biochemical screening in the first trimester is equally sensitive to that of second trimester
c. Inhibin A improves the sensitivity of screening in the second trimester
d. Inhibin A level is reduced in pregnancies affected by trisomy 21

Ans. a. Sensitivity is 76%. (See Dutta's Textbook of Obstetrics, 8th Edition, p. 132). d. Inhibin A level is significantly increased. (See Dutta's Textbook of Obstetrics, 8th Edition, p. 127).

Q.308 As regard to the progress of labor:
a. Vaginal examination is done in every 4 hours
b. For assessment of descent vaginal examination is a must
c. Active phase of labor is from 1 to 10 cm cervical dilatation
d. First stage of labor is divided into latent and active phase

Ans. a and d. Descent of the head is assessed abdominally in **fifths above the brim**. It is more reliable than vaginal examination as it avoids the confusion due to caput formation. Active phase is from 3 to 10 cm (full cervical dilatation).

Q.309 In assessing the progress of labor:
a. Assessment of descent is done abdominally in fifths felt above brim
b. 3–4 contractions with duration of 30–40 seconds are optimum
c. When three-fifths of the head is felt above the brim, it is engaged
d. Normal progress means cervical dilatation remains either on the alert line or to the left of it

Ans. a; b. and d. (*See* Manual of Obstetrics and Gynecology for the Postgraduates Case 9 and 10, p. 20, 22).

Q.310 Regarding systemic lupus erythematosus (SLE) in pregnancy:
a. Flare ups are more likely if the patient was in the remission phase before pregnancy
b. May be associated with thrombocytosis to cause thrombosis
c. Incidence of pre-eclampsia is low
d. Congenital lupus syndromes may occur

Ans. d. *See* Dutta's Textbook of Obstetrics, 8th Edition, p. 340.

Q.311 Concerning single umbilical artery:
a. It is an insignificant observation
b. Equally common in the neonates of diabetic and nondiabetic mothers
c. Predictor of fetal malformation
d. Present in 8–10% of all births

Ans. c. Single umbilical artery occurs in 1% of all singleton neonates, in 2.5% of all abortuses and about 5% of at least one twin. It is significantly raised in neonates of diabetic women. Fetal malformation is as high as 18% and cause high perinatal mortality. This finding is an indication of amniocentesis, cordocentesis, chorionic villus sampling for fetal chromosomal study. (*See* Dutta's Textbook of Obstetrics, 8th Edition, p. 254).

Q.312 Regarding the second stage of labor:
a. Its duration must be strictly adhered as normally stipulated
b. Dorsal position has many advantages
c. Benefits of 'guarding the perineum' is yet to be established
d. Routine episiotomy protects the pelvic floor muscles

Ans. c; a. As long as the maternal and fetal conditions are good and there is progress of labor, there is no reason to rigidly adhere to a stipulated duration of 1 or 2 hours. b. Upright position or lateral tilt is advantageous as the maternal discomfort, pain and perineal trauma are less. However, women can adopt any position of their choice except long periods of lying dorsal supine position. c. Till date evidences are insufficient as regards to its usefulness. However, the result of HOOP (Hands on or Poised) study of Oxford are awaited. d. There is no reliable evidence to support that the procedure protects the fetal head, pelvic floor muscles and prevents SUI.

Q.313 As regard to the maternal positions during the first stage of labor:
a. Supine position is always preferred
b. Lying on one side increases the intensity and efficiency of the uterine contractions

c. Position should be the choice of the woman as long as the head is engaged
d. Women must confine themselves to one position only

Ans. b and c; a. Supine position is preferred only when the membranes are ruptured and the head is not engaged. Otherwise it should be avoided as it causes aortocaval compression. d. Women often change positions as no position is comfortable for her at this stage.

Q.314 *Timing of umbilical cord clamping:*
a. Clamping should be done early in normal birth
b. Late clamping causes hypervolemia and hyperbilirubinemia in the newborn
c. Late clamping prevents iron deficiency anemia in the infant
d. A period of 3–4 minutes following birth is ideal

Ans. c and d. Recent research supports late clamping as it helps in the transfusion of additional 80 mL of blood from the placenta of mother to the infant. b. It is a theoretical possibility.

Q.315 *Regarding anemia in pregnancy:*
a. Hemoglobin 11.0 g/dL is the lowest acceptable level
b. Hemoglobin below 10 g/dL at any time is considered low
c. Hemoglobin should be estimated best at 20 weeks of gestation
d. Investigations should be started when the hemoglobin level is 10 g/dL

Ans. b; a. It was considered in the past and had no scientific justification. Hemoglobin should be estimated early in pregnancy for baseline value and again at 30 weeks (point of maximum hemodilution) to get an accurate picture. Hb of less than 9.0 g/dL requires detailed investigations. **Ref:** Standards of midwifery practice for safe motherhood: Notes on advances in practice; World Health Organization : 1999.

Q.316 *Immediate care of the newborn includes:*
a. To prevent hypoglycemia, the newborn should have early glucose feed
b. Body temperature of neonate rises immediately following delivery
c. 'Kangaroo' method is very effective to protect the newborn
d. Temperature should be taken from the rectum of the newborn

Ans. c. Body temperature of neonates fall significantly immediately following delivery. Hypothermia is associated with hypoglycemia and asphyxia leading to high neonatal mortality and morbidity. Putting the newborn to mother's breast and wrapping them together (skin to skin contact) is an effective method known as kangaroo method. 'Kangaroo' is specially for low birth weight babies. Temperature should be taken in the axilla and not in the rectum. Soon after delivery (within 2 hours) baby should be put near to breast to prevent hypoglycemia as the colostrum is rich in calories. (*See* Dutta's Textbook of Obstetrics, 8th Edition, p. 518).

Q.317 *For fetal lung maturation, all the corticosteroids can be used except:*
a. Betamethasone
b. Dexamethasone
c. Hydrocortisone
d. Methylprednisolone

Ans. d. It is not effective because of poor placental transfer. Betamethasone also the drug of choice.

Q.318 *In relation to recurrent miscarriage these are the genetic consideration except:*
a. Balanced translocations are the most common structural parental chromosomal abnormalities

b. Karyotyping of the abortus has got no prognostic value
c. Inversion is the rarer parenteral chromosomal rearrangement
d. When the first fetus is chromosomally abnormal, the risk for the second fetus to have the same abnormality is 75%

Ans. b; d. is the explanation for b. counseling.

Q.319 *In the developing countries, the following are the targets for 2015 in 'making pregnancy safer' (WHO/UNFPA/UNICEF/World Bank—1999):*
a. Reduction in maternal mortality ratio by 75% between 1990 and 2015
b. Skilled attendants to be present in 60% of births by 2015
c. Reduction of infant mortality below 50 per 1,000 live births by 2015
d. Access to reproductive health services to 50% by 2015

Ans. a and b; c. target is below 35 per 1,000 live births; d. access to all (100%) by 2015.

Q.320 *Changes in the respiratory system in pregnancy:*
a. Vital capacity is increased
b. Subcostal angle remains unchanged
c. Tidal volume remains unaltered
d. Residual volume is decreased

Ans. d. *See* Dutta's Textbook of Obstetrics, 8th Edition, p. 63. (*See* Konar & Dutta's Bedside Clinic, p. 102). Subcostal angle is increased from 68° to 103°. Tidal volume is increased by 40% and vital capacity remains unaltered.

Q.321 *Regarding trophoblast cells, all are correct except:*
a. Can be detected in maternal blood circulation
b. Cells are genetically maternal
c. Produce thyrotropin releasing hormone (TRH)
d. Immunologically active

Ans. b. *See* Dutta's Textbook of Obstetrics, 8th Edition, p. 36, 131. Trophoblast cells are relased in maternal blood circulation and are destroyed in the lung. These cells are genetically fetal in origin and are immunologically active.

Q.322 *Regarding fetal breathing movements in utero, all are correct except:*
a. Can be detected earliest by 11 weeks
b. It increases with increasing gestational age
c. Increased after meals
d. Are increased, is asymmetrical IUGR

Ans. d. *See* Dutta's Textbook of Obstetrics, 8th Edition, p. 48. Fetal breathing movements are detected by real time USG.

Q.323 *As regard the ischial spine in a female bony pelvis, all are correct except:*
a. The obstetric pelvic axis is directed abruptly forward at this level
b. The spines lie between the greater and lesser sciatic notches
c. When the biparietal diameter of the fetal skull is at this level, the head is engaged
d. The internal pudendal nerve runs through its ventral surface

Ans. d. *See* Dutta's Textbook of Obstetrics, 8th Edition, p. 98, 102. The internal pudendal nerve runs through its dorsal surface.

98 Manual of Obstetrics and Gynecology for the Postgraduates

Q.324 Oxytocin:
   a. Is synthesized by the pituitary gland
   b. Stimulates milk formation
   c. Is a steroid hormone
   d. Stimulates myometrial contractile system in labor

Ans. d. Oxytocin and arginine vasopressin are synthesized in the supraoptic and paraventricular nuclei of the hypothalamus and are stored in the posterior pituitary. It stimulates myoepithelial cells (breast) to cause milk ejection and myometrial cells (uterus) in labor. It is a polypeptide hormone (nonapeptide or octapeptide). (See Dutta's Textbook of Obstetrics, 8th Edition, p. 573).

Q.325 In a normal pregnancy:
   a. TSH crosses the placental barrier freely
   b. Levels of free T_3 and T_4 are increased
   c. Fetal thyroid starts functioning from 6th week
   d. Maternal pituitary gland is not essential for maintenance of pregnancy

Ans. d. See Dutta's Textbook of Obstetrics, 8th Edition, p. 62, 70. TSH, T_3 and T_4 cross the placenta very minimally. Fetal thyroid start functioning by the end of first trimester.

Q.326 Human chorionic gonadotropin (hCG):
   a. Is a protein hormone
   b. Is produced by the cytotrophoblast
   c. Doubling time in plasma is 72 hours (See Dutta's Textbook of Obstetrics, 8th Edition, p. 67)
   d. Disappears from circulation within 2 weeks following delivery

Ans. d. See Dutta's Textbook of Obstetrics, 8th Edition, p. 66.

Q.327 Match the following with their recognized side effects:
   When used during pregnancy

a. Methyldopa		1.	Pulmonary edema
b. Terbutaline		2.	Gingival hypertrophy
c. Phenytoin		3.	Postural hypotension
d. Heparin		4.	Thrombocytopenia

Ans. a = 3; b = 1; c = 2; d = 4 (though rare). (See Dutta's Textbook of Obstetrics, 8th Edition, p. 581).

Q.328 Gestational trophoblastic neoplasia (GTN):
   a. Most common chromosomal pattern of a complete mole is 46 XY
   b. In a partial mole the level of hCG is significantly high
   c. Risk of persistent GTN in both (complete and partial) is around 20%
   d. In complete moles, the chromosomes are from the father

Ans. d. 46 XX is the common chromosomal pattern (90%) of a complete mole. Complete mole arises from the fertilization of an empty ovum by a single sperm (23X). The sperm duplicates its own chromosomes to form 46XX. (See Dutta's Textbook of Obstetrics, 8th Edition, p. 230).

Q.329 The second stage of labor:
   a. Starts with maternal bearing down efforts
   b. The membranes usually remains intact

    c. Ends with the separation of placenta
    d. Causes fetal bradycardia with uterine contractions
Ans. d. *See* Dutta's Textbook of Obstetrics, 8th Edition, p. 143, 153, 158, 159.

Q.330 The third stage of labor:
    a. Begins when the cervix is fully dilated
    b. Ends with placental separation
    c. There is retraction of uterine muscle
    d. Uterine activity ceases thereafter
Ans. c. *See* Dutta's Textbook of Obstetrics, 8th Edition, p. 143, 162, 163.

Q.331 All are the contraindications for vaginal birth after previous cesarean except:
    a. Previous classical uterine incision
    b. Previous lower segment transverse cesarean
    c. Presence of inverted 'T' shaped uterine incision
    d. Where facilities for emergency cesareans are not available
Ans. b. Success rate for VBAC-TOL after one cesarean is about 60–80% and after two is about 50–70%. (*See* Dutta's Textbook of Obstetrics, 8th Edition, p. 384).

Q.332 Regarding cesarean hysterectomy—all are correct except:
    a. Morbid adherent placenta is a recognized as an indication
    b. Placenta accreta can be managed conservatively
    c. Women having placenta previa with previous cesarean are at high-risk for cesarean hysterectomy
    d. Subtotal hysterectomy is effective in all the cases
Ans. d. In cases with placenta previa and accreta, total hysterectomy is needed because blood flow via cervical branch of uterine artery remains uncontrolled. The need of cesarean hysterectomy is about 25%. Rarely focal placenta accreta can be managed by over sewing the placental bed.

Q.333 Regarding prenatal genetic diagnosis (PGD) all are correct except:
    a. Blastomere biopsy increases fetal anomaly
    b. Linkage analysis is necessary when gene has not been sequenced
    c. Polar body biopsy cannot assess paternal genotype
    d. Fetal cells recovered from maternal blood can detect fetal chromosomal anomaly
Ans. a. *See* Dutta's Textbook of Obstetrics, 8th Edition, p. 127.

Q.334 Regarding chorionic villus sampling (CVS) all are correct except:
    a. The procedure either transcervical or transabdominal is equally safe
    b. Limb reduction defects (LRD) in CVS could be 1 in 3000 procedures
    c. Optimum time for CVS is between 8 and 10 weeks of gestation
    d. Fetal loss rate in CVS and in genetic amniocentesis are nearly the same at present
Ans. c. CVS should not be performed before 10 weeks of gestation (*See* Dutta's Textbook of Obstetrics, 8th Edition, p. 129). d. Canadian multicenter trial study (1991) reports pregnancy loss rates are not different for both the groups.

Q.335 Concerning obstetric hemorrhage all are correct except:
    a. Loss up to 15% of blood volume needs immediate replacement by crystalloid solution
    b. Systemic vascular resistance increases due to sympathoadrenal stimulation

c. Narrowing of the pulse pressure (difference between systolic and diastolic pressure) indicates class II hemorrhage
d. Urine output 1 mL/minute indicates adequate perfusion of vital organs

Ans. a. Class I hemorrhage rarely exhibit any features of volume deficit and it is restored normally by 24–48 hours. In class II, tube pressure is reduced (*See* Dutta's Textbook of Obstetrics, 8th Edition, p. 700).

Q.336 *Regarding fetal hemoglobin (HbF) all are correct except (Fig. 2.2):*
a. O_2 carrying capacity of HbF is high
b. O_2 dissociation curve is shifted to the right
c. Concentration of 2, 3 DPG in HbF is low
d. At term 30% of fetal hemoglobin is HbA

Ans. b. It is shifted to the left due to lower binding of HbF to 2, 3-diphospho-glycerate. (*See* Dutta's Textbook of Obstetrics, 8th Edition, p. 47).

Q.337 *Regarding acid base changes in pregnancy all are correct except:*
a. PaO_2 (arterial) is increased to 106 mm Hg
b. There is maternal respiratory alkalosis
c. Excretion of (HCO_3^-) is reduced by the kidney
d. $PaCO_2$ (arterial) is decreased

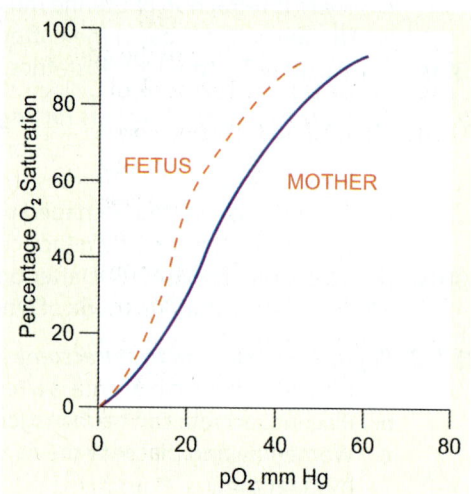

Fig. 2.2: Oxyhemoglobin dissociation curves of maternal and fetal human blood at pH 7.4 and 37°C. Fetal hemoglobin carries more oxygen than adult at any given oxygen tension

Ans. c. Partial renal compensation occurs by increased excretion of bicarbonate. This lowers the plasma HCO_3^- levels to 21 mmol/L and maintains the pH at 7.45. (*See* Dutta's Textbook of Obstetrics, 8th Edition, p. 63).

Q.338 *About the principles of assisted vaginal breech delivery all are correct except:*
a. Never be in a haste
b. Steady pull from below
c. Always keep the back anterior
d. Time interval from delivery of the umbilicus to mouth cavity is 5–10 minutes

Ans. b. Never pull. Encourage the woman to push and the assistant to add fundal pressure. Maternal expulsive efforts are best to maintain flexion and to expedite the delivery. Pull from below and haste to deliver the fetus results in extension of the arms and the head. (*See* Dutta's Textbook of Obstetrics, 8th Edition, p. 441, 442).

Q.339 *Pelvic adequacy is best judged by:*
a. Clinical pelvimetry
b. Erect lateral X-ray pelvimetry
c. Trial of labor
d. Real time ultrasonography

Ans. c. X-ray pelvimetry measures certain pelvic diameters but not the passenger (fetus). Successful birth depends upon the ability of the fetal head to flex, descend and rotate through the bony and soft tissue passage. Therefore, it is true that none of the methods of evaluation (X-ray pelvimetry, clinical pelvimetry, or ultasonography) can reliably predict the pelvic adequacy for final outcome. (*See* Dutta's Textbook of Obstetrics, 8th Edition, p. 406).

Q.340 Regarding shock in obstetrics:
a. Loss of 10% of blood volume causes hypovolemic shock
b. Endotoxic shock is caused by bacterial proteins
c. Tissue hypoxia leads to metabolic alkalosis
d. The circulation of the adrenal gland is not affected unless the shock is severe

Ans. d. See Dutta's Textbook of Obstetrics, 8th Edition, p. 699.

Q.341 Regarding lactation correct statement is:
a. Progesterone promotes growth of ducts rather than alveoli of breast tissue
b. Prolactin causes milk ejection
c. Cry of the baby can initiate let down reflex
d. Pyridoxin therapy enhances milk production

Ans. c. See Dutta's Textbook of Obstetrics, 8th Edition, p. 172.

Q.342 The following hormones are synthesized in the placenta except:
a. Gonadotropin releasing hormone (GnRH)
b. Corticotropin releasing hormone
c. Pregnancy associated plasma protein A (PAPPA)
d. Dehydroepiandrosterone

Ans. d. See Dutta's Textbook of Obstetrics, 8th Edition, p. 66.

Q.343 Regarding placental transfer active transport mechanism is involved in:
a. Oxygen
b. Glucose
c. Histidine
d. Chloride

Ans. c. See Dutta's Textbook of Obstetrics, 8th Edition, p. 40.

Q.344 The following is true about fetal hemoglobin (HbF):
a. HbF is less resistant than HbA to denaturation by acid
b. HbF is less resistant than HbA to denaturation by alkali
c. Consists of 90% of all fetal hemoglobin at 20 weeks of pregnancy
d. Consists of two alpha chains and two delta chains ($\alpha_2\delta_2$)

Ans. c. See Dutta's Textbook of Obstetrics, 8th Edition, p. 47, 371.

Q.345 Natural surfactant contains:
a. Phospholipids 80%
b. Natural lipids 10%
c. Protein 10%
d. All of the above

Ans. d.

Q.346 Fetal lung has got the following proportions of phospholipids except:
a. Phosphatidyl choline 70%
b. Phosphatidyl glycerol 25%
c. Phosphatidyl inositol 2%
d. Phosphatidyl ethanolamine 3%

Ans. b. It is about 5% only.

Q.347 The significant change of pulmonary hemodynamics at birth:
  a. Fall in pulmonary artery mean pressure
  b. Rise in pulmonary blood flow
  c. Drop in pulmonary vascular resistance
  d. All of the above
Ans. d.

Q.348 A forceps rotation of 30° from left occiput anterior (LOA) to occiput anterior (OA) with extraction of the fetus from +2 station is described as which type of forceps delivery:
  a. High forceps
  b. Midforceps
  c. Low forceps
  d. Outlet forceps
Ans. c. See Dutta's Textbook of Obstetrics, 8th Edition, p. 653.

Q.349 Regarding fetal circulation:
  a. Only small amount of blood from right atrium is directed to the left atrium through the foramen ovale
  b. The proximal parts of the umbilical arteries persists as superior vesical arteries
  c. The ductus arteriosus carries blood from pulmonary artery to the ascending aorta
  d. The umbilical vein becomes lateral umbilical ligament after birth
Ans. b. See Dutta's Textbook of Obstetrics, 8th Edition, p. 49. About 75% of blood passes through the foramen ovale from the right to the left atrium. The ductus arteriosus connects the descending aorta. The umbilical vein becomes ligamentum teres.

Q.350 In a normal pregnancy all are correct except:
  a. Serum protein bound iodine (PBI) is increased
  b. Level of aldosterone is increased
  c. There is hyperinsulinism
  d. Levels of all the three estrogens are equally increased
Ans. d. Estriol production surpasses estrone and estradiol.

Q.351 Progesterone:
  a. Placental trophoblast is the only source in pregnancy
  b. Stimulate uterine myometrial activity
  c. Fetal cholesterol is the precursor of synthesis
  d. Excreted mainly as pregnanediol glucuronide in the urine
Ans. d. See Dutta's Textbook of Obstetrics, 8th Edition, p. 69. Progesterone is a steroid hormone, secreted by the luteinized granulosa cells of the corpus luteum. Trophoblasts (in pregnancy) take over progesterone production from corpus luteum of pregnancy (luteal-placental shift) between 7 and 10 weeks. Maternal cholesterol is the major precursor.

Q.352 The anatomical features of a typical female bony pelvis—all are correct except:
  a. The inlet is round in shape
  b. Subpubic angle is wide (85°)
  c. Sacrosciatic notch is deep and narrow
  d. Poses no difficulty for usual mechanism of labor
Ans. c.

Q.353 Regarding amniotic fluid:
   a. Volume increases as the gestational age advances
   b. The fetal contribution is to increase the volume only
   c. Osmolality decreases with advancing gestational age
   d. Level of alpha fetoprotein increases with gestational age

Ans. c. Volume diminishes after 38 weeks, the fetus also decreases the volume by ingestion, and level of α-FP decreases after 14 week.

Q.354 Regarding HIV in pregnancy:
   a. The risk of parent to child transmission is 15–20% in nonbreastfeeding infant
   b. Vertical transmission does not occur when the plasma viral load is less than 500 copies/mL
   c. All newborns of women with HIV should receive antiretroviral therapy for 4–6 months
   d. Viral load in cervicovaginal secretions has been shown to correlate with mother to child transmission

Ans. a and d. (*See* Dutta's Textbook of Obstetrics, 8th Edition, p. 351).

Q.355 All of the following statements related to the management of ruptured tubal ectopic pregnancy are false, except:
   a. Resuscitation should be followed by laparotomy
   b. Blood transfusion is a must prior to laparotomy
   c. Salpingo-oophorectomy is done as a routine
   d. Laparotomy is the preferred surgery compared to laparoscopy

Ans. d. Resuscitation and simultaneous laparotomy should be the principle in acute ectopic pregnancy. Even if blood for transfusion is not available, laparotomy should be done. Salpingectomy is the usual surgery.

SECTION 2

Gynecology

Section Outline

Ch. 3. Objective Structured Clinical Examination (OSCE) in Gynecology
- Case 1: Polycystic Ovarian Syndrome (PCOS)
- Case 2: Endometriosis
- Case 3: Primary Amenorrhea
- Case 4: Secondary Amenorrhea
- Case 5: Pelvic Pain
- Case 6: Infertility
- Case 7: Hematocolpos
- Case 8: Infertility
- Case 9: Hydatidiform Mole
- Case 10: Endometriosis
- Case 11: Cervical Fibroid
- Case 12: Carcinoma Cervix
- Case 13: Carcinoma Endometrium
- Case 14: Carcinoma of the Ovary
- Case 15: Carcinoma Cervix
- Case 16: Menopause and Hormone Replacement Therapy (HRT)
- Case 17: Carcinoma Cervix
- Case 18: Hysterectomy and Oophorectomy
- Case 19: Postmenopausal Bleeding
- Case 20: Inherited Cancers and the Management

Ch. 4. Self-assessment in Gynecology

3 Objective Structured Clinical Examination (OSCE) in Gynecology

CASE 1: POLYCYSTIC OVARIAN SYNDROME (PCOS)

Case Summary

Mrs UC, 30-year-old receptionist, married for 3 years, was seen with the problem of oligomenorrhea-amenorrhea and infertility. She also complained of excess body hair (Fig. 3.1).

Her height was 5'1" and she weighed 80 kg. Her hormone assay done on D-2 of the cycle revealed FSH 5.0 IU/L, LH 13.01 IU/L. Testosterone 3.8 nmol/L prolactin 60 ng/mL; TSH 3.8 mU/L.

Q. What is the likely diagnosis?
Ans. Polycystic ovarian syndrome

Q. What is the current diagnostic criteria for PCOS?
Ans. According to ASRM/ESHRE, 2003 diagnosis of PCOS is based upon the presence of any two of the following three criteria:
1. Oligo and/or anovulation
2. Hyperandrogenism (clinical and/or biochemical)
3. Polycystic ovaries.

Other causes of hyperandrogenic conditions (adrenal) are to be excluded.

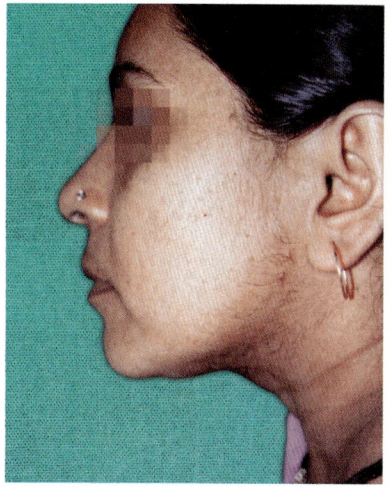

Fig. 3.1: Excess growth of facial (upper lip, cheek, chin and male-pattern beard) hair

Q. What are the symptoms of PCOS?
Ans.
- Obesity
- Infertility
- **Menstrual abnormality:** Oligomenorrhea, amenorrhea, dysfunctional uterine bleeding (DUB)
- Hirsutism
- Characteristic skin changes (acanthosis nigricans)
- Acne
- Hair-AN syndrome (See Dutta's Textbook of Gynecology, 7th Edition, p. 379).

Q. What are the characteristic changes in the ovary of a woman with PCOS? (See Dutta's Textbook of Gynecology, 7th Edition, p. 378).

Ans. Ovaries are enlarged in volume. The capsule is thickened. On cut section multiple (≥ 2) follicular cysts measuring about 2–9 mm in diameter are seen peripherally (Fig. 3.2). There is stromal hyperthecosis. Transvaginal sonography (TVS) can demonstrate the enlarged ovarian volume with peripherally arranged cysts.

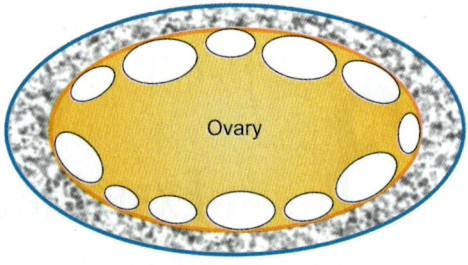

Fig. 3.2: Polycystic ovary

Q. What other investigations would be appropriate for her?

Ans.
- Ultrasound scan (TVS) (Figs 3.3A and B)
- To detect polycystic ovarian changes
- Investigations for other factors for infertility, e.g. tubal patency test and husband's semen analysis.

Q. What is the basic underlying pathology in this condition of PCOS?

Ans. Hyperandrogenic state and chronic anovulation.

Q. What are the biochemical abnormalities seen in a case of PCOS?

Ans.
- Hyperandrogenemia [(↑) testosterone, DHEA, androstenedione)]
- Hyperinsulinemia (insulin resistance)
- Hypersecretion of luteinizing hormone (LH)
- Hyperprolactinemia
- (↑) Serum estrogen
- (↓) Sex hormone-binding globulin (SHBG)
- (↑) Lipids

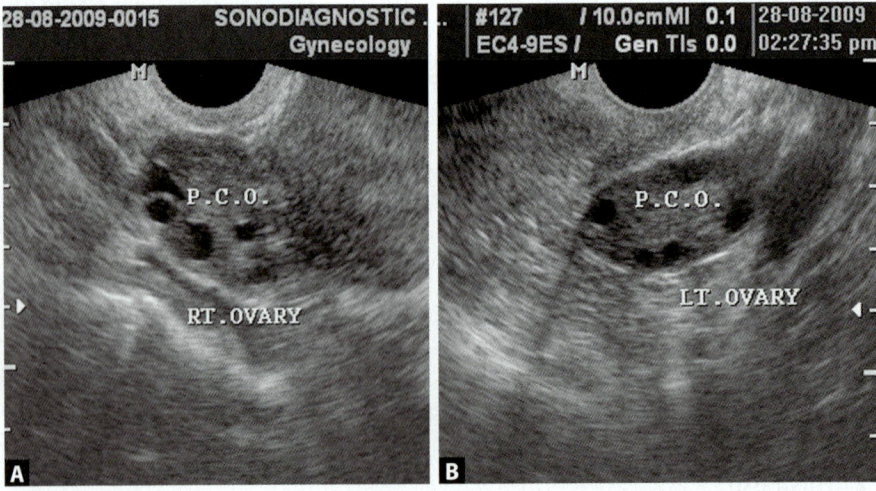

Figs 3.3A and B: **A.** Ultrasonography of the pelvis showing polycystic ovary (right); **B.** Ultrasonography of the same patient showing polycystic ovary (left)

Courtesy: Dr (Mrs) S Ghosh, Prof BN Chakravorty, IRM, Calcutta

Q. How can obesity and hyperinsulinemia cause hyperandrogenism?
Ans.
- **Obesity** → increased insulin resistance and raised insulin level stimulate → ovary (theca cells) → androgens (↑) : **Obesity** → (↓) SHBG → (↑) androgens (free).
- **Hyperinsulinemia** → ovarian theca cells → (↑) androgens: *increased insulin* → (↓) hepatic synthesis of SHBG → more (↑) free androgens.

Q. What are the long-term consequences in a woman suffering from PCOS?
Ans.
- Risk of developing diabetes mellitus due to insulin resistance
- Risk of endometrial carcinoma due to unopposed action of estrogen
- Risk of developing hypertension and cardiovascular disease due to abnormal lipid profile (dyslipidemia).

Q. What is the aim of management of PCOS?
Ans. Aim of treatment is to individualize the patient for her presenting symptoms like infertility, obesity or menstrual abnormality. In obese patients, weight reduction is essential.

Q. How do you treat hyperandrogenemia?
Ans.
- Weight reduction
- GnRH agonists
- Spironolactone
- Combined oral contraceptive pills
- Cyproterone acetate
- Flutamide.

Q. What medical management will improve her fertility status?
Ans. Weight reduction and induction of ovulation. Adjuvant drugs may be needed (e.g. metformin, bromocriptine) depending upon the associated abnormalities.

Q. If the woman is desirous of pregnancy how can you help her?
Ans. Ovulation of induction is to be done as she suffers from chronic anovulation. However, other factors (male factor, tubal patency tests) should be normal.

Q. What drug is commonly used for induction of ovulation?
Ans.
- Clomiphene citrate
- However, clomiphene citrate is to be combined with other drugs when other biochemical abnormalities are associated.
    - Clomiphene citrate + metformin → where there is obesity and hyperinsulinemia.
    - Clomiphene citrate + bromocriptine → where there is associated hyperprolactinemia.

Q. What is the place of insulin sensitizers in the management of women with PCOS desiring for conception?
Ans. Women with PCOS with body mass index more than 25 are often found insulin resistant. Along with weight reduction, treatment with metformin (insulin sensitizer) is found to reduce hyperinsulinemia and hyperandrogenemia. Pioglitazone and rosiglitazone are also being used in cases, resistant to metformin. Metformin is given in a dose 500 mg thrice daily.

Q. What are the different surgical methods?
Ans. Laparoscopic ovarian drilling (LOD) or laser (CO_2) vaporization of the cysts is usually done. LOD reduces systemic and intraovarian androgen levels. The woman ovulates spontaneously following LOD (*See* Dutta's Textbook of Gynecology, 7th Edition, p. 382).

CASE 2: ENDOMETRIOSIS

Case Summary

Mrs PL, 24-year-old lady, married for 1 year, complaining of pelvic pain and deep dyspareunia. She was advised diagnostic laparoscopy which revealed the pathology (Fig. 3.4). She does not wish to become pregnant at present.

Q. What is the likely diagnosis?
Ans. Pelvic endometriosis.

Q. What is endometriosis?
Ans. It is the presence of functioning endometrium (both glands and stroma) in sites other than the uterine mucosa.

Q. What are the common sites of endometriosis?
Ans.
- Ovary
- Uterosacral ligaments
- Rectovaginal septum
- Pouch of Douglas (POD)
- Sigmoid colon
- Abdominal scar.

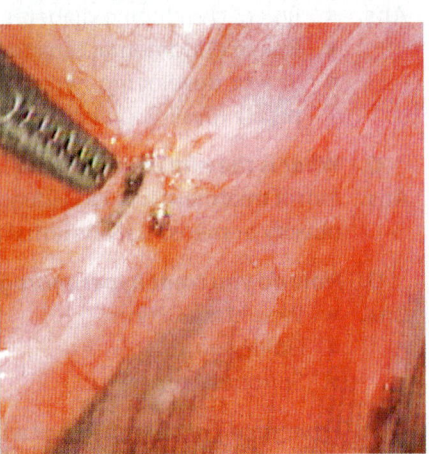

Q. What are the other symptoms?

Fig. 3.4: Pelvic endometriosis

Ans. Abnormal menstruation like menorrhagia, dysmenorrhea (secondary), dyspareunia, pain during defecation, rectal bleeding. She may be asymptomatic.

Q. What is the naked eye appearance of pelvic endometriotic lesions?
Ans. Lesions may appear as:
- Small black dots (powder burns)
- White patches
- Subovarian adhesions
- Ovaries may be involved—chocolate cysts
- White peritoneal areas.
- Red flame shaped areas
- Peritoneal windows
- Puckering of peritoneum

Q. What are the important symptoms of pelvic endometriosis?
Ans.
- Some patients remain asymptomatic (25%)
  - Dysmenorrhea (50%)
  - Abnormal menstruation—menorrhagia, polymenorrhea
  - Infertility (40–60%)
  - Dyspareunia
  - Pelvic pain
  - Abdominal pain
  - Bladder symptoms (dysuria)
  - Bowel symptoms (rectal bleeding)
  - Pain during defecation.

Q. How the diagnosis of pelvic endometriosis is confirmed?
Ans. It is commonly done by diagnostic laparoscopy.

Q. What is the place of serum CA 125 in the diagnosis of pelvic endometriosis?
Ans. Measurement of serum CA 125 levels is not a diagnostic tool because of its low sensitivity (< 50%). It may be used to predict the recurrence of endometriosis after therapy.

Q. What are the causes of infertility in a woman with pelvic endometriosis?
Ans. The possible cause of infertility are:
- **Ovarian dysfunction:** Anovulation, defective folliculogenesis or luteal phase defect
- **Tubal dysfunction:** Pelvic adhesions, causing distorsion of normal tube ovary relationship
- **Others:** Abnormal peritoneal fluid, implantation failure, miscarriage.

Q. What are the endocrine abnormalities associated with endometriosis?
Ans.
- Corpus luteum insufficiency
- Raised prolactin level
- Luteolysis due to increased PGF2α.

Q. What associated condition such a patient may present with?
Ans. Infertility.

Q. What are the complications of endometriosis?
Ans.
- Leakage or rupture of chocolate cyst
- Infection of chocolate cyst
- Infertility
- Obstructive features (ureteral obstruction).

Q. What are the different modalities of therapy for pelvic endometriosis?
Ans.
- Expectant
- Surgery
- Combined surgical and medical
- Medical NSAIDs: Hormonal
- Conservative
- Definitive
- Assisted reproduction (See Manual of Obstetrics and Gynecology for the Postgraduates, p. 388).

Q. What are the factors that determine the type of treatment to a particular woman?
Ans. To an individual woman the determining factors are:
- Age of the woman
- Size and extent of lesion
- Severity of symptoms
- Desire for a child
- Stage of the disease [American Fertility Society (AFS) scoring system—See Dutta's Textbook of Gynecology, 7th Edition, p. 253]
- Results of previous therapy.

Q. What are the different hormones that can be used for the treatment of pelvic endometriosis?
Ans.
- Combine oral contraceptives (COCs) (See Dutta's Textbook of Gynecology, 7th Edition, p. 399)
  - Progestogens
    - Oral:
      - Medroxyprogesterone acetate
      - Dydrogesterone
      - Dienogest

- ♦ Parenteral (IM): Medroxyprogesterone
- ♦ Intrauterine contraceptive device (IUCD): Levonorgestrel intrauterine system (LNG-IUS) (*See* Dutta's Textbook of Gynecology, 7th Edition, p. 392)
- Danazol
- Gestrinone
- GnRH analogs.

Q. What are the important side effects of danazol and GnRH analogs?
Ans.
- **Danazol:** It causes symptoms due to pseudomenopause and it is less tolerated.
- **GnRH analogs:** It works by creating medical oophorectomy compared to danazol, GnRH analogs are well-tolerated.

Q. What are the indications of surgery for pelvic endometriosis?
Ans.
- Symptomatic endometriosis which is not responsive to hormone therapy (*See* Dutta's Textbook of Gynecology, 7th Edition, p. 255).
- Severe endometriosis—to correct the distortion of pelvic anatomy or for improvement of symptoms.
- Chocolate cyst ≥ 4 cm needs ovarian cystectomy and adhesiolysis.

Q. What are the different types of surgery that can be done?
Ans. Either by laparotomy or laparoscopy.

Q. What is meant by conservative surgery?
Ans. Preservation of the reproductive organs and restoration of their anatomy for enhancement of fertility (function).

Q. What is meant by expectant treatment?
Ans. Expectant treatment means doing nothing actively. The woman is kept under observation.

Q. What is the place of expectant treatment?
Ans. Role of any treatment for minimal to mild endometriosis is controversial. Cumulative pregnancy rate is similar following expectant treatment and that after conservative surgery.

Q. Who are the cases for expectant treatment?
Ans. Minimal endometriosis when observed in
- Unmarried women
- Young married woman who is desirous of a baby
- Women approaching menopause.

Q. What type of laparoscopic surgery is commonly done?
Ans. Destruction of endometriotic implants over the peritoneal surface is commonly done. It is done by diathermy or by laser vaporization. Ovarian endometrioma (chocolate cyst) can be resected laparoscopically. Laparoscopic uterosacral nerve ablation (LUNA) is done when pain is very severe.
Division of adhesions (adhesiolysis) can also be done by laparoscopy.

Q. What are the treatment options for this woman (*See* Dutta's Textbook of Gynecology, 7th Edition, p. 253)?
Ans. **Combined oral contraceptive pill** for a period of 6–9 months would be most appropriate for her. Continuous therapy without the usual 7 days break would make her amenorrheic.

This will help regression of the endometriotic deposits. This will also improve her symptoms. At the same time contraception is also provided.

Other options depending on the severity of endometriosis would be:
- **Medical therapy:** Continuous progestogen, danazol or GnRH analogs.
- **Surgical therapy:** Laparoscopic laser or electrodiathermy to ablate the endometriotic implants.

Q. What would be the appropriate management when she desires to conceive?

Ans. Pregnancy itself provides remission to the problem. For this case, following the initial treatment, expectant management would be appropriate for next 6 months. About 60–70% women will become pregnant within a year provided there is no other factor for infertility.

Q. What is the optimum treatment for scar endometriosis?

Ans. Treatment is done by excision. Hormone therapy is ineffective.

Q. What is adenomyosis?

Ans. Adenomyosis is a condition when there is ingrowth of endometrium (both the glands and stroma) directly within the myometrium (*See* Dutta's Textbook of Gynecology, 7th Edition, p. 256).

Q. How does a woman with adenomyosis present?

Ans. Usually the woman is parous, with age above 40 years.

Common symptoms are:
- Menorrhagia
- Dysmenorrhea.

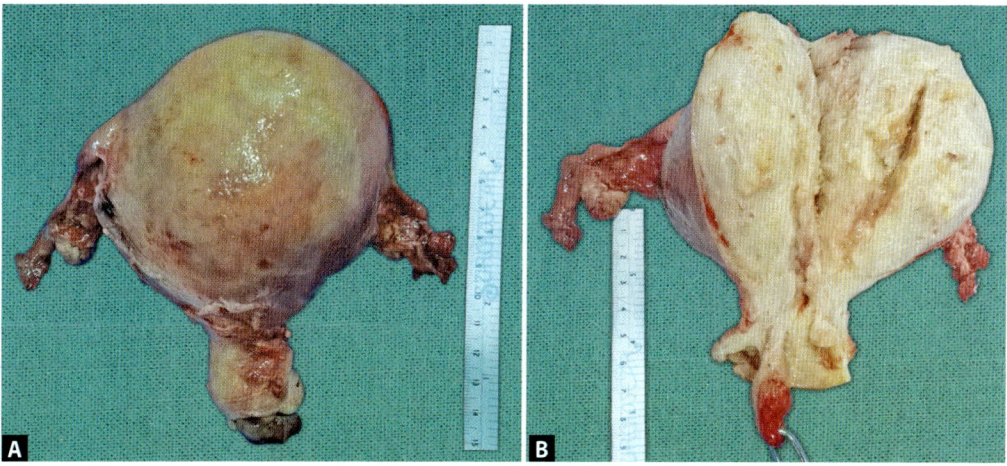

Figs 3.5A and B: **A.** Postoperative specimen of a uterus with tubes and ovaries. Mrs SE, a 46-year-old, parous lady, was admitted for menorrhagia and intractable dysmenorrhea. She did not respond to any medical therapy. She was investigated. She underwent hysterectomy and bilateral salpingo-oophorectomy. The uterus is seen uniformly enlarged; **B.** The specimen of the same patient is cut opened to show myohyperplasia with hemorrhagic spots within the myometrium

Q. How can you differentiate a fibroid uterus from an adenomyosis?
Ans. *See* Dutta's Textbook of Gynecology, 7th Edition, p. 552.

Q. What should be the treatment of adenomyosis in a parous and elderly woman?
Ans.
- Treatment of adenomyosis (Figs 3.5A and B) is predominantly surgical
- Medical management (hormones) is often ineffective
- Conservative surgery includes partial resection of adenomyomata
- Total hysterectomy with or without bilateral salpingo-oophorectomy is the optimum treatment for a woman who is parous and aged.
- Currently, LNG-IUD is being used and found to be effective in improving the symptoms of menorrhagia and pelvic pain.

CASE 3: PRIMARY AMENORRHEA

Case Summary

A 18-year-old school girl has been seen in the gyne clinic due to failure to commence menstruation. Secondary sex characters were well-developed. On systemic examination there was no abnormality. Pelvic examination revealed as shown in the Figure 3.6.

Q. What is most likely the diagnosis?
Ans. A case of vaginal agenesis.

Q. How do you define primary amenorrhea?
Ans. A young girl who has not menstruated by 16 years of age is defined as primary amenorrhea.

Q. When do you start investigations for primary amenorrhea?
Ans.
- No menstruation by the age of 16 years, when other secondary sex characters are normal.
- No menstruation by the age of 14 years when there is absence of growth and/or development of secondary sex characters.

Q. What are the factors essential for the onset and continuation of normal menstruation?
Ans.
- Normal female chromosomal pattern (46XX)
- Coordinated function of the hypothalamopituitary ovarian axis
- Anatomical presence and patency of the outflow tract
- Responsive endometrium
- Active support of thyroid and adrenal gland.

Q. What is cryptomenorrhea?
Ans. It is a condition where the menstrual blood fails to come out from the genital tract due to an obstruction present in the passage.

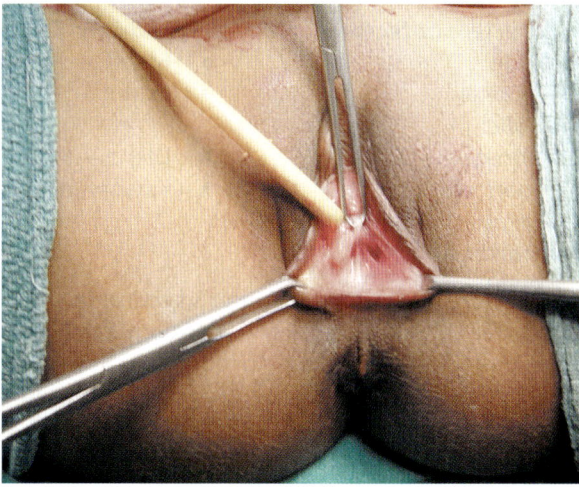

Fig. 3.6: Complete absence of vagina

Q. What are the common causes of cryptomenorrhea?
Ans.
- **Congenital**
  - Imperforate hymen
  - Transverse vaginal septum.
- **Acquired**
  - Cervical stenosis following amputation
  - Vaginal stricture following traumatic (instrumental delivery).

Q. What are the common causes of primary amenorrhea?
Ans.
- **Hypogonadotrophic hypogonadism**
  - Delayed puberty
  - Hypothalamic and pituitary dysfunction (stress, weight loss, anorexia nervosa)
  - Kallmann syndrome
  - CNS tumors—craniopharyngioma.
- **Hypergonadotrophic hypogonadism**
  - Primary ovarian failure
  - Galactosemia.
- **Abnormal chromosomal pattern**
  - Turner's syndrome (45X)
  - Various mosaic states (45X/46XX)
  - Testicular feminization (46XY).
- **Developmental defect of genital tract**
  - Müllerian agenesis (MRKH syndrome)
  - Imperforate hymen
  - Transverse vaginal septum
  - Vaginal agenesis (Fig. 3.6).
- **Thyroid and adrenal disorders**
- **Metabolic disorders (juvenile diabetes)**
- **Systemic illness (tuberculosis)**
- **Others:** Uterine synechiae, unresponsive endometrium (receptor defect).

Q. What are the characteristic features of Mayer-Rokitansky-Kuster-Hauser syndrome?
Ans.
- Stature—average
- Sexual hair—normal
- Breasts—normal
- External genitalia—normal
- **Internal genitalia:**
  - Vagina—absent
  - Ovaries—normal
  - Uterus—absent/rudimentary
  - Karyotype—normal (46XX)
  - IVP—Urinary tract abnormalities (30%)
- Primary amenorrhea.

Q. What are the characteristic features of Turner's syndrome?
Ans.
- Stature—short (*See* Dutta's Textbook of Gynecology, 7th Edition, p. 363, 367, 368).
- Secondary sex character—poorly developed
- Webbing of the neck
- Shield chest
- Wide apart nipples
- Cubitus valgus
- Coarctation of aorta

- 'Streak' gonads
- Serum gonadotrophins—high
- Karyotype: 45XO or 45XO/46XX (Fig. 3.7)
- Primary amenorrhea.

Q. What are the characteristic features of androgen insensitivity syndrome [testicular feminization syndrome (Fig. 3.8)]?

Ans.
- Stature—average (*See* Dutta's Textbook of Gynecology, 7th Edition, p. 364, 367, 368)
- Scanty pubic and axillary hair
- Breast development—normal
- Vagina—short and blind
- Uterus and tubes—absent
- Gonads—at labia or intra-abdominal or at inguinal region
- Gonadal biopsy—testicular tissue
- Serum testosterone—equal to normal males
- Karyotype: 46XY
- Primary amenorrhea.

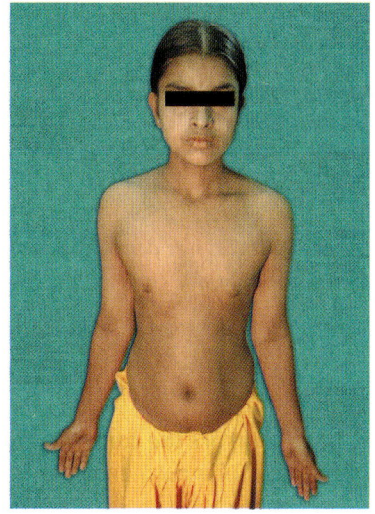

Fig. 3.7: A 19-year-old girl with features of Turner's syndrome. Karyotype: 45XO

Q. What are the characteristic features of adrenogenital syndrome? (See Dutta's Textbook of Gynecology, 7th Edition, p. 362, 366, 367) (Fig. 3.9).

Ans.
- Stature: Average
- Labial fusion
- Uterus: Normal
- Vagina: Normal
- Serum 17-OHP: Elevated
- Primary amenorrhea.
- Phenotypically: Normal female
- Enlargement of clitoris
- Ovaries: Normal
- Karyotype: 46XX
- Urinary pregnanetriol: Elevated

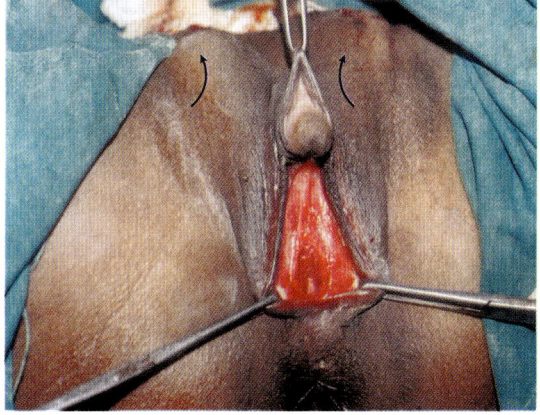

Fig. 3.8: Testicular feminization syndrome showing short and blind vagina, scanty pubic hair, clitoromegaly and labial gonads (arrows)

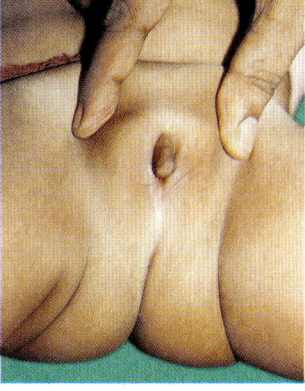

Fig. 3.9: A 14-month-old girl with adrenogenital syndrome showing labial fusion and enlarged clitoris. Congenital adrenal hyperplasia is commonly due to 21-hydroxylase deficiency

CASE 4: SECONDARY AMENORRHEA

Case Summary

Mrs JL, 42-year-old woman, was seen in the gyne clinic with the problem of cessation of menstruation for the last 7 months. Her urine test for pregnancy was negative.

Q. What is her present problem?
Ans. Secondary amenorrhea.

Q. How do you define secondary amenorrhea?
Ans. It is the absence of menstruation for 6 months or more in a woman who has menstruated normally in the past.

Q. What are the common 'uterine factors' that may cause secondary amenorrhea?
Ans.
- Tubercular endometritis
- Synechiae
- Surgical removal (hysterectomy)
- Transcervical resection of endometrium (TCRE).

Q. What are the 'ovarian factors' that may cause secondary amenorrhea?
Ans.
- Polycystic ovarian syndrome
- Surgical removal
- Premature ovarian failure
- Radiation

Q. What are the common 'hypothalamic factors' that may cause secondary amenorrhea?
Ans.
- Stress
- Strenuous exercise
- Infection (tuberculosis)
- Tumors (craniopharyngioma, meningioma).
- Anorexia nervosa
- Trauma
- Psychogenic drugs (phenothiazine)

Q. What are the common causes of secondary amenorrhea?
Ans. See Dutta's Textbook of Gynecology, 7th Edition, p. 378.
- Stress
- Premature ovarian failure
- Drugs (phenothiazine)
- PCOS
- Synechiae (Asherman's syndrome)
- Postpill amenorrhea.

Q. What is PCOS?
Ans. See Dutta's Textbook of Gynecology, 7th Edition, p. 378.

CASE 5: PELVIC PAIN

Case Summary

Mrs CM, 36-year-old lady, had been suffering from lower abdominal pain and severe deep dyspareunia for last 8 months.

Q. What are the common causes of acute pelvic pain in gynecology?
Ans.
- Acute pelvic inflammatory disease (PID)
- Twisted ovarian cyst
- Disturbed tubal ectopic pregnancy
- Ruptured chocolate cyst
- Ruptured corpus luteum cyst
- Ovarian hyperstimulation syndrome.

Q. What are the common causes of chronic pelvic pain?
Ans.
- Dysmenorrhea
- Ovarian remnant syndrome—trapped or residual ovarian syndrome
- Pelvic endometriosis
- Uterine fibroid
- Ovarian cyst
- Premenstrual tension syndrome
- Adenomyosis
- PID (chronic)
- Retroversion or prolapse of the uterus

Q. What are the causes of dyspareunia?
Ans. Superficial
- Narrow introitus
- Tough hymen
- Tender perineal scar
- Vulval infection
- Vulvar vestibulitis syndrome
- Vaginal—septum, infection, agenesis.

Deep
- Pelvic endometriosis
- Chronic PID
- Prolapsed ovary in the polycystic ovarian disease (POD).

Q. Mention some of the important causes of postmenopausal bleeding? (See Dutta's Textbook of Gynecology, 7th Edition, p. 462).
Ans.
- Senile endometritis
- Senile vaginitis
- Dysfunctional uterine bleeding
- Decubitus ulcer
- Genital malignancy:
  - Carcinoma of the cervix, endometrium, vagina, vulva, fallopian tube
  - Uterine sarcoma.
- Retained foreign body—pessary, IUCD (Fig. 3.10)
- Urethral caruncle
- Withdrawal bleeding following estrogen intake.

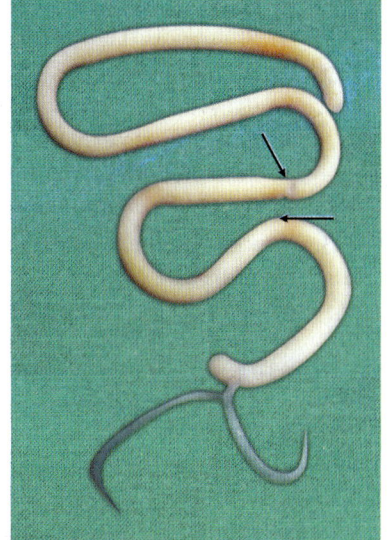

Fig. 3.10: Lippes loop. This has been removed from a 65-year-old lady hysteroscopically. She presented with postmenopausal bleeding. She had this at her age of 27 years. It was embeded within the endometrium and became brittle (arrows)

CASE 6: INFERTILITY

> **Case Summary**
> A 28-year-old woman has been seen for her problem of primary infertility. Her husband's semen analysis was normal. On further investigation she was found to suffer from anovulation. Her tubes were patent.

Q. According to WHO, how the ovulatory disorders are classified?
Ans. **Group I:** Hypothalamic-pituitary failure (hypogonadotrophic hypogonadism)
Group II: Hypothalamic pituitary dysfunction (normogonadotrophic normogonadism)
Group III: Ovarian failure (hypergonadotrophic hypogonadism).

Q. How the problems of anovulatory infertility is treated?
Ans. Induction of ovulation is done. Different drugs are used depending upon the response. Clomiphene citrate is the commonly used drug. It is usually prescribed 50 mg twice daily from D-3 to D-7 (5 days) of the cycle. Ovulation usually occurs 5–7 days after the last day of therapy. For details (See Dutta's Textbook of Gynecology, 7th Edition, p. 199 and Table. 17.8).

Q. What are the indications of gonadotrophin therapy for induction of ovulation?
Ans. Women with infertility due to:
- Hypogonadotrophic hypogonadism (WHO group-I)
- Women who have either failed or are resistant to clomiphene citrate (WHO group II)
- Women with unexplained infertility.

Q. When are GnRH analogs used for induction of ovulation?
Ans.
- Patients who are refractory to gonadotrophins
- Patients with elevated LH
- Patients with premature ovulation due to premature LH surge
- Patients with premature follicular luteinization.

Q. How do you manage the woman with WHO groups I, II or III ovulatory disorders?
Ans. **WHO group I**
- Gonadotropins: Follicle-stimulating hormone (FSH), LH.
- GnRH (pulsatile).

WHO group II
- Clomiphene citrate
- FSH
- For premature LH surges—GnRH agonist/antagonist
- For insulin resistance—insulin sensitizer
- Adrenal androgens—glucocorticoids.

WHO group III
- Cyclic hormone replacement therapy
- Gonadotrophins—high dose (See Dutta's Textbook of Gynecology, 7th Edition, p. 234)
- Chance of spontaneous pregnancy—occasional
- Assisted reproductive technology (ART) (See Manual of Obstetrics and Gynecology for the Postgraduates, p. 388)
- Oocyte donation.

Q. What are the different types of surgery done for the management of infertility?
Ans. Surgery may be needed both for female as well as male factors for infertility.
For female
- Laparoscopic ovarian diathermy (drilling) (LOD).
- Wedge resection of ovary in cases with PCOS (not commonly done).
- Surgery for pituitary prolactinomas (*See* Dutta's Textbook of Gynecology, 7th Edition, p. 201).
- Salpingo-ovariolysis—laparoscopically
- Proximal tubal block: Cannulation and balloon tuboplasty: This is done under hysteroscopic guidance
- Midtubal block: Recanalization procedure (reversal of tubal ligation)
- Distal tubal block:
    - Fimbrioplasty
    - Neosalpingostomy
- Tubal reconstruction (tuboplasty) following sterilization operation.

Q. What is assisted reproductive technology (ART)? What are the different methods of ART?
Ans. ART encompasses all procedures that involve manipulation of gametes and embryos for the treatment of infertility. For the rest (*See* Manual of Obstetrics and Gynecology for the Postgraduates, p. 388).

Q. What are the indications of in vitro fertilization-embryo transfer (IVF-ET)?
Ans.
- Tubal disease
- Endometriosis
- Cervical hostility
- Unexplained infertility
- Male factor infertility
- Failed ovulation induction

Q. What are the indications of intrauterine insemination (IUI)?
Ans.
- Cervical stenosis
- Immunological factors for infertility (male and female)
- Oligospermia or asthenospermia
- Unexplained infertility.

Q. What are the principle steps of an ART cycle?
Ans.
- Down regulation using GnRH analog
- Controlled ovarian stimulation (COS)
- Monitoring of follicular growth
- Oocyte retrieval
- Fertilization *in vitro* [IVF, intracytoplasmic sperm injection (ICSI)]
- Transfer of gametes or embryos
- Luteal support with progesterone.

Q. How is the monitoring of follicular growth done?
Ans. It is done by
- Sonographic (TVS) measurement of follicular diameter
- Serum estradiol level 3 or more follicles more than 18 mm in diameter and serum E_2 levels: 100–150 pg/mL/follicle is optimum. Injection hCG 5000–10,000 IU is given IM. Oocytes are retrieved 36 hours after hCG administration.

Q. What is the procedure for embryo transfer?
Ans. Transfer is done at 4–8 cell stage (48–72 hours later) transcervically. Usually two embryos are transferred.

Q. What is ovarian hyperstimulation syndrome (OHSS)?
Ans. It is characterized by multiple follicular development and ovarian enlargement following hCG stimulation. It may be a serious complication.

It is clinically manifested by bilateral ovarian enlargement, abdominal pain, nausea, vomiting, ascites, hypotension, hemoconcentration, oliguria, disseminated intravascular coagulation (DIC), thrombosis and sometimes adult respiratory distress syndrome.

Q. How can OHSS be prevented and managed?
Ans. See Dutta's Textbook of Gynecology, 7th Edition, p. 437.

Q. How endometrial receptivity could be improved in an IVF cycle?
Ans. Exact understanding of endometrial receptivity is lacking. Importance of many adhesion molecules (integrins) have been considered. However supplemental progesterone therapy is started after oocyte retrieval in all IVF programs as a routine. This is mainly because GnRH analog use and oocyte aspiration impair the secretion of endogenous progesterone from the ovary (corpus luteum).

Q. How is egg retrieval done in an IVF cycle?
Ans. Ultrasound-guided needle aspiration of oocyte through the vagina is done. This is done under IV sedation. The complications may be injury to bowel, bladder or infection.

Q. How can a man without any sperm to ejaculate, father children?
Ans. ICSI is the optimum procedure for this man, if he can produce sperm on testicular biopsy. ICSI is also helpful to men with congenital absence of vas deferens (See Dutta's Textbook of Gynecology, 7th Edition, p. 206).

Q. Should a woman with hydrosalpinx be considered for IVF-ET?
Ans. IVF is considered to bypass the function of the blocked tubes. But presence of hydrosalpinges causes implantation failure with reduced pregnancy rate in IVF cycles. So, it is recommended to remove the tubes (prophylactic salpingectomy) prior to IVF in these women.

CASE 7: HEMATOCOLPOS

Case Summary

Miss LN, 17-year-old young girl, presented in the outpatient clinic with cyclical lower abdominal pain. She had normal physical growth and development of secondary sexual characters. Pelvic examination revealed as shown in the Figure 3.11.

Q. What is the diagnosis?
Ans. Imperforate hymen with hematocolpos.

Q. What other symptoms she might have?
Ans. Urinary retention, dysuria, lower abdominal heaviness.

Q. What investigation you may do for her?
Ans. Ultrasonography of the lower abdomen to ascertain the extent of pathology, e.g. hematocolpos, hematometra.

Q. What would be the appropriate treatment for her?
Ans. Incision (cruciate) and drainage under general anesthesia, antibiotic coverage.

Q. What is the prospect of her future reproductive career?
Ans. Normal.

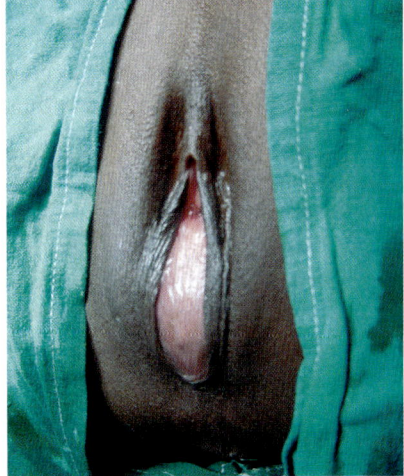

Fig. 3.11: Hematocolpos showing the hymen tense, bluish and bulged

Q. What is the basic underlying abnormality of this condition?
Ans. It is due to failure of disintegration of the central cells of the Müllerian eminence that projects into the urogenital sinus. Depending upon the amount of blood so collected, it may present with hematocolpos (blood in the vagina), hematometra (blood in the uterus) or hematosalpinx (blood within the fallopian tubes).

CASE 8: INFERTILITY

Case Summary

Mrs ZR 26-year-old, $P_{0+0+1+0}$ women presented in the clinic with problems of inability to conceive. Hormone study revealed that she is ovulating and the report of her husband's semen analysis (done recently) was normal. She had an investigation as shown in the Figure 3.12.

Q. What is this investigation?
Ans. Hysterosalpingography.

Q. What is the pathology revealed by the procedure?
Ans. Bilateral hydrosalpinx without any spillage of dye.

Q. What is the basic pathology for this abnormality?
Ans. In majority, it is the sequelae of ascending infection from the lower genital tract. *Chlamydia trachomatis* (85%), *N. gonorrhoeae* and other pyogenic infections (*E. coli*) are responsible. Mixed infections (aerobic and anaerobic) are more common. Infection and inflammation cause destruction of tubal epithelium and pus formation known as **pyosalpinx**. There is peritubal adhesion formation and agglutination of the fimbriae. Gradually when the inflammation subsides, the pus settles down and the tube is filled with a clear fluid called **hydrosalpinx**. The tube is dilated, retort-shaped with closed abdominal ostium.

Q. Is there any other method of evaluation?
Ans. Diagnostic laparoscopy and chromopertubation under general anesthesia. It may reveal tubal edema, hyperemia, dilated tubes (hydrosalpinx), fimbrial adhesion and/or peritubal adhesions.

Q. What are the treatment options that may resolve her problem of infertility?
Ans. Tubal reconstructive surgery (tuboplasty) may be attempted. This may be in the form of releasing the peritubal adhesions (adhesiolysis) and/or opening up the fimbrial end

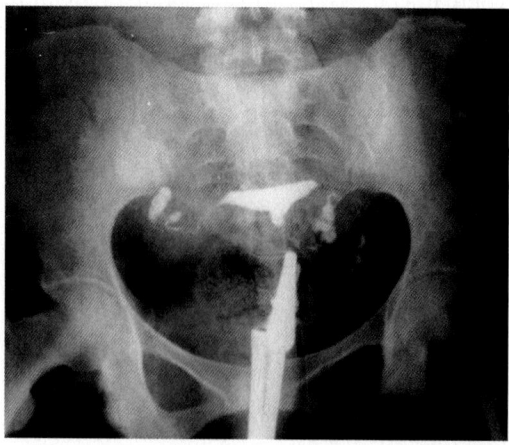

Fig. 3.12: Hysterosalpingogram showing bilateral hydrosalpinx without any spillage of dye

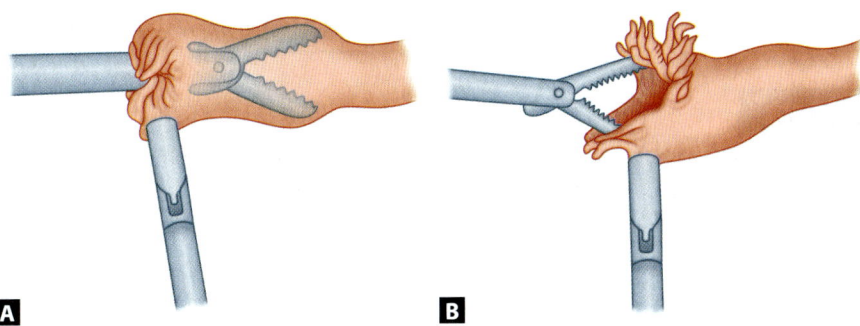

Figs 3.13A and B: A. Laparoscopic fimbrioplasty by introducing the closed forceps within the closed ostium; **B.** The phimotic ostium is opened up and the fimbrial folds are released by opening up the forceps blades

(fimbrioplasty or salpingostomy). As the tubal epithelium is often destroyed, the results of such operations are not always successful. Pregnancy rate following laparoscopic fimbrioplasty is 30–35%. Ectopic pregnancy rate is 5–10% (Figs 3.13A and B).

Q. What other options are left to her?
Ans. Assisted reproduction—IVF-ET.

Q. What are the different methods of assisted reproductive technology that you know? (See Dutta's Textbook of Gynecology, 7th Edition, p. 204)
Ans.

> **IVF–ET:** *In vitro* fertilization and embryo transfer
> **GIFT:** Gamete intrafallopian transfer
> **ICSI:** Intracytoplasmic sperm injection
> **TESE:** Testicular sperm extraction
> **MESA:** Microsurgical epididymal sperm aspiration
> **PESA:** Percutaneous epididymal sperm aspiration

CASE 9: HYDATIDIFORM MOLE

Case Summary

Mrs AL, 24-year-old lady, was admitted in her first pregnancy at 16 weeks of amenorrhea with vaginal bleeding and passage of grape-like structures (See Dutta's Textbook of Obstetrics, 8th Edition, p. 190). On examination she looked pale, uterus was found 20 weeks size. There was no FHS on auscultation.

Q. What is the provisional diagnosis?
Ans. Hydatidiform mole.

Q. What investigations should be done for her?
Ans. Ultrasonography of the uterus (Fig. 3.14) and urine or serum for β-hCG. Once the diagnosis is confirmed, other investigations are complete hemogram, ABO and Rh-grouping, LFT and X-ray chest and thyroid profile.

Q. What is the initial management for this problem?
Ans.
- Correction of anemia with blood transfusion
- To prevent infection
- Suction and evacuation of the uterus with or without oxytocin drip should be done. Tissue should be sent for histological examination.

Q. What are the common complications of this problem?
Ans.
- Hemorrhage
- Infection
- Pre-eclampsia
- Perforation of the uterus
- Respiratory distress due to pulmonary embolization of trophoblastic cells
- Coagulation failure
- Development of choriocarcinoma (2–10% cases).

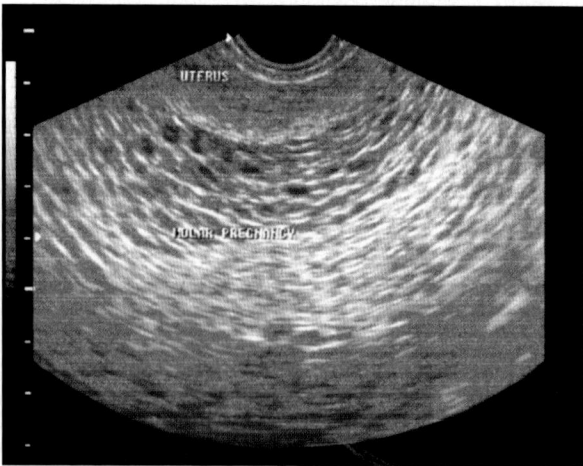

Fig. 3.14: Ultrasonography—snowstorm appearance in hydatidiform mole
Courtesy: Dr (Mrs) S Ghosh, Prof BN Chakravorty, IRM Calcutta

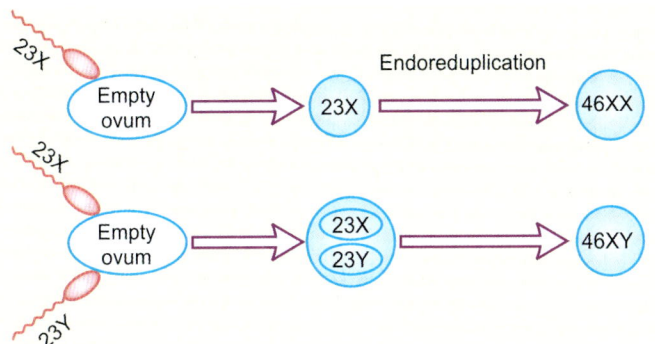

Fig. 3.15: Karyotype pattern of a complete mole—genome is entirely paternal in origin

Q. How should this patient be followed up and for how long?
Ans. Serial urinary β-hCG estimation weekly till negative. Usually, it becomes negative by 4–6 weeks time. Once negative, she is followed up at every month with serum hCG report for 6 months to 1 year.

Q. What precautionary measures she should be advised while on follow-up?
Ans. She should avoid pregnancy for at least 6 months to 1 year. For contraception, she can use barrier methods. Combined oral pills (low dose) may be used following normalization of β-hCG.

Q. What are the reasons that the patient needs to be followed up following initial treatment?
Ans.
- Detection of cases with persistent trophoblastic disease
- Early detection of choriocarcinoma.

Q. What is her prospect of future pregnancy and chance of recurrence of the problem?
Ans. Prospect of future successful pregnancy is high, provided she is followed up. The risk of recurrence is less than 5%.

Q. What is the karyotype pattern of a complete hydatidiform mole and that of a partial mole?
Ans. In complete moles—karyotype pattern in majority is normal—46XX (90%). There is fertilization of 'an empty ovum' by a single sperm carrying 23 chromosomes. The usual 46XX chromosome pattern is the result of doubling of the paternal set of chromosomes (Fig. 3.15).

In about 10% cases, an empty ovum is fertilized by two sperm (dispermy), one carrying X and the other carrying Y chromosome. The chromosomal pattern is 46XY. All the chromosomes are derived paternally.

Partial moles (Fig. 3.16) consist of both the placenta and the fetus. Partial moles usually

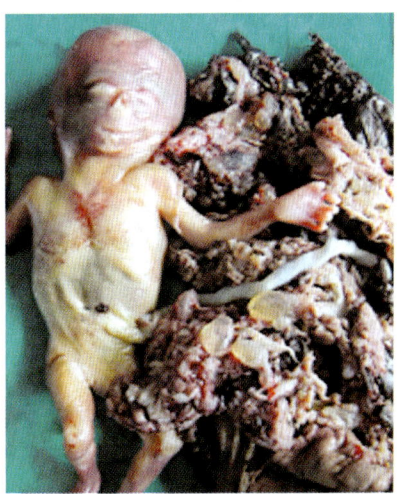

Fig. 3.16: Partial mole with a stillborn baby
Courtesy: Dr S Mitra, Prof, Dept of G and O, MMCH, Midnapore, West Bengal

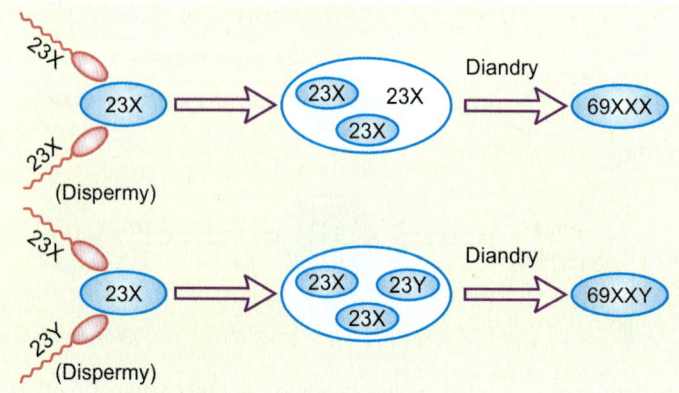

Fig. 3.17: Triploid chromosomal pattern of a partial mole. Genome is both paternal and maternal in origin

(90%) have triploid karyotype (Fig. 3.17). A normal ovum is fertilized by double sperm (dispermy), resulting in 69 chromosomes with sex chromosome configuration of 69XXX, 69XXY and 69XYY. The extra haploid set of chromosomes usually is derived from the father. The fetus is usually triploid, dies in the first trimester or is growth retarded with multiple malformations (syndactyly, hydrocephaly) (*See* Dutta's Textbook of Obstetrics, 8th Edition, p. 230).

CASE 10: ENDOMETRIOSIS

Case Summary

Mrs BK, 24-year-old, married lady has been examined in the outpatient clinic for her pelvic pain which gets worse during menstruation.

Q. What more relevant questions you will ask her to make the provisional diagnosis?

Ans. Regarding the pain, e.g. character of pain, duration, exact relationship with the period, deep dyspareunia and fertility status.

Q. What clinical signs will help you to make the differential diagnosis?

Ans. Pelvic tenderness, nodularity in the pouch of Douglas, fixed retroversion of the uterus, adnexal mass, tenderness and bulky uterus. The differential diagnosis includes pelvic endometriosis, adenomyosis, chronic pelvic inflammatory disease.

Q. To confirm the diagnosis what single investigation would be most valuable?

Ans.
- Diagnostic laparoscopy by double puncture procedure.
- Laparoscopy revealed the diagnosis (Fig. 3.18).

Q. Is this pathology going to affect her future fertility?

Ans. There is an association of pelvic endometriosis and infertility. Amongst the infertile patients, 15% suffer from endometriosis. Whereas patients with endometriosis suffer from infertility in 40–60% cases. The possible explanations are—anovulation, luteal phase defect, luteinized unruptured follicle syndrome, pelvic adhesions, dyspareunia, increased macrophage activity, altered prostaglandin balance and altered immune response.

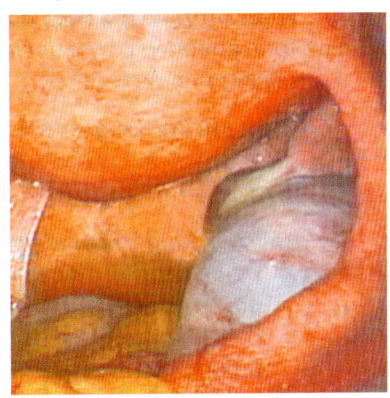

Fig. 3.18: Chocolate cyst of the right ovary

Q. Should a patient with mild endometriosis be treated?

Ans. There is no advantage of any therapy over expectant management in cases with minimal or mild endometriosis. The association of infertility and endometriosis is not absolute unless there is tubal obstruction or extensive pelvic adhesions.

Q. What would be the appropriate treatment for this patient?

Ans. The content of chocolate cysts can be drained and the cavity is to be lavaged with normal saline. The lining of the cyst wall is then separated from the ovarian tissue. This may be done either by laparoscopy or by laparotomy. The principle of surgery is similar to ovarian cystectomy. Bleeding points are electrocoagulated by bipolar diathermy. In a small size chocolate cyst, the contents are aspirated and the cavity is irrigated repeatedly. This may be done under TVS guidance or laparoscopically under anesthesia.

Q. What is the overall result of laparoscopic cystectomy for endometrioma?

Ans. It is effective in relieving pain in about 74% of cases of mild to moderate disease. Pregnancy rate is about 60% in cases with moderate disease. However, improved pregnancy rate is observed within the first 6 months of conservative surgery.

CASE 11: CERVICAL FIBROID

Case Summary

Mrs CR, 40-year-old, had undergone surgery to remove her pathology. The specimen is seen in the Figure 3.19.

Q. What is the diagnosis?
Ans. Posterior cervical fibroid.

Q. With what signs and symptoms she may have presented?
Ans. Vaginal discharge, pressure symptoms:
- **Bowel:** Constipation, incomplete evacuation.
- **Urinary:** Frequency, retention.
- Lateral pelvic wall pressure to cause leg pain or edema.

Q. What surgery had been done for her?
Ans. Total abdominal hysterectomy with bilateral salpingo-oophorectomy.

Q. What are the dangers of this operation?
Ans. Hemorrhage, injury to bladder, rectum and the ureter.

Q. How the dangers could be minimized?
Ans.
- Delineation of the course as well as the proximity of the ureters to the fibroid could be done preoperatively by intravenous urography.
- Ureteric catheterization may be done preoperatively as a precautionary measure.
- Enucleation of the myoma first followed by hysterectomy.
- Preoperative GnRH analog therapy for 3 months may facilitate surgery.

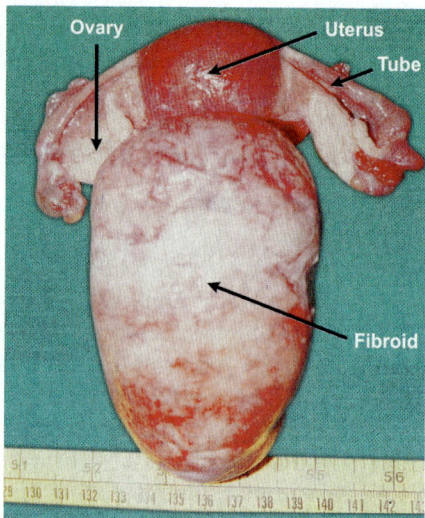

Fig. 3.19: Huge cervical fibroid

CASE 12: CARCINOMA CERVIX

Case Summary

A 47-year-old woman presented with the complaints of postcoital vaginal bleeding and persistent offensive vaginal discharge, pelvic examination revealed an ulcerated tumor arising from the cervix (Fig. 3.20). Biopsy revealed squamous cell carcinoma of the cervix.

Q. Clinically, what are the different types of the lesion?
Ans. (i) Exophytic, (ii) Ulcerative and (iii) Infiltrative.

Q. Histopathologically, what are the different types of carcinoma cervix?
Ans. (i) Squamous cell carcinoma (75–80%), (ii) Adenocarcinoma (20–25%), (iii) Adenosquamous carcinoma, (iv) Neuroendocrine tumors and (v) Others: Lymphomas.

Q. What are the different modes of spread in carcinoma cervix?
Ans.
- Direct extension (parametrium, endocervix, vagina, bladder)
- Lymphatics (pelvic and para-aortic)
- Direct implantation
- Bloodstream (lung, mediastinum, bone, liver).

Q. What are the complications that may arise in a case with carcinoma cervix?
Ans.
- Hemorrhage
- Vesicovaginal fistula
- Uremia
- Pain in the loin due to pyelitis, pyelonephritis
- Rectovaginal fistula
- Sepsis.

Q. What are the advantages of radiotherapy as a primary modality of therapy?
Ans.
- Wider applicability in all stages of carcinoma cervix.
- Survival rate of radiotherapy (85%) is comparable to that of surgery in early stages.
- Less primary mortality or morbidity.

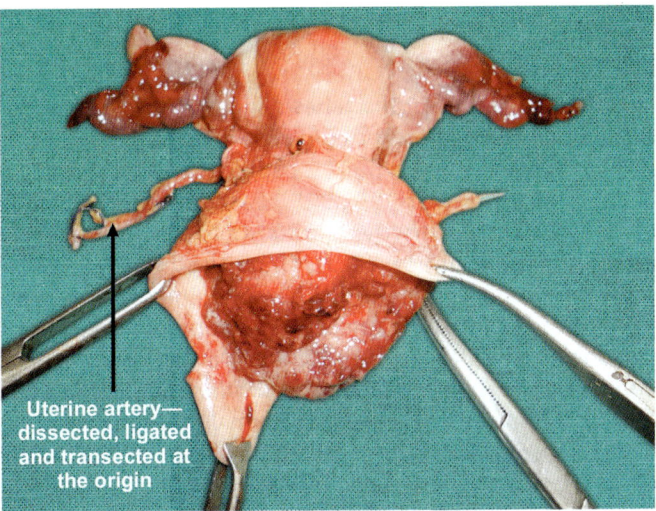

Fig. 3.20: Carcinoma cervix showing an exophytic growth with ulceration

Q. Mention the different types of hysterectomy that can be done for the management of microinvasive and early invasive carcinoma cervix?

Ans. Classification of extended hysterectomy (ACOG–1974).

Rutledge's classification of extended hysterectomy (1974)

Class	Description	Indication
I	Extrafascial hysterectomy; pubocervical ligament is incised, allowing lateral deflection of the ureter	CIN, early stromal invasion
II	Removal of the medial half of the cardinal and uterosacral ligaments; upper third of the vagina	Microcarcinoma post irradiation
III	Removal of the entire cardinal and uterosacral ligaments; upper third of the vagina removed	Stage Ib and stage IIa tumors
IV	Removal of all periureteral tissue, superior vesical artery and three-fourths of the vagina	Anteriorly occurring central recurrences
V	Removal of portions of the distal ureter and bladder	Central recurrent cancer involving bladder and ureter

Q. What are the preventive measures against carcinoma cervix?

Ans. *Primary prevention (See Dutta's Textbook of Gynecology, 7th Edition, p. 268)*
- **Identifying and preventing the high-risk factors:** Preventing human papillomavirus (HPV) infection with HPV vaccine to all school girls (9–15 years).

Other risk factors (cofactors) to avoid are:
- Early sexual intercourse
- Early age of first pregnancy
- Multiple partners
- Too many births and too frequent births
- Poor local hygiene.

Secondary prevention:
- Screening against carcinoma cervix—**cytology (liquid-based cytology), HPV testing** (hybrid capture II), VIA, colposcopy and biopsy.
- 'Down staging screening' by WHO—intends to diagnose the disease early and to minimize cancer death.

Q. What is the role of HPV in the pathogenesis of carcinoma cervix?

Ans. HPV is a DNA virus which is epitheliotropic. High oncogenic risk HPV (types 16, 18, 31, 33, 35, 45, 56) types are responsible in the etiopathogenesis of cancer cervix.

Over 99.7% of patients with CIN and invasive cancer are found to be positive with HPV-DNA. **Infection always starts at the transformation zone (TZ) of the squamocolumnar junction (SCJ).** Once the high-risk oncogenic HPV-DNA integration occurs within human (host) genome (infection), there is overexpression of E6 and E7 oncoproteins. These oncoproteins suppress the tumor suppressor genes [(P-53 and retinoblastoma (Rb)]. This results in neoplastic transformation of the **mitotically active metaplastic epithelium of the 'transformation zone' at the level of SCJ** (See Dutta's Textbook of Gynecology, 7th Edition, p. 262). Normally the tumor suppressor gene P-53 will cause infected **cell death by apoptosis** and thus halting the viral multiplication. But these oncoproteins cause proteolytic degradation of P-53, **resulting in cell immortalization and viral multiplication**. Currently, HPV vaccines are available. Vaccines are very effective in preventing infection with HPV. Vaccines (Cervarix, Gardasil) are approved to all school girls

(9–15 years) and women (16–26 years). Immunity persists for about 5–7.5 years. Vaccines are type specific and effective only when used prophylactically.

Q. What are the advantages of surgery over radiotherapy?

Ans.
- Thorough surgicopathological staging during surgery.
- Accurate prediction of survival rate by para-aortic and pelvic node assessment surgically.
- Preservation of ovarian function when desired.
- Retention of more functional and pliable vagina.
- Transposition of ovaries when needed for consideration of future radiotherapy.
- Psychological benefit of the woman.

Q. What is neoadjuvant chemotherapy and what are the benefits?

Ans. Platinum-based combination chemotherapy is given for three cycles. This is followed by radical hyterectomy and pelvic lymphadenectomy. Neoadjuvant chemotherapy improves the resectibility of bulky (4 cm) disease (stage Ib2 S stage IIa).

Q. What is concurrent chemoradiation?

Ans. It is the combined therapy with radiation and weekly cisplatin-based combination chemotherapy. This therapy is found helpful as a primary treatment for stage IB, IIA or advanced stage (IIB to IVA) disease.

Q. How the radiation dose is calculated in the management of cancer cervix?

Ans. Radiation dose is calculated with respect of radiation received at two arbitary points—point A and point B.
- **Point A** is 2 cm cephalic and 2 cm lateral to the external os. It is the point of crossing of the uterine artery and ureter.
- **Point B** is 2 cm cephalic and 5 cm lateral at the same plane. It is approximately the site of obturator node.
- **Point A** gets about 7000–8000 cGy and **point B** 2000 cgy from radium (brachytherapy). Cancerolytic dose is approximately 7000–75000 cGy. The rest of the dose at Point B is supplemented by external beam radiation.

Q. What is the overall 5 years survival rate following therapy in a woman with carcinoma cervix?

Ans.

Stages	5 years survival rate (%) (International Federation of Gynecology and Obstetrics)	
1A1	98.7	
1A2	95.9	The overall 5 years survival for all the stages is 69.9%.
1B1	88.0	
1B2	78.8	
IIA	68.8	
IIB	64.7	Important prognostic factors are: tumor volume, lymph node metastasis, parametrial invasion and lymphovascular space invasion.
IIIA	40.4	
IIIB	43.3	
IVA	19.5	
IVB	15	

Q. How cervical cancer screening could be organized in a low-resource setting?

Ans. Cytology based cervical cancer screening program (India, Pacific Islands) could not be successful, in many countries of the world, as it requires a number of procedures. Alternative cervical cancer screening strategies in low resource settings can have a consistent and significant impact to improve upon the burden of cancer deaths.

Recommendations (ACOG-2015): The following are the acceptable alternatives where cytology based screening is not feasible or practical.
- HPV testing and follow-up treatment for woman with positive test results. Visual inspection the cervix with acetic acid may or may not be done.
- In settings where HPV-DNA is not available, visual inspection with acetic acid followed by treatment with cryotherapy to be done. Cryotherapy should not be done in women where squamocolumnar junction is not entirely visualized. It has been established with a prospective randomized study in rural India that a single life time HPV-DNA screening test can reduce cervical cancer mortality and late stage disease by about 50%.[1]

Q. What are the aims of palliative treatment? What different palliative treatments can be given to a woman with carcinoma cervix?

Ans. Palliative treatment is aimed to provide comprehensive care for relief of symptoms along with treatment of the cancer, in the advanced stage.

Palliative treatment is given:
- To control vaginal discharge
- To control hemorrhage
- To relief pain.

Discussion continued: *See* Dutta's Textbook of Gynecology, 7th Edition, p. 290.

Reference

1. Sankaranarayan R, Nene BM, Shastri SS, et al. HPV screening for cervical cancer in rural India. N Engl J Med. 2009;360:1385-94.

CASE 13: CARCINOMA ENDOMETRIUM

Case Summary

A 55-year-old obese, hypertensive woman presented with postmenopausal bleeding. Hysteroscopy showed an irregular polypoid mass at the fundus. Biopsy revealed adenocarcinoma of the endometrium [moderately differentiated, Grade 2 (Fig. 3.21)].

Q. What are the important etiological factors for endometrial carcinoma?
Ans.
- Unapposed estrogen stimulation
- Age: 50–60 years
- Parity—nulliparity
- Late menopause
- Corpus cancer syndrome (obesity, hypertension and diabetes)
- Overweight (21–50 pounds overweight increases the risk 3 times)
- Tamoxifen therapy
- Positive family history
- Endometrial hyperplasia.

Q. What is the common histological type of endometrial carcinoma?
Ans. Adenocarcinoma.

Q. What are the high-risk factors for endometrial carcinoma?
Ans.
- Persistent and unopposed estrogen stimulation of endometrium
- Corpus cancer syndrome—obesity, hypertension and diabetes
- Endometrial hyperplasia
- Family history of colon, ovarian or breast cancer.

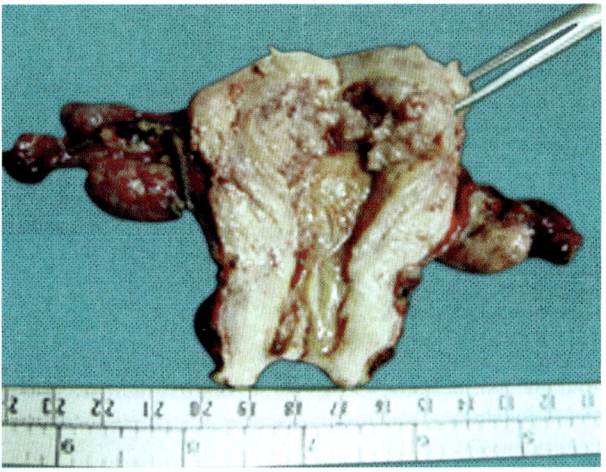

Fig. 3.21: Following surgery, uterus of the same woman is cut open to show a diffused and ulcerated growth at the fundus. The growth is seen to invade the myometrium. Histology confirmed adenocarcinoma

Q. How can be endometrial carcinoma diagnosed?
Ans.
- History and clinical examination: A case of postmenopausal bleeding is considered due to endometrial carcinoma unless proved otherwise.
- Endometrial biopsy (pipelle) diagnostic accuracy is 90–98%.
- Papanicolaou smear (unreliable) as diagnosis accuracy is only 30%.
- Ultrasonography (TVS) including color doppler, endometrial thickness > 4 mm with increased vascularity is suggestive.
- Hysteroscopy helps in detecting polyps or submucous myomas.
- Fractional curettage is the definitive method of diagnosis in case where adequate evaluation is not possible with pipelle biopsy specimen or where bleeding recurs after a negative endometrial biopsy.
- CT and MRI, both can detect myometrial invasion, lymph node involvement and also the spread of the disease. MRI is superior to CT (Figs 3.22A and B).

Q. Describe orderly the steps of fractional curettage?
Ans.
- Endocervical curettage
- Dilatation of internal os
- Introduction of a polyp forceps to remove any polyp
- Uterine curettage
- Specimens, so obtained are sent for histology separately.

Q. Mention the important surgical procedures for the management of a case of endometrial carcinoma?
Ans. *In stage I:* Extrafascial hysterectomy, bilateral salpingo-oophorectomy.

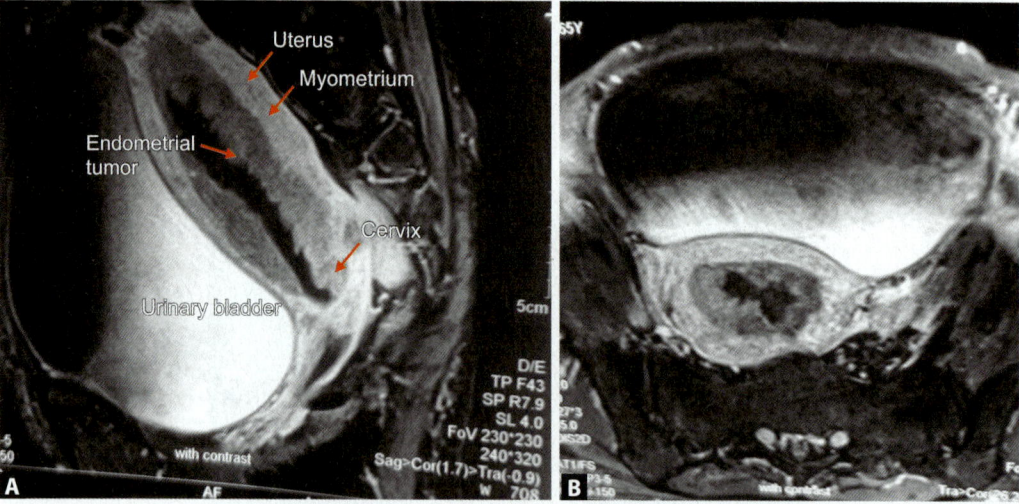

Figs 3.22A and B: A. Magnetic resonance image (MRI) in the sagittal plane of a 65-year-old woman with endometrial carcinoma. Sagittal T_1-weighted image shows endometrial tumor with invasion to the myometrium, more than 50%. There is extension of the cancer to the cervix (*see* arrows), **B.** Magnetic resonance image (MRI) in the axial view of the same woman with endometrial carcinoma. Invasion to the myometrium, more than 50% is seen.

Courtesy: Department of Obstetrics and Gynecology and Department of Radiology, Assam Medical College, Dibrugarh, Assam, India

Procedures
- Incision—longitudinal
- Peritoneal washings for cytology
- Thorough exploration of pelvic and abdominal organs including the pelvic and para-aortic lymph nodes
- Extrafascial hysterectomy (TAH and BSO) is done
- Uterus is cut open in the theater for tumor evaluation (gross examination or frozen section)
- Lymph node sampling—pelvic and para-aortic nodes are done when there is myometrial invasion.

CASE 14: CARCINOMA OF THE OVARY

Q. What are the reasons for failure to improve the outcome of ovarian cancer?
Ans.
- No high-risk factor is known
  - Deep-seated organs—diagnosis is often late
  - No effective preventive measures
  - No preinvasive stage of the disease
  - No effective screening procedure for early detection
  - Spread of the disease is unrelated to the size of the mass slush and or symptoms of the woman
  - Tumor cells move freely within the peritoneal cavity
  - Limitations of cytoreductive surgery, chemotherapy and radiation therapy.

Q. What is the place of screening for ovarian cancer?
Ans. Unfortunately, till date no specific method of screening for early detection of epithelial ovarian cancer is available.

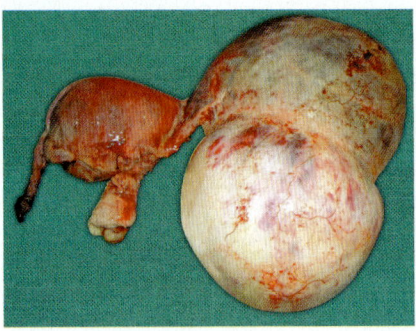

- ***Clinical methods***—bimanual pelvic examination is neither specific nor helpful.
- ***Tumor markers CA 125*** is being done. It is useful but nonspecific.
- ***Ultrasound imaging TVS*** color Doppler imaging has been used to differentiate a benign from a malignant mass (*See* Dutta's Textbook of Gynecology, 7th Edition, p. 354). However, it is not specific also.
- ***Risk of malignancy index (RMI)*** is calculated by U × M × CA 125. The risk of cancer is 75% when the RMI value is greater than 250. When RMI is less than 25 the woman is in the low-risk group. RMI: 25–250 is in the moderate-risk category.

Fig. 3.23: Gross photograph of a surgical specimen showing the uterus with a huge ovarian tumor. The other tube and the ovary are seen. Stretched fallopian tube over the tumor is seen. Histology revealed mucinous adenocarcinoma

- No screening procedure is effective for early detection of ovarian cancer.

Tumor Marker (HE4)
Human epididymis 4 (HE4) protein is derived from the distal epithelium of the epididymis. It is essential for sperm maturation as it is a protease inhibitor.

Levels of serum HE4 is found high in women with serous epithelial ovarian cancer. Unlike serum CA 125, serum levels of HE4 are less affected by other benign pelvic conditions like endometriosis. The sensitivity and specificity of detecting ovarian malignancy with HE4 is high in premenopausal women. This is especially beneficial for early stage ovarian cancer.

The use in combination of serum CA 125 and HE4 was found superior when compared with any other marker alone.

Risk of Ovarian Malignancy Algorithm (ROMA): ROMA is calculation based on the combined results of the CA 125 and the HE4. This algorithm classifies women either as low risk or high risk

Procedures
- Incision—longitudinal
- Peritoneal washings for cytology
- Thorough exploration of pelvic and abdominal organs including the pelvic and para-aortic lymph nodes
- Extrafascial hysterectomy (TAH and BSO) is done
- Uterus is cut open in the theater for tumor evaluation (gross examination or frozen section)
- Lymph node sampling—pelvic and para-aortic nodes are done when there is myometrial invasion.

CASE 14: CARCINOMA OF THE OVARY

Q. What are the reasons for failure to improve the outcome of ovarian cancer?
Ans.
- No high-risk factor is known
  - Deep-seated organs—diagnosis is often late
  - No effective preventive measures
  - No preinvasive stage of the disease
  - No effective screening procedure for early detection
  - Spread of the disease is unrelated to the size of the mass slush and or symptoms of the woman
  - Tumor cells move freely within the peritoneal cavity
  - Limitations of cytoreductive surgery, chemotherapy and radiation therapy.

Q. What is the place of screening for ovarian cancer?
Ans. Unfortunately, till date no specific method of screening for early detection of epithelial ovarian cancer is available.
- **Clinical methods**—bimanual pelvic examination is neither specific nor helpful.
- **Tumor markers CA 125** is being done. It is useful but nonspecific.
- **Ultrasound imaging TVS** color Doppler imaging has been used to differentiate a benign from a malignant mass (*See* Dutta's Textbook of Gynecology, 7th Edition, p. 354). However, it is not specific also.
- **Risk of malignancy index (RMI)** is calculated by U × M × CA 125. The risk of cancer is 75% when the RMI value is greater than 250. When RMI is less than 25 the woman is in the low-risk group. RMI: 25–250 is in the moderate-risk category.
- No screening procedure is effective for early detection of ovarian cancer.

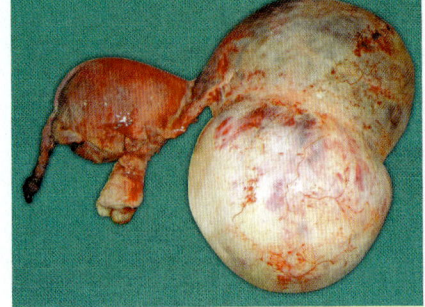

Fig. 3.23: Gross photograph of a surgical specimen showing the uterus with a huge ovarian tumor. The other tube and the ovary are seen. Stretched fallopian tube over the tumor is seen. Histology revealed mucinous adenocarcinoma

Tumor Marker (HE4)

Human epididymis 4 (HE4) protein is derived from the distal epithelium of the epididymis. It is essential for sperm maturation as it is a protease inhibitor.

Levels of serum HE4 is found high in women with serous epithelial ovarian cancer. Unlike serum CA 125, serum levels of HE4 are less affected by other benign pelvic conditions like endometriosis. The sensitivity and specificity of detecting ovarian malignancy with HE4 is high in premenopausal women. This is especially beneficial for early stage ovarian cancer.

The use in combination of serum CA 125 and HE4 was found superior when compared with any other marker alone.

Risk of Ovarian Malignancy Algorithm (ROMA): ROMA is calculation based on the combined results of the CA 125 and the HE4. This algorithm classifies women either as low risk or high risk for malignant disease. Both the tumor markers are related to tumor stage and histological type of serous epithelial ovarian cancer.[1,2]

Reference range for HE4 and CA 125:
   HE4: <70p; **CA125:** <35 IU/L
   ROMA: <7.4% in premenopausal patients
              <25.3% in postmenopausal patients

References

1. Moore RG, Brown AK, Miller MC, et al. The use of multiple novel tumor biomarkers for the detection of ovarian carcinoma in patients with a pelvic mass. Gynecol Oncol. 2008;108(2):402-8.
2. Rafael Malina, Jose M, Jose Auge, et al. HE4 a novel tumor marker for ovarian cancer: Comparison with CA125 and ROMA algorithm in patients with gynecological diseases. International Society of Oncology and Biomarkers (2011).

OVARIAN CANCER

Q. What are the epidemiology and risk factors for epithelial ovarian cancer?
Ans.
- Women of North America and most of the industrialized countries of Europe have high incidence.
  - Pregnancy, breastfeeding and use of combined oral contraceptives are associated with reduced risk.
  - Pregnancy in a women after the age of 35 years is more protective against ovarian cancer.
  - Use of long-acting progestin only contraceptive (DMPA, Provera) has protective effects similar to COCs.
  - Surgery: Tubal ligation (interruption) and hysterectomy can reduce the risk of ovarian cancer.

Q. What is the place of imaging studies in the management of ovarian cancer?
Ans. Computed tomography (CT)/positron emission tomography (PET) scan has been integrated for the diagnosis of ovarian cancer and evaluation of disease recurrence. PET scan has very high sensitivity but low specificity. There are false positive results due to increased FDG uptake in benign but metabolically active tissues and with inflammatory changes. Combined CT/PET scan had high sensitivity of 100% and specificity of 92%. It can detect recurrent disease which is superior to CA 125 or CT/MRI scans used alone.

Magnetic resonance imaging (MRI) is a nonradioactive imaging modality. It has excellent soft tissue contrast resolution. MRI is better than CT or ultrasonography in the diagnosis of small peritoneal metastases. CT imaging is better in identifying omental metastasis in ovarian cancer.

Q. What is the place of lymph node dissection in the managment of ovarian cancer?
Ans. *Lymph node dissection in early ovarian cancer:* Both pelvic and para-aortic lymph nodes should be removed. Lymph node dissection provides important prognostic and staging information for patients with suspected early stage ovarian cancer. This is helpful for the decision of about adjuvant chemotherapy. However, there is no convincing evidence that lymphadenectomy has got any therapeutic survival benefit in advanced ovarian cancer. Enlarged nodes may be removed as a part of debulking procedure.

Q. What is the place of neoadjuvant chemotherapy?
Ans. *Neoadjuvant chemotherapy:* Women with FIGO IIIC or IV ovarian cancers were treated with neoadjuvant platinum-based chemotherapy followed by primary debulking surgery. Subsequently, they were treated with platinum-based chemotherapy. The blood loss during surgery was less. The largest residual tumor could be reduced to less than 1 cm. The operative time was also shorter. For patients with huge tumor burden, ascites and several comorbidities, neoadjuvant chemotherapy is a very reasonable choice. Surgical debulking procedure is the single most important component in the management of ovarian cancer.

CASE 15: CARCINOMA CERVIX

Case Summary

Mrs LM, 42-year-old lady was diagnosed to have squamous cell carcinoma of the cervix, stage IIA. She underwent radical hysterectomy with pelvic lymphadenectomy (Fig. 3.24). Before the operation she wanted to know the following.

Q. What is the stage IIA carcinoma cervix?

Ans. Carcinoma of the cervix extending downwards up to upper two-third of the vagina but not laterally (without parametrial invasion).

It is subdivided into:

IIA1: Clinically visible lesion less than or equal to 4.0 cm in greatest dimension.

IIA2: Clinically visible lesion greater than 4 cm in greatest dimension.

Q. What does this radical hysterectomy mean?

Ans. Removal of the uterus, cervix, upper vagina, parametrium, pelvic lymph nodes and for her the ovaries also. Para-aortic node sampling is also done.

Q. What are the important complications of the operation?

Ans. Anesthetic complications and complications due to surgery: Hemorrhage, injury to bladder, bowel, ureters, infection, intestinal obstruction and lately fistula and lymphocyst formation.

Q. What are the consequences if she refuses the operation?

Ans. Progression of the disease and the problems of bleeding, sepsis, metastases, cachexia and renal failure (uremia).

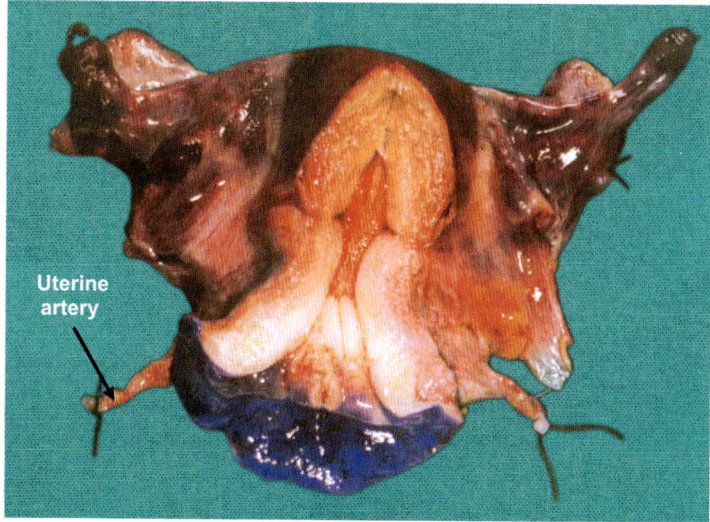

Fig. 3.24: Carcinoma cervix—radical hysterectomy done. Tied ends of uterine arteries are seen as they were dissected out and severed from the origin

Q. What is the long-term outcome following the operation?
Ans. If the nodes are not involved, 5-year survival rate is about 80%. On the other hand 5-year survival rate is about 50% if nodes are involved.

Q. Is there any alternative method of treatment?
Ans. Radiotherapy (combined teletherapy and brachytherapy) has got equal survival rate for this stage. Chemoradiation therapy is also effective. (*See* Dutta's Textbook of Gynecology, 7th Edition, p. 289).

Q. What is the place of fertility-sparing surgery for carcinoma cervix?
Ans. Fertility-preserving surgery for carcinoma cervix is done in highly selected women.
Indication: Woman keen to preserve her fertility and has no other factor for infertility.
Case selection criteria (*See* Manual of Obstetrics and Gynecology for the Postgraduates p. 131, 141, 146)
- Early stage disease
- Woman is strongly motivated for follow-up
- Invasive disease has been excluded on thorough examination
- Tumor is not a highly aggressive histologic subtype (neuroendocrine tumor).

Stage (FIGO) of the disease and the type of operation

Stage (FIGO)	Operation (fertility preservation)

■ Microinvasive carcinoma stage 1A1 (no LVSI)
■ Stage 1A1 with
  ♦ Lymphovascular space involvement (LVSI)
  ♦ Stage 1A2
  ♦ Stage 1A (adenocarcinoma)
  ♦ Stage IB1 (tumor volume ≤ 2 cm)
	■ Cervical conization (cold knife cone)
	■ Radical trachelectomy with lymphadenectomy (laparoscopic robotic assisted)
	■ Radical trachelectomy removes most of the cervix, bilateral parametria and upper vagina
	■ Uterus is preserved for child bearing function. It can be done vaginally or abdominally (laparoscopically or a robotic-assisted laparoscopy)

Q. What are the serum tumor markers of carcinoma cervix?
Ans. Serum tumor markers are valuable for predicting the prognosis, the response to treatment and also the risk of recurrence. In carcinoma cervix, the role of serum tumor markers in predicting 5-year survival rate is limited.
The most commonly studied tumor markers are:
- Squamus cell carcinoma antigen (SCCA)
- Cancer antigen 125 (CA 125)
- Cytokeratin fragment 19 (CYFRA 21.1).

Raised levels of SCCA, CYFRA 21.1 and CA 125 have been observed in 20–88% of women with cervical cancer. Raised levels are correlated with tumor stage, tumor volume, cervical stromal invasion, lymphovascular space invasion, parametrial involvement and lymph node metastasis.

Q. What is the role of radiographic studies in tumor evaluation?
Ans. According to FIGO, radiographical studies such as CT, PET, combined PET/CT and MRI may be used to determine the extent of the disease within the pelvis, lymph nodes, for

evaluation of prognosis and risk of recurrence following of initial treatment. However, these are not mandatory and are not considered integral to formal staging.
- MRI is more accurate to determine tumor diameter, uterine extension and parametrial involvement compared to CT or clinical examination
- PET/CT is more valuable to evaluate nodal metastases
- Dynamic contrast-enhanced MRI can evaluate tumor vascularity and perfusion. [18F] fluorodeoxyglucose PET: PET/CT can evaluate intratumoral metabolic actively. All these can predict response to therapy.

CASE 16: MENOPAUSE AND HORMONE REPLACEMENT THERAPY (HRT)

Case Summary

Mrs VL, 55-year-old school teacher, was seen in the clinic for the problem of postmenopausal bleeding. She did not have any history of pelvic pain, recent weight gain or weight loss. Clinical examination did not reveal any abnormality.

Q. What are the common causes of postmenopausal bleeding?
Ans. Senile vaginitis, senile endometritis, cervical carcinoma, endometrial carcinoma (*See* Dutta's Textbook of Gynecology, 7th Edition, p. 462).

Q. What investigations should you organize for her?
Ans. Ultrasonography to assess endometrial thickness and/or any of the biopsy methods as:
- Pipelle endometrial biopsy
- Hysteroscopy and endometrial biopsy
- Fractional curettage and endometrial biopsy.

Q. What abnormality will guide her to go for hysterectomy?
Ans. Significant endometrial pathology and risks of endometrial carcinoma are as follows:
Type of endometrial hyperplasia and endometrial carcinoma.
Typical
- Simple (cystic without atypia): 1%
- Complex (adenomatous without atypia): 3%.

Atypical
- Simple (cystic with atypia): 8%
- Complex (adenomatous with atypia): 29%
  The risk of malignancy with atypical hyperplasia is high. This may necessitate hysterectomy.
  She is aware of menopause and osteoporosis. She wants to know the following.

Q. Has she got any of the risk factors for osteoporosis?
Ans. Risk factors are:
- Family history
- Early menopause
- Low body weight
- Excess caffeine intake
- Smoking
- Sedentary habit or use of some drugs (corticosteroids).

Q. What preventive measures can she take to prevent osteoporosis?
Ans. Exercise, adequate dietary intake of calcium, vitamin D and nonhormonal treatment (biphosphonate) or HRT (*See* Dutta's Textbook of Gynecology, 7th Edition, p. 49).

Q. What HRT would be appropriate for her?
Ans. If the uterus is intact, combined estrogen and progestin cyclically. Progestin is added for last 12–14 days of each month or she can have low dose estrogen and progestin combined

and continuous. Otherwise, following hysterectomy she should take estrogen only. There is reduction in the risk of osteoporosis, coronary heart disease and colon cancer.

Q. *What other benefits can she have with HRT?*
Ans.
- Improvement of vasomotor symptoms (hot flushes, night sweats)
- Prevention of atrophic changes in the skin, genital and urinary tract epithelium
- Protection against cardiovascular disease
- Reduction in the problems of anxiety, insomnia, irritability and depression.

Q. *Is there any risk for continuing HRT?*
Ans. In a well-selected case, risks are generally less compared to the benefits. In most of the studies (WHO 2003, Million Women Study 2003), there is no increased risk of breast cancer when estrogen is only used (in a hysterectomized woman). Currently low dose estrogen (conjugated equine estrogen 0.3 mg or ethinyl estradiol 1 mg) is recommended. However, the woman needs to be counseled.

But regular breast self-examination (BSE) monthly, clinical breast examination (CBE) yearly and mammography yearly (ACOG-2000) should be carried out as a part of breast screening.

There is an increased risk of deep vein thrombosis (DVT) from 10 to 30 per 10,000 users.

Q. *What are the contraindications of HRT?*
Ans. Contraindications are:
- Undiagnosed genital tract bleeding
- Estrogen-dependent cancer in the body
- Active liver disease
- History of venous thromboembolism
- Gallbladder disease.

Q. *What are different routes through which HRT can be administered?*
Ans. HRT can be administered orally, through the skin as patches, gel, subcutaneous implant or nasal spray. It can also be administered by vaginal route as creams or pessaries. Use of oral route and the first pass liver metabolism has its beneficial effects on the lipoproteins.

Q. *How long can HRT be taken?*
Ans. The optimal duration of use for HRT is currently debatable. Small dose and short-term use for a period of 3–5 years has been recommended for bone protection.

CASE 17: CARCINOMA CERVIX

Case Summary

Mrs LK, a 34-year-old woman $P_{1+0+0+1}$, diagnosed to have carcinoma cervix stage IA. She is admitted for subsequent management. Before that she desired to be counseled with the following.

Q. What is stage Ia carcinoma cervix?
Ans. Carcinoma strictly confined to the cervix and that is in the preclinical stage. It is diagnosed by biopsy only.

Q. Is there any subdivisions of the stage?
Ans. Yes, stage IA1: When there is minimal microscopically evident stromal invasion less than or equal to 3.0 mm in depth and extension of less than or equal to 7.0 mm.
Stage IA2: Microscopically measured stromal invasion more than 3 mm but less than 5 mm with an horizontal spread of not more than 7.0 mm.

Q. What is the significance of such classification?
Ans. It is entirely related to spread of the disease and hence directly related to the prognosis and survival outcome.

Q. What is the approximate rate of lymph node involvement in this stage and 5-year survival rate?
Ans. Pelvic nodes involvement for stage IA1 (< 3 mm) is 0–0.5% and for stage IA2 (3–5 mm) is 5–6%. The risk of para-aortic nodes involvement is 0 and 1%, respectively. 5-year survival rate for stage IA1 is 98.7% and for stage IA2 is 95.9% respectively (*See* Dutta's Textbook of Gynecology, 7th Edition, p. 290).

Q. What are the treatment options for this woman?
Ans. Either extrafascial hysterectomy (type I) or modified radical hysterectomy (type II) should be optimum for her depending on whether she belongs to stage IA1 or stage IA2.

Q. What is meant by type I and type II hysterectomy?
Ans. *Type I:* Extrafascial hysterectomy; the pubocervical ligament is incised allowing lateral deflection of the ureter.
Type II (modified radical): Here medial half of the Mackenrodt's and uterosacral ligaments along with selective (clinically enlarged and palpable) lymph nodes are removed. Upper third of vagina is also removed.

Q. Can she have any surgery preserving her fertility status?
Ans. Yes, such treatment can be provided in exceptional circumstances only. Therapeutic conization is the option that she can have. In that case, she must realize the need of long-term follow-up. She should be followed up with cytology and colposcopy regularly.
Laparoscopic-assisted radical vaginal trachelectomy with pelvic and aortic lymphadenectomy (LARVT) is also recommended currently for early stage (IA2 and IB1) disease. This is done only for a strongly motivated woman who wants to preserve her fertility (*See* Dutta's Textbook of Gynecology, 7th Edition, p. 289).
In either of the above treatment options, the surgical margin must be free of disease.

Q. What is radical trachelectomy?
Ans. It involves removing the cervix, parametria and cuff of vagina. Body of the uterus is preserved for fertility. This procedure is combined with either extraperitoneal or laparoscopic pelvic lymphadenectomy.

Q. What is concurrent chemoradiation?
Ans. Cisplatin-based concurrent chemoradiation is currently recommended as a treatment option of carcinoma cervix. It acts as a radiosensitizer and reduces disease progression. The appropriate cases for this treatment are: (i) Early stage (stages IA2, IB, IIA) disease after radical hysterectomy, (ii) Locally advanced (stages IIB to IVA) disease as a primary therapy.

CASE 18: HYSTERECTOMY AND OOPHORECTOMY

Case Summary
Mrs CJ, 46-year-old, parous, woman had been admitted for hysterectomy due to the problem of multiple fibroid uterus. She had been adequately counseled for this operation. She is further interested to know about the current status of prophylactic-oophorectomy during hysterectomy. You have to discuss with her in this regard.

Q. What are the risks of bilateral oophorectomy during hysterectomy?
Ans. Risks are mainly due to loss of endocrine function of the ovaries. Loss of estradiol function is significant. Moreover, ovarian stroma secretes androgen precursors which are converted to estrogen in adipose tissue (peripheral endocrine organs). Major health hazards following oophorectomy are osteoporosis, fracture and cardiovascular risk. Additional morbidities are due to atrophy of the genital and urinary organs (dyspareunia, dysuria), vasomotor instability (hot flushes) and psychological disturbances (irritability, insomnia, mood swing).

Q. What are the benefits of doing bilateral oophorectomy during hysterectomy?
Ans. Bilateral oophorectomy protects the woman against the risks of developing ovarian cancer (100%) and peritoneal cancer (95%). It reduces residual ovarian syndrome (3–5%) and risks of relaparotomy (5–10%) for any benign or malignant ovarian lesions. It also reduces the risk of breast cancer by 50%. It eliminates the problems of chronic pelvic pain and dyspareunia.

Q. What is the risk of age (46 years in this case) in developing ovarian cancer?
Ans. Yes, this age has its own independent risk. The current information about the age and the risk of ovarian cancer as follows:

> Age < 40 years = infrequent; age 40–45 years = 15–16/100,000; age 60–70 years = 57/100,000 and the median age for ovarian cancer is 63 years.

Q. What are the benefits and risks of hysterectomy alone in relation to ovarian cancer and menopause problems?
Ans. The current information in this regard is, a woman who had undergone hysterectomy alone had a long-term reduced risk of epithelial ovarian cancer. However, hysterectomy is associated with earlier onset of menopause (3.7–4.4 years) even if the ovaries are preserved.

Q. What is familial ovarian cancer and how common it is?
Ans. Mutations of certain genes (BRCA1 and BRCA2) are associated with higher risk of ovarian and breast cancers. However, of all the epithelial ovarian cancers 1 out of 10 is hereditary. Familial ovarian cancer has an earlier onset of disease.

Q. Is there any current guidelines for prophylaxis of oophorectomy during hysterectomy?
Ans. Nothing is specifically recommended till date. It should be based on individual woman's risk and the family history. However, prophylactic oophorectomy during hysterectomy is performed at a median age of 48 years or 5 years before the index case with the family history of ovarian cancer whichever is earlier. Once oophorectomy is done, management of surgical menopause with nonhormonal or hormonal method should be considered.
    All these needs informed consent of the individual concerned.

CASE 19: POSTMENOPAUSAL BLEEDING

Case Summary

Mrs AB, 58-year-old woman presented with postmenopausal bleeding (PMB). She was thoroughly investigated and diagnosed to have endometrial carcinoma. Her clinical staging (FIGO) was stage IB, G2. You are asked to discuss the pros and cons of different risk factors, investigations and the stage of endometrial carcinoma.

Q. What are the common causes of PMB?

Ans. In the developing countries including India genital malignancy particularly carcinoma cervix is the most common cause of PMB. Other causes are:
- Atrophic endometritis
- Endometrial hyperplasia
- Endometrial polyps
- DUB
- Decubitus ulcer
- Retained (forgotten) pessary or IUCD (Fig. 3.25)
- Endometrial carcinoma.

Q. Who are the high-risk women to develop endometrial carcinoma?

Ans.
- Unopposed estrogen stimulation
- Delayed menopause
- Hypertension
- Diabetes
- Overweight (50 pounds overweight increases the risk by 10 times)
- Nulliparity
- PCOS
- Tamoxifen therapy
- Family history of endometrial, breast, ovary or colon carcinoma.

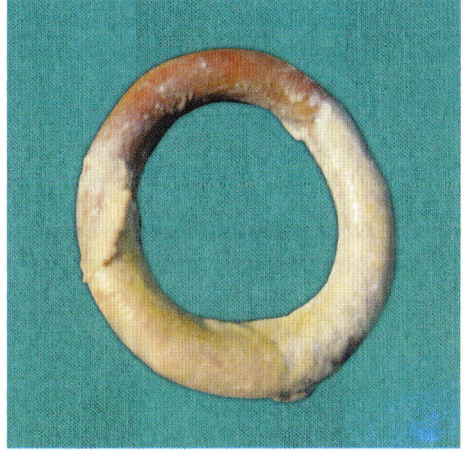

Fig. 3.25: Rubber ring pessary. This had been removed from a 70-year-old woman. She presented with postmenopausal bleeding. She had been using this for last 20 years. This forgotten pessary caused ulceration and infection in the vagina. Crust had been formed on its surface due to its prolonged stay in the vagina

Q. What is the significance of family history?

Ans. Lynch II syndrome is observed in about 2% of all such cases of hereditary cancers. Such families display high incidence of hereditary nonpolyposis colorectal cancer (HNPCC), adenocarcinoma of ovary, endometrium, stomach, small bowel and the urinary tract. It is associated with mutations in the DNA mismatch repair (MMR) genes (MSH2, MLH1, PMS1 or MSH6).

Q. What is the current change in the trends of diagnosis of endometrial cancer?

Ans. Most gynecologists recommend outpatient endometrial biopsy to confirm the diagnosis. Diagnostic accuracy of outpatient endometrial biopsy using pipelle endometrial sampler is 90–98%. Besides pipelle endometrial sampler, Sherman curette, transvaginal ultrasonography, sonohysterography, hysteroscopy and directed biopsy are also used.

Q. What is the place of different procedures in the diagnosis of endometrial carcinoma?
Ans. Fractional curettage is a definite diagnostic procedure for endometrial cancer but it is invasive. Role of hysteroscopy in the diagnosis has certain advantages. To date, there is no universal agreement to the cut off measurement of endometrial thickness to diagnose endometrial cancer. Endometrial thickness less than or equal to mm in a postmenopausal woman is commonly due to atrophy.

- Hysteroscopy is more accurate in detecting polyps or submucous fibroids. It helps to see the pathologic lesion as to take direct biopsy. It also helps to evaluate the endocervical canal.
- Saline infusion sonography (SIS) is helpful in differentiating patients with minimal endometrial tissue from patients with thickened endometrium or polyps.
- Fractional curettage is mandatory if endometrial sampling procedures fail to provide sufficient material for diagnostic evaluation or when the symptoms are persistent in spite of negative endometrial sampling.
- Considering the benefits most clinics prefer to do outpatient (office) endometrial biopsy as a first diagnostic step. When biopsy result is negative and further evaluation is needed, hysteroscopy and biopsy is done.

Q. What are the characteristics of type I and type II endometrial carcinoma?
Ans. *Differentiating features of type I and II endometrial carcinoma*

Clinical characters	Type I	Type II
Risk factor	Unopposed estrogen	Age
Occurrence	Common (85%)	Less common
Predisposing factor	Hyperestrogenic state	No such
Precursor endometrium	Atypical hyperplasia	May be atrophic
Age	Young (perimenopause)	Older (postmenopause)
Endometrial hyperplasia	Present	Absent
Tissue differentiation	Well	Poor
Myometrial invasion	Minimal	Deep
Histology	Endometrioid	Serous, clear
Molecular characters		
Ploidy	Polyploid	Aneuploid
HER2/neu overexpression	No	Yes
P-53	No	Yes
PTEN mutations	Yes	No
Prognosis	Favorable	Not favorable

Q. Are all endometrial cancers due to estrogenic stimulation?
Ans. Currently two pathogenic types of endometrial carcinoma are being observed.[1]
Type I: The majority (75–85%) belong to this group. Women having a persistent stimulation of endometrium with unopposed estrogen either endogenous or exogenous, run the risk of developing type I endometrial carcinoma.

Type II: Women with type II develop endometrial carcinoma without any estrogenic stimulation. Carcinoma develops not from the background of endometrial hyperplasia but may arise from an atrophic endometrium.

Estrogen dependent tumors develop in relatively younger perimenopausal women as opposed to the estrogen independent tumors that occur in older postmenopausal women. Tumors that are estrogen dependent have favorable prognosis compared to estrogen independent tumors. Based on molecular genetic studies, these two types of tumors have different pathogenetic pathways.

Q. What are the limitations and risks of FIGO surgical staging of endometrial cancer?

Ans. Staging laparotomy recommended by FIGO do not specify any well-defined procedures to stage the disease appropriately. Ultimately, it is left to the discretion of the surgeon. It is generally observed that risks of extended staging procedures are greater compared to limited steps for low risk patients. In that case, if survival for high-risk patients is not improved, the purpose of surgical staging is of limited value.

On the other hand surgical staging is faced with immediate and delayed complications. Extended surgical staging laparotomy that involves lymphadenectomy, may end up with injury to the ureter, major vessels or bowel. Moreover, extensive intraperitoneal surgical procedures result in adhesions. Another major concern is the risk of radiation injury to the small bowel as delayed complications in the postoperative phase, should the woman need radiation as an adjuvant therapy.

Q. What is the current situation of TVS, CT and MRI in the evaluation of endometrial cancer?

Ans. MRI is found to be superior to conventional CT in the assessment of depth of myometrial invasion. Studies have shown diagnostic accuracy of TVS is about the same (68–69%) compared to T_2-weighted MRI (68–74%) in evaluating myometrial invasion. However, contrast enhanced MRI is always superior to TVS and is found to be better when compared to CT even.

Multicoil (phased-array) and fast spinecho (FSE) sequences can increase the signal to noise ratio (SNR) in pelvic images and shorten the acquizition time. This is helpful for higher resolution and acquizition in multiple planes. Gadolinium enhancement easily distinguishes vascularized tumor from areas of nonenhanced necrosis or fluid accumulation.

The accuracy of MRI in staging endometrial carcinoma has been reported to be 85% overall. Gadolinium enhanced images significantly improve accuracy.

There are certain clinical situations where assessment of endometrial carcinoma may be difficult (e.g. obesity) or may not be possible (e.g. contraindications for surgical staging or because of tumor spread). In such situations MRI has got distinct advantages to evaluate the disease.

Reference

1. Bokhman JV. Two pathogenic types of endometrial carcinoma. Gynecol Oncol 1983;15:10–7.

CASE 20: INHERITED CANCERS AND THE MANAGEMENT

Case Summary

Ms RT, 44-year-old lecturer, nulligravida was seen for her abnormal uterine bleeding for last 8 months. Family history revealed cancers in the first-degree relatives for three generations. Family cancers included ovarian cancer, endometrial cancer and colorectal cancer—all are confirmed histologically. Her grandmother, mother, maternal uncles, sisters, brothers all are affected. Her thorough investigation including hysteroscopy and biopsy revealed endometrial adenocarcinoma (G-I). Total abdominal hysterectomy (extrafascial) with bilateral salpingo-oophorectomy was done. Histology revealed stage IA GI adenocarcinoma of the endometrium.

Q. Ms RT is keen to know what is inherited or familial cancers. How it could be prevented?
Ans. Familial or inherited cancers are well known. They are more common in relation to ovarian, endometrial, breast and colon cancers. Unfortunately, as regard the diagnosis and prevention, no such specific guidelines are there as yet.

Q. What are the diagnostic criteria for familial cancers?
Ans. Till date no such specific guidelines are there. Amsterdam criteria (1999) has considered the following:
- At least three relations with breast, ovarian cancer and hereditary nonpolyposis colorectal cancer must be there
- One affected person is a first-degree relative of the other two
- At least two successive generations are affected
- At least one person was diagnosed before the age of 50 years.
- Familial adenomatous polyposis had been excluded.
- Tumors have been verified by histopathological examination.

Q. How do BRCA-1, BRCA-2 and mismatch repair genes protect us?
Ans. BRCA-1 and BRCA-2 are the tumor suppressor genes. Others: MLH-1, MSH-2 and MSH-6 are the mismatch repair genes. These genes repair the single base pair mismatches that occur during DNA replication. Mutations in these genes cause cell immortalization, neoplastic proliferation and ultimately cancers.

Q. How familial cancers could be prevented?
Ans. At the moment there are no such guidelines. But following measures could be adopted:
- Family history must be enquired and recorded in all positive cases
- Clinical geneticist must be consulted and family tree should be drawn in a positive case (Amsterdam criteria)
- Molecular screening for detection of gene mutation is not possible at the moment. This is very expensive, time consuming and also labor intensive.
- Screening procedure may be initiated wherever available (e.g. breast cancer, colon cancer)
- Combined oral contraceptives are chemopreventive against ovarian cancer and endometrial cancer. Tamoxifen is chemopreventive against breast cancer.
- Place of prophylactic surgery may be considered. Prophylactic salpingo-oophorectomy/salpingectomy may be done specially while doing hysterectomy for some other reason.

This is an alternative in the high-risk group of women for ovarian cancer (*See* Manual of Obstetrics and Gynecology for the Postgraduates, p. 140).
- Human fertilization and embryology authority (HFEA), UK, has recommended preimplantation genetic diagnosis in cases with familial cancers. Affected blastocysts are removed from the transfer in ART. This may be one way to eliminate the risk of inherited cancers.
- As a prophylaxis to endometrial cancer, LNG-IUS (*See* Dutta's Textbook of Gynecology, 7th Edition, p. 295) is currently being used. Long-term reports are awaited.
- Resequencing chips are being tried, once available molecular diagnosis of gene mutation would be helpful.

Q. *Who are the women that may be considered for molecular screening?*
Ans. At the moment there is no such established criteria. However, women fulfilling the following criteria are the high-risk group for consideration:
- Positive family history following Amsterdam criteria
- Risk scoring more than 10 (Manchester scoring system)
- Tumors positive for microsatellite instability by immunohistochemistry method.

Q. *What is the significance of family history?*
Ans. This is often observed in early age onset (around 45 years).
Lifetime risk of endometrial cancer in women with Lynch II syndrome is 32–60% and that of ovarian cancer is 10–12%.

4
Self-Assessment in Gynecology

SINGLE BEST ANSWER (SBA) AND MULTIPLE CHOICE QUESTIONS (MCQs)

Q.1 The following are hormonal changes during a normal 28 day menstrual cycle except:
  a. The rising LH in the first part of the cycle stimulates estrogen production from theca cells
  b. FSH begins to fall after 7th day
  c. There is sudden rise of estrogen few days prior to ovulation
  d. The estrogen surge results in LH surge and prostaglandin F2α secretion

Ans. a. In the early follicular phase, FSH stimulates appearance of LH receptors on the theca cells. These receptors are activated by LH to produce primarily androstenedione and testosterone. These steroids diffuse into the granulosa cells and are aromatized to estradiol under the influence of FSH. (*See* Dutta's Textbook of Gynecology, 7th Edition, p. 58).

Q.2 The following are related to granulosa cells except:
  a. It has got no blood supply
  b. In the first half of the cycle, it has no steroidogenic function
  c. Granulosa cells produce activin and inhibin
  d. Estrogen stimulates the proliferation of granulosa cells

Ans. b. In the late follicular phase, FSH augmented by estrogen, stimulates the appearance of LH receptors on the granulosa cells. Small amount of progesterone is also produced. (*See* Dutta's Textbook of Gynecology, 7th Edition, p. 58, 69).

Q.3 The following are related to corpus luteum except:
  a. Luteinized granulosa cells produce progesterone
  b. Estrogen continues to be produced by the luteinized theca cells
  c. Luteolysis is due to estrogen, PGF2α and endothelin
  d. The peak steroid production is between 23rd and 25th day

Ans. d. The peak production is between 18th and 22nd day. (*See* Dutta's Textbook of Gynecology, 7th Edition, p. 70).

Q.4 Endometrial carcinoma is related to all except:
  a. Feminizing ovarian tumor
  b. Polycystic ovarian disease
  c. Exogenous estrogen therapy
  d. Early menopause

Ans. d. *See* Dutta's Textbook of Gynecology, 7th Edition, p. 292.

Q.5 The following statement(s) are related to fibroid:
  a. Genetic predisposition of myoma is not known
  b. Menorrhagia is manifested only in submucous fibroid
  c. The environment within the myoma is hyperestrogenic
  d. Corporeal fibroid is too frequently associated with pressure symptoms

Ans. c. In about 40%, myomas show abnormal karyotype. Cervical fibroid produces pressure symptoms. (*See* Dutta's Textbook of Gynecology, 7th Edition, p. 221).

Q.6 The following are related to adenomyosis except:
  a. The incidence is high amongst nulliparous women
  b. It often coexists with fibroid
  c. Posterior wall is commonly affected
  d. It is an estrogen dependent lesion

Ans. a. It is common in parous women. (*See* Dutta's Textbook of Gynecology, 7th Edition, p. 257).

Q.7 The following statements are related to tuberculous salpingitis except:
  a. The abdominal ostium may be patent with eversion of fimbriae
  b. The early lesion may be confused with adenocarcinoma on histology
  c. Genital tuberculosis is always secondary and the tubes are invariably the primary sites
  d. Salpingitis isthmica nodosa is the exclusive pathology to tuberculosis

Ans. d. It is also observed in endometriosis. a. It is called 'tobacco pouch' appearance.

Q.8 The following statements are related to genital tuberculosis:
  a. Ovarian involvement can occur without tubal affection
  b. Infertility is mainly due to anovulation
  c. Acid fast bacilli is identified in 100% cases of tuberculous endometritis
  d. A negative Mantoux test reasonably excludes tuberculosis

Ans. d. Ovaries are involved in following tubal affection. Infertility is mainly due to tubal and endometrial pathology. (*See* Dutta's Textbook of Gynecology, 7th Edition, p. 116).

Q.9 Follicular cysts of the ovary may undergo all these changes except:
  a. Spontaneous resorption   b. Malignant change
  c. Intracystic hemorrhage   d. Rupture

Ans. b. *See* Dutta's Textbook of Gynecology, 7th Edition, p. 236.

Q.10 The following are related to lutein cyst except:
  a. Lutein cyst is always related to pregnancy
  b. May undergo into torsion
  c. Intracystic hemorrhage
  d. Rupture

Ans. a. It is also related to gonadotropin or clomiphene therapy.

Q.11 The following are related to staging of pelvic malignancy, as per FIGO, except:
  a. Cervical carcinoma staging is based on clinical examination which cannot be altered on surgical findings
  b. Staging of ovarian malignancy should be done from clinical, operative and pathologic consideration

c. Staging of carcinoma body of the uterus is based both on clinical as well as surgical findings
d. Vulvar carcinoma staging is based principally on surgery

Ans. d. It is clinical staging. (*See* Dutta's Textbook of Gynecology, 7th Edition, p. 276).

Q.12 The following statements are related to Krukenberg tumor except:
a. It is always secondary
b. The most common primary site is pylorus of the stomach
c. The tumor is bilateral
d. 'Signet ring' looking cells are characteristic

Ans. a. The primary site is not rare and the prognosis is better.

Q.13 Regarding infertility:
a. Fecundability in a healthy couple is 80%
b. Unexplained infertility is about 10–15%
c. Women with amenorrhea, ↓E2, ↓FSH, belong to WHO Group I anovulation
d. Elevated basal FSH indicates poor ovarian reserve

Ans. b and d. Likelihood of pregnancy in an ovulatory cycle in a healthy young couple (fecundability) is 20%. According to WHO, anovulatory states are: **Group I**—(hypogonadotropic hypogonadism) woman with amenorrhea, ↓E2, ↓FSH, ↓LH and with negative progesterone challenge test (hypothalamic cause). Women in; c. belong to **Group I**; **Group III** belongs to hypergonadotropic hypogonadism (ovarian failure group). **Group II** includes women with PCOS (hypothalamic-pituitary dysfunction). Elevated basal FSH (>20%) indicates extremely poor prognosis (or ovarian failure). (*See* Dutta's Textbook of Gynecology, 7th Edition, p. 186, 203, 436).

Q.14 Corpus luteal insufficiency is associated with all except:
a. Recurrent miscarriage
b. Infertility
c. Preterm labor
d. Spontaneous miscarriage

Ans. c. *See* Dutta's Textbook of Gynecology, 7th Edition, p. 188, 194, 201.

Q.15 Corpus luteal insufficiency is observed in:
a. Women above 35 years
b. Clomiphene-induced ovulation
c. Hyperprolactinemia
d. All of the above

Ans. d. *See* Dutta's Textbook of Gynecology, 7th Edition, p. 188.

Q.16 Corpus luteal insufficiency can be diagnosed from all except:
a. BBT chart
b. Endometrial biopsy showing features of at least 2 days out of phase
c. Progesterone assay
d. Estradiol assay

Ans. d. *See* Dutta's Textbook of Gynecology, 7th Edition, p. 194.

Q.17 The following are related to diagnosis of female infertility:
a. Hysterosalpingography has got a definite place in the investigation
b. Sonohysterosalpingography is done in the secretory phase
c. Falloposcopy is done through operating channel laparoscope
d. Serial sonography may replace hysterosalpingography

Ans. a; b. In the proliferative phase; c. It is done through hysteroscope; d. It is for follicular measurement.

Q.18 Cervical intraepithelial (CIN I, II) neoplasia may undergo:
a. Regression in majority
b. Persistence in few cases
c. Progress to invasive carcinoma in majority
d. Recurrence following local treatment is high

Ans. a, c. Progression to CIS is 10–15%. d. It is 3–5%. (*See* Dutta's Textbook of Gynecology, 7th Edition, p. 270).

Q.19 Pelvic lymph node involvement in stage 1 Carcinoma cervix is about:
a. 5%
b. 15%
c. 25%
d. 30%

Ans. b.

Q.20 Theca lutein cyst is associated with all except:
a. Hydatidiform mole
b. Danazol therapy
c. Gonadotropin therapy
d. Clomiphene therapy

Ans. b.

Q.21 Galactorrhea occurs in all except:
a. Pituitary adenoma
b. Hypothyroidism
c. Use of metoclopramide
d. Kallmann syndrome

Ans. d.

Q.22 The most important clinical feature in the diagnosis of PCOS:
a. Oligomenorrhea and/or anovulation
b. Hyperandrogenism (clinical/biochemical)
c. Polycystic ovaries
d. Any two of the above

Ans. d. Presence of any two of the above three criteria (a, b and c) has been considered diagnostic (with exclusion of other etiologies) at a joint meeting of the American Society for Reproductive Medicine (ASRM) and the European Society of Human Reproduction and Embryology (ESHRE) in Rotterdam, 2004.

Q.23 Most common cause of menorrhagia in childbearing period:
a. Fibroid
b. Dysfunctional uterine bleeding
c. Pelvic endometriosis
d. Adenomyosis

Ans. b.

Q.24 The following are related to removal of vaginal cuff along with hysterectomy:
a. Carcinoma *in situ* of the cervix
b. Microinvasive carcinoma of the cervix
c. Carcinoma body of the uterus
d. Radical hysterectomy

Ans. d. Colposcopic evidence of involvement of the vault (carcinoma *in situ*) also requires its removal.

Q.25 The following are the definitive surgeries for microinvasive carcinoma of the cervix:
a. Hysterectomy with or without removal of vaginal cuff
b. Radical hysterectomy
c. Therapeutic conization
d. All of the above

Ans. d. Microinvasion of less than 3 mm beyond the basement membrane along with colposcopic evidence of presence of carcinoma *in situ* in the vault requires removal of cuff along with hysterectomy. Involvement of the lymphatic channels or confluence needs radical hysterectomy. In highly motivated cases with rigid follow-up, therapeutic conization can be done.

Q.26 Primary amenorrhea is most commonly associated with:
  a. Developmental defect of the genital tract
  b. Tuberculosis
  c. Endocrine disorders
  d. Chromosomal abnormality

Ans. d.

Q.27 Secondary amenorrhea is most commonly associated with:
  a. Sheehan's syndrome
  b. Premature ovarian failure
  c. Polycystic ovarian disease
  d. Hyperprolactinemia

Ans. c.

Q.28 The most common site of defect in primary amenorrhea:
  a. Pituitary
  b. Ovary
  c. Endometrium
  d. Chromosomal

Ans. d. Chromosomal abnormality is the most common.

Q.29 The most common site of defect in secondary amenorrhea:
  a. Hypothalamus
  b. Pituitary
  c. Ovary
  d. Thyroid

Ans. c. See Dutta's Textbook of Gynecology, 7th Edition, p. 378.

Q.30 Attempt to induce withdrawal bleeding in amenorrhea is effective in:
  a. Turner's syndrome
  b. Uterine synechiae
  c. Unresponsive endometrium
  d. Triple 'X' syndrome

Ans. a. See Dutta's Textbook of Gynecology, 7th Edition, p. 363.

Q.31 Dysfunctional uterine bleeding is commonly met in all except:
  a. Adolescence
  b. Following childbirth
  c. Premenopausal period
  d. Postmenopausal period

Ans. d.

Q.32 The following statements are related to secondary amenorrhea except:
  a. Pituitary disorder is the most common cause of hypogonadotrophic amenorrhea
  b. In early phase of ovarian failure, FSH level becomes high, LH level may be normal
  c. Ovarian biopsy is not essential to confirm the diagnosis of premature ovarian failure
  d. Hypothalamic dysfunction (psychogenic) is associated with normal levels of FSH and LH

Ans. a. Hypothalamic disorders are the common causes of hypogonadotropic amenorrhea. (See Dutta's Textbook of Gynecology, 7th Edition, p. 387, 388).

Q.33 Causes of premature ovarian failure are all except:
  a. Systemic chemotherapy
  b. Resistant ovarian syndrome
  c. Autoimmune response
  d. Androgenic polycystic ovary

Ans. d.

Q.34 Causes of first trimester abortion include all except:
 a. Luteal phase defect
 b. Chromosomal abnormalities of the fetus
 c. Cervical incompetence
 d. Polycystic ovarian disease
Ans. c.

Q.35 Ovulation is likely to occur, following clomiphene citrate in all except:
 a. Polycystic ovarian disease
 b. Postpill amenorrhea
 c. Recurrent dysfunctional uterine bleeding
 d. Resistant ovarian syndrome
Ans. d.

Q.36 Cryosurgery is effective in all except:
 a. Chronic cervicitis
 b. Squamous intraepithelial lesion (SIL)
 c. Condyloma acuminatum
 d. Cases with severe dysplasia or CIS lesion
Ans. d. See Dutta's Textbook of Gynecology, 7th Edition, p. 269.

Q.37 Exposure of a female fetus to androgen in early embryogenesis may arrest differentiation of:
 a. Müllerian ducts
 b. Ovary
 c. Urogenital sinus
 d. Mesonephric ducts
Ans. c.

Q.38 Subseptate uterus is diagnosed by:
 a. Hysterography
 b. Hysteroscopy
 c. Laparoscopy
 d. Combined hysteroscopy and laparoscopy
Ans. d. To see both the internal and the external architecture of the uterus. (See Dutta's Textbook of Gynecology, 7th Edition, p. 36).

Q.39 Congenital vaginal agenesis is usually associated with all except:
 a. Normal female karyotype
 b. Absence of functioning uterus
 c. Normal secondary sexual characters
 d. Presence of nonfunctional ovaries
Ans. d. Ovaries are not Müllerian structures; so they are normal anatomically and functionally.

Q.40 Agenesis of vagina is usually associated with all except:
 a. Presence of urinary tract anomalies in about one-third
 b. High incidence of gonadal malignancy
 c. Presence of skeletal anomalies of spine in about 10%
 d. Absence of uterus
Ans. b. See Dutta's Textbook of Gynecology, 7th Edition, p. 33, 373.

Q.41 Congenital malformation of the Müllerian ducts may produce all except:
  a. Dyspareunia
  b. Amenorrhea
  c. Infertility
  d. Poor breast development
Ans. d.

Q.42 About the embryology of the urogenital system:
  a. The trigone of the bladder is mesodermal in origin
  b. The rest of the bladder is endodermal in development
  c. The urachal fistula is due to patent allantoic diverticulum
  d. Most of the female urethra is mesodermal in origin
Ans. a, b and c; d. It is developed from the vesicourethral part of the endodermal cloaca.

Q.43 The following statements are related to genital tuberculosis:
  a. Should be treated surgically in the first instance when tubercular TO mass is present
  b. Cervical tuberculosis is mainly sexually transmitted
  c. Is a cause of infertility
  d. Pregnancy outcome is usually successful by following treatment
Ans. c; a. AT drugs must be started before surgery at best for 6 weeks; b. It is rare; d. Pregnancy is rare; if occurs, chance of ectopic is more; if uterine pregnancy occurs, chance of abortion is more and delivery of a live baby is a remote possibility.

Q.44 The following are related to surgical treatment of genital tuberculosis:
  a. Surgery should be preceded by at least 3 months of antitubercular therapy
  b. Abdomen is to be closed if minimal lesion is found accidentally in undiagnosed cases
  c. A negative chest radiograph rules out genital tuberculosis
  d. Surgery poses no special problem
Ans. a and b. Surgery is risky due to adhesions. The adhesions are dense and dissection is likely to produce sinus formation.

Q.45 Vault prolapse is most commonly due to the following:
  a. Vaginal hysterectomy for prolapse
  b. Abdominal total hysterectomy
  c. Subtotal hysterectomy
  d. Extended hysterectomy
Ans. a. The presence of pre-existing anatomical abnormality (laxity of the supporting structures) in spite of effective repair is the responsible factor in recurrence. Pre-existing enterocele, if left uncorrected increases the risk. Vault prolapse is expected to be less following subtotal than total hysterectomy.

Q.46 The following statements are correct in relation to paraovarian cyst except:
  a. It is a true broad ligament cyst
  b. It usually arises from epoophoron
  c. More chance of ureteric injuries during surgical removal
  d. Malignant change is frequent
Ans. d. Malignant alteration is rare. (*See* Dutta's Textbook of Gynecology, 7th Edition, p. 37, 246, 546).

Q.47 The following relations of the ureter are correct except:
  a. Ureter lies anterior to internal iliac artery
  b. Ureter forms the anterior boundary of the ovarian fossa
  c. Ureter crosses the uterine artery from below
  d. Because of dextrorotation of the uterus, the left ureter is more close to the cervix

Ans. b. Ureter forms the posterior boundary. (*See* Dutta's Textbook of Gynecology, 7th Edition, p. 11, 349).

Q.48 The following are related to the hormones in reproduction except:
  a. FSH and LH are secreted from the basophilic cells of the anterior pituitary
  b. Prolactin and thyrotropic hormones are secreted from the acidophilic cells of the anterior pituitary
  c. IGF-II stimulates aromatase activity and granulosa cell proliferation
  d. FSH along with LH is steroidogenic

Ans. b. Thyrotropic hormone is secreted from the basophilic cells.

Q.49 The median time interval for development of invasive carcinoma cervix from CIS:
  a. 5 years
  b. 10 years
  c. 15 years
  d. 20 years

Ans. c. *See* Dutta's Textbook of Gynecology, 7th Edition, p. 264.

Q.50 Testicular feminization syndrome has got the following features except:
  a. Poorly developed breasts
  b. Scanty axillary and pubic hair
  c. Short and blind vagina
  d. Karyotype—46XY

Ans. a. Breasts are large with less glandular tissue. (*See* Dutta's Textbook of Gynecology, 7th Edition, p. 364, 367).

Q.51 Regarding sterilization by the pomeroy method all are correct except:
  a. Is performed with absorbable suture material
  b. Includes crushing of the fallopian tube
  c. Results in two separate ends of the fallopian tubes several months later
  d. Has a higher failure rate, if performed at the time of cesarean section

Ans. b.

Q.52 Regarding placenta accreta:
  a. Ultrasonography can diagnose it antenatally
  b. Color Doppler USG has a specificity > 90%
  c. MRI is reliable to the diagnosis
  d. Internal iliac ligation is effective to control hemorrhage in majority

Ans. b. Sensitivity and specificity of color Doppler are found to be 82% and 97% respectively. Internal iliac ligation has been shown to fail in 40–60% cases.

Q.53 Accidental injury of the ureter during abdominal operation should be managed by all except:
  a. Deligation
  b. End-to-end anastomosis through an ureteric catheter
  c. Implantation into the bladder
  d. Colonic implantation

Ans. d.

162 Manual of Obstetrics and Gynecology for the Postgraduates

Q.54 *Laparoscopic ovarian drilling (LOD) for a woman with PCOS who is clomiphene-resistant:*
   a. Results in higher pregnancy rates compared to that of gonadotropin use
   b. Four punctures per ovary is considered optimum
   c. The women ovulate spontaneously for several years following LOD
   d. Incidence of multiple pregnancy is not changed
Ans. b, c and d.

Q.55 *Regarding the sling procedure for urodynamic stress incontinence (USI):*
   a. Tension-free vaginal tape (TVT) elevates the bladder neck to a retropubic position
   b. TVT is an autologous sling material
   c. Recurrent USI, intrinsic sphincter deficiency are the common indications
   d. Success rate of TVT is low than other retropubic procedures
Ans. c; a. TVT acts by increasing urethral coaptation, kinking the urethra with the rise in abdominal pressure; b. TVT is made from polypropylene (marlex) or polytetrafluoroethylene (Gore tex). Natural sling materials are made from rectus fascia or porcine dermis. These are less antigenic; d. Success rate of sling procedure are over 80% and it can be performed under local anesthetic.

Q.56 *Combined vesicovaginal fistula (VVF) and rectovaginal fistula (RVF) may have to be tackled by:*
   a. Local repair of RVF followed by local repair of VVF in the same sitting
   b. Preliminary colostomy followed 6 weeks later by local repair of VVF and repair of RVF in the same sitting
   c. Ileal bladder and colostomy followed by repair of RVF
   d. Colpocleisis
Ans. b. Repair of VVF should be done first. If RVF is repaired first, the operation field will be constantly contaminated with urine. Moreover, the repaired RVF site will have to be depressed by the posterior vaginal speculum while repairing the VVF.

Q.57 *Complications of sling procedures (TVT) for USI are all except:*
   a. Injury to bladder and wound hematoma
   b. Sling erosion particularly with polytetrafluoroethylene (Gore tex)
   c. Overactive bladder in about 7% cases
   d. Obturator nerve injury is about 10%
Ans. d. It is rare. It is avoided by correct medial needle insertion.

Q.58 *Regarding outpatient hysteroscopy all are correct except:*
   a. Abnormal uterine bleeding is an indication
   b. Normal saline as distension medium can be used
   c. It is less accurate than saline infusion sonography (SIS)
   d. It is not reliable to exclude endometrial carcinoma
Ans. c. Results are comparable. d. Positive hysteroscopy is more reliable than the negative one.

Q.59 *Ureter is commonly injured directly during operation of hysterectomy for all except:*
   a. Broad ligament fibroid
   b. Cervical fibroid
   c. Radical hysterectomy
   d. Endometriosis
Ans. c. In radical hysterectomy, ureter is dissected under direct vision all through. As such, direct injury during operation is a rarity. But avascular necrosis with fistula formation may occur at a later date.

Q.60 Ureteric injury can be prevented during total hysterectomy by the following procedures:
a. Using a lighted ureteral catheter
b. Enucleation followed by hysterectomy in cervical fibroid
c. Direct visualization rather than ureteric catheterization during pelvic surgery
d. Utmost care during clamping the uterine artery in simple hysterectomy

Ans. b and c. Ureter is not injured during clamping of the uterine artery. It is commonly injured while clamping the Mackenrodt's ligament along with descending cervical artery near the vaginal angle. a. It is cumbersome and of no added advantage.

Q.61 The following lymph nodes are removed during radical hysterectomy for carcinoma cervix except:
a. Parametrial
b. Obturator
c. Internal iliac group
d. Presacral group

Ans. d.

Q.62 The most common indication for abdominal hysterectomy for benign lesion:
a. Fibroid
b. Dysfunctional uterine bleeding
c. Endometriosis
d. Tubo-ovarian mass

Ans. b.

Q.63 The following are related to ligation of internal iliac artery:
a. For hemostasis, anterior division is to be ligated
b. Pelvic arteries freely communicate with branches from aorta, external iliac and femoral arteries
c. Hemostasis is effective due to temporary lowering of pulse pressure by 85%
d. All of the above

Ans. d. There is no rationale to tie the posterior division as the same supplies the major collateral circulation from the aorta and femoral vessels.

Q.64 During laparoscopic procedures all are correct except:
a. A volume of 3 litres of CO_2 is sufficient for pneumoperitoneum
b. A minimum intra-abdominal pressure of 15–18 mm Hg is required
c. Transillumination of the abdominal wall for inferior epigastric vessels is needed before secondary trocar insertion
d. Risk of significant complication during diagnostic procedure is about 10 in 1,000

Ans. d. Multicentre observational study mentioned the complication rate of 1.0 per 1,000 for minor and between 8 and 17 per 1,000 for advanced procedures.

Q.65 Subtotal hysterectomy may be indicated in all except:
a. Difficult tubo-ovarian mass
b. Extensive endometriosis involving the rectovaginal septum
c. As a matter of urgency during total hysterectomy
d. To preserve menstrual function

Ans. d. Preservation of the cervix may be done for increased sexual satisfaction not for menstrual function.

Q.66 Regarding sling procedure for urodynamic stress incontinence (USI) all are correct except:
  a. Tension-free vaginal tape (TVT) is placed under the bladder neck to act as a hammock
  b. Voiding disorders are high with TVT
  c. The bladder may become overactive following the TVT procedure
  d. Transobturator tape (TOT) is placed underneath the midurethra
Ans. b. The incidence of voiding dysfunction *seems* to be lower with TVT.

Q.67 To minimize ureteric damage, the following preoperative and operative precautions may be taken except:
  a. Cystoscopy
  b. Direct visualization during surgery
  c. Ureter should not be dissected off the peritoneum for a long distance
  d. Bladder should be pushed downwards and outwards while the clamps are placed near the angles of vagina
Ans. a. It should be intravenous (IV) pyelography.

Q.68 The following are related to ureteral injury:
  a. Majority (75%) occur with abdominal gynecological procedure
  b. Less common with vaginal hysterectomy than with abdominal
  c. Spontaneous resolution and healing are common
  d. Complete ligation of one ureter may cause silent death of that kidney
Ans. a, b and d; c. It is highly unlikely.

Q.69 Urinary symptoms of procidentia:
  a. Frequency of micturition
  b. Retention of urine
  c. Stress incontinence
  d. All of the above.
Ans. d.

Q.70 Regarding radiotherapy for carcinoma of the cervix:
  a. Bowel complications are more compared to urinary tract complications
  b. Large bowel is more sensitive compared to small bowel
  c. Squamous cell carcinoma is more sensitive compared to adenocarcinoma
  d. Presence of pelvic inflammatory disease (PID) affects the prognosis adversely
Ans. a and d.

Q.71 Recurrence sites of malignancy following pelvic surgery are all except:
  a. Carcinoma cervix—lateral pelvic wall and central pelvis
  b. Carcinoma ovary—lung
  c. Chorionepithelioma—suburethral region in anterior vaginal wall
  d. Carcinoma body—vault of vagina
Ans. b. It should be liver.

Q.72 The following statements are related to the treatment of carcinoma cervix stage 1B except:
  a. Surgery and radiotherapy have got almost equal 5-year-survival rate
  b. Surgery has got higher morbidity than radiotherapy
  c. Radiotherapy has got few limitations
  d. In younger age group, radiotherapy is preferred
Ans. d. The treatment of choice is radical surgery with preservation of ovaries.

Self-Assessment in Gynecology

Q.73 The following statements are appropriately related to gynecological surgery except:
  a. Hysterectomy is the operation of choice for symptomatic uterine fibroid unless there is sufficient reason to do myomectomy
  b. Local repair of VVF is the operation of choice unless there is sufficient reason to do urinary diversion operation
  c. In vitro fertilization and embryotransfer (IVF-ET) is the treatment of choice in preference to tubal reconstruction in all cases of tubal infertility
  d. Laparoscopic chromopertubation is not the procedure of choice in preference to hysterosalpingogram (HSG) for all cases of tubal infertility

Ans. c. Considering the cost and success rate of IVF-ET, tubal reconstructive surgery (reversal of sterilization) may be done in selected cases.

Q.74 Granulosa cell tumor of the ovary has the following features:
  a. It may present as postmenopausal bleeding
  b. Known to cause true precocious puberty
  c. Call-exner bodies are pathognomonic.
  d. Follow-up is needed even after hysterectomy and bilateral salpingo-oophorectomy

Ans. a, c and d; a. It is due to unopposed estrogen causing endometrial hyperplasia or endometrial carcinoma; b. It causes precocious pseudopuberty; d. It is of low-grade malignancy and late recurrences (even up to 20 years) have been noted.

Q.75 The following are related to vaginal axis except:
  a. In erect posture, it makes an angle of 45° with the horizontal
  b. In supine position, the angle is 75° with the horizontal
  c. Vaginal axis is almost parallel to the plane of inlet
  d. On cross-section, vagina looks oval

Ans. d. It looks like the letter 'H' in cross-section.

Q.76 Ovarian senescence actually starts:
  a. At 20th intrauterine week
  b. From puberty
  c. After the first childbirth
  d. At menopause

Ans. a. The peak period of follicular development is achieved at 20th intrauterine week, numbering about 20 million. Thereafter, atresia of the follicles starts which ultimately ends in menopause.

Q.77 Primary amenorrhea occurs in:
  a. Testicular feminization syndrome
  b. Estrogen secreting tumors
  c. Paraovarian cyst
  d. Intracranial tumors

Ans. a and d.

Q.78 Regarding gonadotropin-releasing hormone (GnRH) analogs treatment of fibroids:
  a. Should be used routinely before myomectomy
  b. Helps enucleation of myoma easily
  c. Reduces the incidence of recurrence
  d. Enables myomectomy through Pfannenstiel incision

Ans. d. It reduces the uterine size; b. It becomes difficult to shell out due to reduction of vascularity.

Q.79 In testicular feminization syndrome:
a. Buccal smear is chromatin positive
b. Normal breast size is observed
c. Menstruation is scanty and infrequent
d. Familial incidence is recognized
Ans. b and d.

Q.80 Indications of rectal examination in gynecology are all except:
a. In cases with Müllerian agenesis
b. Women having rectal symptoms
c. To differentiate rectocele from enterocele
d. For staging of ovarian malignancy
Ans. d.

Q.81 The following are related to colposcopy except:
a. Colposcopic directed biopsy is ideal in clinically undetected lesion of the cervix
b. It eliminates cytologic examination
c. It eliminates the random use of cone biopsy
d. It eliminates the need of hospitalization
Ans. b. Colposcopic examination is complementary to cytology and as such it cannot replace cytologic examination.

Q.82 The most common site of vulval cancer:
a. Labia majora
b. Labia minora
c. Prepuce of the clitoris
d. Bartholin's gland
Ans. a.

Q.83 The following statements are related to clear cell carcinoma of the vagina except:
a. Common to those whose mothers were given diethylstilbestrol during early pregnancy
b. Vaginal adenosis may progress to this conditions
c. The middle one-third is the most common site
d. May be multicentric and may involve even the cervix as well
Ans. c. The upper one-third is the most common site.

Q.84 The following statements are related to cervical intraepithelial neoplasia (CIN) except:
a. In majority, the changes are located in the transformation zone
b. Squamocolumnar junction (SCJ) is dynamic in relation to the phases of life
c. In severe dysplasia, whole thickness of the epithelium is involved by the undifferentiated neoplastic cells
d. Invasive carcinoma may occur in 5–10 years
Ans. c. It is the carcinoma *in situ* (CIS) or Grade III CIN which involves whole thickness and not severe dysplasia where superficial one or two layers are well differentiated.

Q.85 Primary carcinoma body of the uterus may be of following types except:
a. Adenocarcinoma
b. Adenosquamous carcinoma
c. Adenoacanthoma
d. Large cell keratinizing type
Ans. d.

Q.86 The following are precursors of endometrial carcinoma except:
a. Atypical adenomatous hyperplasia
b. Atrophic endometrium
c. Adenocarcinoma *in situ*
d. Cystic hyperplasia
Ans. b.

Q.87 Regarding polycystic ovarian syndrome (PCOS):
   a. Most common cause of anovulatory infertility
   b. Occurs only in obese women
   c. Associated hyperinsulinemia stimulates androgen secretion by the ovarian stroma
   d. Hirsutism is due to increase in total testosterone levels
Ans. a and c. See Dutta's Textbook of Gynecology, 7th Edition, p. 378.

Q.88 Diagnosis of Sheehan's syndrome is made by all except:
   a. Secondary amenorrhea following a turmoil childbirth
   b. Lactation is not affected
   c. Falling pubic hair
   d. Evidences of hypogonadotropic hypogonadism
Ans. b. Failure of lactation is a constant and important feature.

Q.89 Regarding metformin therapy in polycystic ovary syndrome (PCOS) all are correct except:
   a. Inhibits gluconeogenesis and stimulates peripheral uptake of glucose
   b. Reduces insulin resistance
   c. Causes hypoglycemia in women with PCOS
   d. Improves ovarian hyperandrogenism
Ans. c. It does not provoke hyperinsulinemia and does not precipitate hypoglycemia. It reduces plasma level of luteinizing hormone (LH). Metformin improves menstrual cyclicity and ovulation rate in women with PCOS. (See Dutta's Textbook of Gynecology, 7th Edition, p. 199, 382).

Q.90 The essential substitution therapy in Sheehan's syndrome is by:
   a. Combined estrogen and progestogen preparations
   b. Cortisone followed by thyroid hormone
   c. Gonadotropins for fertility improvement
   d. Combination of all the above drugs
Ans. b. Although there is plurideficiency state, essential substitution therapy includes cortisone and thyroid.

Q.91 The most common organism causing salpingitis:
   a. Gonococcal
   b. Pyogenic
   c. Tubercular
   d. Chlamydial
Ans. d. Gonococcal infection was responsible previously.

Q.92 Regarding Fitz-Hugh-Curtis syndrome:
   a. Characterized by violin string adhesions in the perihepatic region
   b. Primary pathology is hepatitis
   c. Pain is felt in the suprapubic region
   d. Organisms involved are *N. gonorrhoeae* and/or *C. trachomatis*
Ans. a and d; b. Acute salpingitis → acute perihepatitis → perihepatic adhesions; c. Chronic right upper quadrant pain. (See Dutta's Textbook of Gynecology, 7th Edition, p. 107).

Q.93 The gonococcal affection of the genital organs is diagnosed with high specificity by:
   a. Gram staining of endocervical mucus
   b. Culture of endocervical mucus in Thayer-Martin media

c. Enzyme immunoassay (Gonozyme) for antigens
d. Diagnostic laparoscopy

Ans. c. Specificity is 94–99% and is independent of viability of the organisms.

Q.94 Common opportunistic infections in AIDS patient are the following—match them appropriately:
a. Bacteria
b. Fungi
c. Parasites
d. Viruses

1. Cryptococcus carinii
2. Pneumocystis carinii
3. Legionella pneumophila
4. Varicella zoster

Ans. a = 3; b = 1; c = 2; d = 4.

Q.95 Vaginal pH during reproductive period averages:
a. 3.5–3.9
b. 4–5
c. 5.1
d. 6.1–7

Ans. b. Although, there is fluctuation of the vaginal pH during different phases of menstrual cycle and during pregnancy, the average pH is between 4 and 5.

Q.96 Causes of hematosalpinx are all except:
a. Disturbed tubal pregnancy
b. Acute salpingitis
c. Carcinoma of the fallopian tube
d. Tubercular salpingitis

Ans. d.

Q.97 Granulosa cells produces estrogen with the help of the enzyme:
a. Alkaline phosphatase
b. Aromatase
c. Acid phosphatase
d. Glucuronidase

Ans. b.

Q.98 Regarding adenocarcinoma of the cervix:
a. Adenocarcinoma is common in younger women
b. Downward extension of adenocarcinoma of the body to the cervix may occur
c. Adenosquamous tumors may occur
d. On prognostic comparsion adenocarcinoma is a high-risk cell type.

Ans. a, b, c, d.

Q.99 The following are related to menopausal symptoms except:
a. Estrogen deprivation is responsible for the symptoms
b. Low estrogen level and high GnRH pulses are responsible for hot flashes
c. Elevation of prolactin level also contributes to hot flashes
d. Surgical menopause is associated with more symptoms

Ans. c. Prolactin is unrelated to hot flashes.

Q.100 Menstrual pattern preceding menopause are all except:
a. Sudden stoppage following normal periods
b. Gradual hypomenorrhea
c. Increasing oligomenorrhea
d. Period of shorter cycles

Ans. d. Anovulation becomes more prevalent and menstrual cycle length increases.

Self-Assessment in Gynecology

Q.101 *Withdrawal bleeding following administration of progesterone in a case of secondary amenorrhea indicates all except:*
  a. Absence of pregnancy
  b. Production of endogenous estrogen
  c. Endometrium is responsive to estrogen
  d. Defect in pituitary gonadal axis
Ans. d. See Dutta's Textbook of Gynecology, 7th Edition, p. 386.

Q.102 *Gonadotropins in female usually begin to increase:*
  a. Even prior to puberty
  b. At menarche
  c. 1–2 years following menarche
  d. Generally, LH rises initially while follicle stimulating hormone (FSH) rises more slowly
Ans. a. In general, FSH rises initially whereas LH rises more slowly and reaches adult levels in late puberty.

Q.103 *Polycystic ovary syndrome:*
  a. Should be diagnosed by laparoscopy
  b. Could be treated by wedge resection
  c. Produces hypoestrogenism
  d. Is best treated by clomiphene, if pregnancy is desired
Ans. d.

Q.104 *Surest laboratory test to confirm the onset of menopause:*
  a. Estriol assay
  b. Endometrial biopsy
  c. Cytohormonal study
  d. Serum gonadotropin assay
Ans. d. Serum FSH and LH > 40 mIU/mL, three values at weeks interval are needed. Persistent serum estradiol < 20 pg/mL along with raised FSH is also diagnostic.

Q.105 *The following are usually related to primary spasmodic dysmenorrhea except:*
  a. Appears 2–3 years following menarche
  b. Starts 3–5 days prior to the period
  c. Lasts for few hours
  d. Present only in ovulatory cycles
Ans. b. It starts with the onset of period. (See Dutta's Textbook of Gynecology, 7th Edition, p. 147).

Q.106 *The most rare type of primary ovarian malignancy:*
  a. Simple serous cyst adenocarcinoma
  b. Mucinous cyst adenocarcinoma
  c. Papillary cyst adenocarcinoma
  d. Malignant change in dermoid
Ans. d. See Dutta's Textbook of Gynecology, 7th Edition, p. 239.

Q.107 *Regarding imaging of uterine fibroids all are corrrect except:*
  a. Ultrasound is ideal to confirm the diagnosis
  b. Saline infusion sonography (SIS) is more sensitive to detect any submucous fibroid
  c. MRI is superior to USG to identify the exact location of myoma
  d. CT scanning is an alternative to MRI
Ans. d. CT has got limited contrast resolution compared to MRI.

170 Manual of Obstetrics and Gynecology for the Postgraduates

Q.108 **Dysgerminoma with intact capsule (Stage Ia) in a 20-year-old newly married woman should be treated by:**
  a. Unilateral salpingo-oophorectomy
  b. Chemotherapy
  c. Ovarian cystectomy
  d. Radiotherapy
Ans. a.

Q.109 **The development of gonads in relation to embryonic age are—match them appropriately:**
  a. Gonadal ridge
  b. Ovary
  c. Testis
  d. Germ cell migration
  1. 3–4 weeks
  2. 4–6 weeks
  3. 6–8 weeks
  4. 4–5 weeks
Ans. a = 4; b = 3; c = 2; d = 1.

Q.110 **Peak level of plasma progesterone in the luteal phase:**
  a. 5 ng/mL
  b. 10 ng/mL
  c. 15 ng/mL
  d. 30 ng/mL
Ans. c. The value is average normal.

Q.111 **Regarding tubal sterilization procedure:**
  a. A pregnancy test should be performed, when there is a missed period
  b. Routine curettage should be done during the procedure to prevent luteal phase pregnancy
  c. Failure rate is the same as in interval procedure done during MTP
  d. A negative pregnancy test cannot exclude pregnancy reliably
Ans. d. RCOG guidelines recommend universal pregnancy testing for women undergoing tubal occlusion. (b) Routine curettage does not reduce luteal phase pregnancy. (c) Failure rate is high when sterilization is done during MTP.

Q.112 **Regarding reversal of tubal sterilization:**
  a. Falope rings damage the tube less compared to Pomeroy method
  b. Filshie clips damage the tube more than the Falope rings
  c. The rate of ectopic pregnancy is 10%
  d. Chance of successful pregnancy is over 70%
Ans. a and d. Filshie clips damage less (5 mm) compared to Falope rings (2 cm). Rate of ectopic pregnancy is about 3–4%. Success rate following reversal has increased with the use of rings, clips and also due to new surgical procedures for reversal (microsurgery).

Q.113 **The following are related to adrenal gland:**
  a. Adrenal medulla secretes epinephrine and norepinephrine
  b. Zona glomerulosa produces steroid hormone, testosterone
  c. Zona fasciculata mainly produces aldosterone
  d. Zona reticularis produces glucocorticoids
Ans. a. Zona glomerulosa produces aldosterone; zona fasciculata produces glucocorticoids and zona reticularis produces sex steroids, predominantly androgens.

Q.114 **Laparoscopic ovarian surgery (LOS) in women with PCOS:**
  a. All women, who are resistant to clomiphene citrate respond to LOS
  b. Failure of ovulation within 6–8 weeks or conception within 12 months is considered as the failure of LOS

c. LOS makes intrafollicular microenvironment from androgenic to estrogenic
d. The cautery needle should preferably be put close to the ovarian hilum

Ans. b and c. Women resistant to LOS are: BMI > 35 kg/m², serum testosterone > 4.5 nmol/L, free androgen index (FAI) >15 and infertility for > 3 years. The cautery needle should be away from the ovarian hilum to avoid damage to ovarian vessels. Otherwise risk of premature ovarian failure is there.

Q.115 Ovarian causes of hirsutism are all except:
a. Polycystic ovarian disease (PCOS)
b. Sertoli-Leydig cell tumor
c. Luteoma of pregnancy
d. Brenner tumor

Ans. d.

Q.116 Adrenal tumor is differentiated from hyperplasia by all these except:
a. Elevation of serum 17-hydroxy progesterone in hyperplasia
b. Negative dexamethasone suppression test in tumor
c. Marked elevation of adrenocorticotropic hormone (ACTH) in adrenal tumor
d. Tumor has got rapid onset

Ans. c. DHEA-S is markedly elevated in adrenal tumor.

Q.117 Testicular biopsy is indicated in:
a. Azoospermia
b. Oligospermia with high FSH
c. Oligospermia with normal FSH level
d. All of the above

Ans. a and c. It can differentiate obstructive cause of azoospermia from testicular failure. Raised FSH level indicates testicular failure. But in Sertoli cell, only syndrome, focal areas of spermatogenesis may be present. This can help in intracytoplasmic sperm injection (ICSI).

Q.118 Preferred surgery of uterine synechiae:
a. D and C
b. D and C followed by insertion of intrauterine device (IUD)
c. Adhesiolysis through hysterotomy followed by placement of IUD
d. Hysteroscopic adhesiolysis and placement of IUD

Ans. d.

Q.119 The cause of adrenal hyperplasia is due to:
a. Defect in cortisol synthesis
b. Defect in ACTH synthesis
c. Defect in testosterone synthesis
d. None of the above

Ans. a. An enzyme 21-hydroxylase deficiency leads to inadequate cortisol synthesis → by negative feedback leads to excessive secretion of ACTH → excessive stimulation of adrenal → adrenal hyperplasia → excessive secretion of adrenal androgen → virilization.

Q.120 Regarding cervical carcinoma:
a. HIV positive women have an increased risk
b. Staging is surgicopathological
c. Extension to the uterine corpus increase the stage of the disease
d. Adenocarcinoma is less radiosensitive than the squamous cell type

Ans. a; b. It is clinical staging only; c. It is not accounted by FIGO staging; d. Stage for stage, the management is the same, though adenocarcinoma is a high risk cell type. (*See* Dutta's Textbook of Gynecology, 7th Edition, p. 282).

Q.121 Causes of ovulation are all except:
a. LH surge
b. Necrobiosis of the thinned wall of the stigma
c. Contraction of the micromuscles in the theca interna
d. Activation of plasminogen

Ans. c. Contraction of micromuscles lie in theca externa.

Q.122 The following statements are related to choriocarcinoma:
a. It is not a tumor of the uterus but the uterus is secondarily involved
b. Histologic confirmation of diagnosis is a must before chemotherapy
c. The most common site of metastasis is in the anterior wall of the vagina
d. 1–5% of hydatidiform mole develops persistent gestational trophoblastic neoplasia (GTN)

Ans. a. Histological confirmation is neither essential to the diagnosis nor a prerequisite to treatment. A new pregnancy must be excluded, as serum β-hCG is important. The most common site of metastasis is lungs. 15–20% of hydatidiform mole develop persistent GTN.

Q.123 The most common cause of precocious puberty:
a. Constitutional
b. Endocrinal
c. Intracranial lesion
d. Iatrogenic

Ans. a. *See* Dutta's Textbook of Gynecology, 7th Edition, p. 40.

Q.124 Ovarian tumor producing features of thyrotoxicosis:
a. Carcinoid tumor
b. Struma ovarii
c. Dermoid
d. Lipid cell tumor

Ans. b.

Q.125 Best surgical treatment of apparently benign cystic ovarian tumor in a parous patient aged 40 years:
a. Ovariotomy
b. Ovarian cystectomy
c. Total hysterectomy with bilateral salpingo-oophorectomy
d. Ovariotomy followed by immediate frozen section and then formulation of extent of surgery

Ans. c.

Q.126 Carcinoma involving lower two-thirds of vagina should be treated primarily by:
a. Radiotherapy
b. Mitra's operation
c. Chemotherapy
d. Radical hysterectomy, partial vaginectomy and bilateral pelvic lymphadenectomy

Ans. a; d. is when upper vagina is involved.

Q.127 The following are the complications of the ovulation inducing drugs in infertility except:
a. Fetal abnormality
b. Cervical mucus hostility
c. Postural hypotension
d. Ascites

Ans. a. Bromocriptine produces hypotension; clomiphene causes cervical mucus hostility and ascites with gonadotropins in ovarian hyperstimulation syndrome.

Q.128 **The most common type of sarcoma of the uterus:**
a. Endometrial stroma
b. Intramural (myometrium)
c. Mixed mesodermal
d. On pre-existing fibroid

Ans. b. 65%.

Q.129 **The following are related to genital malignancy except:**
a. Overall 20% of patients with molar pregnancies require chemotherapy
b. The most common symptom of the endometrial carcinoma is postmenopausal bleeding
c. Endometrial acanthosis is a premalignant lesion
d. Postcoital bleeding is a recognized symptom of carcinoma cervix

Ans. c. Endometrial acanthosis is not a premalignant condition. Overall 20% develop persistent disease and need chemotherapy.

Q.130 **The following primary tumors are common in the vulva except:**
a. Adenocarcinoma
b. Basal cell carcinoma
c. Choriocarcinoma
d. Squamous cell carcinoma

Ans. c. See Dutta's Textbook of Gynecology, 7th Edition, p. 275.

Q.131 **In 36 days cycle, the ovulation usually occurs on:**
a. 14th day of the cycle
b. 22nd day of the cycle
c. 18th day of the cycle
d. None of the above

Ans. b. Ovulation usually occurs approximately 14 days prior to the expected date of the next period.

Q.132 **The following are related to bromocriptine except:**
a. It is dopamine agonist
b. It may cause multiple pregnancy
c. Cabergoline (dopamine agonist) can be administered vaginally
d. It restores menstruation earlier than stoppage of galactorrhea

Ans. b. It is not associated with multiple pregnancy. Cabergoline, an ergot derivative has low side effects and oral dose is 0.5–3 mg once a week.

Q.133 **The best sutures obliterating the myoma bed during myomectomy:**
a. Continuous interlocking
b. Mattress
c. Interrupted through
d. Interrupted and tier

Ans. d. See Dutta's Textbook of Gynecology, 7th Edition, p. 498.

Q.134 **The ovaries are situated:**
a. 6–8 weeks following birth—abdominal
b. 9 weeks to 7 year—at the pelvic brim
c. 10–13 years—descends to its normal position
d. All of the above

Ans. d.

Q.135 **Position of the patient should be as described except:**
a. Diagnostic laparoscopy—Trendelenburg with about 30° tilt
b. Colposcopy—lithotomy
c. Transvaginal sonography in gynecology—lithotomy with full bladder
d. Hysteroscopy—lithotomy

Ans. c. The position is dorsal with legs drawn up, full bladder is not needed.

174 Manual of Obstetrics and Gynecology for the Postgraduates

Q.136 Major sources of androgen in females are all except:
   a. Adrenals
   b. Ovaries
   c. Peripheral conversion to androgen precursors in the liver, gastrointestinal tract and adipose tissue
   d. Corpus luteum

Ans. d.

Q.137 The biochemical changes in established cases of Stein-Leventhal syndrome are as mentioned except:
   a. Marked elevation of LH in contrast to FSH
   b. Insulin resistance
   c. Elevation of plasma testosterone
   d. Elevation in the level of sex hormone binding globulin (SHBG) level

Ans. d. SHBG level is low in PCOS.

Q.138 Hormone assay findings in the diagnosis of adrenal hyperplasia are all except:
   a. Elevated serum level of ACTH
   b. Elevated excretion of urinary pregnanetriol
   c. Elevated plasma cortisol
   d. Elevated serum level of 17-hydroxyprogesterone

Ans. c. Plasma cortisol level is not elevated.

Q.139 Gynecological symptoms in relation to gross congenital malformation of the uterus include:
   a. Amenorrhea
   b. Menorrhagia
   c. Dysmenorrhea
   d. All of the above

Ans. d.

Q.140 A vesicovaginal fistula is sometimes a complication of all these except:
   a. Hysterectomy
   b. Pelvic radiotherapy
   c. Cervical cancer
   d. Endometriosis

Ans. d.

Q.141 The following are related with vasectomy except:
   a. Leads to immediate sterility
   b. Failure rate is 0.1%
   c. Involves ligation and division of spermatic cord
   d. Partner (wife) may be given DMPA for 3 months

Ans. a. DMPA may be used as an interim contraception before vasectomy is effective. (See Dutta's Textbook of Gynecology, 7th Edition, p. 403).

Q.142 Pyometra in a suspected case of carcinoma body should be tackled by:
   a. Drainage of pus followed immediately by diagnostic D and C
   b. Drainage of pus followed one week later by diagnostic D and C
   c. Hysterectomy with bilateral salpingo-oophorectomy straight way
   d. Hysteroscopy and biopsy

Ans. b. As the uterus is thin and soft, chance of perforation is more during curettage if done in the same sitting. After the pus is drained out, curettage is to be done after 1 week for better diagnosis. Definite surgery should not be done without prior diagnosis. In the presence of pyometra, hysteroscopy is not possible.

Q.143 Regarding puberty and primary amenorrhea:
 a. Precocious puberty is diagnosed when secondary sexual characters appear before the age of ten
 b. Congenital absence of vagina is associated with renal tract abnormality in about 10% of cases
 c. Primary amenorrhea is defined as the absence of menstruation by 14 years of age
 d. Precocious puberty may due to congenital adrenal hyperplasia

Ans. d. *See* Dutta's Textbook of Gynecology, 7th Edition, p. 40, 362; b. Renal tract abnormality in association with the absence of vagina is 30%.

Q.144 Theca lutein cyst is commonly associated with all except:
 a. Hydatidiform mole
 b. Multiple pregnancy
 c. Early normal pregnancy
 d. Gonadotropin or clomiphene citrate therapy

Ans. c. In normal pregnancy, corpus luteal cyst is commonly associated. Theca lutein cyst is rarely observed.

Q.145 Sex cord stromal tumors of the ovary include all except:
 a. Luteomas
 b. Gynandroblastomas
 c. Sertoli-Leydig cell tumors of the ovary
 d. The ca-fibroma

Ans. a. *See* Dutta's Textbook of Gynecology, 7th Edition, p. 316.

Q.146 The following are related to carcinoma fallopian tube:
 a. It is usually primary
 b. Papanicolaou smear is always negative
 c. Should be primarily treated by radiotherapy
 d. 'Hydrops tubae profluens'—may be a presentation

Ans. d. The carcinoma of the fallopian tube is usually secondary following carcinoma of the uterine body or ovary. Histologically, it is always adenocarcinoma. The diagnosed case should be treated by surgery. Papanicolaou smear may be positive without any cervical or endometrial pathology.

Q.147 The following are related to theca cell tumor except:
 a. It is a cause for postmenopausal bleeding
 b. It is usually associated with Brenner tumor
 c. It may be associated with ascites and hydrothorax
 d. Either conservative or radical surgery gives excellent result

Ans. b. It is usually associated by granulosa cell tumor.

176 Manual of Obstetrics and Gynecology for the Postgraduates

Q.148 Regarding the surgical treatment for urodynamic stress incontinence (USI) all are correct except:
   a. Burch colposuspension is superior to Marshall-Marchetti-Krantz (MMK) on 5-year follow-up
   b. Midurethrel tape procedures (TOT) are considered as Grade A
   c. Following colposuspension long-term voiding disorders are seen in about 10% of women
   d. Enterocele is more common after the suburethral sling procedures

Ans. d. It is more common with following colposuspension.

Q.149 The following statements are related to congenital adrenogenital syndrome in the female newborn except:
   a. The most common variety is due to 21-hydroxylation deficiency
   b. Palpable gonads in the inguinal canal or labial fold excludes the diagnosis
   c. Karyotype is 46 XX
   d. Normal excretion of urinary pregnanetriol

Ans. d. In adrenogenital syndrome, the gonads are placed in normal position. Urinary pregnanetriol excretion is markedly elevated.

Q.150 Ambiguous sex in a newborn can be classified as:
   a. Female intersex is due to adrenogenital syndrome or hormone induced masculinization
   b. Male intersex is due to androgen receptor defect
   c. True hermaphroditism is also due to chromosomal defect
   d. All of the above

Ans. d.

Q.151 Fetal testis has got the following functions except:
   a. Masculinization of the external genitalia
   b. Suppression of the Müllerian structures
   c. Enhancement of Wolffian structures
   d. Differentiation of the gonad

Ans. d. Differentiation of the biopotential gonad is done by SRY gene, located on the Y chromosome.

Q.152 The following statements are related to intersex except:
   a. Female intersex patients are potentially fertile with normal internal genitalia
   b. Male intersex and hermaphrodite patients are unlikely to be fertile but can have a normal sexual life
   c. Dysgenetic gonadal tissue should be removed in the presence of Y chromosome
   d. External genitalia inconsistent with sex assignment should not be changed

Ans. d. It should be surgically changed or modified. Conversion of male to female is convenient.

Q.153 The following are related to Paget's disease of vulva except:
   a. It arises from the apocrine glands of labia majora
   b. Paget's disease of the vulva is much more common than its breast counterpart
   c. The presence of Paget's cells (large cells with clear cytoplasm) within the epidermis is diagnostic
   d. Simple vulvectomy is the optimum treatment

Ans. b. Paget's disease of the breast is more common than its vulvar counter part. Multiple biopsies must be taken to exclude associated adenocarcinoma, which if present needs bilateral lymph node dissection.

Q.154 Bromocriptine is used in all except:
a. Inappropriate lactation
b. Inhibition of lactation
c. Induction of ovulation
d. Hypothyroidism

Ans. d.

Q.155 The following statements are related to bromocriptine therapy except:
a. It is used in cases with galactorrhea and amenorrhea
b. Resumption of ovulation is earlier than cessation of galactorrhea
c. Galactorrhea is commonly observed with irregular menses and with high prolactin level
d. In most of the cases, there is reduction in prolactin level and pituitary adenoma size

Ans. c. Galactorrhea is commonly observed with regular menses and with normal prolactin level.

Q.156 A huge ovarian tumor in a patient aged 18 years should best be removed by:
a. Removal of the intact tumor through an adequate abdominal incision
b. To make a small abdominal incision and to reduce the tumor size by aspiration followed by its removal
c. A vertical incision should be the choice
d. Tumor should be removed by a transverse suprapubic incision for the young girl

Ans. a and c. The ovarian tumor should be removed intact. Tapping of the tumor is avoided as the nature of the tumor is unknown—may be malignant or infective. Vertical incision is always indicated. However, a cystic tumor (benign) may be removed laparoscopically by aspiration followed by its removal.

Q.157 Endometrial curettage in a suspected case of genital tuberculosis should be done:
a. In the proliferative phase
b. In the secretory phase
c. Following antitubercular drug for 1 week in secretory phase
d. All of the above

Ans. b. The tubercle bacilli are expected to come more towards the surface with the thickness of the endometrium as in secretory phase. Prior antitubercular therapy prevents dissemination.

Q.158 The following are related to ectopy except:
a. It is due to the downward movement of the squamocolumnar junction with high level of estrogen
b. It is not in the true sense, an ulcer
c. It is only cured by cauterization or cryotherapy of the cervix
d. Nabothian follicles are formed during the process of healing

Ans. c. The physiological erosion is too often cured spontaneously.

Q.159 Pelvic endometriosis may produce infertility by all except:
a. Dyspareunia
b. Anovulation, luteal phase defect
c. Reduced macrophage activity
d. Defective ovum pick up

Ans. c. It is increased macrophage activity with sperm phagocytosis.

Q.160 *Basic investigations of an infertile couple include:*
   a. Semen analysis
   b. Detection of ovulation (BBT/Folliculometry)
   c. Detection of tubal patency (HSG/Laparoscopy)
   d. All of the above
   Ans. d.

Q.161 *Pick up the correct statements:*
   a. "Strawberry" look of the ectocervix in monilial cervicitis
   b. "Tobacco pouch" appearance of the fallopian tube is due to tubercular salpingitis
   c. "Match stick spots" in the pelvic peritoneum is in toxic shock syndrome
   d. "Retort shape" fallopian tube is due to unruptured tubal ectopic
   Ans. b. Strawberry look is peculiar to trichomonal vaginitis. Retort shape is due to large hydrosalpinx of the tube. 'Match stick spots' are characteristic of pelvic endometriosis.

Q.162 *The following statements are related to recent complete perineal tear (CPT):*
   a. The most common cause is a short perineum
   b. Routine episiotomy can prevent CPT
   c. The operative steps are like those of repair of old CPT
   d. End-to-end sphincter approximation is done
   Ans. d. The most common cause is mismanaged 2nd stage of labor. CPT is observed more in those centers where episiotomy is practised as a routine. The operative steps are unlike those of old CPT in the sense that flaps are not separated. No overlapping of sphincter margins is needed (*See* Dutta's Textbook of Gynecology, 7th Edition, p. 353, 356).

Q.163 *Turner's syndrome (45 XO) is characterized by:*
   a. Low serum gonadotropin levels   b. Absent vagina
   c. Coarctation of aorta   d. Premature menopause
   Ans. c and d. Other features are short stature, ovarian dysgenesis, neck webbing, broad chest, cubitus valgus, renal anomalies, raised gonadotropins and primary amenorrhea.

Q.164 *Choriocarcinoma is differentiated from invasive mole (chorioadenoma destruens) by:*
   a. Presence of high titer of urinary chorionic gonadotropin
   b. Presence of cannon ball shadow in the lungs
   c. Absence of villi structure on histological examination of the lesion
   d. All of the above
   Ans. c. High titer of urinary chorionic gonadotropin and cannon ball shadow in the X-ray lungs are found in both the conditions.

Q.165 *Causes of deep dyspareunia are all except:*
   a. Fixed retroverted uterus
   b. Prolapsed ovary
   c. Endometriosis on rectovaginal septum
   d. Vaginal atrophy in menopause
   Ans. d. It causes superficial dyspareunia.

Q.166 *As regard the PCOS and hyperinsulinemia:*
   a. Hyperinsulinemia is observed in about 40–80% of women with PCOS
   b. Hyperinsulinemia stimulates hepatic synthesis of SHBG

c. Metformin causes hypoglycemia in normoglycemic women
d. Metformin has many other health benefits

Ans. a and d. Insulin resistance and compensatory hyperinsulinemia is observed in about 40% of women with normal weight and 80% obese women with PCOS. Hyperinsulinemia results in decreased hepatic synthesis of SHBG and increased ovarian androgen biosynthesis. Metformin reduces fasting insulin levels, blood pressure and LDL cholesterol. Metformin does not cause hypoglycemia either with normoglycemic or with diabetic individuals. (*See* Dutta's Textbook of Gynecology, 7th Edition, p. 378, 380).

Q.167 The following are the contraindications of tubal reconstructive surgery:
a. Tubal damage following sterilization operation
b. Patients over 30 years of age
c. Pelvic tuberculosis
d. Active pelvic inflammatory disease

Ans. c and d. Reversal of tubal sterilization is more successful where tubal damage is less as following laparoscopic procedures. Age over 30, is not a contraindication, though age-related fertility is reduced.

Q.168 The following are related to estrogen secretion from the ovary:
a. Theca cells and granulosa cells are interlinked in the secretion of estrogen
b. Granulosa cells takes no part in the secretion
c. Estrogen is solely secreted from theca cells
d. Luteinized granulosa cells are the source

Ans. a. LH acts on theca cells to produce androgen precursors (*See* Dutta's Textbook of Gynecology, 7th Edition, p. 58). When activated by FSH and IGF-II, the receptors on the granulosa induces aromatase enzyme activity. This converts thecal androstenedione and testosterone to estradiol. A small amount of progesterone is also produced by the granulosa cells in the proliferative phase. IGF-II stimulates granulosa cell proliferation, aromatase activity and progesterone synthesis.

Q.169 The following are the ovarian cancer markers—match them appropriately:
a. CA 125　　　　　　　　　　　　　1. Ovarian germ cell tumor
b. Carcinoembryonic antigen　　　　2. Choriocarcinoma of ovary
c. Alpha fetoprotein　　　　　　　　3. Serous, endometrioid cancer
d. High serum hCG　　　　　　　　4. Epithelial malignancy

Ans. a = 4; b = 3; c = 1; d = 2.

Q.170 As regard the principles of screening:
a. It aims to make a diagnosis　　　　b. It guides to treatment protocol
c. It is used to select those at risk　　　d. This test is to apply to everyone

Ans. c. Screening is systematic attempt to select the high-risk group from the apparently healthy individuals. It is not essential that everyone must be included.

Q.171 The following are related to cloaca:
a. The gut caudal to the allantois widens to form the cloaca
b. The cloaca divides into a dorsal hindgut and a ventral urogenital sinus
c. The external opening of the ventral cloaca is the urogenital ostium
d. All of the above

Ans. d.

Q.172 In the female, the following structures are developed from the urogenital sinus:
a. Urinary bladder and urethra
b. Lower part of vagina
c. Bartholin's glands
d. All of the above

Ans. d.

Q.173 The contents of the mesosalpinx are:
a. Fallopian tube
b. Utero-ovarian anastomosis vessels
c. Parovarium—a vestigial structure derived from the mesonephros
d. All of the above

Ans. d. Parovarium derived from Wolffian duct (mesonephros).

Q.174 Vestigial structures derived from the Wolffian duct are:
a. Kobelt's tubules
b. Paraovarian cyst
c. Gartner's cyst
d. All of the above

Ans. d.

Q.175 The following are the features of anovular menstruation except:
a. The only symptom may be failure of conception
b. It is usually associated with painless periods
c. May be associated with premenstrual syndrome
d. May be associated with DUB

Ans. c. PMS is associated with ovulatory menstrual cycle.

Q.176 The following are related to differentiation of external genitalia except:
a. Dihydrotestosterone from fetal testis cause male differentiation of external genital organs from cloaca
b. In the absence of fetal testosterone, external genitalia of either sex fails to differentiate
c. Once the female genitalia develop, even a heavy dose of exogenous testosterone cannot alter the genital structure to male
d. Differentiation in male is earlier than female

Ans. b. In the absence of fetal testosterone, the female external genitalia will form.

Q.177 The following are X-linked inherited conditions except:
a. Stein-Leventhal syndrome
b. Congenital adrenal hyperplasia
c. True hermaphroditism
d. Male pseudohermaphroditism

Ans. b. Congenital adrenal hyperplasia is considered to be an autosomal recessive inherited condition.

Q.178 Subnuclear vacuolation in the endometrial glands appears (in a regular ovular menstrual cycle) on:
a. 14th day
b. 17th day
c. 20th day
d. 23rd day

Ans. b.

Q.179 Mortality rate per 10,000 procedures is highest in:
a. Vaginal hysterectomy
b. Abdominal hysterectomy
c. Cesarean hysterectomy
d. Cesarean section

Ans. c. Overall mortality per 10,000 cases are for — (a) 2.7; (b) 8.6; (c) 71; (d) 10.

Q.180 Causes of isosexual (true) precocious puberty are all except:
   a. Constitutional
   b. Juvenile hypothyroidism
   c. Albright's syndrome
   d. Granulosa cell tumor

Ans. d. Isosexual is synonymous with true precocious puberty. In this condition, sexual maturation occurs due to premature precocious maturation of hypothalamo-pituitary-ovarian axis. Granulosa cell tumor produces pseudoprecocious puberty. There is no premature ovarian maturation and the serum gonadotropins are not elevated.

Q.181 Regarding primary peritoneal adenocarcinoma (PPA):
   a. In PPA, the ovaries are either absent or normal in size
   b. The tumor is predominantly of the serous type histologically
   c. FIGO staging for ovarian carcinoma is currently being used for PPA
   d. Prophylactic oophorectomy is protective against PPA

Ans. a, b and c. PPA is thought to be a separate clinical entitity from papillary serous ovarian carcinoma (PSOC). Clinical presentation of cases with PPA and PSOC are similar and the prognosis of patients with PPA is poor. Prophylactic oophorectomy is not protective against PPA.

Q.182 Regarding gamete intrafallopian transfer (GIFT):
   a. Indicated in cases with nonfunctioning fallopian tube
   b. Unexplained infertility is an indication
   c. Controlled ovarian hyperstimulation (superovulation) is needed
   d. Gametes are transferred through a hysteroscope

Ans. b and c. Fallopian tubes must be patent. Collected oocytes and motile sperm are transferred to the tubes (fimbrial end) through laparoscope.

Q.183 The following are related to herpes genitalis except:
   a. Herpes genitalis is chiefly caused by herpes simplex virus type-1
   b. It is related to carcinoma of the vulva and cervix
   c. It tends to recur
   d. Neonatal risk is more with primary infection in pregnancy

Ans. a. Herpes simplex virus type-2 is most common (85%) and not the type-1.

Q.184 The biochemical effects of FSH are all except:
   a. Increases synthesis of its own receptors
   b. Inhibits LH receptor synthesis
   c. Induces aromatase enzyme system
   d. Stimulates plasminogen activator

Ans. b. FSH stimulates LH receptor synthesis.

Q.185 The refrigerants used in cryosurgery include:
   a. Freon (– 60° C)
   b. Carbon dioxide (– 60° C)
   c. Nitrous oxide (– 80° C)
   d. All of the above

Ans. d.

Q.186 Criteria for high-risk metastatic trophoblastic disease include all except:
   a. Metastasis of brain or liver or both
   b. Initial serum hCG more than 40,000 mIU/mL
   c. Duration of disease more than 1 year from the termination of the preceding pregnancy
   d. Failure of prior chemotherapy

Ans. c. It should be 4 months and not 1 year.

Q.187 *The following are related to danazol therapy in endometriosis except:*
  a. Plasma estradiol level is significantly depressed
  b. Inhibition of pituitary secretion of both FSH and LH
  c. Elevates the level of sex hormone binding globulin (SHBG)
  d. Menopausal symptoms may occur

Ans. c. Level is low as the hepatic synthesis is depressed. Level of free testosterone is raised which causes atrophy of the endometrium.

Q.188 *Female genital tuberculosis:*
  a. Genital tract involvement results from lymphatic spread
  b. Premenstrual endometrial biopsy is diagnostic
  c. Polymerase chain reaction (PCR) techniques have got higher sensitivity in detection
  d. Reproductive outcome following antituberculous chemotherapy is satisfactory

Ans. c. Genital tuberculosis is usually secondary to primary infection (lungs, bones, lymph nodes). It is by hematogenous spread leading to endosalpingitis. Caseous granulomatous lesions with giant cells on histology are suggestive of TB but is not diagnostic as it can be seen in fungal infection and sarcoidosis. PCR can detect even less than 10 organism in a clinical specimen compared to 10,000 necessary for smear positivity. Reproductive outcome even after treatment is poor. Pregnancy rate is about 20%, livebirth rate is only 7%. Risk of miscarriage and ectopic pregnancy are high.

Q.189 *The following are related to chromosomal abnormality except:*
  a. Nondisjunction is the most common chromosomal error in offsprings
  b. Down's syndrome is the most common aneuploidy in livebirths
  c. Turner's syndrome is the only human monosomy compatible with survival
  d. Chromosomal translocations are not related to miscarriage

Ans. d. Structural chromosomal abnormality—translocations (reciprocal) are most commonly responsible for recurrent miscarriages.

Q.190 *All the statement are correct except:*
  a. Presence of the ovary is essential for female genital tract differentiation
  b. Two normal "X" chromosomes seem to be essential for normal ovarian function
  c. A loss of even a portion of one of the "X" chromosomes results in gonadal dysgenesis
  d. Apart from SRY, autosomal genes are essential for gonadal differentiation

Ans. a. Ovaries do not play any part in the embryological development of the genital tract.

Q.191 *Definite diagnostic procedure to detect invasive carcinoma cervix:*
  a. Colposcopy
  b. Wedge biopsy
  c. Cone biopsy
  d. Cervical cytology

Ans. c.

Q.192 *Preferred conservative surgery for CIN lesion of cervix:*
  a. Cone biopsy
  b. Cryosurgery
  c. Carbon dioxide laser beam
  d. Large loop excision of the transformation zone

Ans. d. Tissue is available for biopsy and it is a simple procedure.

Q.193 Regarding carcinoma of the cervix:
   a. High-risk human papilloma virus (HPV) are responsible for most cases
   b. Use of contraceptive pill in HPV positive women increases the risk of cancer
   c. Progesterone only pill increases the risk of cancer
   d. Women with abnormal smears are contraindicated for pill use

Ans. a and b. HPV oncogenic subtypes HPV 16, 18 is responsible for cervical cancers; c. No relationship has been found between POP use and cervical cancer; d. Pills uses is not contraindicated for women with abnormal smears. However, women with high grade CIN lesion may have alternative contraception.

Q.194 Regarding the use of selective estrogen receptor modulators (SERMs) in postmenopausal women:
   a. Tamoxifen decreases the risk of endometrial cancer
   b. Raloxifene reduces the vasomotor symptoms
   c. Raloxifene elevates the level of low density lipoproteins
   d. Raloxifene has no effect on the development of endometrial pathology

Ans. d and a. Tamoxifen has both estrogenic and antiestrogenic activity. It stimulates endometrium and increases the risk of endometrial cancer; b. Raloxifene does not improve vasomotor symptoms of menopause; c. Raloxifene reduces total cholesterol and LDL and increases cardioprotective fraction of HDL.

Q.195 Absolute contraindications of laparoscopy are:
   a. Diaphragmatic hernia
   b. Generalized peritonitis
   c. Patient on anticoagulant therapy
   d. Previous incomplete laparoscopy

Ans. a, b and c. Previous incomplete laparoscopy is an indication for repeat laparoscopy for detailed evaluation.

Q.196 For effective pneumoperitoneum, the veress needle can be introduced into the peritoneal cavity through:
   a. Subumbilical fold
   b. Left subcostal (Patner's) point
   c. Left McBurney's point
   d. All of the above

Ans. d.

Q.197 For operative hysteroscopy, the preferred substance to distend the uterine cavity:
   a. Carbon dioxide at the rate of 80–150 mL/minute
   b. Saline or dextrose solution in rapid drip
   c. Heavy dextran (70%)
   d. Glycine 1.5%

Ans. d. Glycine is commonly used because blood is not miscible with glycine. As such, the view is better and it does not conduct electricity.

Q.198 The following are related to pseudoprecocious (peripheral) puberty in female except:
   a. There is always presence of any organic lesion either in the hypothalamo-pituitary-gonadal axis or in the adrenal
   b. Isolated development of sexual characteristics of puberty

c. Ovulation occurs usually
d. None of the above
Ans. c. Ovulation fails to occur.

Q.199 Causes of pseudoprecocious (GnRH independent) puberty are all except:
a. Congenital adrenal hyperplasia
b. Cushing's syndrome
c. Granulosa cell tumor
d. Juvenile hypothyroidism
Ans. d. Juvenile hypothyroidism produces true (GnRH dependent) one.

Q.200 The most common indication for diagnostic laparoscopy in gynecology:
a. Chronic pelvic pain
b. Infertility work-up
c. Genital malformation
d. Gonadal abnormality
Ans. a.

Q.201 To achieve pneumoperitoneum for operative laparoscopy, the gas used is:
a. Nitrous oxide
b. Carbon dioxide
c. Oxygen
d. Air
Ans. b. *See* Dutta's Textbook of Gynecology, 7th Edition, p. 508.

Q.202 The following are related to androgen:
a. The term hyperandrogenemia implies virilism and hirsutism
b. The most potent androgen is dihydrotestosterone followed by testosterone
c. In normal women, about 1% of testosterone is free
d. Pilosebaceous units in the skin are sensitive to androgens and their number increases with androgen level
Ans. b and c. Sebaceous glands and hair follicles together comprise pilosebaceous unit. Total number of hair follicle per unit area of skin is fixed by 22 weeks of gestational age. (*See* Dutta's Textbook of Gynecology, 7th Edition, p. 473).

Q.203 The following statements are related to development of female genital organs except:
a. In the absence of anti-Müllerian hormone (AMH), the urogenital sinus develops towards female
b. The development of the female genital tract organs is due to the absence of testis
c. AMH gene mutation may cause persistence of uterus and tubes in a male
d. AMH is secreted by the Leydig cells
Ans. d. AMH is secreted by the Sertoli cells.

Q.204 The following are the relations of the ovarian fossa except:
a. Superiorly, to the external iliac artery
b. Posteriorly, the ureter and internal iliac vessels
c. Laterally, the obturator vessels and nerves
d. Medially, coils of intestine
Ans. a. The ovarian fossa is related superiorly to external iliac vein. External iliac artery is still beyond it.

Q.205 The following are related to pelvic ureter except:
a. The ureter enters the pelvis behind the root of the mesentery on the right side
b. Its length is about 13 cm

c. The mucous layer is lined by columnar epithelium
d. It is crossed by uterine artery anteriorly

Ans. c. The mucous coat is lined by transitional epithelium.

Q.206 The following are the contents of deep perineal pouch except:
a. Deep transverse perinei (paired)
b. Sphincter urethrae
c. Blood vessels and nerves
d. Bartholin's gland

Ans. d. Bartholin's gland is situated in the superficial perineal pouch.

Q.207 The following are related to round ligament except:
a. Developmentally, it corresponds to the gubernaculum testis
b. It is attached to the uterine cornu anterior to uterine tube
c. It courses medial to the inferior epigastric artery
d. It terminates at the upper border of labium majus

Ans. c. Round ligament courses lateral to the artery and through the deep ring.

Q.208 Lymphatics of the body of the uterus drain primarily into the following glands except:
a. Para-aortic
b. Deep inguinal
c. Internal iliac
d. External iliac

Ans. b. Lymphatics from the cornu of the uterus drain into the superficial group of inguinal glands.

Q.209 Superficial inguinal glands receive lymphatics from the following except:
a. Cornu of the uterus
b. Labia majora
c. Glans of clitoris
d. Bartholin's gland

Ans. c. Glans of the clitoris directly drains into the pelvic nodes.

Q.210 Sensory component of pudendal nerve supplies the following structures except:
a. Skin of the vulva
b. Lower half of the anal canal
c. Clitoris
d. Whole of urethra

Ans. d.

Q.211 The following are related to the course of pudendal nerve except:
a. The nerve leaves the pelvis through greater sciatic foramen between piriformis and coccygeus muscle
b. The nerve re-enters the pelvis curling the ischial spine through lesser sciatic foramen
c. Pudendal canal is at the medial wall of the ischiorectal fossa
d. The dorsal nerve to the clitoris is a content of the deep perineal pouch

Ans. c. The pudendal canal, which is a fascial tunnel, is situated at the lateral wall of the ischiorectal fossa about 2.5 cm above the ischial tuberosity.

Q.212 Regarding pneumoperitoneum during laparoscopic surgery:
a. CO_2 is less soluble in blood than air
b. CO_2 is not easily excreted by the lungs
c. CO_2 is buffered by formation of bicarbonate
d. Insufflation pressures of 10–15 mm Hg are well-tolerated

Ans. c and d. CO_2 is twenty times more soluble in blood than air and it is easily excreted by the lungs. It is nontoxic and does not support combustion. It is thus preferred in laparoscopic surgery. (*See* Dutta's Textbook of Gynecology, 7th Edition, p. 508).

Q.213 The following are in relation to Bartholin's gland except:
a. It is a compound racemose gland
b. It measures about 5 mm
c. It lies deep to the urogenital diaphragm
d. Its duct measures about 20 mm

Ans. c. Bartholin's gland lies superficial to urogenital diaphragm, in the superficial perineal pouch. (*See* Dutta's Textbook of Gynecology, 7th Edition, p. 2).

Q.214 The following are related to female pelvic ureter except:
a. It enters the pelvis on the left side behind the apex of mesosigmoid
b. It forms the posterior boundary of the ovarian fossa
c. It lies between the ovary and external iliac artery—as it courses in lateral pelvic wall
d. It changes its course forwards and medially at the level of ischial spine

Ans. c. The ureter lies between the ovary and internal iliac artery as it courses in the lateral pelvic wall.

Q.215 The following are related to ovarian structures except:
a. The earliest primordial follicles are found in the outermost part of the ovarian cortex
b. The follicular cells are derived from the coelomic epithelium
c. Cytologically, the hilus cells are identical to testicular leydig cells
d. The characteristic stroma of the cortex does not appear until several years after birth

Ans. a. The earliest primordial follicle are present in the corticomedullary junction.

Q.216 The following are few branches of anterior division of internal iliac artery except:
a. Uterine
b. Vaginal
c. Superior gluteal
d. Middle rectal

Ans. c. Superior gluteal artery is a branch of posterior division of internal iliac artery.

Q.217 The following are related to fallopian tube except:
a. It is developed from paramesonephric duct
b. Its widest part is infundibulum and the longest part is the isthmus
c. The mucous lining is columnar
d. The blood supply is from uterine and ovarian

Ans. b. The maximum diameter of the infundibulum measures about 6 mm and the ampulla is the longest part, measuring 5 cm.

Q.218 The following are related to levator ani except:
a. Viewed from above, it slopes downwards, forwards and medially
b. The inferior surface is related to the anatomical perineum
c. It is entirely innervated by pudendal nerve
d. Its important function is to support the pelvic organs

Ans. c. Apart from the pudendal nerve (S2, S3), the levator ani is supplied directly by the S4 from the pelvic surface.

Self-Assessment in Gynecology 187

Q.219 Arterial supply to the vulva is from the following except:
   a. Internal pudendal
   b. Superficial external pudendal
   c. Deep external pudendal
   d. Inferior epigastric

Ans. d.

Q.220 The following are related to internal iliac artery except:
   a. It measures about 2 cm
   b. Internal iliac vein lies anteriorly
   c. One of its visceral branches is middle rectal
   d. One of its parietal branches is inferior gluteal

Ans. b. Internal iliac vein lies posterior to the artery.

Q.221 The following are related to development of genital organs except:
   a. Bartholin's gland is developed from the urogenital sinus
   b. Clitoris is developed from genital tubercle
   c. Labia minora is developed from the urogenital sinus
   d. Endometrium is developed from the coelomic epithelium

Ans. c. Labia minora is developed from the urogenital folds.

Q.222 The following are related to development of ovary except:
   a. Ovary is developed from the gonadal ridge
   b. The germ cells are endodermal in origin from the yolk sac
   c. The bipotential gonad develops into an ovary about two weeks before the testicular development
   d. At birth, the ovaries are situated at or above the pelvic brim

Ans. c. The bipotential gonad develops into an ovary about two weeks after the testicular development.

Q.223 In female, the following structures are developed from the urogenital sinus except:
   a. Urethrovesical unit
   b. Vestibule
   c. Bartholin's gland
   d. Anal canal

Ans. d. The anal canal is not developed from the urogenital sinus. It develops from the cloaca—an endodermal structure.

Q.224 The following are related to differentiation of external genitalia except:
   a. Dihydrotestosterone from fetal testis causes male differentiation of external genital organs
   b. In the absence of fetal testosterone, the female external genitalia will form
   c. Testicular development is by active gene (SRY) control and expression
   d. In the absence of gonad, male external genitalia will develop

Ans. d. In the absence of gonad, female external genitalia will form and the individual is phenotypically female.

Q.225 Clinical presentations of hematometra following cervical atresia are all except:
   a. Amenorrhea
   b. Periodic pain in lower abdomen
   c. Urinary complaints to the extent of retention
   d. Lump in the lower abdomen

Ans. c. Hematometra following cervical atresia will not produce any urinary symptoms. Urinary symptoms are predominant in hematocolpos.

Q.226 *Regarding oligoasthenoteratozoospermia (OAT) syndrome:*
   a. Testicular biopsy can differentiate obstructive from testicular cause of oligospermia
   b. The biopsied tissue should be sent in formal saline
   c. Congenital absence of vas deferens is observed in Young's syndrome
   d. The number of sperms required for IVF and ICSI are the same

Ans. a. Testicular biopsy can detect spermatogenic disorder; the tissue should be sent in either Bouin's, Zenker's or in buffered glutaraldehyde solution. Formaline solution is avoided because it causes destruction of seminiferous tubular structures. 95% of men with cystic fibrosis have congenital absence of vas. IVF needs 50,000–100,000 sperm for insemination of the eggs, whereas ICSI is performed with essentially one sperm for one egg (*See* Dutta's Textbook of Gynecology, 7th Edition, p. 190, 206).

Q.227 *The following are related to hypothalamopituitary secretions except:*
   a. Gonadotropin-releasing hormone (GnRH) is a decapeptide
   b. Thyrotropin-releasing hormone (TRH) is a tridecapeptide
   c. Corticotropin-releasing hormone (CRH) is a tetradecapeptide
   d. Oxytocin is a nonpeptide

Ans. b. TRH is a tripeptide and not tridecapeptide.

Q.228 *The following are the control of neurotransmitters and neuromodulators on GnRH secretion except:*
   a. Norepinephrine exerts stimulatory effect
   b. Dopamine exerts inhibitory effect
   c. Serotonin exerts stimulatory effect
   d. Endogenous opioids inhibits the release

Ans. c. Serotonin exerts inhibitory effects on GnRH secretion.

Q.229 *The following are the actions of FSH except:*
   a. It is involved in multiplication of granulosa cells
   b. It synthesizes its own receptors in the granulosa cells
   c. It converts androstenedione to estradiol
   d. It stimulates resumption of meiosis with extrusion of first polar body

Ans. d. It is the LH which stimulates resumption of meiosis probably by interfering oocyte maturation inhibitory factor (OMI) present in the antral fluid.

Q.230 *The following are the actions of LH except:*
   a. It predominantly synthesizes its own receptor in the granulosa cells
   b. It induces luteinization of the granulosa cells to secrete progesterone
   c. It synthesizes prostaglandins
   d. It helps in formation and maintenance of corpus luteum

Ans. a. FSH synthesizes its own receptors and also the receptors for LH (*See* Dutta's Textbook of Gynecology, 7th Edition, p. 57).

Q.231 *The ovarian sites of secretion of androgens are all except:*
   a. Stroma
   b. Theca interna
   c. Theca externa
   d. Granulosa cells

Ans. c. *See* Dutta's Textbook of Gynecology, 7th Edition, p. 58, 61.

Q.232 Regarding ovarian cancer:
  a. Combined oral contraceptive pill reduces the risk of ovarian cancer
  b. Mutation in BRCA genes account for about 80% of all ovarian cancers
  c. Prophylactic salpingo-oophorectomy has no effect on the risk of breast cancer
  d. Prophylactic salpingo-oophorectomy reduces the risk of ovarian cancer
Ans. a and d. BRCA gene mutation group account for only 10% of all ovarian cancers. Prophylactic oophorectomy reduces the incidence of breast cancer by 50%.

Q.233 The following are the approximate time interval of hormonal events prior to ovulation except:
  a. Onset of estradiol rise—about 84 hours
  b. Onset of LH rise—about 72 hours
  c. Estradiol peak—about 24 hours
  d. LH peak—about 16 hours
Ans. b. Onset of LH surge occurs about 32–36 hours before ovulation.

Q.234 The following are related to prostaglandins in relation to menstrual bleeding and pain except:
  a. $PGF2\alpha$ causes myometrial contraction and vasoconstriction
  b. PGE_2 produces myometrial contraction but causes vasodilatation
  c. Leukotrienes and endothelins causes myometrial relaxation and vasoconstriction
  d. The bleeding and pain are related to the relative proportion of different prostaglandins
Ans. c. They cause myometrial contraction and vasoconstriction.

Q.235 The following subjects may be excluded from routine cervical cancer screening program except:
  a. Women who had never been sexually active
  b. Women over the age of 60 who had negative smears in the past
  c. Women who had hysterectomy for benign lesion
  d. Women on oral pill
Ans. d. Oral pill users should be included in the routine screening program.

Q.236 The risk factors of acute pelvic inflammatory disease (PID) are the following except:
  a. Menstruating teenagers who have multiple sex partners
  b. IUD users
  c. Women with monogamous partner who had vasectomy
  d. Previous history of acute PID
Ans. c. It is infact a protective factor.

Q.237 The following embryonic and adult structures are related:
  a. Mesonephric tubules   1. Labia minora
  b. Mesonephric duct   2. Urethra
  c. Urogenital sinus   3. Duct of Gartner
  d. Urogenital folds   4. Epoophoron
Ans. a = 4; b = 3; c = 2; d = 1.

Q.238 The following are the clinical presentations of genital tuberculosis in Indian context except:
a. Infertility is present in about 70% cases of pelvic tuberculosis
b. About 10% infertile women have got genital tuberculosis
c. There may not be any menstrual abnormality
d. Menorrhagia is the late manifestation

Ans. d. Menorrhagia is the early manifestation due to endometrial hyperemia.

Q.239 The following are the primary sites of acute gonococcal infection except:
a. Urethra
b. Bartholin's gland
c. Skene's gland (paraurethral glands)
d. Ectocervix

Ans. d. Ectocervix covered by squamous epithelium, resistant to gonococcal infection. The endocervical glands are the primary sites of infection.

Q.240 The following are related to herpes genitalis infection except:
a. The causative organism is *herpes simplex* virus type 2
b. The entity is possibly linked with cervical carcinoma
c. Women should have annual cervical smear
d. A primary infection in the genital tract in late pregnancy can have safe vaginal delivery

Ans. d. Primary HSV infection in the genital tract in late pregnancy should have a delivery by abdominal route to minimize fetal affection from the birth canal during vaginal delivery. The delivery should be completed within 4 hours of rupture of the membranes.

Q.241 The following are related to function of testis except:
a. Seminiferous tubules are the site of spermatogenesis
b. Leydig cells are the site of production of testosterone
c. Sertoli cells produce androgen binding protein
d. Inhibin is synthesized by the leydig cells

Ans. d. Inhibin is synthesized from the sertoli cells of the testis in response to FSH.

Q.242 Regarding uterine artery embolization (UAE) for the treatment of uterine fibroids:
a. Polyvinyl particles are used for the procedure
b. It is an alternative to myomectomy in infertile women
c. It causes amenorrhea in 25% of the women
d. Pregnancy outcome is uneventful following the procedure

Ans. a. RCOG and NICE have stated that UAE should not be offered to women who desirous of future childbearing. Avascular necrosis of myometrium makes it prone to rupture during pregnancy. Amenorrhea occurs in 1% of women and often it is transient.

Q.243 The following are related to SHBG except:
a. It is a glycoprotein
b. The circulatory level is directly related to weight
c. Increased circulatory levels of insulin lower its level
d. Danazol decreases its level

Ans. b. The circulatory level of SHBG is inversely related to weight. In obese, the SHBG level decreases.

Self-Assessment in Gynecology

Q.244 The following are related to increased circulatory SHBG except:
a. Pregnancy
b. Hyperthyroidism
c. Combined steroidal contraceptives users
d. Hirsutism

Ans. d. In hirsutism, SHBG is decreased resulting in increased free testosterone to act on the target cells—hair follicles. SHBG is a glycoprotein. 69% of estradiol and 80% of testosterone are bound to SHBG and only 30% and 19% respectively, are bound to albumin, only about 1% of testosterone are unbound and free. Hyperthyroidism, pregnancy and estrogen administration increase SHBG levels whereas corticosteroids, androgens and progestogens decrease SHBG. The circulatory level of SHBG is inversely related to weight. Hyperinsulinemia lowers the SHBG levels.

Q.245 The following are related to inhibin except:
a. It is secreted from the granulosa cells
b. FSH controls its secretion
c. It preferentially stimulates FSH
d. When the follicle grows—level of activin declines and levels of inhibin and follistatin increase

Ans. c. Inhibin inhibits FSH.

Q.246 The following are related to excretory channel of adult testis except:
a. Vas deferens measures 30–35 cm in length
b. Seminiferous tubules, if stretched, measures about 70 cm
c. Epididymis is about 5–6 meters long
d. The first part of the semen contains seminal vesicle secretion

Ans. d. The last part of the semen contains seminal vesicle secretion. First part of semen contains highest concentration of sperm.

Q.247 Derivatives of embryonic urogenital structures in male and female are all except:
a. Ventral aspect of penis corresponds to labia minora
b. Prostatic utricle corresponds to vagina
c. Ductus epididymis corresponds to Gartner's duct
d. Seminiferous tubules corresponds to ovarian follicle

Ans. c. Ductus epididymis corresponds to duct of epoophoron in female.

Q.248 Regarding the viral infections true statements are:
a. Human papilloma virus (HPV) infection is associated with koilocytic atypia on cervical cytology
b. Nosocomial exposure is a mode of spread for HIV
c. The carrier neonate of hepatitis B virus may suffer from hepatocellular carcinoma
d. Patients with anti-HBe ('e' antibodies) are of high-risk for transmitting the infection

Ans. a and c. Patients with HBeAg ('e' antigen) are high-risk for transmitting the infection, but presence of 'e' antibodies is protective against transmission. Koilocytes have irregular hyperchromatic cells surrounded by clear cytoplasm. Certain HPV types are strongly associated with some genital cancers.

Q.249 The major contribution to the human seminal fluid is from:
a. Testes
b. Seminal vesicles
c. Prostate
d. Bulbourethral and urethral glands

Ans. b. The seminal vesicle contributes 60% and prostate about 30% of the seminal fluid.

Q.250 Regarding Paget's disease of the vulva all are true except:
   a. It is a special type of VIN
   b. Cells are large with abundant pale cytoplasm
   c. Incidence of associated carcinoma (breast, cervix, ovary) is about 30%
   d. Prognosis is always poor

Ans. d. Prognosis is good unless associated with dermal invasion or other carcinomas. (See Dutta's Textbook of Gynecology, 7th Edition, p. 261).

Q.251 As regard the use of laser in gynecology, all are correct except:
   a. Management of CIN, VIN, VaIN
   b. Laser laparoscopy for ectopic pregnancy
   c. Laser hysteroscopy for presacral neurectomy
   d. It acts by tissue cutting, vaporization or coagulation

Ans. c. Laser hysteroscopy is used for endometrial ablation and septum resection. Presacral neurectomy is done by laser laparoscopy.

Q.252 Laser properties are all except:
   a. Spot size is the point of convergence of the laser beams
   b. Power density is the degree of concentration of the laser beams
   c. Smaller the spot size greater the power density
   d. Laser-tissue interaction results in cell explosion and vaporization

Ans. b. It is the measure of laser effects on tissues (Watts/cm^2). (See Dutta's Textbook of Gynecology, 7th Edition, p. 103).

Q.253 As regard the endoscopic visualization procedures match the following:

a.	Laparoscopy	1.	Endometrial cavity
b.	Hysteroscopy	2.	Cervix, vagina, vulva
c.	Salpingoscopy	3.	Peritoneal cavity
d.	Colposcopy	4.	Tubal mucosa

Ans. a = 3; b = 1; c = 4; d = 2.

Q.254 Regarding Asherman's syndrome all are true except:
   a. May occur following myomectomy
   b. Always associated with amenorrhea
   c. Progesterone challenge test is negative
   d. Hysteroscopy or hysterography can be diagnostic

Ans. b. There may also be hypomenorrhoea or Oligomenorrhea depending on the extent. (See Dutta's Textbook of Gynecology, 7th Edition, p. 378).

Q.255 Genuine stress incontinence (GSI) is due to all of these except:
   a. Dysfunction of the intrinsic bladder sphincter
   b. Descent of the bladder neck and proximal urethra below the urogenital diaphragm
   c. Hypermobility of the urethra
   d. Increase in intraurethral pressure

Ans. d. There is decrease in intraurethral pressure.

Q.256 Retention of urine in association with gynecologic lesion—match the following:

a.	Postoperative	1.	Uterine fibroid impacted in POD
b.	Cryptomenorrhea	2.	Hematocolpos

c. Secondary amenorrhea
d. Menorrhagia
3. Most common cause of retention
4. Retroverted gravid uterus

Ans. a = 3; b = 2; c = 4; d = 1.

Q.257 As regard ovulation all are correct except:
   a. Ovulation occurs 24–36 hours after the estradiol peak
   b. Ovulation occurs 24 hours after the LH peak
   c. Ovulation occurs 32–36 hours after the onset of LH surge
   d. A threshold of LH surge should persist for 24 hours

Ans. b. It is 10–16 hours after the LH peak.

Q.258 Regarding female sterilization all are true except:
   a. Postpartum sterilization has lower failure rate compared to interval procedure
   b. Failure may be due to technical error or formation of tuboperitoneal fistula
   c. Risks of ectopic pregnancy is increased
   d. Laparoscopic method is contraindicated in the puerperium

Ans. a.

Q.259 Regarding CIN III all are correct except:
   a. It is same as CIS and HSIL
   b. Usually treated by LLETZ
   c. Pelvic lymph node involvement is about 2%
   d. May extend into the vagina

Ans. c. It is not a carcinoma so no node is involved. (*See* Dutta's Textbook of Gynecology, 7th Edition, p. 262).

Q.260 Regarding cervical cancer all are correct except:
   a. Radiotherapy is ineffective in adenocarcinomas
   b. IVP is required for FIGO staging
   c. Stage for the prognosis of adenocarcinoma and squamous cell cancers are the same
   d. In stage Ib, pelvic lymph node involvement is about 18%

Ans. a. Adenocarcinoma is not radioresistant and both are treated similarly.

Q.261 Indications of diagnostic conization are all except:
   a. Entire squamocolumnar junction is not seen
   b. Normal colposcopy with persistent abnormal cytology
   c. Cytology, colposcopy and biopsy revealed CIN lesion
   d. Colposcopically directed biopsy revealed microinvasion

Ans. c. *See* Dutta's Textbook of Gynecology, 7th Edition, p. 487.

Q.262 In microinvasive cancer of the cervix all are true except:
   a. Belongs to Stage IA
   b. Microscopically, measured depth of invasion should not be more than 5 mm
   c. Can be diagnosed by colposcopy
   d. Can be treated by cone biopsy

Ans. c. Depth of invasion is measured only by biopsy. (*See* Dutta's Textbook of Gynecology, 7th Edition, p. 282).

Q.263 Regarding cervical cytology screening all are correct except:
a. Screening programs have failed to reduce the mortality from cervical cancer
b. A dyskaryotic cell often reverts back to normal
c. Papanicolaou's grade V smear suggests malignancy
d. A dyskaryotic cell shows pleomorphism and multinucleation

Ans. a. Mortality has steadily declined due to Papanicolaou smear screening programs.

Q.264 As regard to endometrial carcinoma all are correct except:
a. Serous cell histology has poorer prognosis compared to endometrioid type
b. Prognostically depth of myometrial invasion is important
c. Squamous metaplasia on histology has worst prognosis
d. Ovarian metastasis is about 3–5%

Ans. a. Adenoacanthoma has similar prognosis as that of adenocarcinoma. Serous cell type has worst prognosis.

Q.265 As regard the functions of LH and FSH all are true except:
a. FSH rescues follicles from apoptosis
b. FSH stimulates production of androgen precursors from theca cells
c. Aromatase in granulosa cells make the follicular microenvironment estrogenic
d. Ovarian steroidogenesis is by two cell two gonadotropin mechanism

Ans. b. LH acts on theca cells to produce androsterone, androstenedione and testosterone (*See* Dutta's Textbook of Gynecology, 7th Edition, p. 58, 59).

Q.266 As regard the rising incidence of endometrial carcinoma all are true except:
a. More awareness to diagnosis
b. Increased life expectancy
c. Injudicious use of estrogen as HRT
d. Prolonged use of combined oral pills

Ans. d. It is protective to endometrial carcinoma.

Q.267 Increased incidence of endometrial carcinoma is observed in women with:
a. Cigarette smoking
b. Premature menopause
c. Members of the Lynch type-II family
d. Women using DMPA as contraception

Ans. c.

Q.268 Regarding sarcoma botryoides:
a. Usually occurs around the age of 18
b. It is an embryonal rhabdomyosarcoma
c. It is not sensitive to chemotherapy
d. It is a tumor of the uterine body

Ans. b. Embryonal rhabdomyosarcoma is a highly malignant tumor, seen commonly below the age of 5, arising from the cervix or vagina (lower end of Müllerian tubercle) and is sensitive to chemotherapy. (*See* Dutta's Textbook of Gynecology, 7th Edition, p. 323).

Q.269 Regarding neoplasms of the ovary:
a. Stromal invasion is commonly present in ovarian tumors of borderline malignancy
b. Lymphocytic infiltration is characteristic to dysgerminoma

c. Presence of ascites and pleural effusion in Brenner tumor indicates poor prognosis
d. Endometrioid carcinoma of the ovary may coexist with endometrial adenocarcinoma

Ans. b and d. Stromal invasion is absent. The epithelium shows multilayering, cellular atypia, pleomorphism and mitotic activity. Brenner tumor may present with the features of Meigs' syndrome and treatment prognosis is satisfactory. 20% of ovarian endometrioid carcinoma is associated with endometrial carcinoma.

Q.270 Concerning fibroids:
a. Use of GnRH analogs cause permanent reduction in size
b. Pregnancy following myomectomy is about 80%
c. Recurrence rate following myomectomy is about 30%
d. Growth factors (IGF-1, EGF) stimulates myoma to grow

Ans. d; a. Regrowth of myoma occurs often after 3 months of therapy; b. It is about 50–60%; c. It is about 1–10% depending on the number.

Q.271 Regarding polycystic ovarian syndrome (PCOS) all are true except:
a. Hirsutism is directly related to the level of 5α-reductase activity
b. Reduced level of sex hormone binding globulin (SHBG)
c. Acanthosis nigricans
d. Decreased pulse frequency of GnRH

Ans. d. Increased pulse frequency of GnRH with preferential secretion of LH.

Q.272 Regarding PCOS:
a. Characterized by increased insulin sensitivity
b. Most common cause of anovulatory infertility
c. Hyperandrogenism is an inconsistent observation
d. Polycystic morphology of the ovaries is characteristic to the diagnosis

Ans. b; c. Hyperandrogenism is characteristic to the diagnosis and polycystic ovaries are observed in about 20% normal women in reproductive period with ultrasonography.

Q.273 Concerning PCOS:
a. PCOS increases the risk of type I diabetes mellitus
b. Levonorgestrel-releasing IUS is a management option
c. Metformin decreases insulin secretion
d. Insulin therapy is a management option

Ans. b. Women with PCOS have an increased risk of developing type-2 diabetes and gestational diabetes. LNG-IUS gives endometrial protection against hyperplasia and carcinoma due to unopposed estrogen action. Such women are insulin resistant due to abnormalities of the insulin receptor. Metformin is used to improve sensitivity to insulin like other strategies that includes diet, exercise, lifestyle changes. Metformin improves hyperandrogenism, fertility and lipid profile. However, it has some gastrointestinal adverse effects (anorexia, nausea, diarrhea, flatulence).

Q.274 Regarding bacterial vaginosis, all are true except:
a. Homogeneous vaginal discharge with pH 5.0–6.0
b. Positive KOH—with fishy odor
c. Positive clue cells in 100% of cases
d. It is due to *Gardnerella vaginalis*

Ans. c. Clue cells are diagnostic but about 40% patients may not have clue cells.

Q.275 These organisms cause vaginitis—match them appropriately:
- a. Trichomonas vaginalis
- b. Candida albicans
- c. Gardnerella vaginalis
- d. Mobiluncus

1. Gram-negative rod
2. Stippled desquamated epithelial cells
3. Gram-positive fungus
4. 'Strawberry' cervix

Ans. a = 4; b = 3; c = 2; d = 1.

Q.276 Regarding prolactinomas:
- a. Often progresses from microadenoma to macroadenoma
- b. In men, it causes oligospermia
- c. Surgical excision completely cures the patient on long-term basis
- d. Women with normal prolactin level can have prolactinomas

Ans. d; a. Not necessarily all microadenomas progress to macroadenoma. b. In men it causes impotence, decreased libido. c. Cases may recur even following surgery or may develop panhypopituitarism.

Q.277 Regarding sex hormone binding globulin (SHBG):
- a. 25% of circulating testosterone in female is bound to SHBG
- b. Combined oral pill lowers its level
- c. Low level predicts development of type II diabetes mellitus
- d. SHBG binds 70% of circulating progesterone

Ans. c. SHBG is a glycoprotein. 69% of E2 and 80% of T are bound to SHBG and only 30% and 19% respectively are bound to albumin leaving only about 1% unbound and free. Hyperthyroidism, pregnancy and estrogen administration increase SHBG levels whereas corticosteroids, androgens and progestins decrease SHBG. The level of SHBG is inversely related to weight. Hyperinsulinemia lowers the SHBG levels; d. 79% progesterone is bound to albumin.

Q.278 Regarding craniopharyngioma all are correct except:
- a. May cause secondary amenorrhea
- b. Leads to hypogonadotropic hypogonadism
- c. May cause hyperprolactinemia
- d. It is a tumor of the meninges

Ans. d. It is a cyst derived from the remnants of Rathke's pouch. Severity of pathology varies depending upon the extent of pituitary stalk involvement.

Q.279 Regarding endocrinology of normal menstrual cycle all are correct except:
- a. In the follicular phase, level of FSH is higher than that of LH
- b. GnRH pulse frequency is more in the follicular phase but pulse amplitudes are higher in luteal phase
- c. The time difference between estradiol peak and LH peak is about 12 hours
- d. Follicular recruitment is always monofollicular

Ans. d. It is always multiple follicular but final maturation is unifollicular.

Q.280 Regarding male infertility all are true except:
- a. Chromosomal abnormality is associated with 2% of cases
- b. Testicular volume of 20 mL indicates testicular atrophy

c. Chronic sinusitis and bronchitis suggests Young's syndrome
d. ICSI is possible in a case of sertoli cell only syndrome

Ans. b. Normal testicular volume is 20 mL. d. With the concept of 'focality' from areas of normal spermatogenesis, sperm for ICSI could be obtained.

Q.281 Hypogonadism is observed in all except:
a. Primary ovarian failure
b. Turner's syndrome
c. Stein-Leventhal syndrome
d. Laurence-Moon-Bardet-Biedl syndrome

Ans. c.

Q.282 Gonadotropin levels are raised in all except:
a. Turner's syndrome
b. Premature ovarian failure
c. McCune-Albright syndrome
d. Androgen insensitivity syndrome

Ans. c. Serum level of LH is elevated in androgen insensitivity syndrome.

Q.283 Conditions in relation to male fertility—match the following:
a. Hyperprolactinemia
b. Diabetes mellitus
c. Kartagener syndrome
d. Absence of fructose in semen

1. Retrograde ejaculation
2. Seminal vesicle agenesis
3. Impotence
4. Asthenozoospermia

Ans. a = 3; b = 1; c = 4; d = 2.

Q.284 Kallmann's syndrome is characterized by all except:
a. State of hypogonadotropic hypogonadism
b. Anosmia, color blindness are associated
c. Deficient secretion of GnRH
d. Abnormal female karyotype

Ans. d. See Dutta's Textbook of Gynecology, 7th Edition, p. 383.

Q.285 Regarding the peptides derived from the granulosa cells all are true except:
a. FSH stimulates the synthesis of these peptides
b. Follistatin stimulates FSH activity
c. Activin stimulates FSH release from the pituitary
d. Inhibin inhibits FSH secretion

Ans. b. It suppresses FSH activity.

Q.286 Regarding follicle stimulating hormone and luteinizing hormone (FSH and LH) all are correct except:
a. LH is high in androgen insensitivity syndrome
b. FSH stimulates spermatogenesis from sertoli cells of the testis
c. FSH level is raised when long-term GnRH agonist is used
d. LH stimulates testosterone secretion from leydig cells of the testis

Ans. c. Level is suppressed.

Q.287 In relation to precocious puberty in girls all are true except:
a. It is the development of secondary sexual characters before the age of 8
b. Most common cause is idiopathic

c. GnRH analogs is an useful treatment for all cases
d. Premature adrenarche is a cause

Ans. c. It is useful only when it is gonadotropin dependent.

Q.288 Regarding GnRH analogs all are correct except:
a. Plasma half-life is about 10 minutes
b. There is significant reduction of trabecular bone density after 6 months of use
c. Benefits of antagonists are the same as that of agonists
d. Can be used as a diagnostic test for premenstrual tension syndrome

Ans. a. Plasma half-life is more than 2 hours.

Q.289 As regard the gonadotropin releasing hormone all are true except:
a. It is a decapeptide
b. It is secreted from the arcuate nucleus of the hypothalamus
c. Plasma half-life is about 30–40 min
d. Endogenous opioids suppress its release

Ans. c. It is 2–4 minutes.

Q.290 Regarding adrenogenital syndrome:
a. Treated by low-dose combined oral pill
b. It is inherited as an autosomal dominant mode
c. 17-OHP is elevated in 3β hydroxysteroid dehydrogenase deficiency
d. Majority of the IIβ hydroxylase deficient patients become hypertensive

Ans. d; a. Treatment is low-dose dexamethasone; b. It is an autosomal recessive condition; c. Blood levels of DHA and DHES are markedly increased.

Q.291 Regarding Asherman's syndrome all are correct except:
a. Is a cause of recurrent miscarriage
b. May be due to uterine schistosomiasis
c. Despite treatment, prospect of pregnancy is poor
d. Hysteroscopic adhesiolysis is preferred to D and C

Ans. c. Successful pregnancy following treatment is approximately 70–80%.

Q.292 Regarding male pseudohermaphroditism all are true except:
a. It is due to failure of virilization
b. The individual is a male genetically (46 XY)
c. Testosterone level is within normal female range
d. The individual is reared up as a female and the gonads are removed

Ans. c. It is normal or slightly elevated male range.

Q.293 Regarding congenital adrenal hyperplasia all are true except:
a. Characterized by masculinized external genitalia
b. Enzyme defects in cortisol synthesis is 21-hydroxylase P450c21 mainly (95%)
c. Prenatal diagnosis and treatment is yet to develop
d. Testosterone is the major circulating androgen

Ans. c. Chorionic villus biopsy and DNA probe can make the diagnosis. Treatment includes pregnancy termination or dexamethasone therapy.

Q.294 Concerning premature ovarian failure:
   a. Most of the patients present with primary amenorrhea
   b. Overall incidence is 10%
   c. It may be associated with hypothyroidism
   d. Chance of spontaneous pregnancy is absent

Ans. c; a. It is the secondary amenorrhea; b. Incidence is about 1%; d. Spontaneous pregnancy has been observed though rare (*See* Dutta's Textbook of Gynecology, 7th Edition, p. 382).

Q.295 Induction of ovulation with clomiphene citrate:
   a. Indicated in hypothalamopituitary dysfunction
   b. Multiple pregnancy rate is approximately 15%
   c. Indicated in patients with premature ovarian failure
   d. Indicated in hypothalamopituitary failure

Ans. a.

Q.296 Regarding luteal phase defect (LPD):
   a. Is an established cause of infertility
   b. Is diagnosed by ultrasonography
   c. Defective follicular maturation may be a cause
   d. The basal body temperature (BBT) chart is monophasic

Ans. c. LPD is due to deficient function of the corpus luteum with insufficient progesterone production. Whether it is an established cause of infertility, remains controversial. BBT can be biphasic but the duration of temperature rise is short. Diagnosis of luteal phase defect is made by BBT chart, estimation of serum progesterone and accurate dating of endometrial sampling is extremely important. USG is not helpful in this regard.

Q.297 Concerning female sexual development all are correct except:
   a. Lack of SRY gene
   b. Absence of testosterone
   c. Absence of anti-Müllerian hormone (AMH)
   d. SRY gene is located on the long arm of Y chromosome

Ans. d. SRY gene is located on the short arm of the Y chromosome.

Q.298 Regarding premenstrual syndrome (PMS):
   a. Symptoms occur during the midmenstrual phase
   b. Mostly occurs in the non-ovulatory cycle
   c. Suppression of ovarian cycle always brings improvement
   d. Pathology is due to high level of serotonin

Ans. c; a. It is in the luteal phase; b. It is the ovulatory cycle; d. Exact pathology is obscure.

Q.299 Risk factors that increases osteoporosis are:
   a. Heparin on long-term use
   b. Sedentary habit
   c. Tamoxifen therapy
   d. Tibolone use

Ans. a and b.

Q.300 Contraindications of HRT are:
   a. Undiagnosed vaginal bleeding
   b. Active liver disease
   c. Gallbladder disease
   d. History of endometrial carcinoma
Ans. a, b and c. *See* Dutta's Textbook of Gynecology, 7th Edition, p. 50.

Q.301 Concerning laparoscopy, hysteroscopy and ultrasonography:
   a. In the diagnosis of pelvic infection, ultrasonography is superior to laparoscopy
   b. Vaginal sonography is superior to hysteroscopy or laparoscopy in the diagnosis of fibroids
   c. Vaginal sonography is superior to hysteroscopy and biopsy in the diagnosis of endometrial carcinoma
   d. In the diagnosis of uterine malformation, combined laparoscopy and hysteroscopy is superior to vaginal sonography
Ans. b and d.

Q.302 Regarding the surgery for hysterectomy:
   a. In vaginal hysterectomy—the uterosacral and cardinal ligaments are clamped and cut separately
   b. Oophorectomy is not routinely done in vaginal procedure
   c. Ovarian ligament should be cut if oophorectomy is to be done in abdominal procedure
   d. Ureteric injury is most common during uterine artery clamping in abdominal procedure
Ans. b; a. both are taken together as they are atrophic; c. It is the infundibulopelvic ligament; d. It is at the angle of vagina.

Q.303 Regarding atrophic vaginitis:
   a. Reflects deficient estrogen state
   b. Occurs only after menopause
   c. Vaginal cytology is not diagnostic
   d. May cause postmenopausal bleeding
Ans. a and d; b. May occur before menarche and during lactation; c. It is diagnosed by large number of parabasal cells and by absence of superficial squamous cells.

Q.304 Regarding transcervical resection of endometrium (TCRE):
   a. Resectoscope must remove the basal layer of endometrium
   b. Prior hysteroscopic assessment is recommended
   c. Uterine size is not a consideration
   d. Success rate is nearly 100%
Ans. a and b; c. Large uterine size is a contraindication; d. It is about 80%. (*See* Dutta's Textbook of Gynecology, 7th Edition, p. 159).

Q.305 Effectiveness of combined oral pills is reduced by all except:
   a. Phenobarbitone
   b. Rifampicin
   c. Sodium valproate
   d. Spironolactone
Ans. c.

Q.306 Complications of hysteroscopic surgery:
a. Electrothermal injury
b. Fluid overload
c. Injury to intra-abdominal organs
d. Cerebral edema

Ans. a, b, c and d.

Q.307 Features of Turner's syndrome include:
a. Kyphoscoliosis
b. Lymphedema
c. Cystic hygroma
d. Absent menstruation

Ans. a, b and c. In mosaic (45, X/46, XX) variety, menstruation and conception can occur.

Q.308 Regarding Mifepristone:
a. It is an antiestrogen
b. Used for medical termination of pregnancy
c. Can be used up to 63 days of pregnancy
d. Failure rate is about 5%

Ans. b and c; a. Antiprogesterone; d. It is only 1%.

Q.309 In relation to pelvic infection:
a. Laparoscopy should be used for diagnosis in all cases
b. 'Violin string' adhesions suggest chlamydial infection
c. Ultrasonography is superior to laparoscopy
d. Salpingitis isthmica nodosa is one form of tubal endometriosis

Ans. b and d.

Q.310 The ovarian ligament has the following characteristics:
a. Is attached medially to the uterus
b. Contains the ovarian vessels
c. Is attached laterally to the pelvic wall
d. Is homologous to the gubernaculum testis in male

Ans. a and d.

Q.311 The following are the correlations with the types of epithelium and the organ:
a. Cervix and the columnar epithelium
b. Urethral meatus and the transitional epithelium
c. Vagina and the stratified squamous epithelium
d. Uterine body and the ciliated epithelium

Ans. c.

Q.312 As regard the karyotype and the diagnosis—match the following:
a. 45 XO
b. 46 XY
c. 47 XXY
d. 47 XXX

1. Androgen insensitivity syndrome
2. Turner's syndrome
3. Super female
4. Klinefelter's syndrome

Ans. a = 2; b = 1; c = 4; d = 3.

Q.313 These are the names with associated conditions—match the following:
a. Henry Turner
b. John Tanner

1. Repair of bladder fistula
2. Primary amenorrhea with delayed secondary sex characters

c. Marion Sims
d. Joe Meige
3. Surgery for carcinoma cervix
4. Staging of puberty changes

Ans. a = 2; b = 4; c = 1; d = 3.

Q.314 Causes of vulval pain are due to all except:
a. Neuralgia of the genitofemoral nerve
b. Behçet's disease
c. Vulvar vestibulitis syndrome
d. Lichen sclerosus

Ans. d.

Q.315 The following ovarian tumors are malignant:
a. Brenner tumor
b. Dermoid cyst
c. Krukenberg tumor
d. Granulosa cell tumor

Ans. c and d.

Q.316 Regarding cervical cytology screening:
a. Primary aim of cytology is to detect cervical cancer
b. WHO advocates cervical cytology screening specially in the developing world
c. There is a significant difference in the reduction of cervical cancer between 3 and 5 yearly screening
d. Liquid-based cytology is superior to conventional smears

Ans. c and d; a. The primary aim of cervical cytology screening is to prevent deaths from cervical cancer by preventing the disease. This is done by **detecting and treating the precancerous condition**; b. WHO advocates **downstaging** in developing countries where resources and infrastructure are limited; c. Five yearly screening of women (aged between 20 and 65 years) could reduce the incidence of cervical cancer by 84%, whereas by 3 yearly it is 91% and by annual screening it is 93%; d. Liquid-based cytology can reduce the number of unsatisfactory smears and false-negative smears. It increases the sensitivity. **Liquid-based cytology (LBC):** Smear is taken with a plastic device. The device is rinsed in a buffered methanol solution. Cells are separated by centrifugation. Thin layer smears are then made. LBC can reduce the number of unsatisfactory and false-negative smears. It increases the sensitivity also. (See Dutta's Textbook of Gynecology, 7th Edition, p. 90, 91).

Q.317 Regarding postmenopausal osteoporosis:
a. Bone density in the proximal forearm is generally measured to assess the bone mineral content
b. Single photon absorptiometry is the investigation of choice to detect lumbar spine mineral content
c. Average bone mineral loss every year is 5%, postmenopausally
d. Estrogen therapy even after fracture, prevents further bone loss

Ans. a and d; b. Dual energy X-ray absorptiometry (DEXA) is the most accurate method; c. Average bone mineral loss in the first year is 3%, thereafter it is 1% annually.

Q.318 With regard to metabolic changes in menopause and HRT:
a. Level of low density lipoprotein (LDL) cholesterol is reduced
b. Level of high density lipoprotein (cholesterol) is raised

c. Calcium and vitamin D provide no significant protection against osteoporosis
d. Asian women run high-risk for osteoporosis

Ans. a, b and d.

Q.319 With regard to postmenopausal hormone replacement therapy:
a. Risk of ischemic heart disease is reduced
b. Risk of cerebrovascular accident is not altered
c. Estrogen is an antioxidant and prevent oxidation of LDL
d. Risk of endometrial cancer is increased even with combined HRT

Ans. a and c; b. Risk is significantly reduced after 5 years of use; d. Combined HRT is protective against endometrial and ovarian cancer.

Q.320 Hormone replacement therapy (HRT) and menopause:
a. Estrogen is ideal for a woman who has intact uterus
b. Progestins in HRT should be given for 12–14 days per cycle
c. Continuous estrogen and progestin therapy protects bone loss equally
d. HRT is to be continued for 10 years or more as desired

Ans. b and c; a. Women with intact uterus should have combined HRT either cyclical or continuous; d. HRT is currently recommended for a short period of time, preferably for 5 years.

Q.321 As regard the development of the vagina all are correct except:
a. Develops partly from the urogenital sinus and mainly from the Müllerian ducts
b. May be completely absent even when the uterus is present
c. May be absent even when the ovaries are present
d. Vaginal plate is completely canalized by 16 weeks

Ans. d. It is completely canalized by 20 weeks postconception (*See* Dutta's Textbook of Gynecology, 7th Edition, p. 33).

Q.322 Regarding uterine sarcoma all are true except:
a. Endometrial stromal sarcoma is of high-grade malignancy
b. Tumor is heterologous when tissue elements are not native
c. Rarely arises from the pre-existing benign leiomyoma
d. Usually, metastasis via lymphatics

Ans. d. It is by hematogenous.

Q.323 As regard the three swab test for urinary fistula—match the following:

a. Uppermost swab soaked but unstained with dye and lower two swabs remain dry	1. Vesicovaginal fistula
b. Lower swab stained with dye and upper two swabs dry	2. Ureterovaginal fistula
c. Middle swab stained with dye and upper and lower swab dry	3. Stress incontinence
d. Swabs dry but dye leaks from urethral meatus	4. Urethrovaginal fistula

Ans. a = 2; b = 4; c = 1; d = 3. *See* Dutta's Textbook of Gynecology, 7th Edition, p. 345.

Q.324 The first choice of surgical treatment for stress urinary incontinence is:
a. Cystourethroplasty or colposuspension
b. Sling procedure (TVT, TVT–O)

c. Salvage procedure
   d. Raj or Stamey procedure especially in a young woman
Ans. b. *See* Dutta's Textbook of Gynecology, 7th Edition, p. 332.

Q.325 Regarding interstitial cystitis all are true except:
   a. It presents with dysuria, frequency, hematuria
   b. Cause is obscure
   c. Cystoscopy reveals normal bladder mucosa
   d. Management is unsatisfactory
Ans. c. Bladder mucosa is ulcerated.

Q.326 Urge incontinence is characterized by:
   a. Absence of urge prior to urine leak
   b. Amount of urine loss is always small
   c. Detrusor is hypersensitive to infection or calculi
   d. Cystourethroscopy is always normal
Ans. c; a. Urge is always present; b. Amount of loss is large; d. Usually informative. (*See* Dutta's Textbook of Gynecology, 7th Edition, p. 334).

Q.327 Genuine stress urinary incontinence (GSI) is characterized by all except:
   a. Occurs usually in parous lady
   b. Escape of urine occurs during coughing, laughing (stress)
   c. Amount is always large
   d. Micturition is normal
Ans. c. It is always small in amount. (*See* Dutta's Textbook of Gynecology, 7th Edition, p. 328, 329).

Q.328 Detrusor overactivity is characterized by:
   a. Leakage of urine due to detrusor overactivity
   b. Patient can voluntarily inhibit it
   c. Cystometry reveals normal detrusor pressure
   d. It is usually observed when the bladder is full. (*See* Dutta's Textbook of Gynecology, 7th Edition, p. 334).
Ans. a; b. Patient cannot control it; c. Detrusor pressure is increased on cystometry; d. It occurs at a much lower bladder filling.

Q.329 Regarding urinary incontinence and urodynamic investigation all are correct except:
   a. Normal bladder capacity is in the range of 400–600 mL
   b. Detrusor overactivity can be accurately diagnosed by these investigations
   c. Midstream specimen of urine must be cultured in all cases of incontinence
   d. Normal voiding is affected by sympathetic control of bladder
Ans. d. It is the parasympathetic nerve control. (*See* Dutta's Textbook of Gynecology, 7th Edition, p. 326, 329, 334).

Q.330 The burch colposuspension includes all except:
   a. Is the operation for genuine stress incontinence
   b. 5 years success rate is about 90%
   c. May be complicated by detrusor instability after the operation
   d. Involves suturing the vagina to the rectus sheath
Ans. d. Suturing is done to the ipsilateral iliopectineal ligament.

c. Calcium and vitamin D provide no significant protection against osteoporosis
d. Asian women run high-risk for osteoporosis

Ans. a, b and d.

Q.319 *With regard to postmenopausal hormone replacement therapy:*
a. Risk of ischemic heart disease is reduced
b. Risk of cerebrovascular accident is not altered
c. Estrogen is an antioxidant and prevent oxidation of LDL
d. Risk of endometrial cancer is increased even with combined HRT

Ans. a and c; b. Risk is significantly reduced after 5 years of use; d. Combined HRT is protective against endometrial and ovarian cancer.

Q.320 *Hormone replacement therapy (HRT) and menopause:*
a. Estrogen is ideal for a woman who has intact uterus
b. Progestins in HRT should be given for 12–14 days per cycle
c. Continuous estrogen and progestin therapy protects bone loss equally
d. HRT is to be continued for 10 years or more as desired

Ans. b and c; a. Women with intact uterus should have combined HRT either cyclical or continuous; d. HRT is currently recommended for a short period of time, preferably for 5 years.

Q.321 *As regard the development of the vagina all are correct except:*
a. Develops partly from the urogenital sinus and mainly from the Müllerian ducts
b. May be completely absent even when the uterus is present
c. May be absent even when the ovaries are present
d. Vaginal plate is completely canalized by 16 weeks

Ans. d. It is completely canalized by 20 weeks postconception (*See* Dutta's Textbook of Gynecology, 7th Edition, p. 33).

Q.322 *Regarding uterine sarcoma all are true except:*
a. Endometrial stromal sarcoma is of high-grade malignancy
b. Tumor is heterologous when tissue elements are not native
c. Rarely arises from the pre-existing benign leiomyoma
d. Usually, metastasis via lymphatics

Ans. d. It is by hematogenous.

Q.323 *As regard the three swab test for urinary fistula—match the following:*

a. Uppermost swab soaked but unstained with dye and lower two swabs remain dry	1. Vesicovaginal fistula
b. Lower swab stained with dye and upper two swabs dry	2. Ureterovaginal fistula
c. Middle swab stained with dye and upper and lower swab dry	3. Stress incontinence
d. Swabs dry but dye leaks from urethral meatus	4. Urethrovaginal fistula

Ans. a = 2; b = 4; c = 1; d = 3. *See* Dutta's Textbook of Gynecology, 7th Edition, p. 345.

Q.324 *The first choice of surgical treatment for stress urinary incontinence is:*
a. Cystourethroplasty or colposuspension
b. Sling procedure (TVT, TVT–O)

c. Salvage procedure
d. Raj or Stamey procedure especially in a young woman

Ans. b. *See* Dutta's Textbook of Gynecology, 7th Edition, p. 332.

Q.325 Regarding interstitial cystitis all are true except:
a. It presents with dysuria, frequency, hematuria
b. Cause is obscure
c. Cystoscopy reveals normal bladder mucosa
d. Management is unsatisfactory

Ans. c. Bladder mucosa is ulcerated.

Q.326 Urge incontinence is characterized by:
a. Absence of urge prior to urine leak
b. Amount of urine loss is always small
c. Detrusor is hypersensitive to infection or calculi
d. Cystourethroscopy is always normal

Ans. c; a. Urge is always present; b. Amount of loss is large; d. Usually informative. (*See* Dutta's Textbook of Gynecology, 7th Edition, p. 334).

Q.327 Genuine stress urinary incontinence (GSI) is characterized by all except:
a. Occurs usually in parous lady
b. Escape of urine occurs during coughing, laughing (stress)
c. Amount is always large
d. Micturition is normal

Ans. c. It is always small in amount. (*See* Dutta's Textbook of Gynecology, 7th Edition, p. 328, 329).

Q.328 Detrusor overactivity is characterized by:
a. Leakage of urine due to detrusor overactivity
b. Patient can voluntarily inhibit it
c. Cystometry reveals normal detrusor pressure
d. It is usually observed when the bladder is full. (*See* Dutta's Textbook of Gynecology, 7th Edition, p. 334).

Ans. a; b. Patient cannot control it; c. Detrusor pressure is increased on cystometry; d. It occurs at a much lower bladder filling.

Q.329 Regarding urinary incontinence and urodynamic investigation all are correct except:
a. Normal bladder capacity is in the range of 400–600 mL
b. Detrusor overactivity can be accurately diagnosed by these investigations
c. Midstream specimen of urine must be cultured in all cases of incontinence
d. Normal voiding is affected by sympathetic control of bladder

Ans. d. It is the parasympathetic nerve control. (*See* Dutta's Textbook of Gynecology, 7th Edition, p. 326, 329, 334).

Q.330 The burch colposuspension includes all except:
a. Is the operation for genuine stress incontinence
b. 5 years success rate is about 90%
c. May be complicated by detrusor instability after the operation
d. Involves suturing the vagina to the rectus sheath

Ans. d. Suturing is done to the ipsilateral iliopectineal ligament.

Q.331 Symptoms suggestive of detrusor overactivity include all except:
a. Frequency
b. Urgency
c. Nocturia
d. Hematuria

Ans. d. See Dutta's Textbook of Gynecology, 7th Edition, p. 334.

Q.332 Regarding the human semen volume contribution—match the following:
a. Sperm
b. Seminal vesicles
c. Prostate
d. Bulbourethral of glands

1. 5%
2. 30%
3. 60%
4. 5%

Ans. a = 4; b = 3; c = 2; d = 1.

Q.333 Regarding ovarian follicular development:
a. Time required for a follicle to achieve preovulatory status is about 120 days
b. Dominant follicle is selected by 5–7 days of the cycle
c. Midfollicular rise in estradiol exerts a negative feedback to FSH and positive feedback to LH
d. FSH stimulates activin and inhibin production by granulosa cells

Ans. b, c and d; a. Time required is about 85 days. (See Dutta's Textbook of Gynecology, 7th Edition, p. 68).

Q.334 Regarding spermatogenesis:
a. FSH stimulates leydig cells
b. Sertoli cells produce androgen binding protein (ABP) and inhibin B
c. Spermatogenesis requires very high local androgen concentration
d. Sertoli cells are analogous to theca cells of the ovary

Ans. b and c; a. FSH stimulates spermatogenesis and sertoli cells. d. Sertoli cells are analogous to granulosa cells and the leydig cells to theca cells of the ovary. (See Dutta's Textbook of Gynecology, 7th Edition, p. 187).

Q.335 Regarding gestational trophoblastic disease (GTD):
a. Complete moles show chromosomal pattern 46 XY in majority
b. Any plateau or re-elevation of hCG level during follow-up, suggests persistent GTD
c. Presence of pre-eclampsia increases the risk for persistent GTD
d. While on chemotherapy, drop of hCG < 25%, suggests a repeat course of the drug

Ans. b and c. Complete moles have a chromosomal complement of 46 XX in majority (90%) and both are paternally derived (See Manual of Obstetrics and Gynecology for the Postgraduates, p. 334). Partial moles are often with a fetus and triploidy (69 XXX or XXY). b. This condition is for careful review and for chemotherapy. c. Risk is as high as 80%. d. This suggests resistance and change in the chemotherapeutic regimen and not to repeat the same drug.

Q.336 Regarding hyperthyroidism:
a. Menstrual abnormality is absent
b. In subclinical hyperthyroid state, TSH level is normal
c. Subclinical hyperthyroidism should be treated
d. Thyroid hormone increases bone mineral resorption and predisposes to osteoporotic fracture

Ans. c and d; a. Abnormality includes oligomenorrhea to amenorrhea. c. It should be treated to prevent cardiac complication and fracture.

Q.337 Concerning thyroid function and reproduction:
　　a. Elevated TSH with normal T_4 level suggests a subclinical hypothyroid state
　　b. Patients on long-term thyroid hormone should not stop taking the drug
　　c. Subclinical hypothyroidism should not be treated
　　d. Response to TSH with thyroid hormone therapy is slow
Ans. a. and d; b.Patient may stop taking medication as there is chance of recovery of hypothalamic-pituitary axis; c. This state should be treated to prevent development of goiter.

Q.338 Regarding toxic shock syndrome:
　　a. May occur at any age group
　　b. Often the patient presents with hypothermia
　　c. Exotoxin liberated by *Staphylococcus aureus* is the causative factor
　　d. Mortality may be as high as 30%
Ans. c; a. Common in menstruating women (15–30 years of age); b. Fever is common; d. Mortality is 5–10%. (*See* Dutta's Textbook of Gynecology, 7th Edition, p. 136).

Q.339 Regarding ectopic pregnancy:
　　a. The incidence of ectopic pregnancy is declining
　　b. The use of IUD is protective against ectopic pregnancy
　　c. It may coexist with an intrauterine pregnancy
　　d. The use of low-dose combined pills increases the risk
Ans. c; a. Incidence is rising; b. IUDs increases the risk; d. It is protective.

Q.340 Regarding cancer of the female genital organs:
　　a. Combined oral pills reduces the risk of ovarian carcinoma
　　b. Obesity increases the risk of endometrial carcinoma
　　c. Breastfeeding increases the risk of ovarian cancer
　　d. Late menopause increases the risk of breast carcinomas
Ans. a, b and d; c. It is protective.

Q.341 Carcinoma of the vagina:
　　a. Commonly occurs as a primary lesion
　　b. Most common site is the anterior and upper third vaginal wall
　　c. Usually is an adenocarcinoma
　　d. Inguinofemoral lymph nodes are involved
Ans. d; a. Primary vaginal carcinoma is rare 1–2% of all genital malignancies; spread from adjacent organs or metastasis is common; b. It is posterior and upper third vaginal wall; c. It is squamous cell carcinoma in 90% of cases. (*See* Dutta's Textbook of Gynecology, 7th Edition, p. 278).

Q.342 Regarding choriocarcinoma:
　　a. Characterized by snowstorm pattern on uterine ultrasonography
　　b. Histological examination reveals absence of chorionic villi
　　c. Lymph node metastases are common
　　d. Commonly, it is preceded by a hydatidiform mole or miscarriage
Ans. b and d; a. It is common in hydatidiform moles. Estimation of hCG, is the most reliable parameter for diagnosis and therapy; c. Lymph node and bone metastases are rare. Metastasis of lungs (60–95%),

vagina (40–50%), vulva/cervix (10–15%), brain (5–15%) and liver (5–15%) are common; d. Choriocarcinoma develops following hydatidiform mole (50%), term pregnancy (15%) and following abortion or ectopic pregnancy (25%). Trophoblastic disease following a normal pregnancy is either choriocarcinoma or PSTT and not a benign mole. (*See* Dutta's Textbook of Gynecology, 7th Edition, p. 300).

Q.343 Vulvodynia:
   a. It is commonly due to fungal infection
   b. Associated with dyspareunia
   c. Clinical examination reveals vulvar erythema
   d. Amitriptyline is the first choice of treatment
Ans. d. *See* Dutta's Textbook of Gynecology, 7th Edition, p. 215.

Q.344 *Regarding androgen metabolism in female:*
   a. Rapid progression of hirsutism suggests Cushing's syndrome
   b. 90% of dehydroepiandrosterone sulfate is of adrenal origin
   c. GnRH analogs decrease hepatic synthesis of SHBG
   d. GnRH analogs can inhibit adrenal androgen secretion
Ans. b. Rapid progression of hirsutism suggests ovarian or adrenal tumor. GnRH analogs neither affect hepatic synthesis of SHBG nor can inhibit adrenal androgen synthesis. (*See* Dutta's Textbook of Gynecology, 7th Edition, p. 474).

Q.345 *Regarding endometriosis:*
   a. Endometriosis is always a progressive disease
   b. Minimal or mild endometriosis must be treated when diagnosed in any subfertile patient
   c. Danazol acts by increasing the hepatic synthesis of SHBG
   d. Cumulative pregnancy rate (CPR) or monthly fecundity rate (MFR) is important in the evaluation of infertility treatment
Ans. d. Endometriosis is usually progressive but spontaneous regression may occur. Danazol suppresses the midcycle LH and FSH surges and inhibits ovarian steroidogenesis. It inhibits the hepatic synthesis of SHBG. Management (conservative laparoscopic or medical) of minimal or mild endometriosis is controversial. CPR after 5 years without therapy is 90% with minimal or mild endometriosis. CPR or MFR is more scientific and is preferred to simple or crude pregnancy rate. In minimal or mild endometriosis, there is no place of ovulation suppression by medical treatment. During diagnostic laparoscopy, ablation of endometriotic lesion may be considered (Marcoux, et al. 1997). Treatment should be individualized depending on woman's age and duration of infertility.

Q.346 *The endometrium of a normal menstrual cycle:*
   a. Regeneration of endometrium starts after the menstruation ceases
   b. Subnuclear vacuolation indicates ovulation is imminent
   c. The endometrium regresses 1 or 2 days prior to menstruation
   d. The postovulatory endometrial changes are due to estrogen
Ans. c. *See* Dutta's Textbook of Gynecology, 7th Edition, p. 72, (subnuclear vacuolation of gland epithelium usually occurs 24–36 hours after ovulation).

Q.347 About the inguinal canal:
   a. The anterior wall is formed by the external oblique aponeurosis
   b. Posterior wall is formed by the internal oblique muscle
   c. The deep ring is situated in transversus abdominis muscle
   d. The superficial ring is situated on the pubic crest

Ans. d. Inguinal canal is oblique and extends from deep inguinal ring, a gap in the fascia transversal to the superficial inguinal ring, a gap in the external oblique aponeurosis. Anterior wall is formed also by internal oblique laterally. So, also the posterior wall by fascia transversalis and conjoint tendon.

Q.348 In relation to labia majora all are correct except:
   a. Developmentally, it is homologous to scrotum in male
   b. Lymphatic systems are separate on each side
   c. It is supplied by the branches of internal and external pudendal arteries
   d. Abnormal fusion is most commonly seen in testicular feminization

Ans. d. Abnormal fusion of labioscrotal swelling is most common due to congenital adrenal hyperplasia.

Q.349 The femoral triangle:
   a. Femoral nerve lies in the lateral compartment of the femoral sheath
   b. Base of the femoral triangle is formed by fascia transversalis
   c. Branch of genitofemoral nerve is a content of femoral sheath
   d. Femoral ring lies between the artery and the vein

Ans. c. Base of femoral triangle formed by the inguinal ligament. Femoral sheath is formed by the fascia transversalis in front and fascia iliaca behind. The femoral sheath has three compartments.
   1. Femoral artery, femoral branch of the genitofemoral nerve
   2. Femoral vein in the intermediate compartment
   3. Femoral canal lies in the medial compartment. Mouth of the femoral canal is called femoral ring.

Q.350 The labia minora:
   a. Contain sebaceous glands
   b. The lower ends fuse to form the posterior commissure
   c. Developmentally similar to labia majora
   d. Contains few hair follicles

Ans. a. The lower end fuse each other to form fourchette. Labia minora is developed from the genital folds whereas labia majora from the genital swellings. Labia minora do not contain hair follicles.

Q.351 Primary dysmenorrhea:
   a. Usually, there is a primary cause underneath
   b. Often associated with anovulation
   c. Pain usually begins a week before the menstruation
   d. Oral contraceptive pills are effective to relieve the pain

Ans. d. *See* Dutta's Textbook of Gynecology, 7th Edition, p. 146.

Q.352 McCune-Albright syndrome:
   a. Puberty is delayed but menarche is early
   b. Associated with endocrinopathies
   c. It is GnRH dependent
   d. The condition affects boys more than the girls
Ans. b. *See* Dutta's Textbook of Gynecology, 7th Edition, p. 41. There is precocious puberty including premature menarche. Girls are affected more than the boys.

Q.353 Regarding ovulation in a normal menstrual cycle:
   a. Biphasic BBT indicates ovulation is imminent
   b. LH surge occurs immediately following ovulation
   c. Disappearance of cervical mucus ferning is suggestive of ovulation
   d. Vaginal cytology, shift of maturation index (MI) to the right indicates ovulation
Ans. c. *See* Dutta's Textbook of Gynecology, 7th Edition, p. 93, 193. Biphasic BBT indicates ovulation in retrospect. LH surge is prior to ovulation and secretion of progesterone from corpus luteum following ovulation causes shift of MI to the left in vaginal cytology.

Q.354 Regarding ambiguous (DSD) genitalia:
   a. In a girl with congenital adrenal hyperplasia—uterus will be absent
   b. Uterus will be present in a case with 'testicular feminization syndrome (46 XY)'
   c. Ovaries are absent in a case with Mayer-Rokitansky-Küster-Hauser syndrome
   d. In Turner's syndrome, secondary sex characters are poor
Ans. d. *See* Dutta's Textbook of Gynecology, 7th Edition, p. 363, 366.

Q.355 Regarding Turner's syndrome all are correct except:
   a. The patient usually presents with primary amenorrhea
   b. The Karyotype is 45 XO
   c. The patient usually have mental retardation
   d. Breast development is poor
Ans. c. Usually there is no mental retardation. (*See* Dutta's Textbook of Gynecology, 7th Edition, p. 363, 367).

Q.356 Regarding development of gonads all are correct except:
   a. The bipotential gonad differentiate by 6–7 weeks time
   b. Ovarian differentiation occurs 2 weeks later than the testis
   c. SRY gene of Y chromosome controls the differentiation of ovary
   d. The germ cell number in the ovary is maximum at 20th week
Ans. c. *See* Dutta's Textbook of Gynecology, 7th Edition, p. 30.

Q.357 Regarding development of genital organs all are correct except:
   a. The Müllerian tubercle is formed at the dorsal wall of the urogenital sinus
   b. The hymen is developed at the junction of the sinovaginal bulbs and the urogenital sinus
   c. The paramesonephric duct crosses the mesonephric duct anteriorly
   d. The paramesonephric ducts begin to fuse with each other at 12th week
Ans. d. *See* Dutta's Textbook of Gynecology, 7th Edition, p. 27. The paramesonephric ducts begin to fuse each other by 7–8 weeks and it is completed by 12th week.

Q.358 All are the mesonephric (Wolffian) remnants except:
a. Gartner's duct
b. Ovarian ligament
c. The epoophoron
d. The paroophoron

Ans. b. *See* Dutta's Textbook of Gynecology, 7th Edition, p. 27. Ovarian ligament is development from the proximal part of gubernaculum. The distal part remains as round ligament.

Q.359 Concerning the development of the genital organs:
a. The ova (germ cells) arise from the germinal epithelium of the ovary
b. Presence of ovary, controls the development of the paramesonephric ducts
c. In fetal life, the ratio of cervix and body of the uterus is 1 : 2
d. Differentiation of external genitalia is completed by 16th week of fetal at life

Ans. d. *See* Dutta's Textbook of Gynecology, 7th Edition, p. 30, 40. The germ cells are endodermal in origin. They migrate from the yolk sac to the genital ridge. Testosterone from testis is essential for differentiation of Wolffian duct. Development of external genitalia occurs around 9–16 weeks in male (earlier) and 10–18 weeks in female. (*See* Dutta's Textbook of Gynecology, 7th Edition, p. 26).

Q.360 Indications of prophylactic chemotherapy in molar pregnancy are all except:
a. When hCG level following evacuation fails to become normal by 6–9 weeks time
b. In a woman with number of high-risk factors for malignant change
c. Preferably as a routine to all cases following evacuation
d. In cases where there is re-elevation of hCG level following its initial normalization

Ans. c. Routine use of cytoxic drugs prophylactically is not recommended considering their toxicity. (*See* Dutta's Textbook of Gynecology, 7th Edition, p. 302).

Q.361 Choriocarcinoma:
a. Antecedent term pregnancy is a low-risk factor
b. About 25% develop following hydatidiform mole
c. Villus pattern is usually present
d. May follow an ectopic pregnancy

Ans. d. *See* Dutta's Textbook of Gynecology, 7th Edition, p. 299.

Q.362 Regarding hCG all are correct except:
a. Reaches its peak level between 60 and 70 days of pregnancy
b. Level is increased in hydatidiform mole
c. It can be used as a tumor marker
d. It is needed for the differentiation of female external genitalia

Ans. d. hCG stimulate leydig cells of the male fetus to produce testosterone. It is helpful for the development of male external genitalia.

Q.363 Granulosa cell tumors of the ovary:
a. Is a common germ cell tumor of younger age
b. May cause true isosexual precocious puberty
c. Characterized histologically by Call-Exner bodies
d. May cause endometrial carcinoma in about 50% cases

Ans. c. *See* Dutta's Textbook of Gynecology, 7th Edition, p. 316. Risk of endometrial carcinoma is 5–10%.

Q.364 Vulvar intraepithelial neoplasia (VIN):
a. The average age of the women is over 50 years
b. If left untreated, progresses often to invasive disease
c. Carcinomas of other organs may be associated in 30% cases
d. The rete ridges are blunt and koilocytes are absent

Ans. c. See Dutta's Textbook of Gynecology, 7th Edition, p. 260.

Q.365 Serum FSH level is raised in:
a. Postmenopausal women
b. Turner's syndrome
c. Sheehan's syndrome
d. A woman using combined oral contraceptives

Ans. a and b. See Dutta's Textbook of Gynecology, 7th Edition, p. 388.

Q.366 Regarding tubal ectopic pregnancy:
a. Interstitial part of the fallopian tube is the most common site
b. Tubal rupture is common with interstitial implantation
c. Pregnancy can continue to term
d. Arias Stella reaction is strikingly due to progesterone effect

Ans. d. See Dutta's Text book of Obstetrics, 8th Edition, p. 210. Rarely secondary abdominal pregnancy may continue to term—not in tubal.

Q.367 The round ligament:
a. It measures 24 cm in length
b. It is attached to the cornu of the uterus below and behind the fallopian tube
c. It runs posterior to the obturator artery
d. It traverses through the inguinal canal

Ans. d. See Dutta's Textbook of Gynecology, 7th Edition, p. 18.

Q.368 The round ligament:
a. It contains striated muscle
b. It passes medial to the inferior epigastric artery
c. It is homologous to the gubernaculum testis
d. It is inserted in the inguinal ligament

Ans. c. See Dutta's Textbook of Gynecology, 7th Edition, p. 18.

Q.369 The uterine artery:
a. Purely supplies the uterus
b. Is a branch of the posterior division of internal iliac artery
c. Passes below the ureter in the tunnel of the Mackenrodt's ligament
d. It supplies the round ligament through utero-ovarian anastomosis

Ans. d. See Dutta's Textbook of Gynecology, 7th Edition, p. 20.

Q.370 The ovary:
a. Receives its blood supply mainly from the internal iliac artery
b. Ovarian veins drain into the inferior vena cava
c. Ligament of ovary is attached at its lateral pole
d. It is attached to posterior leaf of the broad ligament

Ans. d. See Dutta's Textbook of Gynecology, 7th Edition, p. 8.

Q.371 Regarding the fallopian tube the correct statement is:
  a. It is entirely lined by ciliated columnar epithelium
  b. The abdominal ostium is narrower than the uterine ostium
  c. It undergoes cyclical changes during the menstrual cycle
  d. Fimbria ovarica is attached to the lateral pole of the ovary

Ans. d. The abdominal ostium is 2 mm whereas uterine ostium is 1 mm in diameter. (*See* Dutta's Textbook of Gynecology, 7th Edition, p. 8).

Q.372 The vagina:
  a. Is lined by single layer of squamous epithelium
  b. Is endodermal in origin
  c. Is developed from the mesonephric duct
  d. Complete agenesis of vagina is often associated with absence of uterus

Ans. d. *See* Dutta's Textbook of Gynecology, 7th Edition, p. 3, 28, 33.

Q.373 Germ cell tumors of the ovary:
  a. Majority are malignant
  b. Dysgerminoma is the most common malignant germ cell tumor
  c. Endodermal sinus tumor is the least common malignant germ cell tumor
  d. Dysgerminomas are usually bilateral

Ans. b. *See* Dutta's Textbook of Gynecology, 7th Edition, p. 314. Germ cell tumors constitute about 15–20% of all ovarian neoplasm and around 2–3% of them are malignant. Cystic teratomas or dermoids are the most common benign germ cell tumor. Dysgerminoma is the most common malignant germ cell tumor. Endodermal sinus tumor is the second common malignant germ cell tumor. Dysgerminomas are bilateral in 10–15% cases only.

Q.374 In a postmenopausal woman all are correct except:
  a. Vaginal acidity is reduced
  b. Any vaginal bleeding is alarming
  c. Gonadotropin secretion is reduced
  d. Treatment with estrogen is helpful

Ans. c. *See* Dutta's Textbook of Gynecology, 7th Edition, p. 47. Gonadotropin secretion is increased.

Q.375 Regarding arterial supply of the pelvis all are true except:
  a. Posterior trunk of the internal iliac supplies the gluteal muscles
  b. Median sacral artery arises from the aorta
  c. Inferior vesical artery arises from the posterior trunk of internal iliac artery
  d. Inferior rectal artery is a branch of internal pudendal artery

Ans. c. *See* Dutta's Textbook of Gynecology, 7th Edition, p. 20, 25.

Q.376 All are true about acquired immunodeficiency syndrome (AIDS) except:
  a. The infection is caused by DNA virus
  b. The virus binds to the CD4 molecule of the T cells
  c. Transplacental transmission to fetus is about 14–25%
  d. The virus can be transmitted by artificial insemination

Ans. a. *See* Dutta's Textbook of Gynecology, 7th Edition, p. 126.

Q.377 Regarding Müllerian duct:
 a. Develops medial to the Wolffian duct
 b. Is also known as mesonephric duct
 c. Starts to differentiate at 5–6 weeks of embryonic life
 d. The blind end projects into the urogenital sinus as Müllerian tubercle
Ans. d; c. Differentiation starts after 8 weeks. Before that, both the Müllerian and Wolffian ducts coexist in all embryos. (*See* Dutta's Textbook of Gynecology, 7th Edition, p. 27).

Q.378 Laparoscopic ovarian drilling (LOD) for a woman with PCOS:
 a. Monopolar coagulation current is used for 5 seconds
 b. Power setting is at 30 W
 c. The needle is pushed within the capsule to a depth of 6–8 mm
 d. The ovary is irrigated with normal saline at the end of the procedure
Ans. a, b, c and d.

Q.379 Laparoscopic ovarian surgery (LOS) for a woman with PCOS:
 a. For LOS, laser is found superior to electrocautery
 b. LOS restores regular ovulation in about 70% cases
 c. Cumulative rates of conception and miscarriage are high
 d. There is persistent fall in circulating androgens and continued improvement in insulin sensitivity.
Ans. b. Electrocautery is found more effective in achieving ovulation and pregnancy. Cumulative rates of conception are high (75%) but miscarriage rates are similar to general population. Following LOS, the levels of androgens (testosterone, androsterone) fall rapidly. But there is no improvement of insulin sensitivity and lipid abnormalities.

Q.380 Failure rates of different contraceptive methods per 100 women year
Ans. *See* Dutta's Textbook of Gynecology, 7th Edition, p. 392.

Intrauterine contraceptive devices (IUCDs)		Laparoscopic sterilization electrocoagulation	
■ CuT 380 A	0.8–0.6	■ Unipolar method	0.75%
■ LNG-IUS	0.1	■ Bipolar method	2.1%
Implanon	0.01	*Ring*	
Tubal sterilization (Pomeroy)	0.15–0.5	■ Falope ring	1.77%
		■ Filshie clip	0.1%

Q.381 Unsatisfactory colposcopy means:
 a. Failure to visualize cervix
 b. Failure to visualize transformation zone
 c. Failure to visualize squamous epithelium
 d. Failure to visualize columnar epithelium
Ans. b. *See* Dutta's Textbook of Gynecology, 7th Edition, p. 266.

Q.382 Virilizing tumors of the ovary are:
 a. Arrhenoblastoma
 b. Adrenal tumors of the ovary
 c. Leydig cell tumor

d. Gynandroblastoma
e. All of the above

Ans. e. *See* Dutta's Textbook of Gynecology, 7th Edition, p. 316.

Hormone producing tumors of the ovary (*See* Dutta's Textbook of Gynecology, 7th Edition, p. 316)

Male hormone	Female hormone	Mixed tumor
▪ Sertoli cell tumor ▪ Leydig cell tumor	▪ Granulosa cell tumor ▪ Theca cell tumor	Gynandroblastoma contains both Sertoli-leydig cell (androgenic) and granulosa cell (estrogenic component)

Q.383 *Feminizing tumors of the ovary are:*
  a. Granulosa cell tumor
  b. Theca cell tumor
  c. Dermoid cyst
  d. Serous cystadenoma

Ans. a and b. *See* Dutta's Textbook of Gynecology, 7th Edition, p. 316.

Q.384 *Anencephaly is best diagnosed at 12 weeks by:*
  a. Serum alpha fetoprotein
  b. Ultrasonography
  c. Radiography
  d. Amniography

Ans. b. *See* Dutta's Textbook of Obstetrics, 8th Edition, p. 471, 734.

Conditions associated with elevated maternal serum alpha fetoprotein level (*See* Dutta's Textbook of Obstetrics, 8th Edition, p. 128)

▪ Neural tube defects ▪ IUFD ▪ Multiple pregnancy ▪ Renal agenesis ▪ Polycystic kidney disease ▪ Placental abnormalities ▪ Hemangiomas of placenta ▪ Retroplacental hemorrhage	▪ Placental abruption ▪ Gastroschisis ▪ Omphalocele ▪ Esophageal or duodenal atresia ▪ Fetal hydrops or ascites ▪ Cystic hygroma ▪ Sacrococcygeal teratoma ▪ Oligohydramnios

Low levels of maternal serum alpha fetoprotein (*See* Dutta's Textbook of Obstetrics, 8th Edition, p. 128)

▪ Chromosomal trisomies	▪ Gestational trophoblastic neoplasia	▪ Inaccurate gestational age

Q.385 *Call-Exner bodies is seen with:*
  a. Granulosa cell tumor
  b. Pseudomucinous cystadenoma
  c. Papillary cystadenoma
  d. Dermoid

Ans. a. *See* Dutta's Textbook of Gynecology, 7th Edition, p. 316.

Specific histological features that are used as in the diagnostic criteria (*See* **Dutta's Textbook of Gynecology, 7th Edition, Ch 21 and 24**)
- *Psammoma bodies* in papillary serous cystadenoma of the ovary (p. 238)
- *Signet ring cells* for Krukenberg tumor (metastatic ovarian carcinoma) (p. 319)
- *Call-Exner body* in granulosa cell tumor of the ovary (p. 316)
- *Reinke's crystal* in hilus cell ovarian tumor
- *Hobnail cells* in clear cell carcinoma of the ovary
- *Keratin pearls* in squamous cell carcinoma of the cervix (p. 280)
- *Struma ovarii,* presence of thyroid tissue in ovarian teratoma (p. 240)
- *Schiller-Duval body* in endodermal sinus cell tumor of the ovary (p. 315)
- *'Coffee bean' nuclei* in granulosa cell tumor of the ovary (p. 239)

Q.386 **Which of the following feature of second trimester ultrasound is not a marker of Down's syndrome:**
   a. Single umbilical artery
   b. Choroid plexus cyst
   c. Aplasia Cutis
   d. Duodenal atresia

Ans. c. *See* Dutta's Textbook of Obstetrics, 8th Edition, p. 568.
Abnormalities associated with Down's syndrome (Trisomy 21) (*See* Dutta's Textbook of Obstetrics, 8th Edition, p. 568)
It is the most common autosomal chromosomal syndrome. Its relationship with maternal age is: 1 in 952 by the age of 30 and 1 in 106 by the age of 40 years. 95% cases are due to maternal nondisjunction, usually in meiosis-I.
The characteristic features are: Brachycephaly, epicanthal folds, broad nasal bridge, a protruding tongue, small and low set ears, hypotonia, broad short fingers, clinodactyly, wide space between the first two toes (sandle gap), single palmar crease (30%), cardiac lesions, duodenal atresia, diaphragmatic hernia, single umbilical artery. Cardiac defects (ASD, VSD), hypoechoic bowel, short humerus and femur, thickened nuchal fold and hydrocephalus. The risk of recurrence in subsequent pregnancy is 1%. Females with Down's syndrome are fertile and the risk of having Down baby for them is about 30%. Males are usually sterile.

Q.387 **Chorionic villus sampling done before 10 weeks may result in:**
   a. Fetal loss
   b. Fetomaternal hemorrhage
   c. Oromandibular limb defects
   d. Sufficient material not obtained

Ans. c. *See* Dutta's Textbook of Obstetrics, 8th Edition, p. 129.
CVS of the developing trophoblast is done in the first trimester of pregnancy. Indications are similar to amniocentesis for the purpose of molecular (DNA analysis), cytogenetic and biochemical studies. **CVS** is done between 10 and 12 completed weeks of pregnancy. Chorion frondosum is sampled as it contains the most mitotically active cells. CVS is done either by transcervical or transabdominal route. Prior ultrasound evaluation is done to detect fetal viability gestational age and placental location.

Procedure
- **Transcervical CVS:** A polythene catheter with a malleable obturator is passed through the cervix under ultrasound guidance. Placental trophoblast is aspirated into a 20 mL syringe containing the tissue culture medium.
- **Transabdominal CVS:** A 19 or 20 gauge needle with a stylet is directed into the thickest part of the placenta under the ultrasound guidance. The stylet is withdrawn and a syringe containing tissue culture medium is attached to the hub of the needle and suction is applied as the needle is moved up and down until an adequate amount of tissue is obtained. The sample is inspected to ensure that 20–40 mg of villus material is obtained.

Selection of method for CVS: CVS can be performed by any of the two routes and it is safe and effective. *Transcervical approach* is preferred when the placenta is located posteriorly and the uterus is retroverted. *Transabdominal route* is preferable in anterior location of placenta, anteverted uterus and with fundal position.

Contraindication of transcervical approach: Local infection (cervix and vagina), genital tract bleeding, uterine fibroid, cervical polyps, (mechanical hindrance) and markedly retroverted uterus.

Q.388 Congenital anomalies are most severe in:
a. Rubella infection
b. Mumps
c. CMV
d. Toxoplasma

Ans. a. *See* Dutta's Textbook of Obstetrics, 8th Edition, p. 348. Fetal **malformations with maternal rubella infection:** Risks of congenital rubella infection is about 54% in first trimester, 25% at the end of second trimester. The **common manifestations of congenital rubella syndrome (CRS) are:** IUGR, sensorineural hearing loss, hepatosplenomegaly, cardiac lesion (ductus arteriosus), eye defects (cataracts, glaucoma, retinitis, microphthalmia), microcephaly, cerebral palsy, mental retardation. Following congenital rubella infection, infant may shed virus up to 1 year after birth.

Q.389 Chorionic villus sampling is not done before 9 weeks of gestation age because of:
a. Fetomaternal hemorrhage
b. Fetal limb defect
c. Inadequate tissue is obtained for diagnosis
d. High incidence of abortion

Ans. b. *See* Dutta's Textbook of Obstetrics, 8th Edition, p. 129 and 130.

Safety of CVS

Pregnancy loss: CVS is a safe and effective procedure provided properly done by an experienced person. Pregnancy loss presently has decreased from 2.35 to 1.16%. The pregnancy loss rates between CVS and amniocentesis are not significantly different at present. Limb reduction defects are not observed when CVS was done after 9 weeks of gestation.

Confined placental mosaicism may be observed in some cases where the fetus does not carry the mosaic cell line but it is present in the placenta. In such a case, amniocentesis should be performed to determine whether the fetus is affected or not.

Q.390 Most common ovarian tumor below 20 year of age is:
 a. Epithelial cell tumor
 b. Sertoli call tumor
 c. Leydig cell tumor
 d. Germ cell tumor

Ans. d. *See* Dutta's Textbook of Gynecology, 7th Edition, p. 314.

> **Occurrence of ovarian tumors** (*See* Dutta's Textbook of Gynecology, 7th Edition, p. 237, 314)
> - **Common in all ages:** Epithelial tumors of the ovary
> - **Common in young woman:** Germ cell tumors
> - **Common epithelial ovarian tumor:** Serous cystadenoma
> - **Pseudomyxoma peritonei:** Mucinous cyst tumor
> - **Tumor causing Meigs syndrome:** Fibroma, thecoma, brenner and granulosa cell tumor of ovary
> - **Common germ cell tumor:** Dermoid
> - **Common malignant germ cell tumor:** Dysgerminoma.

Q.391 Anencephaly can be diagnosed by ultrasound at:
 a. 14–18 weeks of gestation
 b. 20–24 weeks of gestation
 c. 24–37 weeks of gestation
 d. 10–12 weeks of gestation

Ans. d. *See* Dutta's Textbook of Obstetrics, 8th Edition, p. 736.

Q.392 All are used in treatment of endometriosis except:
 a. Progesterone
 b. Danazol
 c. GnRH
 d. Estrogen

Ans. d. *See* Dutta's Textbook of Gynecology, 7th Edition, p. 296. Uses of Danazol (*See* Dutta's Textbook of Gynecology, 7th Edition, p. 254): (i) Pelvic endometriosis, (ii) Dysfunctional uterine bleeding, (iii) Fibrocystic breast disease, (iv) Gynecomastia, (v) Precocious puberty, (vi) Symptomatic fibroid uterus, (vii) Premenstrual tension syndrome, (viii) Prior to hysteroscopic endometrial ablation (to suppress endometrial growth).

Q.393 Regarding bilateral ligation of internal iliac arteries:
 a. Ligation is done on the main trunk of the artery
 b. Artery is transected between the ties
 c. Collateral circulation established between superior rectal with middle and inferior rectal arteries
 d. Bleeding is always controlled with this procedure

Ans. c; a. Ligation should be done on its anterior division; b. Artery should not be transected; d. At times, bleeding may fail to stop even after ligation due to venous bleeding or presence of aberrant vessels. (*See* Manual of Obstetrics and Gynecology for the Postgraduates, Case 13, p. 29 and Dutta's Textbook of Gynecology, 7th Edition, p. 25).

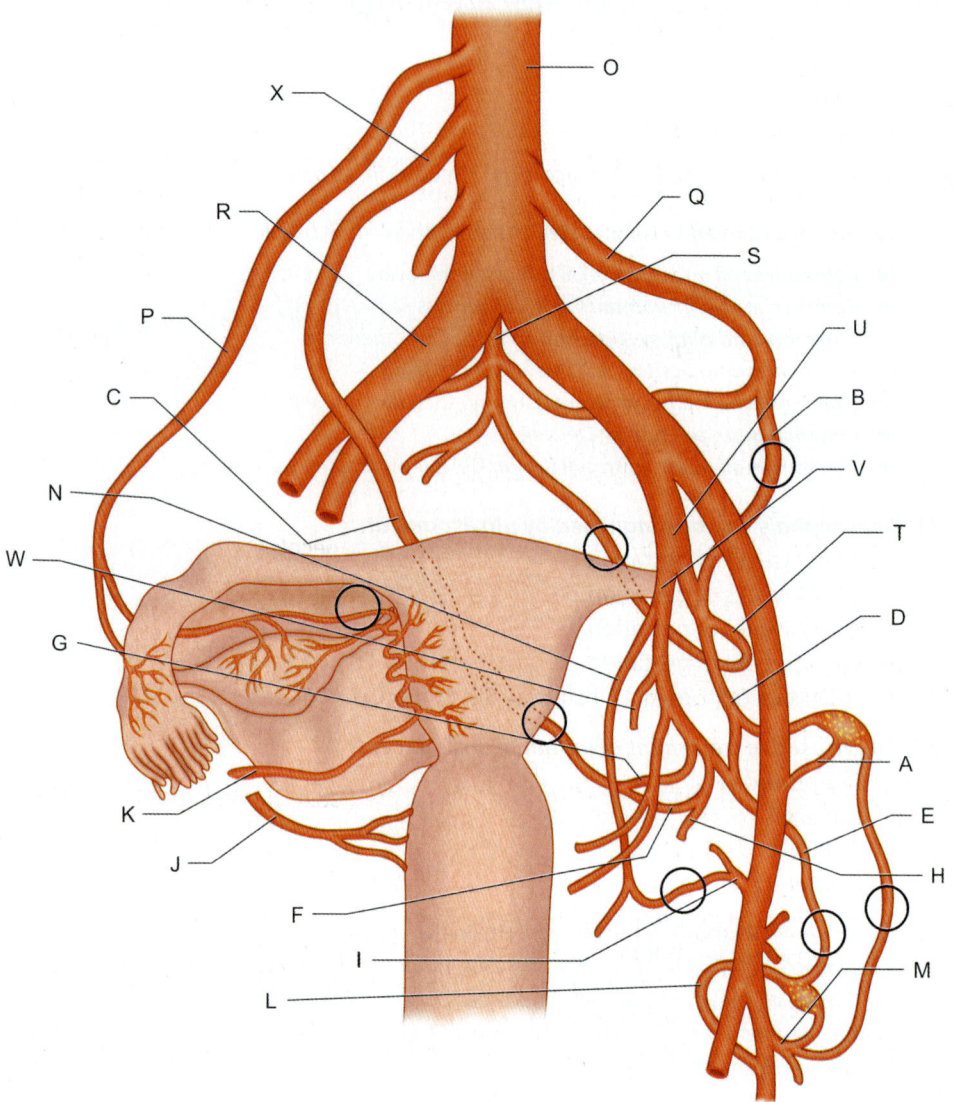

Fig. 4.1: Pathways of collateral circulation after bilateral ligation of hypogastric arteries. **A.** Deep circumflex iliac, **B.** Iliolumbar, **C.** Superior rectal, **D.** Superior gluteal, **E.** Inferior gluteal, **F.** Inferior rectal, **G.** Middle rectal, **H.** Internal pudendal, **I.** Inferior epigastric, **J.** Vaginal, **K.** Uterine, **L.** Medial circumflex femoral, **M.** Lateral circumflex femoral, **N.** Obturator, **O.** Aorta, **P.** Ovarian, **Q.** Lumbar, **R.** Common iliac, **S.** Middle sacral, **T.** Lateral sacral, **U.** Hypogastric, **V.** Anterior division, **W.** Umbilical, **X.** Inferior mesenteric

MODELS FOR MULTIPLE CHOICE QUESTIONS (MCQs)

Q.1 The pudendal nerve:
  a. Derives its fibers from the 2nd, 3rd and 4th sacral segments.
  b. Leaves the pelvis below the pyriformis through the greater sciatic foramen.
  c. The pudendal artery lies on its lateral side when it lies on the ischial spine.
  d. The inferior rectal nerve arises from it.
  e. Dorsal nerve of the clitoris is a branch.
Ans. a, b, d, e = True; c = False.

Q.2 In a postmenopausal woman:
  a. Vaginal pH is increased
  b. Level of total estradiol falls
  c. Level of gonadotropin falls
  d. Treatment with GnRH is often beneficial
  e. Occasional vaginal bleeding is common
Ans. a, b = True; c, d, e = False. (*See* Dutta's Textbook of Gynecology, 7th Edition, p. 47).

Q.3 The following substances are safe in pregnancy:
  a. Aspirin
  b. Rubella vaccination
  c. Varicella vaccination
  d. ACE inhibitors
  e. Paracetamol
Ans. a, e = True; b, c, d = false. (*See* Dutta's Textbook of Obstetrics, 8th Edition, p. 348, 588).

Q.4 The urinary bladder:
  a. The trigone develops from the urogenital sinus
  b. The bladder base remains fixed even when the bladder is distended
  c. The mucous membrane is lined by transitional epithelium
  d. Lower end of the mesonephric ducts are incorporated within the bladder
  e. The inferolateral surfaces are related to the space of Retzius
Ans. b, c, d, e = True, a = False. (*See* Dutta's Textbook of Gynecology, 7th Edition, p. 11).

Q.5 The female breast:
  a. Is made up of 15–20 lobes
  b. Lies over the fascia covering the pectoralis major muscle
  c. 30–40 lactiferous ducts open in the nipple
  d. Lymphatics drain to the axillary nodes
  e. Supplied by the internal mammary arteries
Ans. a, b, d, e = True; c = False. (*See* Dutta's Textbook of Gynecology, 7th Edition, p. 464 and 465).

Q.6 The rectum and the anal canal:
  a. The anal canal measures 2.5 cm in length
  b. Rectum starts at the level of S_1 vertebra
  c. Rectum is covered with peritoneum entirely

d. Uterosacral ligaments are related lateral to the rectum
e. All the lymphatics of the anal canal drain into the internal iliac lymph nodes

Ans. a, d = True; b, c, e = False. (*See* Dutta's Textbook of Gynecology, 7th Edition, p. 12).

Q.7 Regarding thyroid hormones:
a. Thyrotropin-releasing hormone (TRH) is nonapeptide
b. T3 or T4 is formed by iodination of amino acid tyrosine
c. Nearly, 99.5% of circulating thyroid hormones are bound to thyroxin-binding albumin
d. 90% of T3 is derived by peripheral deiodination of T4
e. The ratio of T4:T3 in blood is approximately 20:1

Ans. a, c = False; b, d, e = True. TRH is a tripeptide. 99.5% of circulating thyroid hormones are protein bound of which 75% are bound to thyroxin-binding globulin.

Q.8 Causes of delayed puberty are:
a. Constitutional
b. Craniopharyngioma
c. Hypogonadotropic hypogonadism
d. Cystic fibrosis
e. Androgen insersitivity syndrome

Ans. a, b, c, d, e = True.

Q.9 Risk-factor for osteoporosis are:
a. Caffeine intake
b. Increased body mass index
c. Hyperthyroidism
d. Kallman syndrome
e. Corticosteroid use

Ans. a, b = False; c, d, e = True.

Q.10 Factors for shifting to the right for oxygen dissociation curve are the followings:
a. Decreased temperature
b. Increased blood pH
c. Increased 2,3-diphosphoglycerate
d. Increased CO_2
e. Higher partial pressure of oxygen

Ans. a, b = False; c, d, e = True.

Q.11 In relation to functions of the liver:
a. Procoagulants are synthesized in the liver
b. Kupffer cells are progocytic
c. Alkaline phosphatase is decreased
d. Physiological jaundice in newborn is due to failure of conjugation
e. Hepatic transaminases are raised in pregnancy

Ans. a, b, d = True; c, e = False.

Q.12 Regarding a sample with a normal distribution:
a. It is described as a Gaussian distribution
b. The mode lies at the centre of the distribution
c. The median is the middle value in a ranked set of data
d. Normal distribution may be bimodal also
e. 60% of the data set lies within two standard deviations from the mean

Ans. a, b, c, d, = True; e = False. The standard deviation (SD) is a measure of the spread of the data set around the mean. Approximately 68% of the data set in a Gaussian distribution sits within one SD from the mean. Approximately 95% of the data set sits within two SDs from the mean.

Q.13 Regarding shock:
   a. Associated with metabolic alkalosis
   b. Cellular hypoxia is characteristic
   c. Hypokalemia is common
   d. Respiratory distress may be associated
   e. Capillary permeability is reduced due to endothelial damage

Ans. a, c, e = False; b, d = True.

Q.14 Thyroid function during pregnancy:
   a. Maternal serum iodine levels fall
   b. Levels of thyroid-binding globulin is raised
   c. Gestational transient thyrotoxicosis is due to high levels of TSH
   d. Maternal free T4 levels are raised
   e. Total T3 and T4 levels are unchanged

Ans. a, b = True; c, d, e = False. Gestational transient thyrotoxicosis is due to thyrotropic effect of hCG and there is actually some fall in the level of serum TSH in the first trimester. Total T3 and T4 levels are increased.

Causes of Fetal Heart Rate Abnormalities

Tachycardia	*Bradycardia*	*Reduced baseline variability*
■ Fetal distress	■ Fetal hypoxia	■ Fetal hypoxia
■ Fetal infection	■ Fetal acidosis	■ Fetal sleep
■ Fetal anemia	■ Drugs to mother	■ Fetal congenital malformations
■ Drugs to mother	♦ Pethidine	■ Drugs to mother
♦ β-adrenergic	♦ Methyldopa	♦ Sedatives, $MgSO_4$, antihypertensives
♦ Isoxsuprine	♦ $MgSO_4$	■ Maternal acidosis
■ Maternal infection	■ Epidural analgesia	
	■ Fetal heart conduction defect (SLF)	

SECTION 3

Obstetric Discussion

Section Outline

- Ch. 5. Preterm Birth and Management Issue
- Ch. 6. Gestational Diabetes Mellitus
- Ch. 7. Obesity in Pregnancy
- Ch. 8. Monochorionic Twin Pregnancy
- Ch. 9. Prenatal Screening for Fetal Abnormalities
- Ch. 10. Severe Pre-eclampsia and Eclampsia
- Ch. 11. HELLP Syndrome
- Ch. 12. Cesarean Section
- Ch. 13. Placenta Previa, Placenta Previa Accreta and Vasa Previa
- Ch. 14. Perimortem Cesarean Section
- Ch. 15. Puerperal Sepsis
- Ch. 16. Maternal Near Miss
- Ch. 17. Cesarean Delivery on Maternal Request
- Ch. 18. Classification of Evidence and Grades of Recommendation

5 Preterm Birth and Management Issues

PRETERM BIRTH

Preterm birth (birth before 37 completed weeks or <259 days) is associated with high perinatal mortality and morbidity. More than 70% of perinatal deaths are due to preterm births. **Preterm birth affects infants' survival as well as quality of life when they survive.**

Perinatal survival is much lower when the birth occurs very preterm (before 32 weeks). Perinatal mortality for infants born very preterm (<32 weeks) is significantly high (144/1,000 live births). Infants born preterm, often suffers from visual and hearing impairment, chronic lung disease, bronchopulmonary dysplasia, respiratory distress syndrome (RDS), intraventricular hemorrhage (IVH), necrotizing enterocolitis (NEC), cerebral palsy, retinopathy of prematurity and delayed development. Risk factors and pathophysiology for preterm birth (*See Dutta's Textbook of Obstetrics, 8th Edition, p. 365*) are not always clearly understood.

MANAGEMENT ISSUES

Main Objectives in the Management of Preterm Birth

- **Antenatal transfer of the mother with fetus in utero** to a center equipped with neonatal intensive care unit.
- **Antenatal administration of glucocorticoids** to the mother to enhance fetal pulmonary maturity.
- **Antibiotics** administration to prevent neonatal infection with Group B Streptococcus.

Maternal transfer to a center equipped with neonatal intensive care unit (NICU) is an advantage to improve the survival of the infant born especially before 32 weeks.

Antibiotics for woman with preterm labor are to prevent neonatal infection with Group B Streptococcus. Ampicillin or penicillin or erythromycin is recommended.

Antenatal corticosteroids are associated with significant reduction of neonatal deaths and are safe to the mother.

Dose schedule and route of administration: Two doses of 12 mg betamethasone, given IM at 24 hours apart or four doses of dexamethasone, 6 mg IM, every 12 hours apart is recommended. However, it is reasonable to use 24 mg of either drug within a period of 24–48 hours period. In that case, any dosing regimen can be used.

Q. What are the benefits of antenatal corticosteroids?
Ans. It prevents neonatal—(i) respiratory distress syndrome, (ii) NEC, (iii) patent ductus arteriosus, (iv) bronchopulmonary dysplasia and (v) intraventicular hemorrhage.
  Randomized controlled trials and meta-analysis, confirmed the improvement of neonatal survival with the use of antenatal corticosteroids. Benefits of antenatal corticosteroids are usually for 18 days.

Q. How long after administration of corticosteroids delivery should occur?
Ans. Neonatal complications are mostly prevented when delivery occurs 24 hours after and up to 7 days of administration of second dose of antenatal corticosteroids. However, it should still be given even if delivery is to occur within 24 hours.

Q. At what period of gestation, women should be given antenatal corticosteroids?
Ans. Women with preterm birth occurring up to 34 weeks of gestation should be given antenatal corticosteroids. However, women planned to be delivered by elective cesarean section, prior to 38 completed weeks should be given antenatal corticosteroids.

Q. Is there any contraindication for antenatal corticosteroids?
Ans. Corticosteroids suppress the immune system. This may cause flaring up of any systemic infections (latent). However, there is no such evidence in this respect when used with this dose schedule. One should take cautious attitude in presence of sepsis (tuberculosis, chorioamnionitis or fungal infection). Presence of diabetes is not a contraindication for antenatal corticosteroids. Women should be given additional dose of insulin for glycemic control.
  Repeat course of corticosteroids is not found to have any added benefit. It may be considered (with caution) in cases where first course was given at less than 26 weeks of gestation.

Q. What are the different methods for prevention of preterm labor?
Ans. Prevention of preterm labor (PTL) has been attempted with several means:
- Tocolysis
- Cervical cerclage
- Treatment of specific cause (when present).

Rational use of tocolysis
The following are the clinical situations where tocolytics are used:
- Intrapartum fetal distress due to hyperstimulation of the uterus
- Impaired fetal growth to improve uteroplacental circulation
- To facilitate external cephalic version
- To arrest preterm labor.

Medications used to arrest uterine contractions (tocolytics)
- β agonists (isoxsuprine, ritodrine)
- Calcium channel blockers
- Oxytocin receptor antagonists (atosiban)
- Nitric oxide donors
- $MgSO_4$.

Q. What are the most important issues in the use of tocolytics?
Ans.
- **Effectiveness** of any tocolytic drug in prolonging labor

- **Safety** of the drug in terms of maternal and fetal health
- **Cost-effectiveness** of the drug and the outcome.

Q. Who are the women most likely to benefit from tocolytics?
Ans.
- Women with very PTL (<32 weeks)
- Time needed to transfer the mother to a center with NICU facilities
- To buy time for completion of a full course of corticosteroid.

Not all women with PTL should be recommended for tocolytics.

Q. What are the contraindications in the use of tocolytic drugs?
Ans.
- Fetal factors
  - Lethal congenital malformations
  - Chromosomal defect
  - Fetal compromise or death
  - Non-reassuring cardiotocography (CTG)
  - Intrauterine growth restriction (IUGR)
- Placental insufficiency
- Chorioamnionitis
- Placental abruption
- Severe pre-eclampsia
- Advanced cervical dilatation.

> Women with preterm birth up to 34 weeks and pregnant women for planned cesarean delivery prior to 38 completed weeks should be given antenatal corticosteroids.

Based on evidences, use of tocolytics can arrest preterm labor when compared to placebo.

Tocolytics can reduce preterm birth <24 hours (OR: 0.47; CI: 0.29–0.77) whereas it can reduce preterm birth <7 days with (OR: 0.60; CI: 0.38–0.95) less number of women with preterm birth.

However, use of tocolytic drugs did not show any significant benefit in reducing perinatal or neonatal mortality or morbidity (OR: 1.22; 95% CI: 0.84–1.78).

Commonly used tocolytics: Atosiban (oxytocin receptor antagonists) when compared with β agonists, there was no difference in outcome.
- **Cycloxygenase (COX) inhibitors**: Indomethacin, rofecoxib are not effective in reducing preterm labor. Moreover, COX-2 inhibitors have got significant adverse effects on fetal renal function and the ductus arteriosus.
- **Nitroglycerine** (nitric oxide donor) did not have any clear effect on preterm birth.
- **MgSO$_4$**: There is no evidence that MgSO$_4$ reduces the risk of preterm birth. However, MgSO$_4$ can reduce the risk of neonatal cerebral palsy.[1,2]

Regarding superiority of one tocolytic drug over the other:
- **Nifedipine and atosiban** have comparable effectiveness.
- Compared to β agonists, nifedipine has improved neonatal outcome, although no long-term data available as yet. Calcium channel blocker (nifedipine) reduces the risk of RDS, NEC and IVH (RR 0.63; CP:0.46–0.88). Nifedipine has not been compared with atosiban.
- **Nifedipine** has certain advantages that it has low purchase price and it can be given orally.
- **Atosiban** has no clear advantage over other tocolytics. Moreover, atosiban is associated with increased neonatal death. This may be due to fetal vasopressin

receptor blocked by atosiban. This causes change in the amniotic fluid volume. This also leads to changes in fetal renal and lung development.
- **COX-2 inhibitors:** Fetal adverse effects are premature closure of ductus arteriosus, NEC and IVH.

Q. What are the effects of tocolytics on preterm babies?
Ans. There is no such long-term follow-up study. Drugs having adverse effects are: COX-2 inhibitors and atosiban (see above).
Cost-effectiveness of tocolytic drugs: Compared to atosiban, the other drugs like nifedipine and β agonists have low purchase price. Moreover, nifedipine and β agonists could be used orally.

Q. What is the place (based on evidence) of tocolytics to prevent preterm labor in women with multiple pregnancies?
Ans. There is no evidence to support the use of tocolytics in PTL for women with multiple pregnancies.

Q. What is the place of maintenance therapy of tocolytics?
Ans. Maintenance therapy of tocolytics for PTL is not recommended.[3]

Q. What is the recommended dose schedule of tocolytics?
Ans.
- **Nifedipine** is given orally. The recommended dose schedule is 20 mg initial dose followed by 10–20 mg 3–4 times a day. Dose is adjusted according to uterine activity.
- **Atosiban:** IV bolus dose 6.75 mg over 1 minute followed by atosiban infusion 18 mg/hour for 3 hours, then 6 mg/hour for 45 hours. Atosiban is used mainly in UK.
- Use of $MgSO_4$ for prevention of preterm birth was associated with increased fetal, neonatal or infant death. It is better not to use it.

Q. What should be the tocolytic of choice for prevention of preterm labor?
Ans. Best choice for tocolytic drug should be the one which is most effective and at the same time has fewer adverse effects.

Q. Should multiple tocolytics be used for prevention of preterm labor?
Ans. Using multiple tocolytic drugs is associated with a higher risk of adverse effects. It is recommended not to use multiple tocolytic drugs.

Adverse Effect of Tocolytics[4]
- β agonists has got high side effects
- Others
  - Nifedipine ⎫
  - Atosiban ⎬ Fewer side effect
  - COX inhibitors ⎭

Common Adverse Effects of β agonists
- Palpitation
- Hypokalemia
- Pulmonary edema
- Chest pain
- Headache
- ARDS
- Dyspnea
- Tremor
- Nausea, vomiting
- Hypotension
- Hypoglycemia

β agonists reduce preterm birth within 48 hours. They have efficacy similar to other tocolytics. These drugs are widely used tocolytics in India, UK and some parts of the world. β agonists have been most thoroughly evaluated in trials. β agonists have some side effects that may be life threatening (see above). One systematic review reported one case of pulmonary edema in 425 women treated with β agonists.

Q. What are the perinatal outcomes of using tocolytics for prevention of preterm labor?

Ans. Tocolysis is not associated with a clear reduction of perinatal mortality[5] (OR: 1.22; CI: 0.84–1.78) or neonatal morbidity (OR: 0.82; CI: 0.64–1.07).

Q. What is the place of tocolytics in preterm labor based on evidence?

Ans. There is no clear evidence that use of tocolytic drugs which improve the perinatal outcome. So, it is reasonable not to take them.

Q. What are the evidence-based observations and recommendations for tocolytics in preterm labor?

Ans.
- There is **no reduction** in perinatal mortality and morbidity.
- Tocolytics may be used for selected women to buy time for 48 hours to 7 days (see earlier).
- Nifedipine and atosiban have comparable effectiveness and fewer side effects.

Unfortunately, there is no reliable test to detect preterm labor early with high predictive value; though fetal fibronectin detection and cervical length (USG measurement) have been tried.

References

1. Doyle LW, Crowther CA, Middleton P, et al. Magnesium sulphate for women at risk of preterm birth for neuroprotection of the fetus. Cochrane Database Syst Rev. 2009;(1):CD004661.
2. Papatsonis D, Flenady V, Cole S, et al. Oxytocin receptor antagonists for inhibiting preterm labour. Cochrane Database Syst Rev. 2005;(3):CD004452.
3. Dodd JM, Crowther CA, Dare MR, et al. Oral betamimetics for maintenance therapy after threatened preterm labour. Cochrane Database Syst Rev. 2006;(1):CD003927.
4. Anotayanonth S, Subhedar NV, Garner P, et al. Betamimetics for inhibiting preterm labour. Cochrane Database Syst Rev. 2004;(4):CD004352.
5. Gyetvai K, Hannah ME, Hodnett ED, et al. Tocolytics for preterm labor: a systematic review. Obstet Gynecol. 1999;94(5 Pt 2):869-77.

6

Gestational Diabetes Mellitus

Q. Regarding gestational diabetes mellitus (GDM).
   a. GDM differs from type 2 diabetes mellitus
   b. GDM is controlled by diet only
   c. IADPSG recommends one step 75 g oral GTT at 24–28 weeks of gestation
   d. BMI > 30 kg/m² is a high-risk factor.

> GDM may be an early type 2 diabetic state or it is the same disease with a different name.

Ans. a. F   b. F
       c. T   d. T

GESTATIONAL DIABETES MELLITUS (GDM)

Diagnosis and Management

Gestational diabetes mellitus is a state of carbohydrate intolerance of variable severity with onset or first recognition during pregnancy. This entity usually presents late in the second or third trimester of pregnancy. The **definition is not changed irrespective of its presence at 6 weeks of postpartum, though GTT comes down to normal following delivery in majority**.

The definition, however, needs further clarification. Millions of type 2 diabetic women remain undiagnosed and they are recognized for the first time during pregnancy. These women are all categorized as GDM. Thus, GDM actually represents a group of women who have had abnormal carbohydrate tolerance test results in pregnancy and also have undiagnosed type 2 diabetes.

Prevalence of GDM is in direct proportion to the prevalence of type 2 diabetes in a given population, ethnic group or geographic area. In India, prevalence of GDM ranges from 3.8 to 21% according to Diabetes in Pregnancy Society of India (DIPSI) compared to US, it ranges from 1–14%.

It is therefore observed that a good number of undiagnosed type 2 diabetic women are masked in the GDM population. So, GDM may be an early type 2 diabetic state or it is the same disease with a different name. As such substitute nomenclature 'pregnancy induced glucose intolerance' seems appropriate.

GDM and type 2 diabetes have many similarities in terms of endocrine and metabolic abnormalities and the risk factors in pregnancy. Thus, basically they are the same disease of varying severity.

Pathophysiology of GDM and Type 2 Diabetes

- Declining β cell functioning
- Insulin resistance in peripheral tissues
- Impaired hepatic glucose production.

Optimization of glycemic profile is the ultimate goal of treatment for pregnant or nonpregnant diabetic women.

Therapeutic Strategies Include

- Diet control
- Exercise
- Use of pharmacological agents.

These include insulin or oral antidiabetic drugs. Pharmacological interventions are used when glycemic control cannot be achieved by diet and exercise.

There has been a controversy in screening and diagnosis of GDM. Universal screening in pregnancy for GDM has not been recommended by National Institute for Health and Clinical Excellence (NICE-2002). There are several fetal adverse outcomes like macrosomia, shoulder dystocia and stillbirth due to maternal hyperglycemia. Therefore, screening program has been recommended for women with high-risk factor [NICE-2008, (Box 6.1)] only.[1] **Considering the high-risk group (see below) the women of Asian origin are recommended for universal screening for GDM.** Subsequently other studies, Hyperglycemia and Adverse Pregnancy Outcome (Multinational HAPO) study[2,3] and International Association of Diabetes and Pregnancy Study Groups (IADPSG) observed the relationship between maternal glucose and fetal growth and the related fetal adverse outcomes.[4] It was also observed that fetal growth and adverse outcomes can be modified by glucose-lowering therapies. These include diet, lifestyle intervention and also with pharmacological intervention when needed. It is now clear that treatment of women with GDM can improve adverse outcomes. **There is significant reduction of perinatal death, shoulder dystocia, bone fracture and nerve palsy from 4 to 10% [Australian Carbohydrate Intolerance Study (ACHOIS-2005) in pregnant women].**

Box 6.1: Risk factors for GDM: National Institute for Health and Clinical Excellence (NICE)-2008

- BMI > 30 kg/m^2
- Previous macrosomic baby weighing ≥ 4.5 kg
- Previous GDM
- Family history of diabetes (1st degree relatives)
- Family origin with a high prevalence of diabetes:
    - South Asian (India, Pakistan, Bangladesh)
    - Black Caribbean
    - Middle Eastern (Saudi Arabia, United Arab Emirates, Iraq, Syria, Jordon, Oman, Qatar, Kuwait, Lebanon and Egypt).

Significance of 2-hour Plasma Glucose Level > 140 mg/dL (> 7.8 mmol/L)

Increased maternal carbohydrate intolerance in pregnant women is associated with progressively increased adverse maternal and perinatal outcomes. The cumulative risk of developing type 2 diabetes in the offspring (at the age of 24 years), born to a mother who had plasma glucose level between 120 and 139 mg/dL in the third trimester, was 19%. The same study revealed that the cumulative risk of 30% in the offspring, born to a woman who had 2-hour plasma glucose > 140 mg/dL.[5] The development of fetal macrosomia is a process of continuum as the 2-hour plasma glucose rises from 120 mg/dL. Hence, it is wise to level 2-hour plasma glucose value > 140 mg/dL as GDM and that of ≥ 120 mg and ≤ 139 mg as gestational glucose intolerance (GGI).

Woman with fasting plasma glucose ≥ 126 mg/dL and 2 hours post 75 g glucose, plasma glucose ≥ 200 mg/dL HbAIC > 6 or random plasma glucose ≥ 200 mg/dL are considered diabetic.

Treatment for GDM (Based on New Evidence)

Lifestyle interventions including dietary modification and exercise are the primary intervention for all women diagnosed with GDM. This is helpful for majority of women. However, 7–20% women will fail to achieve glycemic control with diet and exercise alone. Oral hypoglycemic agents or insulin will be needed to control their hyperglycemic state.

Both metformin and glibenclamide are effective in the treatment of GDM. However, about 20–30% women may need insulin despite that they are being treated with glibenclamide or metformin due to inadequate glycemic control.

Maternal complications (e.g. pre-eclampsia) are also reduced following treatment of GDM.

Metformin and glibenclamide cross the placenta but no immediate risks to fetus have been demonstrated. However, any potential long-term effects remain under investigation.

International Association of Diabetes and Pregnancy Study Groups had redrawn the diagnosis of GDM (Table 6.1), based on international consensus for screening and diagnosis. *IADPSG recommends a one step 75 g oral GTT for all women (not known to be diabetic) at 24–28 weeks of gestation.* GDM is diagnosed when any one of following plasma glucose value is exceeded: fasting ≥ 5.1 mmol/L, 1 hour ≥ 10.0 mmol/L and 2 hours ≥ 8.5 mmol/L.

These diagnostic levels are set at the level of maternal blood glucose at which the rates of key pregnancy outcomes, e.g. macrosomia, cord blood **C-peptide** (a stable marker of fetal insulin) > 90th percentile, percentage of newborn body fat > 90th percentile are increased by 1.75-fold over the mean for HAPO study population. According to IADPSG system of screening, the incidence of GDM is over 16% compared to current level of 3.5%. It is a major change in terms of obstetric practice.

Table 6.1: Diagnostic criteria for GDM with 75 g oral glucose tolerance

	ADA	NICE	IADPSG*	DIPSI	WHO (2013)
Fasting	≥ 5.1 mmol/L (92 mg/dL)	≥ 7.0 mmol/L (126.7 mg/dL)	≥ 5.1 mmol/L (92.3 mg/dL)	< 100 mg/dL	5.1–6.9 mmol/L (>92 mg/dL)
1 hour	>10 mmol/L (180 mg/dL)	–	≥ 10.0 mmol/L (181 mg/dL)	–	≥10.0 mmol/L (180 mg/dL)
2 hours	≥ 8.5 mmol/L (153 mg/dL)	≥ 7.8 mmol/L (141.1 mg/dL)	≥ 8.5 mmol/L (153.85 mg/dL)	≥ 7.8 mmol/L (≥ 141.1 mg/dL)	8.5–11.0 mmol/L (>153 mg/dL)

Note: Values are for venous plasma samples; *one value is sufficient for diagnosis

Diabetes in Pregnancy Society of India, recommends a one step 75 g oral GTT for all women (not known to be diabetic) attending the antenatal clinic at 24–28 weeks of gestation (Box 6.2).[6]

This is irrespective of time of day and last meal. *GDM is diagnosed when 2-hour plasma glucose value is ≥ 140 mg/dL. Diabetes is diagnosed when women with fasting and blood glucose value is ≥ 126 mg/dL and 2-hour value is ≥ 200 mg/dL.*

Box 6.2: Benefits of one-step procedure of screening

- Women need not keep fast in pregnancy
- No loss of working hours as in two-step procedure
- Avoids dropout rate (23%) for two-step procedure
- One time test for both screening and diagnosis
- It correlates well with perinatal outcome.

Q. *Regarding management of gestational diabetes mellitus (GDM)*
  a. Fasting plasma glucose > 105 mg/dL despite diet control indicates pharmacological intervention
  b. Approximately 10% women with GDM need pharmacologic therapy
  c. Glibenclamide cross the placenta significantly
  d. Metformin stimulates insulin secretion.

Ans. a. T   b. F
      c. F   d. F

Pharmacological Interventions in the Management of GDM

Questions remained to be answered are:
A. Who should be given the medication?
B. How long the therapy to be continued?
C. When should a patient be evaluated for glycemic profile?

The cut off values for initiation of pharmacological agents despite of diet controls are:
A. Fasting plasma glucose ≥ 95 mg/dL or 105 mg/dL
B. Postmeal 2-hour plasma glucose ≥ 120 mg/dL.

Based on these criteria about 30–50% women with GDM will need pharmacologic therapy when diet and exercise fail to control glycemic levels adequately.

Oral Hypoglycemic Agents in GDM

There is a similarity in the pathogenesis of type 2 DM and GDM. These drugs are found to be successful, less invasive, more patient friendly, less expensive and provides similar perinatal outcomes.

Sulfonylureas

Sulfonylureas have been used to treat type 2 DM. It enhances insulin secretion. Enhanced insulin secretion suppresses the production of hepatic glucose as it is the main contributor to fasting hyperglycemia. It improves insulin secretion thus reduces postprandial hyperglycemia. Glibenclamide (Glyburide) is extensively metabolized in liver and the metabolites are excreted in the bile and urine. Half-life is about 10 hours. The main side effect of glibenclamide is hypoglycemia. *The ideal patients for this therapy are individuals having β-cell exhaustion and insulin resistance. This drug does not significantly cross the placenta.* Fetal concentrations are not more than 1–2% of maternal concentrations. Studies could not establish any association between oral hypoglycemic agents and congenital malformations. The outcomes of treatments, when glyburide is compared with insulin, are similar, in respect of complications like pre-eclampsia, macrosomia, cesarean section rate and hyperglycemia.

Biguanides

Metformin is an insulin sensitizer. It reduces insulin resistance and basal plasma insulin levels.

Various Metabolic Effects of Metformin

- It suppresses hepatic glucose output
- Increases insulin mediated glucose uptake
- Decreases fatty acid oxidation
- Improves lipid profile by decreasing LDL, fatty acids, triglycerides and it increases HDL cholesterol
- Decreases intestinal absorption of glucose
- It does not stimulate insulin secretion
- At cellular level, it increases insulin sensitivity.

It may cause lactic acidosis (0.03/1,000 patient years). Metformin is eliminated unchanged in the urine and it is not metabolized in liver. Plasma half-life is 2–5 hours. Renal clearance of metformin occurs more by tubular secretion than by glomerular filtration. It binds minimally to plasma proteins. On the other hand, glibenclamide is cleared by the liver and kidneys. 99.8% of glibenclamide is bound to plasma proteins. Metformin started gradually 500 mg/day or 850 mg/day with increments to a maximum effective dose of 2,000 mg/day. Women with renal disease are contraindicated for metformin therapy (Table 6.2).

Metformin crosses the placenta and is categorized as a class B drug. However, there is minimal effect on transplacental flux. ***Its use in GDM is past the first trimester, after the period of organogenesis. However, the cumulative available data suggest that the cause of anomalies is the level of hyperglycemia and not the use of oral hypoglycemic drugs.*** Metformin is secreted minimally in human milk. Lactation in patients using metformin is not contraindicated. This drug may be an alternative to insulin in the management of GDM in women. However, it is not needed to continue metformin throughout pregnancy in woman with PCOS when she conceives, unless she develops GDM.

Thiazolidinediones (rosiglitazone, pioglitazone) are classified as pregnancy category C. One needs to be careful while using these drugs.

Oral hypoglycemic agents act upon different mechanism of action. Oral monotherapy such as glibenclamide or probably metformin may be started. Glibenclamide (glyburide) is currently the only drug shown either minimal or not to cross the placenta. It has been studied with randomized controlled trials (RCTs).

Table 6.2: Optimum levels of capillary blood glucose levels while on therapy (self-monitored)

Specimen	Level (mg/dL)
Fasting	≤ 95
2-hour PP	≤ 120
Mean	≤ 100
HbA1C	≤ 6

Source: (ACOG Practice Bulletin 60, Washington DC, 2005)

Gestational Diabetes Mellitus

Q. Is the association between GDM and adverse pregnancy outcomes are independent of other risk factors such as age, BMI and weight gain during pregnancy?

Ans. There is a clear relationship between the rising plasma glucose levels during pregnancy and adverse pregnancy outcomes. The HAPO study (2008) was an international multicenter cohort of 25,505 pregnant women tested with a 2-hour 75 g OGTT **and then followed through pregnancy to detect primary and secondary outcomes**. After adjustment for multiple potential cofounders, the study demonstrated the progressive rising relationship between plasma glucose levels and adverse pregnancy outcomes. However, these associations were independent of other known risk factors.

Q. Can treatment for GDM reduce adverse pregnancy outcomes?[7]

Ans. It is established in a quantified term that the relationship between the levels of hyperglycemia in GDM and adverse pregnancy outcomes are directly proportional.

Effect of treatment for GDM depends on the spectrum of hyperglycemia and the type of intervention offered. These interventions were lifestyle changes (like nutritional counseling and exercise) and/or medical therapy (oral hypoglycemic agents or insulin), when necessary.

It has been observed with several studies that treatment of GDM produced statistically significant relative risk reductions for most of the adverse maternal and perinatal outcomes.

> There is decrease in relative risks of macrosomia, large for gestational age, shoulder dystocia, significant relative risk reductions for pre-eclampsia, hypertensive disorders and cesarean section rates. There was also risk reductions for perinatal mortality, neonatal intensive care admission, birth trauma and respiratory distress syndrome.

Q. What is the current opinion as regard to the management of gestational diabetes mellitus and overt diabetes?

Ans. Hyperglycemia first detected at any time during pregnancy should be classified as either
- Diabetes mellitus in pregnancy or
- GDM

The large multinational HAPO study, excluded women with fasting glucose level > 5.8 mmol/L (104 mg/dL) and 2-hour post glucose levels >11.1 mmol/L (200 mg/dL) from the diagnostic criteria of GDM.[3] ACHOIS study excluded women with the fasting plasma glucose (F >126 mg/dL and 2-hour PG > 200 mg/dL) cut off values of plasma glucose from the diagnostic criteria of GDM.

Currently, consensus has moved in favor of distinguishing between overt diabetes from lesser degree of glucose intolerance (GDM). Current opinion: WHO 2006.

However, following issues are resolved in this respect.
- Diabetes in pregnancy whether symptomatic or not is associated with significant risk of adverse pregnancy outcome.[3,8]
- Some differences in approach to management is important for women with diabetes in pregnancy as compared to GDM.
- Detailed assessment for diabetes related complications is recommended when diabetes is diagnosed. This is particularly important for the management of complications like retinopathy, nephropathy, hypertension and coronary artery disease, which affect pregnancy adversely. Moreover pregnancy can worsen the disease condition.

- More intensive monitoring and treatment of hyperglycemia during pregnancy is recommended. Pharmacotherapy is required more frequently to control hyperglycemia.
- Following delivery, women need to be followed up. Women with diabetes need to be monitored and treated for the rest of their lives.

References

1. National Institute for Health and Clinical Excellence (NICE) guideline for diabetes in pregnancy, 2008.
2. HAPO Study Cooperative Research Group. Hyperglycemia and adverse pregnancy outcome (HAPO) Study: associations with neonatal anthropometrics. Diabetes. 2009;58:453-9.
3. HAPO Study Cooperative Research Group, Metzger BE, Lowe LP, et al. Hyperglycemia and adverse pregnancy outcomes. N Engl J Med. 2008;358(19):1991-2002.
4. International Association of Diabetes of Pregnancy Study Groups Consensus Panel, Metzer BE, Gabbe SG, et al. International association of diabetes and pregnancy study groups recommendations on the diagnosis and classification of hyperglycemia in pregnancy. Diabetes Care. 2010;33(3):676-82.
5. Franks PW, Looker HC, Kobes S, et al. Gestational glucose tolerance and risk of type 2 diabetes in young Pima Indian offspring. Diabetes. 2006;55(2):460-5.
6. Seshiah V, Sahay BK, Das AK, et al. Gestational diabetes mellitus—Indian guidelines. J Indian Med Assoc. 2009;107(11):799-802, 804-6.
7. Crowther CA, Hiller JE, Moss JR, et al. Effect of treatment of gestational diabetes mellitus on pregnancy outcomes. N Engl J Med.2005;352(24):2477-86.
8. Landon MB, Spong CY, Thom E, et al. A multicenter, randomized trial of treatment for mild gestational diabetes. N Engl J Med. 2009;361(14):1339-48.

7
Obesity in Pregnancy

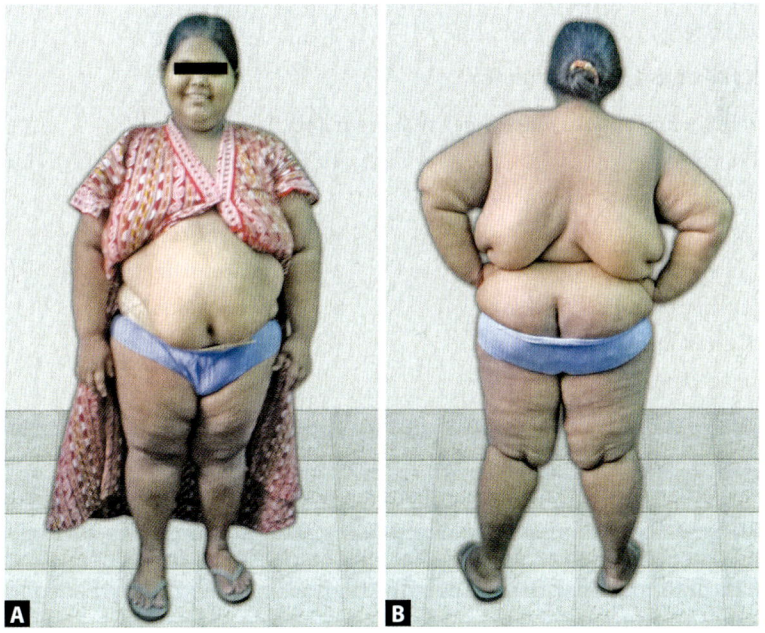

Figs 7.1A and B: Mrs M, a 20-year-old female in her 3rd day of puerperium following cesarean delivery. She weighed 123 kg. Her BMI was 48.1 kg/m²
Courtesy: Department of Obstetrics and Gynecology, CNMCH, Kolkata

Q. Regarding obesity in pregnancy:
    a. Obesity in pregnancy is not a problem in India
    b. Vitamin supplementation should be withheld for obese pregnant women
    c. Pregnancy complications are increased
    d. Intrapartum care is the central important issue

Ans. a. F   b. F
       c. T   d. F

Obesity in pregnancy is a known risk factor. A pregnant women with a BMI of 30 kg/m² or more, detected at the first antenatal visit (1st trimester) is considered obese. Prevalence of obesity in pregnancy is increasing even in India.

Q. What is the prevalence of obesity in India?

Ans. Prevalence of obesity in India is increasing specially in the urban areas compared to the rural residents.[1,2]

Generalized obesity (GO): BMI > 25 kg/m², abdominal obesity (AO): waist circumference > 80 cm (female)/(women). **Combined obesity (CO)** is defined when an individual has both the criteria. Urban women with obesity is highest in Tamil Nadu (23.5%), followed by Maharashtra (18.1%).[1]

Classification of obesity based on BMI

Obesity	BMI (kg/m²)
Class 1	30.0–34.9
Class 2	35.0–39.9
Class 3	≥ 40
Morbid obesity	

$$BMI = \frac{\text{Weight in kilogram (kg)}}{\text{Height in meter (m}^2\text{)}}$$

Effects of obesity in pregnancy

Obstetric complications due to obesity in pregnancy	
▪ Miscarriage	▪ Dysfunctional labor
▪ Fetal congenital anomaly	▪ Increased cesarean delivery
▪ Macrosomia	▪ Anesthetic complication
▪ Stillbirth	▪ Postpartum hemorrhage
▪ Neonatal death	▪ Thromboembolism
▪ Gestational diabetes	▪ Wound infections
▪ Pre-eclampsia	▪ Lactation failure
▪ Ischemic heart disease	▪ Increased risk of maternal mortality

Q. How care should be organized for an obese woman?

Ans. Obese woman should have prepregnancy counseling. The significance of obesity and the increased association of complications in pregnancy should be discussed. The woman should be encouraged to optimize her weight ideally before pregnancy. She should be given the information with regards to the body weight, diet, lifestyle and family planning measures to improve the outcome.

Q. Should women with obesity need to be additionally advised for nutritional supplementation?

Ans.
- Women with obesity BMI ≥ 30 kg/m² are at increased risk of fetal congenital malformations like neural tube defects (NTD) compared to a healthy weight woman. Maternal folic acid deficiency is associated with fetal congenital malformations. Periconceptional use of folic acid (4 mg/day) reduces the risk of NTD. Women with BMI >30 kg/m², should be recommended folic acid (5 mg) supplementation daily. She should start this atleast 1 month before conception and continue to take this during the 1st trimester of pregnancy.
- Obese women (BMI ≥ 30 kg/m²) are also advised to take 10 µg of vitamin D supplementation daily during pregnancy and lactation. Women with obesity (BMI ≥ 30 kg/m²) have vitamin deficiency as compared to a healthy weight woman (BMI < 25 kg/m²).

Q. How the obese woman should be supervised during pregnancy?
Ans.
- Women with booking BMI ≥ 30 kg/m² have an increased risk of pre-eclampsia. They should have blood pressure measurement with appropriate size of the arm cuff. They may need early referral to a specialist care unit.
- All women with booking BMI ≥ 30 kg/m² should be screened for gestational diabetes mellitus (GDM).
- Obesity increases the risk of GDM by 3-fold as compared to a healthy weight woman. All such women should have 2 hours 75 g glucose tolerance test (GTT) at 24–28 weeks by using the WHO criteria.

Q. What are the risks of an obese woman (BMI ≥ 30 kg/m²) during labor and delivery?
Ans. *Intrapartum complications are high:*
- Slow and/or dysfunctional labor
- Shoulder dystocia
- Emergency cesarean delivery
- Difficulties in cesarean delivery
- Complications during anesthesia are
  - Aspiration of gastric contents during general anesthesia
  - Difficulty in tracheal intubation
  - Difficulties in intravenous access and sitting regional anesthesia.
- Monitoring fetal well-being [fetal heart rate (FHR) auscultation]
  Such women should be delivered under direct supervision of consultants. Multidisciplinary team approach should be made. Operative vaginal or abdominal delivery should be performed by an experienced obstetrician involving the senior anesthetist
- All such woman (BMI ≥ 30 kg/m²) should be recommended to have active management of the third stage of labor to prevent postpartum hemorrhage (PPH)
- Obese women run the risk of increased wound infection following either cesarean section or operative vaginal delivery. They should be given prophylactic antibiotics
- Obese women should have suturing of the subcutaneous fatty layer of tissues as this layer is often > 2 cm thick. This procedure reduces the risk of wound infection
- Venous thromboembolism (VTE).

Q. What are the important management issues in the postpartum period?
Ans.
- Obese women should be encouraged for breastfeeding as breastfeeding initiation and maintenance rates are low
- Women diagnosed to have GDM should have GTT after 6 weeks postpartum. They should be followed up regularly. They should be screened for the development of type 2 diabetes.

Q. What are the measures that can minimize the risk of thromboembolism?
Ans. Maternal obesity increases the risk of VTE during antenatal as well as postnatal period.[3] Therefore, measures to be taken are:
- Early mobilization
- Use of compression stockings
- Women with BMI ≥ 30 kg/m², who also has ≥ 2 additional risk factors for thromboembolism (as discussed later), should be considered for prophylactic low molecular weight heparin (LMWH) antenatally.

- All women receiving LMWH; once started, antenatally, should continue the same (LMWH) until 6 weeks postpartum.

Q. How thromboprophylaxis is done in the puerperium for such a woman?
Ans. *Pharmacological thromboprophylaxis according to maternal weight:*[4]

Maternal weight (kg)	Pharmacological agent	Dose	Route
91–130	■ Enoxaparin ■ Dalteparin	60 mg/day 7,000 units/day	SC SC
131–170	■ Enoxaparin ■ Dalteparin ■ Tinzaparin	80 mg/day 10,000 units/day 9,000 units/day	SC SC SC
> 170	■ Enoxaparin ■ Dalteparin ■ Tinzaparin	0.6 mg/kg/day 75 units/kg/day 75 units/kg/day	SC SC SC

Q. Who are the woman with high-risk factors for VTE?
Ans. *Risk factors for VTE are:*

- Previous VTE
- Obesity (BMI ≥ 30 kg/m^2)
- Parity > 4
- Age > 35 years
- Thrombophilia
  ♦ Inherited
  ♦ Acquired
- Surgical intervention (cesarean delivery)
- Dehydration
- Severe infection
- Prolonged labor
- Prolonged immobilization
- Ovarian hyperstimulation syndrome (OHSS)

Q. What other antithrombotic agents are used?
Ans.
- **Low dose aspirin:** It is an antiplatelet agent and is commonly used in cases with antiphospholipid syndrome.
- **Warfarin:** It is a vitamin K antagonist (VKA). It inhibits the synthesis of vitamin K dependent clotting factors (II, VII, IX and X). It crosses the placenta and carries the risk of fetal congenital abnormalities (warfarin embryopathy). Its use is restricted in the 1st trimester of pregnancy. Warfarin embryopathy is observed to be dose-dependent. Risks are more when the woman is taking >5 mg/day.
- **Unfractionated heparin (UFH):** It can be used around the time of delivery where the risk of thrombosis is high. It has a short half-life. Heparin induced thrombocytopenia is more with UFH composed to LMWH.

Q. What are the contraindications to the use of LMWH?
Ans. Women having the risk of bleeding with heparin should be avoided. Women in this group are:
- Active bleeding in the antenatal or postpartum period
- Increased risk of major hemorrhage (placenta previa)
- Women with disseminated intravascular coagulation (DIC)
- Thrombocytopenia
- Comorbid medical conditions, e.g. renal or hepatic disease, uncontrolled hypertension.

Q. Should the women with warfarin or UFH or LMWH feed their baby with breast milk?

Ans. Women with LMWH or UFH during puerperium can feed their baby with breast milk without any problems. Warfarin can be safely used following delivery. Breastfeeding is not contraindicated.

References

1. Pradeepa R, Anjana RM, Joshi SR, et al. Prevalence of generalized & abdominal obesity in urban & rural India- the ICMR-INDIAB Study (Phase-I) [ICMR - INDIAB-3]. Indian J Med Res. 2015;142(2):139-50.
2. Dasgupta A, Harichandrakumar KT, Habeebullah S. Pregnancy Outcome among Obese Indians–A Prospective Cohort Study in a Tertiary Care Centre in South India. International Journal of Scientific Study. 2014; 2(2):13-8.
3. National Institute for Health and Care Excellence (NICE). (2010). Venous thromboembolism: reducing the risk for patients in hospital. NICE guidelines—acute and chronic conditions. [online]. Available from www.nice.org.uk. [Accessed June, 2016].
4. Royal College of Obstetrics and Gynecology (RCOG). (2004). Thromboprophylaxis during pregnancy, labor and after vaginal delivery. RCOG Guideline. [online] Available from www.rcog.org.uk. [Accessed June, 2016].

8 Monochorionic Twin Pregnancy

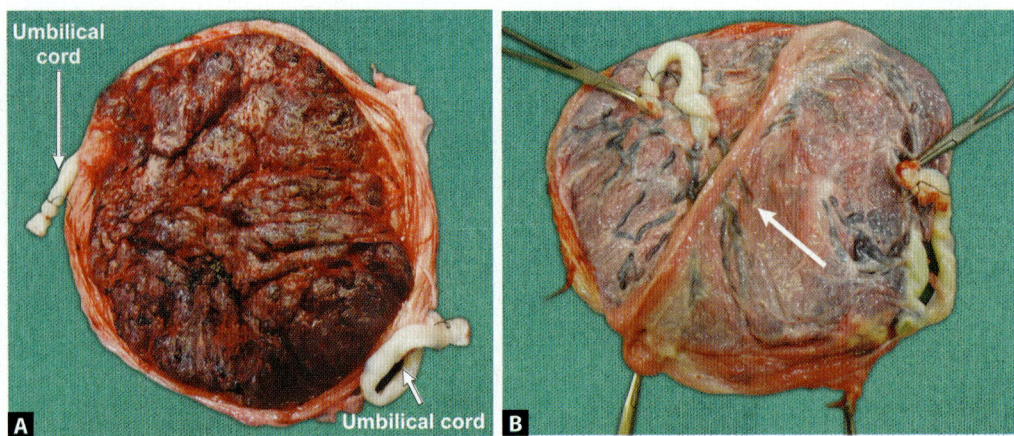

Figs 8.1A and B: *Placenta of monochorionic twin pregnancy.* **A.** Single placental mass with two umbilical cords (*see* arrows); **B.** Vascular communications beneath the amnion (*see* arrow)

SINGLE BEST ANSWER (SBA) AND MULTIPLE CHOICE QUESTIONS (MCQs)

Q. Regarding diagnosis and management of twin-to-twin transfusion syndrome (TTTS):
  a. Placenta appears as a single mass
  b. Presence of critically abnormal Doppler studies in either twin is classified as Quintero stage III
  c. Amnioreduction, septostomy or laser ablation is the recommended intervention
  d. Often delivery of the twins is considered at 34 weeks

Ans. a. T b. T
 c. F d. T
  c. Laser ablation is preferred rather than amnioreduction or septostomy. Eurofetus trial with TTTS to either laser ablation or amnioreduction was prematurely terminated. Results of NICHD trial of amnioreduction versus laser ablation are awaited.

Q. Regarding monochorionic (MC) twin pregnancies (MCTPs), (Figs 8.1A and B):
  a. All types of multiple pregnancies are increased recently
  b. Placental vascular anastomoses are universal

c. Monoamniotic twins have higher risks
d. Co-twin fetal death is a known complication

Ans. a. T b. T
c. T d. T

Q. Regarding twin-to-twin transfusion syndrome:
a. Unidirectional anastomoses are more likely
b. It is more common in monochorionic diamniotic (MCDA) pregnancies
c. Presence of twin peak sign on ultrasonography suggests dichorionic placenta
d. Fetal survival is better in artery-vein anastomosis

Ans. a. T b. T
c. T d. F

Q. What is the importance of zygocity and chorionicity?

Ans. In multifetal gestation, zygocity refers to the genetic make-up of pregnancy whereas chorionicity indicates pregnancy membrane status. Complications of pregnancy are predominantly related to chorionicity.

> Monoamniotic twins comprise about 1% of all monozygotic twins. They have high fetal death rate due to congenital anomaly, cord entanglement, TTTS, and twin reverse arterial perfusion (TRAP), (Fig. 8.2).

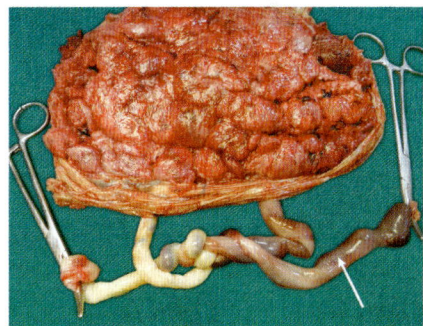

Fig. 8.2: Monoamniotic twins placenta showing entanglement of the umbilical cords. One cord is seen thrombosed (*see arrow*) and this fetus suffered intrauterine death. The other fetus was alive

Q. What is the importance of prenatal diagnosis of MCTP?

Ans. Ultrasound examination at 10–13 weeks of twin gestation should be done. Benefits are to detect fetal viability, chorionicity, nuchal translucency and major congenital malformations.

Nuchal translucency measurements in MCTPs should be done for fetal aneuploidy screening.

Q. How monochorionicity is diagnosed?

Ans. **Chorionicity is best diagnosed by ultrasound before 14 weeks**. Sonography reveals membrane placenta interface as **'lambda' or 'twin peak' sign making the diagnosis of dichorionic placenta**. Presence of **T-sign indicates monochronic one** (sensitivity 89.8% and specificity 99.5%).

Q. What are the pathophysiological changes in monochorionic twins?

Ans. Pathology unique to monochorionic twins are due to single shared placenta. Vascular communications are almost always found in monochorionic gestations. The vascular communication may be artery to artery, vein to vein or artery to vein. The artery-artery and vein-vein communications are end to end anastomosis that occurs at the placental surface. On the other hand in artery-vein anastomosis, an artery enters the capillary bed of a cotyledon and it drains into the venous system of the c-twin. Artery-artery communications are more common.

Placental vascular anastomosis in monochorionic twins is a characteristic feature. Most vascular anastomoses are hemodynamically balanced and safe. Once major hemodynamic shunts are developed within the placental vessels, circulatory imbalances are created. TTTS, acardiac twins, single fetal death are the known problems (see below).

MONOCHORIONIC TWIN PREGNANCY

Management Issues

Monochorionic twin pregnancy share a single placenta. There is a placental vascular anastomosis that connects the umbilical circulations of both fetuses.
Special issues in the management of MCTP are:
- Twin-to-twin transfusion syndrome
- Single fetal death in twin pregnancy
- Fetal abnormalities
- Twin reverse arterial perfusion
- Conjoint twins
- Monochorionic monoamniotic twin pregnancy
- Growth discordance
- Selective fetal reduction

- All types of multiple pregnancies are increasing
- Placenta vascular anastomosis is universal in monochorionic twins
- Monochorionic twins have higher perinatal complications
- Chorionicity is more important compared to zygocity.

Twin-to-twin Transfusion Syndrome

Pathology: In TTTS (10–15% of all monochorionic pregnancies), the blood flow is commonly unidirectional (artery-vein) and less often it is bi-directional (artery-artery). Fetal survival is better when artery-artery anastomosis is present. TTTS is more common in MCDA than monochorionic-monoamniotic pregnancies.

Blood is transferred from the donor to the recipient twin in a situation where major placental vascular (artery to artery, artery to vein) shunts are developed. The unidirectional flow results in hemodynamic imbalance between the fetuses. Deoxygenated blood from the donor twin is pumped into the recipient through the shared placenta. The donor twin becomes—anemic, hypovolemic, hypotensive and oliguric. There is oligohydramnios in the donor sac.

The recipient twin becomes—polycythemic, plethoric, hypervolemic and polyuric. There is polyhydramnios in the recipient sac.

The donor twin becomes a 'stuck twin' as this twin is prevented from any movement due to oligohydramnios. **This polyhydramnios-oligohydramnios** or **Poly-Oli** syndrome is associated with many complications.

The complications are: Donor twin suffers fetal growth restriction, pulmonary hypoplasia, hypotension, cerebral palsy, microcephaly, neurological damage. Death of the affected twin causes acute hypotension of the surviving twin. This is due to transfusion through the placental anastomotic vessels from the high pressure zone of the living twin to the low pressure vessels of the dead twin. It leads to ischemic brain damage of the living twin. This acute nature of TTTS makes the survival of the living twin impossible.

TWIN-TO-TWIN TRANSFUSION SYNDROME

Diagnostic Criterias of TTTS Based on Ultrasound
- Single placental mass
- Fetuses with concordant gender
- Oligohydramnios in one sac [maximum vertical pocket (MVP) <2 cm]
- Polyhydramnios in other sac (MVP ≥ 8 cm)
- Discordant bladder filling
- Hemodynamic instability and cardiac compromise.

Q. What is the perinatal outcome of monochorionic compared to dichorionic twin pregnancy?

Ans. Monochorionic twin pregnancies have higher perinatal loss compared to dichorionic (DC) twins. Neurodevelopmental morbidity is also high in MCTPs.

> Monochorionic twins have more perinatal mortality and morbidity compared to dichorionic twins. Perinatal outcome of monozygotic dichorionic twins and the dizygotic twins are the same. Hence, chorionicity is more important as compared to zygocity.

Q. What is the place of ultrasonography in monochorionic twins?

Ans. All women with twin pregnancy should have ultrasound examination at 10–13 weeks (before 14 weeks) of pregnancy. The information obtained with this have both diagnostic and prognostic values:
- Fetal viability
- Chorionicity
- Nuchal translucency for aneuploidy screening
- Twin-to-twin transfusion syndrome and its severity
- Echocardiography (cardiac abnormalities and functional compromise)
- Growth profile (fetal biometry).

Ultrasonographic assessment should be continued at an interval of 2–3 weeks or earlier if indicated.

Grading for Severity of TTTS

The **Quintero system** of grading TTTS has got some prognostic value.[1]

Quintero system of classification (1999)

Grades	Classifications
I	• Discrepancy in amniotic fluid volume—oligohydramnios (MVP ≤ 2 cm) in one sac and polyhydramnios (MVP ≥ 8 cm) in other sac • The bladder of the donor twin is visible; Doppler studies are normal
II	The bladder of the donor twin is not visible (over 1 hour of observation) but Doppler studies are not critically abnormal
III	Doppler studies are critically abnormal in either twin (abnormal or reversed end diastolic flow in umbilical artery, reverse flow in ductus venosus or pulsatile umbilical venous flow)
IV	Presence of ascites, pericardial or pleural effusion, scalp edema or overt hydrops
V	One or both babies are dead

Management of TTTS

Management should be done in a fetal medicine center

Treatment options available are:
- Serial amnioreduction
- Laser ablation of the connecting vessels[2]
- Septostomy—making a hole in the dividing septum, so that the amniotic fluid volume in donor's sac improves. However, perinatal outcome did not improve with this measure significantly.

Laser ablation may not be effective for deep seated vessels and in few cases anastomosis may be missed. Therefore, the risk of recurrence of TTTS (up to 14%) has been observed.

Time and Mode of Delivery in a Woman with Monochorionic Twin Pregnancy

Management of a woman with MCTP depends mainly with the fetal growth profile and the presence or absence of TTTS.

Monochorionic Twin Pregnancy without any Intrauterine Growth Restriction (IUGR) and TTTS

- **Vaginal delivery** may be allowed when there is no specific clinical indication for cesarean section.
- **Optimum time of delivery** should be at 36–37 weeks of gestation.
- **Earlier delivery** is indicated when there is specific indication (IUGR, TTTS fetal compromise).
- **Cesarean delivery** is indicated in cases with noncephalic first fetus, prior cesarean delivery, monoamniotic-monochorionic twin or TTTS with fetal compromise.

Growth Discordance in Twins (Discordant Twins)

Difference in weight of the twin fetuses is common. The higher the weight difference, the more is the perinatal mortality. The more early the discordance starts, the higher the risk of fetal demise. The etiology of growth discordance is not always clear.

In monochorionic twin gestation, the hemodynamic instability arising out of placental vascular anastomosis is an important cause. Fetal abnormalities are also responsible for growth discordance.

In dizygotic twin fetuses, the placentas are separate. Suboptimal placental implantation due to lack of space is an important factor for discordant fetal growth.

Diagnosis: Fetal growth discordance can be diagnosed by sonographic weight estimation of each fetus. The weight difference between the fetuses is calculated. Weight discrepancy of more than 25–30% is associated with poor perinatal outcome.

Management: Factors to be consider in the management are: (a) Degree of growth discordance, (b) Gestational age and (c) Fetal surveillance report. Once growth discordance is diagnosed with sonographic parameters, close fetal surveillance is maintained. Presence of oligohydramnios is an important observation associated with adverse perinatal outcome.

Delivery is the option in majority of the cases when growth discordance is >25% and the gestational age is more than 34 weeks.

Fetal Malformations and Morbidity in Twin Pregnancy

Risks of congenital malformations and morbidity are almost double as compared to a singleton pregnancy. The increased risks are mainly confined to the monozygotic twins.

Q. What are the different types of malformations and associated morbidity in MCTP?

Ans.
- Morbidity due to twining itself
  - Neural tube defects
  - Cardiac anomaly
  - Holoprosencephaly
  - Conjoint twins
- Anomalies due to placental vascular anastomoses resulting in hemodynamic instability
  - Microcephaly
  - Renal cortical necrosis
  - Multicystic encephalomalacia
  - Aplasia cutis
- Abnormalities due to compression effects within the uterus
  - Talipes equinovarus
  - Congenital dislocation of hip

SINGLE FETAL DEATH IN TWIN PREGNANCY

- This is more common than singleton pregnancy (10–20%).
- Majority are dichorionic, following *in vitro* fertilization pregnancy.
  Single fetal death in a monochorionic twin pregnancy results in damage to the surviving twin. The possible pathologies are:
  - Acute hemodynamic changes at the time of death
  - The surviving twin bleeds part of its circulatory blood volume into the circulation of the dying twin. The surviving twin suffers
  - Persistent hypotension
  - Low perfusion of vital organs
  - Ischemic damage of vital organs
  - Ischemic damage of organs, particularly the brain.

Management Issues

Assessment for the wellbeing of the surviving fetus.
- **Cardiotocography (CTG):** To note the changes due to hypoxia
- **Ultrasound Doppler study** for fetal anemia and abnormal middle cerebral artery peak systolic velocity (MCA-PSV).
- **Fetal magnetic resonance imaging (MRI)**—for brain to detect any neurological damage. Situations where the survival of the fetus is found compromised, termination of pregnancy is an option. However, fetal survival depends upon fetal gestational age. Antenatal corticosteroids should be given before preterm delivery.

Prognosis of the living twin depends upon the following factors:
- Gestational age at the time of demise of the co-twin
- Chorionicity
- Length of time between the fetal demise and delivery of the surviving twin.

Dichorionic twins: Usually have favorable outcome. Main risks are miscarriage or preterm delivery. Conservative management is commonly done with sonographic follow-up.
Monochorionic twins: (i) Double intrauterine fetal demise (IUFD) (10–25%) and (ii) Miscarriage.
Maternal disseminated intravascular coagulation (DIC) may rarely develop in twin pregnancy following single fetal IUFD. DIC is due to release thromboplastin from the placenta of the dead

fetus. It may occur following its retention for more than 5 weeks. Heparin therapy and urgent delivery is indicated in such a case.

Actual Management: Situations where the survival of the fetus is found to be compromised, termination of pregnancy is an option. However, fetal survival depends upon fetal gestational age and weight.

Antenatal corticosteroid should be given before preterm delivery.

- *Early fetal death (≤14 weeks):* 'Vanishing twin' the dead twin is vanished and it does not affect the surviving fetus.
- *Late fetal death:*
  - In monochorionic twins—neurological abnormality of the surviving twin is high (18%). Conservative management of the living fetus may be done with continued fetal surveillance till the fetal viability.
  - In dichorionic twins usually the outcome in favorable.

TWIN REVERSED ARTERIAL PERFUSION (TRAP)

It is a rare complication (1 in 35,000 births) of monochorionic twins. The recipient twin has no heart (acardius) whereas the donor twin suffers from high output cardiac failure. There is a large artery to artery placental vascular anastomosis. There may be vein to vein shunt also. The recipient twin receives reverse blood (deoxygenated arterial blood) flow from the donor co-twin. This used arterial blood supplies to the lower part of the body of the recipient twin. Criterias to be fulfilled for development of a TRAP sequences are:

- Arterio-arterial anastomosis
- Discordant development of the fetuses to allow reversal of blood flow.

The blood from the donor enters the recipient acardiac twin via umbilical artery and aorta. Little oxygen is present when the blood reaches the upper part of the body. So upper body structures are poorly developed. Due to combined failure of heart and head development, the recipient twin is known as **acardius acephalus** or **acardius amorphus** (Fig. 8.3). The donor twin suffers the problem of cardiomegaly and high output failure. The mortality rate of the donor or 'pump' twin may as high as 75%.

Management options depend on
- Relative size of the 'acardiac' twin to that of the pump twin
- Degree of cardiac dysfunction of the 'pump' twin.

Diagnosis is made by ultrasonography. Doppler study can detect reverse arterial perfusion.

Management options are
- Coagulation of the cord of the recipient twin using bipolar diathermy
- Intrafetal laser ablation
- Fetoscopic ligation of the umbilical cord of the recipient twin is done to stop the blood flow from the donor.

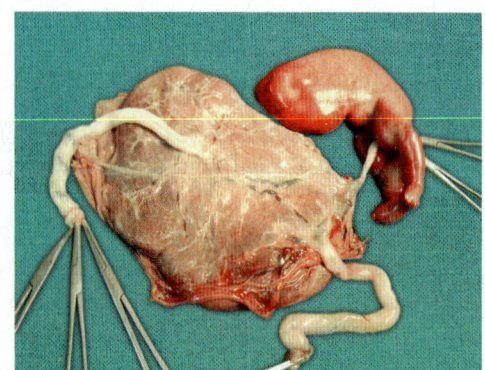

Fig. 8.3: Acardius acephalus fetus

CONJOINT TWINS

Diagnosis and Management

Incidence of conjoined twins (Fig. 8.4) are around one in 90,000–100,000 pregnancies.

Delivery: When the cases are diagnosed prenatally they are delivered by elective cesarean section. Cases that remained undiagnosed till labor, deliver vaginally. The risks of vaginal delivery are: prolonged labor, dystocia and even rupture of the uterus.

Antenatal diagnosis of conjoined twin can be made even in early (10–12 weeks onwards) pregnancy. **Ultrasonography** using B-mode, Doppler, color Doppler and 3D imaging techniques are informative. Detailed assessment of cardiovascular anatomy should be done. **Prenatal diagnosis** of conjoint twins is of much value in assessing the prognosis as well as planning the management.

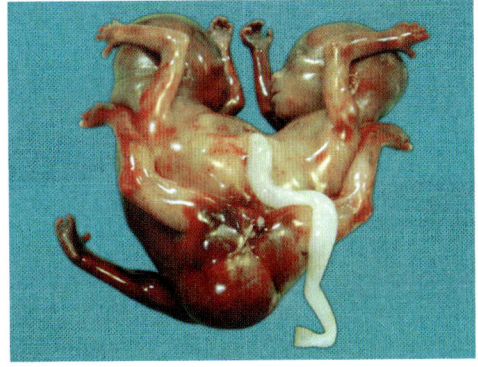

Fig. 8.4: *Conjoint twins:* Omphalopagus and pygopagus fetuses

MONOCHORIONIC MONOAMNIOTIC (MCMA) TWIN PREGNANCY

Nearly 1% of monozygotic twins are monoamniotic. In MCMA twin pregnancy, the main risks to the fetuses are due to cord entanglement causing death of one or both the fetuses. Best time to deliver such fetuses are at 32 weeks electively. Mode of delivery is by cesarean section. Mother should be given corticosteroids to accelerate fetal pulmonary maturity.

Selective Fetal Reduction

Multifetal pregnancy is often associated with adverse perinatal outcome. Multifetal gestation is more common with assisted reproductive technologies (ART). In order to improve the survival rate of the fetuses, selective reduction of fetus(es) in multichorionic multifetal gestation may be done. It is commonly done by transabdominal route. It is done between 10 and 13 weeks when the fetuses are evaluated sonographically. The fetus(es) who is smallest and/or anomalous are chosen for reduction. Potassium chloride is injected into the heart or thorax of each selected fetus under sonographic guidance. Generally pregnancies are reduced to twins. The risk of pregnancy loss rate varies with operator skill and experience. It may vary from 4.5–12%.

Selective Fetal Termination

Presence of fetal structural or genetic abnormalities are considered for selective termination.

Selective feticide by injection of potassium chloride into the heart is not done in multiple chorionic pregnancies. This is because of the presence of vascular anastomoses between the fetuses. Coagulation of the cord by bipolar diathermy or intrafetal laser ablation is done.

References

1. Quintero RA, Morales WJ, Allen MH, et al. Staging of twin-to-twin transfusion. J Perinatol. 1999;19:550–5.
2. Roberts D, Nellson JP, Kilby MD, et al. Interventions for the treatment of twin-to-twin transfusion syndrome. Cochrane database Syst Rev. 2008.

9 Prenatal Screening for Fetal Abnormalities

Prenatal screening is recommended for aneuploidy, to all women before 20 weeks of gestation.[1] Background risks for aneuploidy (deviation from exact multiple of haploid number of chromosomes) depend on maternal age, family history and previously affected pregnancy (Table 9.1). **Trisomy** (13, 18 or 21) increases with maternal age. **Monosomy** (45, X) and **triploidy** [extra set of chromosomes (69)] remain at a constant rate.

Table 9.1: Indication of parental and prenatal genetic screening

Parental risk factors	*Prenatal risk factors*
■ Maternal age ≥ 35 years at delivery	■ Oligohydramnios
■ Previous baby born with chromosomal anomaly	■ Polyhydramnios
■ One or both the parents, carry sex-linked or autosomal traits	■ Severe symmetrical intrauterine growth restriction (IUGR)
■ One parent is known to carry a balanced translocation	■ Presence of soft tissue markers for chromosomal anomaly on USG (Table 9.2)
■ Parental aneuploidy	■ Abnormal maternal serum screening

Table 9.2: Common sonographic abnormalities

Trisomy 18	Trisomy 13
Edwards' syndrome (Fig. 9.1)	*Patau syndrome*
■ Cardiac defects	■ Cardiac defects
■ Choroid plexus cyst	■ Microcephaly
■ Strawberry-shaped skull	■ Holoprosencephaly
■ Neural tube defects	■ Cystic hygroma
■ Micrognathia	■ Facial clefts
■ Clenched hands	■ Neural tube defects (*See* Manual of Obstetrics and Gynecology for the Postgraduates, p. 40)
■ Rocker bottom feet	■ IUGR
■ IUGR	
■ Abnormal cerebellum	

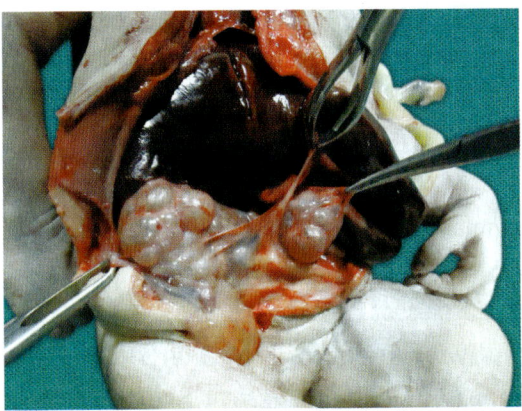

Fig. 9.1: Multiple malformations (cardiac, urinary and genital organs, bowel) in a fetus with trisomy of chromosome 18 (Edwards' syndrome)

FIRST TRIMESTER SCREENING

Combined: Nuchal Translucency + Serum Tests

- Nuchal translucency (NT)
- Free β-human chorionic gonadotrophin (β-hCG)
- Pregnancy-associated plasma protein A (PAPP-A)

> Detection rate of trisomy 21 was 92%, invasive testing rate was 5.2%.

Free fetal DNA (ffDNA); *See* Manual of Obstetrics and Gynecology for the Postgraduates, p. 521.

Nuchal Translucency

- It is the appearance of fluid space (detected by ultrasound), between the fetal skin and underlying soft tissue at the region of the cervical spine.
- It appears as an echolucent fluid space.
- It is measured between 10 and 14 weeks of gestation (Table 9.3).
- Crown rump length (CRL) of fetus should be 38–84 mm.

Fetuses with NT of ≥ 3 mm may need screening combined with serum biochemical markers (as stated above). Fetuses with NT ≥ 4 mm may not need the combined screening for serum biochemical markers (↑ β-hCG and ↓ PAPP-A).

Table 9.3: Anomalies associated with increased NT > 95th centile at 11–14 weeks

■ Chromosomal abnormalities	■ Abdominal wall defect
■ Hydrocephalus	■ Neck lipoma
■ Thanato dysplasia	■ Cardiac defect
■ Duodenal atresia	■ Diaphragmatic hernia
■ Parvovirus B19 infection	■ Nuchal defect
■ Body stalk anomaly	

In the first trimester: Two most important discriminatory biochemical analyzes for anomaly screening are serum β-hCG and PAPP-A.

Nasal bone (NB): Fetal NB can be seen by ultrasound, starting at about 11 weeks pregnancy. NB hypoplasia or aplasia is commonly observed in fetuses with trisomy 21. 73% of trisomy 21 fetuses in the first trimester ultrasound scan, were found to have absent NB with a false-positive rate (FPR) of 0.5%.[2]

However, when absent NB was added to other sonographic markers for aneuploidy the sensitivity of genetic sonography increased to 90%. Dr Down while describing the physical features, identified the nose being small in these children.

SECOND TRIMESTER SCREENING

Genetic Ultrasonography for Aneuploidy Marker(s)

- Nuchal fold thickness (≥ 6 mm)
- Echogenic bowel
- Choroid plexus cysts (≥ 10 mm)
- Cardiac anomalies (four chamber, outflow tract)
- Short femur (< 10th percentile)
- Short humerus (< 10th percentile)
- Fetal hydrops
- Cystic hygroma (*See* Manual of Obstetrics and Gynecology for the Postgraduates, p. 44)
- Duodenal atresia
- Two vessel umbilical cord
- Wide space between first and second toe (sandal gap)
- Clenched hands
- Club feet
- Rocker bottom feet
- Pyelectasis (renal pelvis thickness ≥ 4 mm)
- Neural tube defects
- Absent NB.

Eighty-five percent of fetuses with trisomy 21 had at least one abnormal finding on ultrasound.[3] Genetic sonography is ideally performed between 18 and 20 weeks. It is a targeted examination for fetal aneuploidy to see fetal structural anomalies. Risk of fetal aneuploidy increases with detection of increased number of markers. **Genetic sonography** reduces the invasive tests without any compromise for accuracy of detection. **Three dimensional sonography** imaging is more useful for evaluation of fetal malformations as most anomalies are better visualized with 3D rather than 2D conventional imaging.

INTEGRATED AND SEQUENTIAL SCREENING (FLOWCHART 9.1)

First and Second Trimester Evaluation of Risk (FASTER) Trial for Trisomy 21

Integrated Screening (Wald, et al. 1999)

First and second trimester screening is used to provide a single risk estimate for trisomy 21.[4] It is a two step protocols. First trimester evaluation (NT + PAPP-A) is done. The woman returns in

Flowchart 9.1: Integrated and sequential screening

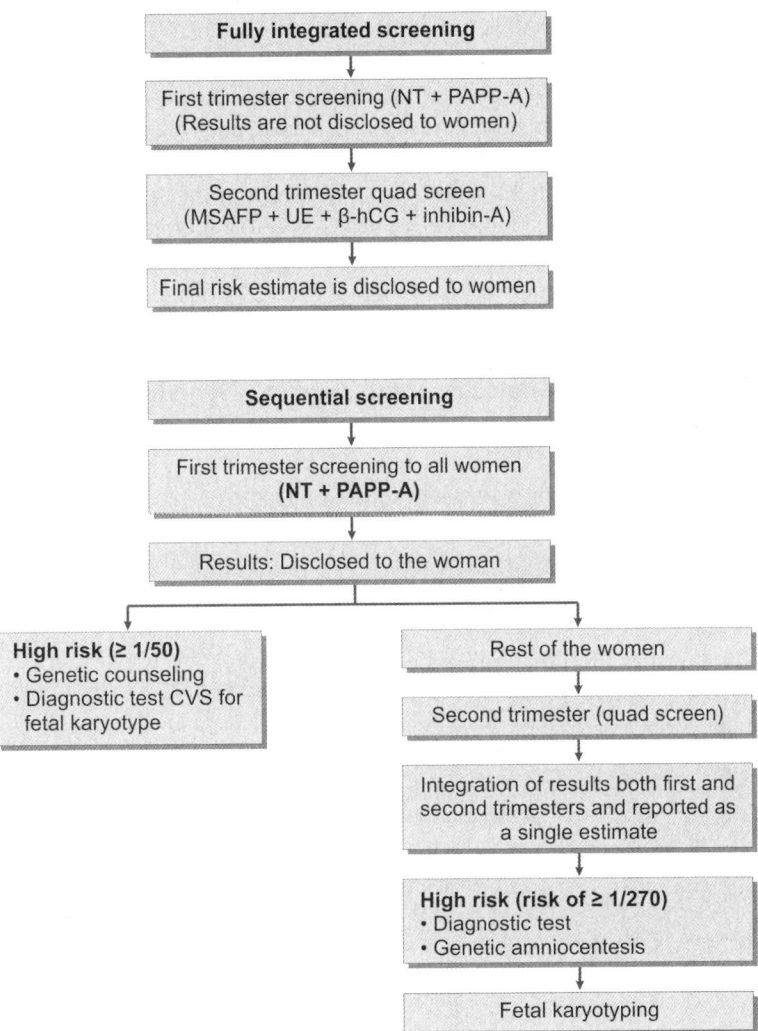

Abbreviations: CVS—Chorionic villus sampling, NT—Nuchal translucency, PAPP-A—Pregnancy-associated plasma protein A, β-hCG—β-human chorionic gonadotrophin, UE—Unconjugated estriol

the second trimester for serum test for ***quad screen*** (↓MSAFP+↓UE3+↑β-hCG+↑inhibin-A). The results of first and second trimesters are integrated and a final risk estimate is given to the woman. Detection of trisomy (using cut off value 1 in 120 or greater) is 85% and FPR 0.9%.[5]

Disadvantages of Integrated Screening
- The woman does not have the screening results done in the first trimester.
- The fetuses at high-risk of trisomy 21 are not identified until the second trimester.
- Moreover, many women (20%) do not comply with the second trimester screening.

Alternative Protocols

To avoid these limitations, alternative protocols used are:
- ***Sequential screening:*** First trimester results are disclosed to the woman above a cut off value (e.g. ≥ 1/50). The woman with substantial risk can be referred for genetic counseling and diagnostic test chorionic villus sampling (CVS) for karyotype evaluation in early pregnancy. The rest of women are not identified in the high-risk group undergo a ***quad screen*** in the second trimester. In these women, risks of both first and second trimester results are integrated and reported as a single number. Those with a risk of 1/270 or higher are offered diagnostic test (genetic amniocentesis) following genetic counseling for karyotype evaluation.
- ***Contingent screening:*** Women with high-risk (e.g. ≥ 1/50) based on first trimester screening are offered diagnostic tests (CVS) while those with very low risk (< 1/1500) are not offered any additional screening, because they are unlikely to become screen positive (Flowchart 9.2). Those women having an intermediate risk (between ≥ 1/50 and < 1/1500) go on the second

Flowchart 9.2: Contingent screening

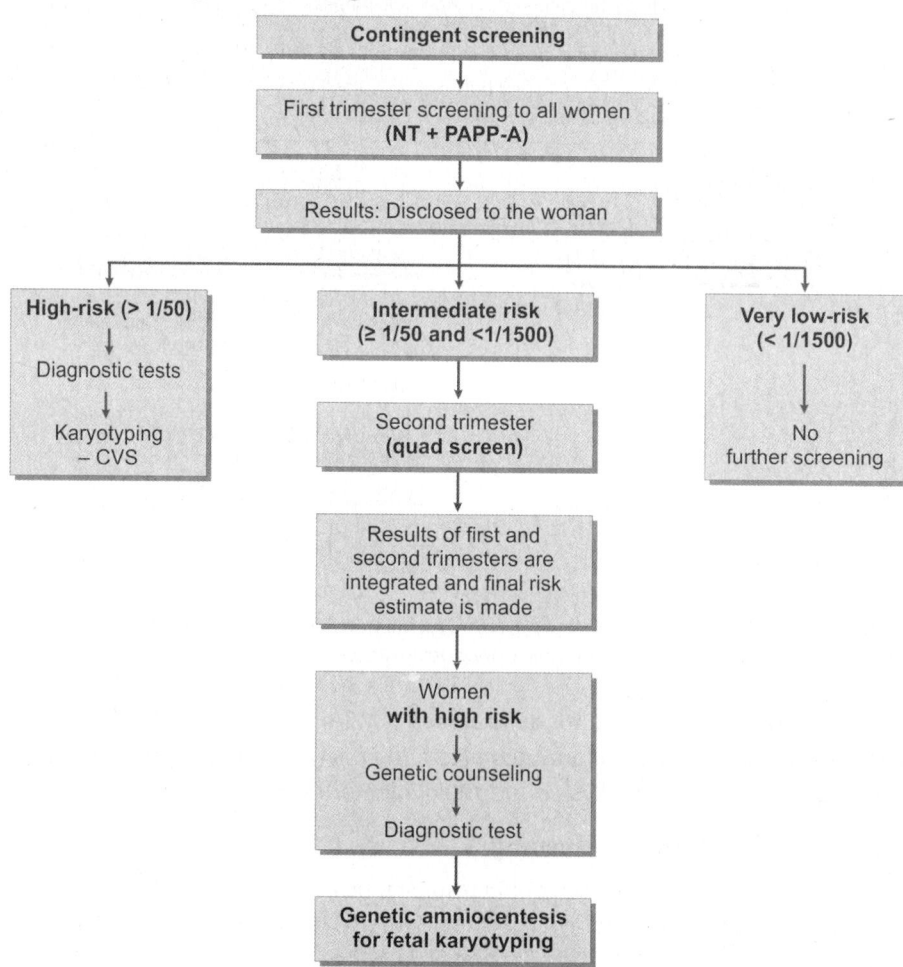

trimester screening (quad screening). In these intermediate group, the results of first and second trimesters are integrated and a final risk estimate is reported. Those women with a risk of 1:270 or greater are offered genetic counseling and diagnostic test (genetic amniocentesis) and karyotyping. Contingent screening identifies 91% of fetuses with trisomy 21 with a FPR of 4.5% (Tables 9.4 and 9.5).[6]

Table 9.4: Prenatal genetic screening tests

Screening Test	Period of Gestation		Follow-up
	11–14 weeks	14–20 weeks	
Combined	↑NT, ↑hCG, ↓PAPP-A		Results disclosed to the woman
Quadruple (Quad screen)		↑β-hCG, ↓MSAFP; ↓UE3, ↑inhibin-A	Results disclosed in second trimester
Fully Integrated	↑NT, ↓PAPP-A	Quad screen	Results are integrated and disclosed as a single risk estimate at the end of screening in second trimester
Serum Integrated	↓PAPP-A	Quad screen	Results are integrated and disclosed as a single risk estimate at the end of screening in second trimester
Stepwise Sequential	NT, ↑β-hCG ↓PAPP-A	Quad screen	Results disclosed after the first part of test. Risk: High → Diagnostic test → CVS; All others → Quad screening
Contingent Sequential	NT, ↑β-hCG ↓PAPP-A	Quad screen	Results are revealed after first part of test. Risk: High → Diagnostic test → CVS; Risk: Intermediate → Quad screening; Risk: Low → No further tests

Abbreviations: NT—Nuchal translucency, MSAFP—Maternal serum alpha fetoprotein, UE3—Unconjugated estriol, PAPP-A—Pregnancy associated plasma protein–A, CVS—Chronic villus sampling

Table 9.5: Detection rate and False-positive rate (FPR) for trisomy 21

Test	False-positive rate (FPR) (%)	Detection rate (%)
MA+NT (10–14 weeks)	5	77
MA + combined test (NT + β-hCG + PAPP-A)	5	85–92
MA + fully integrated (see above)	0.9	85
MA + serum integrated (see above)	2.7	85
MA + stepwise sequential (see above)	5.1	92
MA + contingent sequential (see above)	4.5	91
MA + quad screen (see above)	5	81
MA + NT + NB + β-hCG + PAPP-A	5	97

Abbreviations: MA—Maternal age, NT—Nuchal translucency; β-hCG—β-human chorionic gonadotrophin, PAPP-A—Pregnancy-associated plasma protein A; NB—Nasal bone

MCQs

Q.1 As regard the prenatal tests:
a. Screening and diagnostic tests are the same and are used interchangeably
b. Screen positive fetuses always have the disease
c. Screen positive fetuses are always at increased risk of the disease in future
d. Screen negative fetuses are presumed to be free of disease
e. Screen positive fetuses need further diagnostic tests.

Ans.
a. F   b. F
c. F   d. T
e. T

Q.2 Validity of any test is expressed as:
a. Sensitivity is the ability of the test to correctly identify those who have the disease
b. Specificity in the ability to detect those who do not have the disease
c. False-negative means a subject declared negative when actually having a disease
d. False-positive means a subject declared positive for a disease when actually not having that disease
e. Any test having a high number of false-positives indicates good quality of the test.

Ans.
a. T   b. T
c. T   d. T
e. F
e. High false-positive tests creates more anxiety. It needs further tests which involve, more cost.

Q.3 Regarding prenatal chromosomal abnormalities:
a. Combined test is done in the second trimester
b. Quadruple test includes β-hCG, AFP, UE3 and inhibin-A
c. Detection rate of trisomy 21 with NT alone is 90%
d. Nasal bone is absent in 73% fetuses with trisomy 21, in first trimester screening done with ultrasonography
e. Short femur, pyelectasis are the sonographic markers for trisomy 21

Ans.
a. T   b. T
c. F   d. T
e. T

Q.4 Regarding screening of trisomy 21:
a. In stepwise sequential screening, the high-risk woman are offered CVS for karyotype
b. Fully integrated screening has few advantages
c. In contingent sequential screening, the low-risk women are offered quad screen
d. Detection rate in stepwise sequential is 92%
e. Chorion villus sampling is performed between 9 and 10 weeks of gestation.

Ans.
a. T   b. F
c. F   d. T
e. F

References

1. American College of Obstetricians and Gynecologists: Prenatal diagnosis of fetal chromosomal abnormalities 2003;547-57.
2. Vintzileos A, Walters C, Yeo L. Absent nasal bone in the prenatal detection of fetuses with trisomy 21 in a high-risk population. Obstet Gynecol. 2003;101:905-8.
3. Down, J. Langdon H. Observation on an ethnic classification of idiots. London: London Hospital, Clinical Lecture Reports, 1866. [Online]. Available from: http://home.vicnet.net.au/~dealcc/Downs.htm [Accessed June, 2016].
4. Malone FD, Canick JA, Ball RH, et al. First-trimester or second-trimester screening, or both, for Down's syndrome. N Engl J Med. 2005;353(19):2001-11.
5. Wald NJ, Watt HC, Hackshaw AK. Integrated screening for Down's syndrome on the basis of tests performed during the first and second trimesters. N Engl J Med. 1999;341(7):461-7.
6. Cuckle HS, Malone FD, Wright D, et al. Contingent screening for Down syndrome: results from the FASTER trial. Prenat Diagn. 2008;28(2):89-94.

10. Severe Pre-eclampsia and Eclampsia

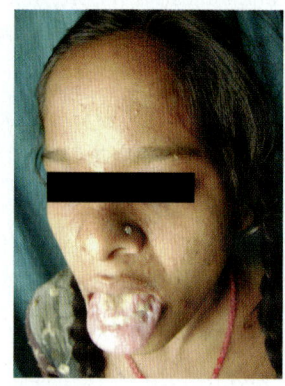

Fig. 10.1: Eclampsia with severe tongue bite. This woman ultimately was diagnosed to be a case of tuberous sclerosis

SINGLE BEST ANSWER (SBA) AND MULTIPLE CHOICE QUESTIONS (MCQs)

Q. Management of severe pre-eclampsia:
   a. Conservative management till fetal maturity
   b. Regular antenatal checkup
   c. Most women respond to antihypertensive drugs
   d. Domiciliary management may be allowed

Ans. a. F b. F
       c. F d. F

Q. What are the complications of severe pre-eclampsia?

Ans. Severe pre-eclampsia has the following complications:
- Placental abruption
- Cerebrovascular hemorrhage
- Pulmonary edema
- Adult respiratory distress syndrome
- Fetal growth restriction
- Preterm delivery (prematurity)
- Intrauterine fetal death
- Subcapsular liver hematoma
- Convulsions (eclampsia)
- Maternal death
- Acute renal failure
- Retinal detachment

To prevent the complications woman at times may need to be delivered early even before the time of fetal maturity. This is purely to prevent maternal mortality.

Regular antenatal checkup is good to detect the early onset of pre-eclampsia but it cannot prevent the onset of the disease. **Etiopathological basis of the disease is still unknown and it is thought to be multifactorial in origin.**

Woman with pre-eclampsia when hospitalized and treated conservatively may have some beneficial response in terms of improvement of hypertension. **But these women are not cured.** Nearly 90% of such women develop hypertension again either before or during labor. **Delivery (termination of pregnancy) is the cure.**

Domiciliary or outpatient management in a case with severe pre-eclampsia, worsens the outcome in terms of maternal and fetal health. Outpatient management may be advised as long the disease process does not worsens the maternal health and jeopardize fetal outcome. **It may be an option for the management of a case with mild pre-eclampsia.** Frequent monitoring of blood pressure at home and urine protein in such cases may be done. They need to be seen in the clinic at a frequent intervals of 2–3 weeks.

Q. What is a place of antihypertensive therapy in a woman with severe pre-eclampsia?
   a. Control of mild hypertension prevents severe pre-eclampsia
   b. Antihypertensive therapy should only be started once diastolic blood pressure is over 110 mm Hg
   c. Diastolic BP is important for mother's health
   d. Moderate hypertension does not need any antihypertensive

Ans. a. F   b. F
     c. F   d. F

Systolic hypertension needs to control for the prevention of maternal stroke. Diastolic hypertension reduces organ perfusion including placental circulation. **Diastolic hypertension** may result in maternal oliguria and compromised fetal well-being. **Antihypertensive therapy** should be considered even at lower degree of hypertension when the woman develops other markers of potentially severe disease (*See* Dutta's Textbook of Obstetrics, 8th Edition, p. 265).

Management of severe pre-eclampsia and eclampsia (PE and E) and antihypertensive therapy. Management principles of severe PE and E are based on:

- Careful assessment of maternal and fetal condition
- Stabilization of woman's health (controling blood pressure) and preventing convulsions
- Continued monitoring (fetal and maternal health)
- Consideration of delivery at an optimum time and selecting best mode of delivery.

Q. What are the common causes of maternal death in eclampsia?

Ans. Severe pre-eclampsia and eclampsia are the leading causes (20–30%) of maternal mortality in India[1] (Konar et al). It is an avoidable factor for maternal deaths.

Common causes are—(a) cardiac failure, (b) pulmonary edema (ARDS), (c) aspiration pneumonia, (d) cerebral hemorrhage, (e) acute renal failure, (f) pulmonary embolism, (g) postpartum shock and (h) puerperal sepsis.

Place of Antihypertensive Therapy

Antihypertensive therapy should be started with a blood pressure of 160 mm Hg systolic or 110 mm Hg diastolic (ACOG 2011, NICE 2010, RCOG 2011, SOGC 2008). **Women with other markers** *of severe disease, antihypertensive therapy should be considered even at a lower degree of hypertension* (SOGC 2008, ACOG 2011). Systolic HTN needs to be controlled for prevention of maternal stroke, diastolic HTN reduces placental perfusion (fetal risk).

Markers of severe pre-eclampsia

Symptoms	Signs
▪ Severe headache	▪ Papilledema
▪ Visual disturbances	▪ Clonus
▪ Confusion/sleeplessness	▪ Liver tenderness
▪ Epigastric pain	▪ Platelet count < 100,000/L
▪ Vomiting	▪ Raised liver enzymes
▪ Right upper quadrant pain	ALT or AST > 70 IU/L
Pain (subcapsular liver hematoma)	▪ HELLP syndrome
▪ Oliguria/anuria	▪ Massive proteinuria
▪ Respiratory distress (pulmonary edema)	

Q. How should seizures be prevented?

Ans. **MAGPIE trial (2002)** has demonstrated that magnesium sulphate reduces the risk of eclampsia.[2] Unfortunately 30–85% of cases of eclampsia remained unpreventable. However, $MgSO_4$ is the drug of choice and should be used as antiseizure prophylaxis. *Therefore, $MgSO_4$ should be considered for women with severe PE when the risk of eclampsia is high or imminent*. This is usually done in a case of severe PE once the delivery decision has been made. Once $MgSO_4$ is given, it should be continued for 24 hours following delivery or 24 hours after the last seizure whichever is the later, unless there is a clinical reason to continue for a longer time. Woman should be monitored when she receives $MgSO_4$.

Monitoring parameters are: Urine output (> 30 mL/hour, presence of tendon reflexes, respiratory rate (>12/min) and oxygen saturation. Therapeutic level of serum $MgSO_4$ is 4–7 mEq/L.

Q. What is the definitive therapy in a case with severe pre-eclampsia?

Ans. Etiology of PE is hitherto elusive. *It is certain that placenta is the cause*. Fetus is not needed as development of PE, observed in a case with molar pregnancy. Lowering BP does not ameliorate the cause of PE. *Delivery is the cure and is the definitive therapy*.

Q. What are the antihypertensive drugs used in a case with severe PE?

Ans. **Drugs commonly recommended are:**[3]
Labetalol—RCOG (1996)
Labetalol—NICE (2010)
Labetalol or hydralazine—ACOG (2011)
Labetalol, nifedipine capsules or hydralazine—SOGC (2008)
Combination of drugs may be necessary
However, **cochrane collaboration** does not support the choice of any one antihypertensive (mentioned above) over the other.
Choice and route of pharmacological agents depend on clinician's experience, local availability and also on the cost of the drug (WHO-2011).

Q. Selection of antihypertensive drug in the management of severe pre-eclampsia?
   a. Labetalol may be given intravenously
   b. Methyldopa should be given PO 4 g a day
   c. Nitroprusside IV should be the drug of first choice
   d. Enalapril in the postpartum period is contraindicated

Ans. a. T b. F
  c. F d. F

Both nifedipine and labetalol are effective and well-tolerated.

In cases with mild to moderate hypertension (BP: 140–159/90–109 mm Hg), lowering BP, using antihypertensive drug, may compromise fetal well-being. *It should not be used for mild hypertension (WHO–2011).*

In moderate hypertension, it may be used with the experience of the clinician involved. Treatment may be needed for prolongation of pregnancy.

Methyldopa and/or labetalol are the commonly used drugs. Methyldopa and labetalol have been proved safe in long-term follow-up. There are some benefits of labetalol also. Labetalol can be given by mouth and as well as IV if needed in a case with severe hypertension.

ANTIHYPERTENSIVE DRUGS IN THE POSTPARTUM PERIOD

Drugs that can be used are:
- Long-acting nifedipine
- Labetalol
- Methyldopa
- Hydrochlorothiazide
- Captopril
- Enalapril

Breastfeeding is not contraindicated with the use of these drugs. **Labetalol (given orally or intravenously), nifedipine (given orally) or hydralazine (intravenously)** can be used for the actue management of severe hypertension (RCOG 2006). Nifedipine should be given orally not sublingually (RCOG 2006).

Q. What are antihypertensives, used in hypertensive crisis?

Ans. Drugs used are—labetalol (IV); hydralazine (IV); nifedipine (PO); nitroglycerine (IV); and sodium nitroprusside (IV). (*See* Dutta's Textbook of Obstetrics, 8th Edition, p. 581).

ANTIHYPERTENSIVE DRUGS CONTRAINDICATED IN PREGNANCY

The following drugs should not be prescribed in pregnancy:
- ***Atenolol*** (fetal growth restriction)
- ***Angiotensin converting enzyme*** (ACE) inhibitors (fetal renal tubular dysgenesis, malformations)
- ***Angiotension receptor-blocking drugs*** (ARB) (fetal malformations)
- ***Diuretics*** (avoided unless pulmonary edema)
- ***Labetalol*** should be avoided in a woman known to suffer from bronchial asthma
- ***Nitroprusside*** preferably to be avoided as it may cause fetal cyanide toxicity.

Q. What are the changes in current concept of hypertension in pregnancy?
Ans. Changes in diagnostic criteria and management:
The diagnosis of severe pre-eclampsia is no longer dependant on the presence of proteinuria.
- Massive proteinuria (>5 g) has been eliminated from consideration of severe pre-eclampsia.
- Fetal growth restriction (FGR) has been removed as a finding indicative of severe pre-eclampsia.
- Not to delay management of pre-eclampsia in the absence of proteinuria.
- NSAIDS may contribute to increase BP and should be replaced by other analgesics in women with hypertension.

Q. What are the risks of cardiovascular disease in women with prior pre-eclampsia?
Ans. Such women are at increased risk of cardiovascular disease in later life. The risk increase may be up to eightfold to ninefold. Recommendations for such women are lifestyle modification for maintaining a healthy weight, increased physical activity, to avoid smoking and yearly assessment of lipid and blood glucose.

References

1. Konar H, Chakroborty AB: Maternal mortality in India—a multicenter FOGSI. Study; Jr Obstet Gynaec India. 2013:63(2):88-95.
2. Magnesium sulphate for prevention of eclampsia (MAGPIE Trial Collaboration Group 2002).
3. Which anticonvulsant for women with eclampsia? Evidence from the Collaborative Eclampsia Trial. Lancet 1995;345:1455(7)–63; Erratum in Lancet 1995;346:258.

11

HELLP Syndrome

SINGLE BEST ANSWER (SBA) AND MULTIPLE CHOICE QUESTIONS (MCQs)

Q. Basic pathology of hemolysis elevated liver enzymes low platelet count (HELLP) syndrome:
a. Microangiopathic hemolytic anemia (MAHA)
b. Periportal necrosis of liver
c. Intrahepatic hemorrhage
d. Subcapsular hematoma of the liver
e. Intravascular aggregation of platelets and fibrin deposition.

Ans. a. T b. T
  c. T d. T
  e. T

Q. What is the diagnostic criteria of HELLP syndrome?
- **Hemolysis:**
  - Abnormal peripheral blood smear (schistocytes, echinocytes)
  - Raised serum bilirubin > 1.2 mg/dL.
- **Elevated liver enzymes:**
  - Raised SGOT ≥ 70 IU/L
  - Raised LDH > 600 IU/L
- **Thrombocytopenia: <100,000/mm^3**

Q. Classification of HELLP syndrome:

Ans. HELLP has been classified by Martin, et al. (Mississippi classification) according to the severity of thrombocytopenia (mainly) along with the level of hepatic enzyme.[1]

Class I
- Platelet count ≤ 50,000/mm^3
- AST/ALT ≥ 70 IU/L; LDH ≥ 600 IU/L

Class II
- Platelet count between >50,000 and <100,000/mm^3
- AST/ALT ≥ 70 IU/L
- LDH ≥ 600 IU/L

Class III
- Platelet count above >100,000 and <1,50,000 mm^3
- AST/ALT ≥ 40 IU/L
- LDH ≥ 600 IU/L

Q. Regarding management of HELLP syndrome:
   a. Renal failure is more in HELLP syndrome compared to hepatic pathology
   b. Abnormal peripheral blood smear is characteristic
   c. Liver enzymes are the important diagnostic and prognostic criteria
   d. Unlike pre-eclampsia recurrence risk is low.

Ans. a. F   b. T
          c. F   d. F

Q. What are the maternal complications of HELLP syndrome?

Ans. Maternal complications are many and they are severe enough to cause high maternal mortality.[2]

Important complications are as follows:
- Pulmonary edema (8%)
- Acute renal failure (8%)
- Disseminated intravascular coagulopathy (15–20%)
- Abruptio placenta (9%)
- Liver pathology:
  - Subcapsular hematoma
  - Hepatic rupture
  - Infarction
  - Hepatic failure
- Acute respiratory distress syndrome (< 1%)
- Sepsis (< 1%)
- Stroke
- Wound hematoma
- Laryngeal edema
- Severe ascites.

Overall maternal mortality of HELLP syndrome is 1% and perinatal mortality varies from 7–20%.

Q. What are the important management issues in HELLP syndrome?

Ans. Similar to the management of pre-eclampsia and eclampsia the definitive management is delivery.[3]

However, there are different other therapeutic modalities to prevent the complications. These are as follows:
- Plasma volume expansion with the use of
  - Crystalloids and/or
  - Colloids
- Antithrombotic agents like heparin or low dose aspirin
- Immunosuppressive agents—use of steroids
- **Others**
  - Fresh frozen plasma (FFP)
  - Hemotherapy—either in the form of packed cell transfusion and/or platelet transfusion.

Q. What are the important issues in the intrapartum management of such a patient?

Ans.
- Seizure prophylaxis—with $MgSO_4$
- Control of hypertension: Nearly 80% of such women will need urgent control
- **Drugs commonly used are** labetalol, nifedipine or hydralazine
- Stabilization of maternal health
- Delivery.

Q. How delivery should be organized in a case with HELLP syndrome?

Ans. It depends on the condition of the mother and the fetus based on the parameters of assessment both clinical and investigations. **Steroid therapy** should be given for a woman with gestational age between 24 and 34 weeks. Regarding the mode of delivery, vaginal delivery is preferred. Though rare, cesarean delivery may have to be performed.

Q. What are the important issues in the management during labor and delivery?

Ans.
- **Hemotherapy:** Need of packed cells, FFP and/or platelet transfusion should be considered.[4]
  Platelet transfusion should be given
  - Prior to spontaneous vaginal delivery when the count is < 20,000/cumm.
  - Prior to cesarean delivery when the count is < 50,000/cumm.
- **Special precautions** when cesarean delivery is required.
  - General anesthesia is preferred
  - Vertical skin incision should be made as there may be need of exploration of upper abdomen organs
  - Manual removal of placenta should be avoided
  - Drains (subfascial and peritoneal) should be used
  - Subcapsular liver hematoma should preferably be managed conservatively (packing or drain, rarely lobectomy). Maternal mortality may be as high as 50%
  - Patient often needs **admission in intensive care unit** with multidisciplinary management.

Q. How the woman should be managed in the postpartum period?

Ans. Patient needs close monitoring to assess the progress.
- Patient may be given dexamethasone therapy. It is safe and effective to reduce the problems of respiratory distress syndrome. It also improves the renal perfusion and urine output.
- Best markers for follow-up are:
  - Sustained rise in platelet count
  - Sustained fall in LDH levels
  - Urine output > 100 mL/hour for 2 consecutive hours without diuretics
  - Decrease in systolic BP ≤ 150 mm Hg and diastolic BP < 100 mm Hg
  - Overall clinical improvement in the health of women.

Q. What is the risk of HELLP syndrome in terms of recurrence in future pregnancy?

Ans.
- For pre-eclampsia and eclampsia—it is nearly 40–45%
- For HELLP syndrome it is about 20–30%.

References

1. Martin JN, Thigpen BD, Rose CH, et al. Maternal benefit of high dose intravenous corticosteroid therapy for HELLP. Am J Obstet Gynecol. 2003;189(3):830-4.
2. Haddad B, Barton JR, Livingston JC, et al. Risk factors for adverse maternal outcomes among women with HELLP syndrome. Am J Obstet Gynecol. 2000;183(2):444-8.
3. Sibai BM, Ramadan MK, Usta I, et al. Maternal morbidity and mortality in 442 pregnancies with hemolysis, elevated liver enzymes, and low platelets (HELLP syndrome). Am J Obstet Gynae. 1993;169(4):1000-6.
4. Audibert F, Friedman SA, Frangieh AY, et al. Clinical utility of strict diagnostic criteria for the HELLP syndrome. Am J Obstet Gynecol. 1996;175(2):460-4.

12
Cesarean Section

Q.1 Regarding indications and place of cesarean section (CS):[1]
   a. Women suspected to have morbidly adherent placenta
   b. Women on HAART with a viral load < 400 copies/mL
   c. Category 2 cesarean section means delivery should be done by next 75 minutes
   d. Walking during labor reduces cesarean delivery
   e. Planned cesarean delivery should be done at 37 weeks.

Ans. a. T
   b. F
   c. T
   d. F
   e. F

   a. **Morbidly adherent placenta**
      Diagnosis can be made
      ♦ Color flow Doppler ultrasound
      ♦ MRI has got improved accuracy and is safe in pregnancy.
   b. **MTCT of HIV**
      Women on highly active antiretroviral therapy (HAART) with a viral load < 400 copies/mL or women on any antiretroviral therapy with a viral load < 50 copies/mL, the risk of MTCT of HIV is same for CS or a vaginal birth.

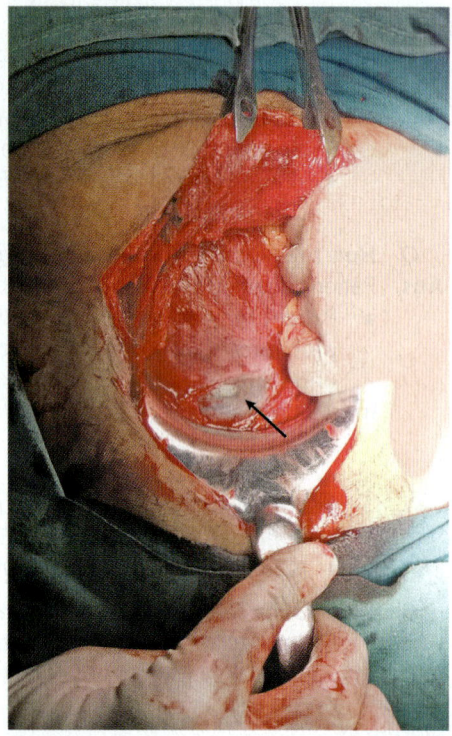

Fig. 12.1: Intraoperative photograph of cesarean delivery. Lower segment of the uterus is shown using the Doyen's retractor. Scar dehiscence is seen as there is: disruption of part of the scar (*see* arrow). Amniotic membrane is seen bulging out and it is intact. Bleeding is almost absent or minimal

Decision-to-delivery interval for cesarean section (CS)

Category	Definition	Decision to delivery intervals
	Classification based on urgency in doing CS	
1	**Immediate threat** to the life of woman or the fetus	Within 30 minutes
2	Maternal or fetal compromise is present but this is not **immediately** life threatening	Within 30 and 75 minutes
3	There is no maternal or fetal compromise but needs **early delivery**	
4	Delivery is **planned with time** to suit woman and/or the staff	

PLANNED CESAREAN SECTION

Common Indications

- Women with prior cesarean delivery are not selected for vaginal birth after cesarean (VBAC) trial of labor
- Women with singleton breech presentation at term for whom external cephalic version is contraindicated or has failed
- Multiple pregnancy (twins) at term when first twin is noncephalic
- Women suspected to have morbidly adherent placenta
- Women with cephalopelvic disproportion in labor
- Women with HIV
  - Not receiving any antiretroviral therapy (ART)
  - Having ART with a viral load ≥ 400 copies/mL.

Timing of Planned Cesarean Section

The risk of neonatal respiratory morbidity is increased by CS delivery. This risk decreases significantly after 39 weeks. **Therefore planned CS should not be done routinely before 39 weeks (ACOG).**
Planned CS: When done before 38 weeks, women should be given corticosteroids (*See* Dutta's Textbook of Obstetrics, 8th Edition, p. 367) to reduce neonatal morbidity.[2]

Types of incision and closure of tissues in different techniques of cesarean section (Table 12.1):
The benefits of the Misgav Ladach technique are: Duration of the operation 10–11 minutes compared to 14–15 minutes in the others; similarly the mean blood loss, the postoperative pain, and the need of analgesia were also less in the Misgav Ladach technique.

When a women requests for CS, reasons for such request are to be discussed and explored. When there is no other indication, women should be given the accurate information as regard to the risks and benefits of CS compared to that of vaginal birth. She should be given evidence-based information, support for her fear and anxiety, given support of other members of the obstetric team (midwife, anesthetist, and pediatrician). Her requests for CS because of anxiety or fear should be taken care with other healthcare professionals for perinatal mental health support.

After discussion and even with the support of perinatal mental support, if vaginal birth is not accepted, she should be offered planned CS.

Table 12.1: Different techniques of cesarean section

Steps	Munro Kerr's Technique with Pfannenstiel incision	Misgav Ladach technique with Joel-Cohen incision
Skin incision	Transverse, sharp	Joel-Cohen (straight incision below the line joining the anterior superior iliac spines), above Pfannenstiel
Subcutaneous tissue	Cut with scalpel/scissors	Blunt, separated digitally
Rectus sheath	Cut with scalpel and scissors, sharp dissection	Incision in the midline (2–3 cm) is made on the rectus sheath
Rectus muscle	Rectus sheath is separated from the rectus muscle by sharp dissection	The cut margins of the sheath is then stretched for blunt separation
Parietal peritoneum	It is cut/incised sharp, longitudinal with scissors	Peritoneum is stretched digitally and a window is created. The space is enlarged by stretching the peritoneum craniocaudally
Uterine incision	Low, transverse with the scalpel and the scissors	Low, transverse, cut with the scalpel for 2 cm in the middle and enlarged with digital separation laterally
Closure uterine muscle	Done in two layers continuous	Single layer continuous
Rectus muscle suturing	No	No
Rectus sheath	Continuous or interrupted	Continuous
Skin suture	Interrupted or continuous intracutaneous	Two or three mattress sutures

FACTORS THAT REDUCES THE LIKELIHOOD OF CS

- Continuous support during labor from women of her choice or from her partner (labor companion)
- Induction of labor for women with uncomplicated pregnancy beyond 41 weeks
- Partographic monitoring of labor with a 4-hour action line
- Involvement of consultant obstetrician
- Fetal blood sampling (scalp blood pH) for confirmation of fetal acidosis in cases with abnormal CTG. However, **there is no good evidence** that during labor, walking, nonsupine position, water birth, epidural analgesia influence the likelihood of CS.

PREOPERATIVE TESTS AND PREPARATION FOR CS

- Hemoglobin estimation (ABO and Rh grouping if not done earlier in antenatal clinic).
- Pregnant women having CS for APH (placental abruption, placenta previa), morbidly adherent placenta, and uterine rupture should have the **arrangement of blood transfusion as they bleed more (> 1L)**.
- Pregnant women who are healthy and who have no complication do not routinely need the following tests before CS:

- ♦ Crossmatching of blood
- ♦ Clotting screen.
- Women should be given **antacids and drugs (H_2) receptor antagonists** or **proton pump inhibitors**, to reduce gastric volume and acidity before CS. This is essential to reduce the risk of **aspiration pneumonitis**.
- **Anesthesia for CS:** Pregnant woman should be given the information on different types (regional, general) of anesthesia.
- Operating table for CS should have the facility of lateral tilt of 15° and this reduces maternal hypotension.
- ***Important issues while performing CS for a woman suspected to have morbidly adherent placenta*** (See Manual of Obstetrics and Gynecology for the Postgraduates, p. 267, 268)
  - ♦ Involvement of a consultant obstetrician and a consultant anesthetist.
  - ♦ Presence of an experienced pediatrician
  - ♦ Availability of blood depending on the need
  - ♦ Availability of a bed in critical care unit
  - ♦ A senior hematologist for advice when needed.

MORBIDLY ADHERENT PLACENTA

Diagnosis and management (See Manual of Obstetrics and Gynecology for the Postgraduates, p. 266).

PROCEDURE OF CESAREAN SECTION

Abdominal Wall Incision for CS

Transverse abdominal incision is commonly used. This causes less postoperative pain. It has improved cosmetic effect. (See Dutta's Textbook of Obstetrics, 8th Edition, p. 669).

Joel-Cohen incision is an incision of advantage.

Steps of Joel-Cohen Incision

- It is a straight skin incision made 3 cm above the symphysis pubic. The subcutaneous tissues are separated bluntly with surgeon's fingers and are not cut, this reduces bleeding. Thus, it differs from Pfannenstiel incision.
- Once the incision is completed, the scalpel is used to open the rectus sheath in the midline. This incision is extended laterally by digital separation, on either side of the midline up to the extent of skin incision.
- The rectus muscles are separated and the opening is stretched craniocaudally to make a space. The rectus muscles are retracted sideways separating them from the peritoneum.
- Intact veins are retracted and are not cut to avoid bleeding.
- The parietal peritoneum is opened digitally with further stretching. A classic Joel-Cohen incision avoids the use of retractors.
- Exposure is obtained by stitching the peritoneum to the skin in the midline and laterally.
- The visceral peritoneum is then incised in the midline just superior to the bladder reflection and the bladder flap is created with blunt dissection.
- The rest of the steps are usual (described above).

Advantages of Joel-Cohen Incision

- Shorter operating time
- Improved postoperative comfort
- Less bleeding
- Fewer wound complications.

IMPORTANT ISSUE IN THE STEPS OF CESAREAN SECTION (NICE, 2011)

Skin incision: Use of separate surgical knives to incise the skin and deeper tissues in CS is not recommended. This method does not decrease wound infection.

Extension of the uterine incision: Following uterine incision in the midline, muscle layers are separated with blunt extension rather than sharp incision. This reduces blood loss. Fetal laceration may occur in about 2% of cases. Forceps should only be used at CS, if there is difficulty in delivering the baby's head.

Exteriorization of the uterus during repair: It is not recommended. This is associated with more pain and does not improve operative outcomes such as hemorrhage and infection.

Usually uterine incision should be sutured in two layers.

Neither the visceral nor the parietal peritoneum should be sutured during CS. This reduces the operating time and the need of postoperative analgesia. It improves maternal satisfaction.

Closure of subcutaneous tissue: Routine closure of subcutaneous tissue should not be done. It should be done when the woman has more than 2 cm subcutaneous fat.

Timing of antibiotic administration: Prophylactic antibiotics are given to reduce the risk of infection (8%). Antibiotics are used to prevent endometritis, urinary tract and wound infections. ***Prophylactic antibiotics are given at CS before skin incision. This has got no effect on the baby.***

Thromboprophylaxis for CS: It should be given in high-risk women to prevent venous thromboembolism. The methods of prophylaxis include graduated stockings, hydration, early mobilization and low molecular weight heparin (LMWH). (*See* Manual of Obstetrics and Gynecology for the Postgraduates, p. 432)

Length of hospital stay: Women who are recovering well, are apyrexial and do not have any complication following CS, may go home after 3–4 days compared to a woman with vaginal birth (1–2 days). This mostly depends on each hospital protocol and that with woman's recovery.

References

1. National Institute for Health and Care Excellence (2011). Fertility, pregnancy and childbirth (NICE guidelines—Intrapartum care). [online] Available from https://www.nice.org.uk/guidance/conditions-and-diseases/fertility--pregnancy-and-childbirth/intrapartum-care [Accessed June 2016].
2. Robert SD, Daiziel SC. Antenatal corticosteroids for accelerating fetal lung maturation for women at risk of preterm birth. Cochrane Database Syst Rev. 2006;(3):CD004454.

13 Placenta Previa, Placenta Previa Accreta and Vasa Previa

SINGLE BEST ANSWER (SBA) AND MULTIPLE CHOICE QUESTIONS (MCQs)

Q.1 *Regarding placenta previa accreta:*
   a. Its occurrence is inversely related to the number of previous cesarean section (CS).
   b. MRI is the choice of first investigation.
   c. 3D power Doppler ultrasound has got high diagnostic sensitivity and specificity.
   d. During CS baby should preferably be delivered without disturbing the placenta.

Ans. a. F   b. F
         c. T   d. T

Q.2 *Regarding vasa previa:*
   a. Accurate diagnosis can be made by examining the blood hemoglobin.
   b. Clinical significance of vasa previa and placenta previa is the same.
   c. Vasa previa with bleeding worsens maternal prognosis.
   d. Placental anomalies may be associated.

Ans. a. F   b. F
         c. F   d. T

PLACENTA PREVIA, PLACENTA PREVIA ACCRETA

Management Issues

Antenatal sonographic imaging can be complemented with magnetic resonance imaging (MRI) when needed to diagnose placenta accreta. MRI should be used to confirm the diagnosis of placenta accreta when there is difficulty in definitive diagnosis with USG. 3D power Doppler ultrasound is best to make the diagnosis (sensitivity 100%; specificity 85%).

Overall incidence of vasa previa varies between 1 in 2,000 and 1 in 6,000 pregnancies. Unlike placenta previa, vasa previa carries no major maternal risk but fetal risk is significant.

Placental anomalies (bilobed placenta, succenturiate lobe) may be associated.

Q. *What are the diagnostic features of placenta previa and accreta with imaging studies?*
Ans. ■ Grey Scale
   ♦ Either absent or irregular retroplacental sonolucent zone
   ♦ Thinning or disruption of the hyperechoic serosa bladder interface

- Invasion of urinary bladder with focal exophytic masses
- Abnormal placental lacunae.
- **3D Power Doppler**
  - Diffuse vessels (vascular lakes) all through the uterine serosa–bladder junction
  - Hypervascularity.
- **MRI**
  - Uterine bulging
  - Dark intraplacental bands on T2-weighted imaging.

Essential Issues in the Management of Placenta Previa Accreta[1]
- Direct involvement of consultant obstetrician
- Direct involvement of consultant anesthetist
- Ready availability of blood and blood products
- Involvement of multidisciplinary team
- Patient counseling for possible interventions (mentioned below)
- Availability of bed in critical care (level 2) unit.

Women with placenta previa should be counseled regarding possible interventions like cesarean section, blood transfusion and hysterectomy as the risk of massive obstetric hemorrhage is high.

Case Summary

Mrs AR, 27-year-old, admitted as an emergency with vaginal bleeding due to placenta previa (USG confirmed). She had the history of prior cesarean delivery 3 years back. Emergency cesarean delivery followed by peripartum hysterectomy had to be done due to uncontrolled hemorrhage. Placenta increta was detected over the entire placentation site (Fig. 13.1).

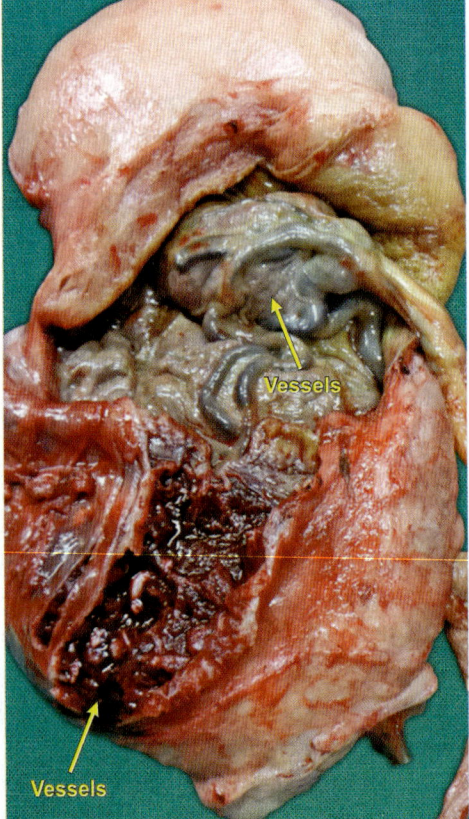

Fig. 13.1: Postoperative specimen of a gravid uterus, cut opened to show the morbidly adherent placenta (*see* arrow).

Courtesy: Dr Manas Saha, Asst Prof, Dept Obstetrics and Gynecology. CNMCH, Kolkata

Q. What is the place of interventional radiology in the management of placenta previa accreta?

Ans. Interventional radiology is lifesaving for the treatment of massive postpartum hemorrhage. Uterine artery embolization in cases of massive hemorrhage due to placenta accreta can be lifesaving as well as uterus sparing. Place of prophylactic catheter placement for balloon occlusion or embolization is not yet routinely recommended.

Relationship of previous cesarean section and placenta previa and accreta

Number of previous cesarean section(s)	Risk of placenta previa and accreta
0	3%
1	11%
2	40%
3	61%
≥ 4	67%

Surgery in the Presence of Morbid Adherent Placenta

- During operation when placenta previa accreta is suspected, surgeon should make the uterine incision at a site away from the placenta. The baby should be delivered without disturbing the placenta. This may be helpful for conservative management of placenta accreta.
- Otherwise elective hysterectomy could be performed following delivery of the baby in a parous woman, if placenta accreta is confirmed.
- Delivery by cutting through the placenta may cause massive hemorrhage and the chance of hysterectomy is high in that case.

Choice of Incision

- Skin
- Uterine

Low transverse skin incision is commonly done. It is acceptable, if the upper margin of the anterior placenta does not extend into the upper segment of the uterus. However, the placenta is anterior and extends towards the level of the fundus, *a midline vertical skin incision is preferred and to perform a classical cesarean section*. Preoperative ultrasound scan should always be done to map out the area of placenta.

Q. What should be the management options, if there is no placental separation after delivery of the baby?

Ans. The options for management are:
- **Conservative management:** The placenta is left in situ when there is no bleeding. The uterus is closed. This is specially done when uterine preservation is needed.
- **Hysterectomy:** When bleeding continues, the placenta is left undisturbed, and the uterus is closed. Thereafter, hysterectomy is done.

The advantages of the two surgical procedures:
- Any attempt of placental separation results in massive obstetric hemorrhage and ultimately ends in hysterectomy in about 100% of cases. Therefore, it is illogical.

- There is significant reduction of short-term morbidity in terms of hemorrhage, blood transfusion, intensive care unit admission and urological injury.
- Emergency hysterectomy in such a situation is associated with all the morbidities discussed above.
- When the placenta separates partly (partial accreta), the separated portion is removed. The adherent portion of placenta can be left in place. The blood loss is to be replaced.
- The use of uterotonic drugs should be continued (*See* Dutta's Textbook of Obstetrics, 8th Edition, p. 481). Other advanced techniques (bimanual compression, aortic compression) or uterine devascularization procedures may be used (*See* Manual of Obstetrics and Gynecology for the Postgraduates, p. 25).

Q. How the massive hemorrhage could be effectively managed?

Ans. Management outline is similar to as described in (*See* Dutta's Textbook of Obstetrics, 8th Edition, p. 481).

Management outlines are:
- Volume replacement by crystalloids, blood and blood products
- Use of uterotonics, oxytocin, prostaglandins (PGF2α, PGE$_1$)
- Bimanual compression/aortic compression
- Balloon tamponade
- B-lynch suture
- Vertical compressions suture
- Suturing the bleeding placental bed
- Isthmic-cervical suture
- Uterine and internal iliac artery ligation
- Intervention radiology techniques and uterine artery embolization to preserve the uterus
- Hysterectomy may be needed with early decision in few cases.

Q. How do you follow-up of women following conservative management of placenta accreta?

Ans. The woman needs to be followed up as there is the risk of vaginal bleeding and discharge. Antibiotic should be given to reduce infection. Routine use of methotrexate or arterial embolization is not recommended. The woman is followed up using ultrasonography to check the resolution of placental mass weekly. Serum β-hCG estimation is done and its falling levels are reassuring.

VASA PREVIA

Differentiation of fetal and maternal blood in a case of suspected vasa previa is difficult and not always clinically possible. Kleihauer-Betke test, hemoglobin electrophoresis or alkali denaturation (Apt test) test have been tried. All these have been found to be complicated and not clinically applicable.

Color Doppler ultrasound (TVS) has been found to be useful for the accurate diagnosis of vasa previa (Figs 13.2A and B).

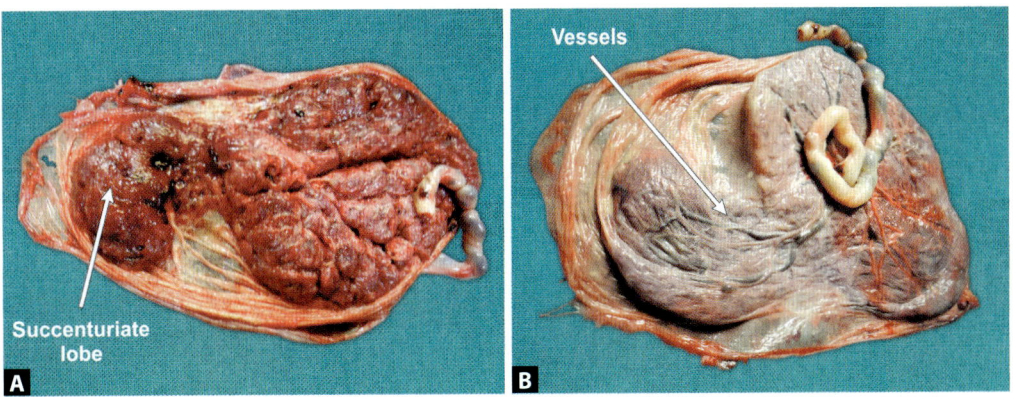

Figs 13.2A and B: Placenta succenturiata. **A.** Maternal surface, **B.** Fetal surface. Leash of blood vessels are seen to run from the main lobe to the small lobe

Courtesy: Dr Manas Saha, Asst Prof Dept Obstetrics and Gynecology. CNMCH, Kolkata

Management Issues

- Vasa previa with bleeding and signs of fetal compromise, delivery should be done by emergency (category 1) cesarean section (*See* Manual of Obstetrics and Gynecology for the Postgraduates, p. 267).
- Vasa previa at term without bleeding, delivery should be done by elective cesarean section. This is due to the risk of fetal hemorrhage in labor as the placental vessels rupture.

Reference

1. Eller AG, Porter TF, Soissan P, et al. Optimal management strtegies for placenta accreta. BJOG. 2009;116(5):648–54.

14 Perimortem Cesarean Section

Q.1 Regarding perimortem cesarean section:
a. It should be done following resuscitation of the mother
b. It is done under general anesthesia with added precautions
c. Chest compression in pregnancy improves pulmonary ventilation
d. It is carried without consent.

Ans. a. F b. F
c. F d. T

PERIMORTEM CESAREAN SECTION

Clinical Issues

Q. What are the special issues that need to be considered while managing a case with obstetric collapse?

Ans. A. The effect of aortocaval compression in pregnancy is an important issue. The implications of this physiological change are:
- It reduces (↓) cardiac output
- It causes supine hypotension
- Reduces efficacy of chest compression during cardiopulmonary resuscitation (CPR) due to mechanical factors (gravid uterus, chanes in pulmonatry function)
- Intubation is difficult due to laryngeal edema
- Mendelson syndrome may occur due to the incompetence of the lower esophageal sphincter.

B. **Other physiological changes in pregnancy results in significant changes in all the body systems.**
There is increase in plasma volume (40–50%), cardiac output (40%), pulse rate (10–15 beats/min) and placental blood flow (10% of cardiac output). There is decrease in systemic vascular resistance and venous return [due to pressure of the gravid uterus on the inferior vena cava (IVC)]. In the respiratory system, respiratory rate (slight) and the tissue oxygen consumption is increased (20%).There is decrease in residual capacity (25%) and arterial PCO_2. The resultant effects of these changes are—dilutional anemia, potential for rapid and massive hemorrhage when any hemorrhage occurs, rapid development of hypoxia and risk of developing acidosis more rapidly. There is decreased gastrointestinal tract (GIT) motility, relaxation of the lower esophageal

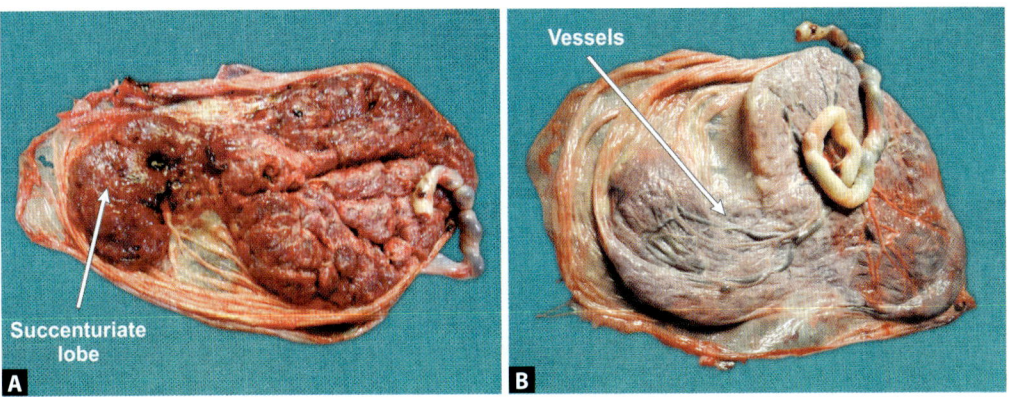

sphincter and splinting effects on the diaphragm due to the gravid uterus. At times endotracheal intubation becomes difficult (*See* Dutta's Textbook of Obstetrics, 8th Edition, p. 63, 596). Mechanical position of the uterus and increased weight gain in pregnancy make the effort of CPR and ventilation more difficult.

Q. *Outline the optimal management of a case of maternal collapse:*
Ans. Resuscitation Council (UK) Guidelines: (A = Airway, B = Breathing, C = Circulation)
- *Left lateral tilt*—15°
- *Airway* is to be maintained. Aspiration should be prevented. Intubation and ventilation whenever needed, is done immediately
- *Breathing* (bag and mask) with supplemental (100%) oxygen ventilation, until intubation
- *Circulation:* Volume should be maintained specially when there is blood loss which is common in obstetrics
- *Chest compression* is performed at a ratio of 30:2 until intubated
- *Wide bore (two), cannulas* are to be sited
- *Early delivery* is to be done
- *Volume replacement* is essential as early as possible
- *Defibrillation* (shock therapy is not contraindicated in pregnancy) energy could be used as in a nonpregnant patient. Fetal electronic monitors are to be removed before shock therapy. **Multidisciplinary team approach in management is to be done.**

Q. *What are the issues regarding the place of perimortem cesarean section (When, Why, Where, How)?*

(i) When it is to be done?
Ans.
- Cardiopulmonary resuscitation has been done correctly for 4 minutes but without any effects
  - When pregnancy (uterus) is >20 weeks. As the resuscitation procedure is ineffective due to the position of the gravid uterus.

(ii) Why it should be done?
Ans. It is done primarily to assist and to improve the maternal resuscitation.

(iii) How and where it should be done?
Ans.
- This procedure does not need any anesthetic
  - There is no need of any consent for this procedure
  - Perimortem cesarean section is done in the resuscitation place. There is no need of any operating theater. Mid line vertical skin incision and a classical uterine incision is preferred as it saves time.

Maternal collapse in pregnancy with cardiopulmonary arrest needs urgent cardiopulmonary resuscitation (CPR). When there is no response with CPR performed correctly for a period of 4 minutes of maternal collapse, delivery should be done.[1] This is to assist maternal resuscitation. **Perimortem cesarean section should be a resuscitative measure for the interest of the mother.**[2] However, delivery within 5 minutes of maternal collapse improves neonate's survival. **Perimortem cesarean section should be done in the same site where**

resuscitation is taking place. No anesthesia is needed. The doctrine of '***the best interest of the patient***' would apply to this procedure. It is carried out without consent.

This time scale of management is based on the fact that pregnant woman becomes hypoxic more quickly than nonpregnant woman. Irreversible brain damage can occur within 4–6 minutes. Aortocaval compression due to the gravid uterus results reduced venus return and reduced maternal cardiac output. Delivery of the fetus improves venous return, cardiac output and reduces oxygen consumption. Chest compression through diaphragm is more effective and pulmonary ventilation is also improved.

Following delivery, with successful resuscitation patient is shifted quickly to an intensive care unit for appropriate management where control of hemorrhage, blood transfusion, etc. could be continued.

References

1. Katz VL, Dotters DJ, Droegemueller W. Perimortem cesarean delivery. Obstet and Gynecol. 1986;68(4):571-6.
2. Morris S, Stacey M. Resuscitation in pregnancy. BMJ. 2003;327(7426):1277-9.

15

Puerperal Sepsis

SINGLE BEST ANSWER (SBA) AND MULTIPLE CHOICE QUESTIONS (MCQs)

Q.1 Regarding puerperal pyrexia:
  a. Maternal diabetes is a high-risk factor.
  b. Group A β-hemolytic streptococcus is a known pathogen.
  c. Patient may present with features of pneumonia.
  d. Infection is monomicrobial in majority.
  e. Reactivation of pulmonary tuberculosis may be a cause in tropics.

Ans. a. T b. T
c. T d. F
e. T

Q.2 Regarding treatment of puerperal sepsis:
  a. β-lactamase producing organisms should be treated with co-amoxiclav IV.
  b. Broad-spectrum antibiotics should be started after microbiological report is available.
  c. Piperacillin/tazobactam (Tazocin) are nephrotoxic.
  d. Clindamycin covers most streptococci and staphylococci.
  e. IVIG is effective against gram-negative sepsis.

Ans. a. F b. F
c. F d. T
e. F

Q.3 Regarding the clinical features suggestive of puerperal sepsis (one or more):
  a. Tachycardia (pulse rate > 90 bpm)
  b. Leukopenia (WBC count < 4 × 10^9/L)
  c. Raised serum lactate ≥ 4 mmol/L
  d. Urine output > 1 mL/kg/hr
  e. WBC count > 12 × 10^9/L

Ans. a. T b. T
c. T d. F
e. T

Rise in temperature 100.4°F (38°C) or more (measured orally), on two separate occasions at 24 hours apart (excluding the first 24 hours) within the first 10 days following delivery is called **puerperal pyrexia**. This definition is based on traditional criteria following UK febrile morbidity. In US, the threshold temperature is 100°F (37.8°C). Whether these rounded numbers are selected for the sake of convenience or for any scientific reason, is not understood. First 24 hours are excluded, as the incidence of pyrexia due to noninfective reasons (labor process) may be there.

Q. What are the maternal risk factors for puerperal sepsis?
Ans.
- Anemia
- Chorioamnionitis
- Prolonged labor/obstructed labor
- Prolonged rupture of membranes
- Traumatic vaginal delivery
- Diabetes
- Impaired glucose tolerance
- Cesarean section
- Retained products of conception
- Immunocompromized state (HIV).

Q. What are the common microbial organisms in the pathogenesis of puerperal sepsis?
Ans.
- Group A β-hemolytic streptococcus (*Streptococcus pyogenes*)
- *Escherichia coli*
- *Staphylococcus aureus*
- Methicillin-resistant *S aureus* (MRSA)
- Mixed infections (aerobics and anaerobics)
- Anaerobic organisms: *Peptostreptococcus, Bacteroides*.

Beta-lactamase producing gram-negative bacteria are resistant to co-amoxiclav and cephalosporins group of antibiotics.

Q. What are the other organs that may be affected in puerperal sepsis?
Ans.
- ***Breasts:*** Mastitis, breast abscess, necrotizing mastitis
- ***Urinary tract:*** Cystitis, pyelitis, pyelonephritis
- ***Lungs:*** Pneumonia, recrudescence of tuberculosis
- ***Skin and soft tissue:*** Cesarean section and episiotomy wound infection, necrotizing fasciitis, cellulitis
- ***Blood vessels:*** Deep vein thrombosis, thrombophlebitis
- ***Others:*** Pharyngitis, gastroenteritis.

Q. What are indications of admission in hospital for a woman with puerperal sepsis?[1]
Ans.
- Woman generally looking ill
- Temperature > 38°C (> 100.4°F)
- Tachycardia (pulse > 90 bpm)
- Breathlessness (respiratory rate > 20/min)
- Abdominal pain, tenderness
- Cough, chest pain
- Dysuria, loin pain.

Q. What are the investigations to be done for a woman with puerperal sepsis?
Ans.
- ***Blood:*** Full blood count (FBC), blood cultures, urea, electrolytes, serum lactate, C-reactive protein (CRP).
- ***Swabs:*** From the sites of infection (genital tract), woman with pharyngitis-throat swab should be taken.

- **Urine:** Midstream specimen for routine examination, culture sensitivity.
- **Imaging studies:** X-ray chest, pelvic ultrasonography.

Q. How a case of puerperal sepsis could be managed?

Ans. Principles of management: The source of infection is diagnosed. Uterus may need evacuation. Drainage of pus from the peritoneal cavity, drainage of breast abscess or pelvic abscess is to done. **Broad-spectrum antibiotics** are started after initial workup of the patient and sending the samples for laboratory tests.

Some patients may need **intensive care unit (ICU)** management (dialysis for renal failure).[2]

Management

Broad-spectrum antibiotics are started in high dose, preferably within an hour, without waiting for the microbiological report to come.

- **Antibiotic regimens are as follows (Table 15.1):**
    - A combination of either piperacillin-tazobactam or a carbapenem plus clindamycin has the broadest range antimicrobial coverage for **severe sepsis**.
    - Woman having MRSA infection needs to be given vancomycin or teicoplanin till sensitivity report is available.
    - In situation with extended-spectrum of beta-lactamase (ESBL) producing organisms, piperacillin/tazobactam may be ineffective.

Table 15.1: Selection of antimicrobials in the management of *puerperal sepsis*

■ Piperacillin/tazobactam or meropenem + clindamycin	♦ Covers most organisms ♦ Does not cover ESBL procedures ♦ Not nephrotoxic
■ Metronidazole	♦ Covers only anaerobes
■ Gentamicin (3–5 mg/kg single dose)	♦ Can be used provided renal function is normal
■ Clindamycin	♦ Covers most streptococci and staphylococci including MRSA
■ Co-amoxiclav	♦ Does not cover MRSA, pseudomonas or ESBL producing organisms
■ Vancomycin or teicoplanin or linezolid	♦ May be used for MRSA positive women, anerobes, Streptococcus group A and B

Abbreviations: ESBL—Extended-spectrum beta-lactamase, MRSA—Methicillin-resistant *Staphylococcus aureus*

Q. What is the place of intravenous immunoglobulin (IVIG) as a part of therapy in puerperal sepsis?

Ans. When other modalities of therapy have failed, IVIG is recommended for severe invasive (streptococcal or staphylococcal) infection. High dose IVIG has been used in the management of shock due to exotoxin producing organisms (streptococci and staphylococci). IVIG neutralizes bacterial exotoxins and inhibits production of tumor necrosis factors (TNFs) and interleukins (ILS). IVIG may not be effective in gram-negative (endotoxin) sepsis.

NECROTIZING FASCIITIS (HOSPITAL GANGRENE)[3]

Necrotizing fasciitis is the result of polymicrobial synergistic infection. It is most commonly due to streptococcal (group A, β-hemolytic) in combination with staphylococcus, *E. coli*, bacteroides or clostridium. Mixed infection with aerobic or anaerobic bacteria or with gas gangrene producing *Clostridium perfringens* may also occur. Strains of MRSA that produce the Panton-Valentine leukocidin (PVL) is known to cause necrotizing fasciitis. Other organisms involved are *E. faecalis, S. aureus group A and Enterobacteriaceae* (Table 15.2).

Criteria for Diagnosis of Necrotizing Fasciitis

- Microvascular thrombosis with no major vessel block
- Extensive superficial tissue necrosis
- Clostridial infection is absent
- No involvement of muscles
- Exaggerated infiltration of WBC in necrotic wound
- Systemic toxicity (moderate to severe).

Risk factors for necrotizing fasciitis
- Atherosclestic heart disease
- Diabetes mellitus
- Obesity
- Debilitating disease
- Older age
- Smoking
- Radiation therapy

Table 15.2: Classification of operative wounds and risk of infection (Culver et al. 1991)[4]

Classification	Description	Infection risk
Clean wounds	<ul><li>Uninfected operative wound</li><li>No acute inflammation</li><li>No entry to genitourinary, alimentary or respiratory tract</li><li>No break in aseptic technique</li></ul>	< 2%
Clean contaminated wounds	<ul><li>Entry to GU, alimentary or respiratory tract was there but no significant spillage of contents</li><li>No evidence of infection or major break in aseptic technique</li></ul>	< 10%
Contaminated wounds	<ul><li>Entry to internal organs with inflammation or spillage of contents</li></ul>	15–20%
Dirty wounds	<ul><li>Purulent, inflammation present, intraperitoneal abscess formation or visceral perforation</li></ul>	40%

Microorganisms involved in necrotizing fasciitis are: *Escherichia coli, Enterococcus faecalis, Staphylococcus aureus,* group A β-*hemolytic streptococci,* Bacteroides and the *Enterobacteriaceae.*

Pathology: Early infection starts deep in the tissues. Early necrotizing fasciitis may not have any visible skin changes. The necrotizing process ascends to the skin in a late phase when skin blisters and necrosis could be seen. It is a surgical emergency. Initially the patient may be febrile and tachycardic, progression to shock may be very rapid. **Radiographs** may show air in the tissues.

Antibiotics to be used for group A streptococcal necrotizing fasciitis are: clindamycin 600–900 mg IV 6–8 hourly plus second-generation cephalosporin or Penicillin G 4 million units IV 4 hourly.

HEMODYNAMIC CHANGES AND ORGAN DYSFUNCTION DUE TO SEVERE PUERPERAL SEPSIS

- Hypotension: Mean arterial pressure <70 mm Hg
- Serum lactate: ≥ 4 mmol/L
- PaO_2 (partial pressure of oxygen in arterial blood)/FiO_2 (fraction of inspired oxygen) < 40 KPa
- Oliguria (urine output < 0.5 mL/kg/hr for 2 hours).
- Serum creatinine >176 μmol/L
- Abnormal coagulation profile (INR >1.5 or APPT > 60 seconds)
- Thrombocytopenia (platelet count <100,000/mL)
- Hyperbilirubinemia (plasma bilirubin >70 mmol/L)

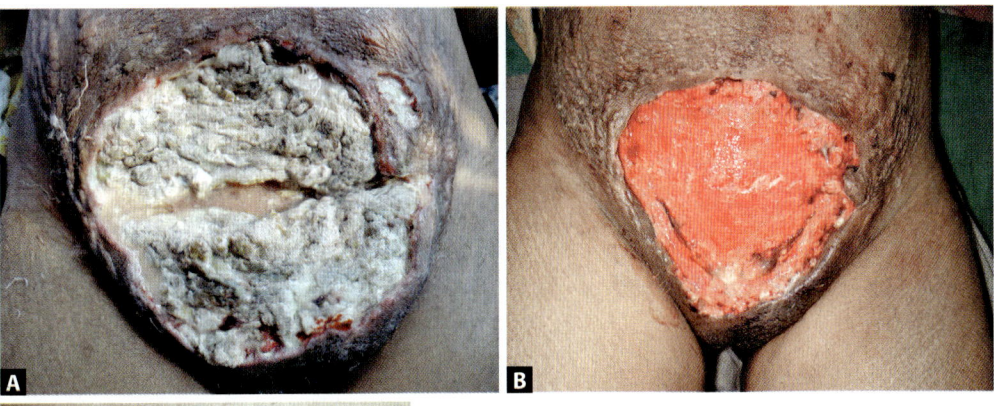

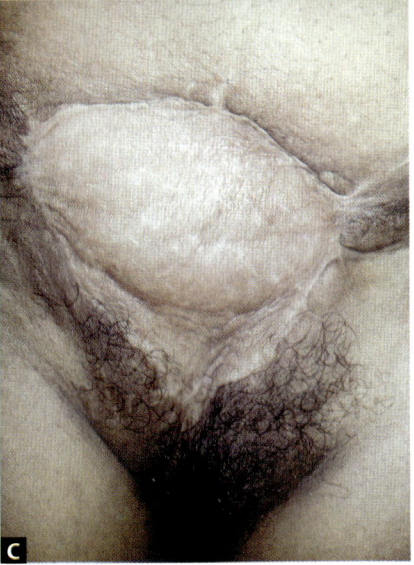

Figs 15.1A to C: *Necrotizing fasciitis in a woman due to wound sepsis following cesarean delivery:* **A.** Necrotizing process involving the rectus sheath and up to skin, **B.** Healthy tissues are seen following wound debridement, **C.** Same wound following skin grafting

- Paralytic ileus (absent bowel sounds)
- Pulmonary edema
- Hypothermia
- Decreased consciousness levels.

Majority of these patients need ICU management. Women with respiratory distress syndrome or with persistent hypotension and oliguria or with multiorgan failure, are admitted in ICU for management. Involvement of anesthetic and critical care teams is essential to initiate early management and ICU transfer.

References

1. Centre for Maternal and Child Enquiries (CMACE) Saving mother's lives: Reviewing maternal deaths to make motherhood safe 2006-08. The eighth report on confidential enquiries into Maternal Deaths in the United Kingdom. BJOG. 2011;118:1-203.
2. Levy MM, Fink MP, Marshall JC, et al. 2001 SCCM/ESICM/ACCP/ATS/SIS International Sepsis Definitions Conference. Crit Care Med. 2003;31(4):1250-6.
3. Morgan MS. Diagnosis and management of necrotizing fasciitis and multiparametric approach. J Hosp Infect. 2010;75(4):249-57.
4. Culver DH, Horan TC, Gaynes RP, et al. Surgical wound infection rates by wound class, operative procedure, and patient risk index. National Nosocomial Infections Surveillance System. Am J Med. 1991;91(3B):152S-157S.

16 Maternal Near Miss

Q.1 Regarding maternal near miss (MNM):
   a. Refers to a woman who died due to obstetric complications but could have been saved
   b. MNM is used to analyze the quality of emergency obstetric care
   c. Severe acute maternal morbidity is based on strict criteria
   d. Higher the mortality index (MI), higher is the quality of care.

Ans.
   a. F
   b. F
   c. T
   d. F

In resource poor setting, maternal mortality is an important health indicator of the country. For improvement of maternal deaths, it is essential to identify the weakness or failure within the system and to take corrective action.

But women who experienced and survived a severe health condition during pregnancy, childbirth or postpartum are considered as ***maternal near miss (MNM) or severe acute maternal morbidity (SAMM) cases***. The terminology ***near miss*** has been borrowed from airline industry. ***MNM refers to a condition where a woman experienced a severe complication and she nearly died but survived***. Near miss and SAMM are the two terms used interchangeably. It best reflects the situation of 'Nearly dying but surviving'.

It appears a diverse situation to define the condition with an uniform criteria to identify MNM/SAMM.

International Statistical Classification of Disease (ICD) and related health problem reconciled the definition in relation to 'maternal death'.[1] Therefore, a MNM is defined as: ***A woman who nearly died but survived a complication that occurred during pregnancy, childbirth or within 42 days of termination of pregnancy.***

Q. How to identify cases with MNM or SAMM?

Ans. Three approaches to identify a MNM (criteria selected must be locally usable and relevant).

   1. ***Clinical criteria to a specific disease entity:*** Specific diseases are used as the starting points and then for each disease, morbidity is defined, e.g. pre-eclampsia is the disease entity and the complications; eclampsia, renal failure, pulmonary edema and disseminated intravascular coagulation (DIC) are used to define severe morbidity.
   2. ***Intervention-based criteria:*** Intervention such as admission to an intensive care unit (ICU), the need for an emergency hysterectomy, the need for blood transfusion, cesarean section are used as the marker of MNM.

3. ***Organ system dysfunction-based criteria:*** This system is based on the concept that there is a sequence of events leading from good health to death. The sequence is **clinical insult**, followed by a systemic inflammatory response syndrome, organ dysfunction, organ failure and finally death. MNM cases would be those women with organ dysfunction and organ failure who survive. The criteria for defining a MNM are defined per organ system. Markers for organ system dysfunction or failure are specific.

Advantages and Disadvantages

Clinical criteria related to a specific disease entity

Advantages: Data obtained from the case notes can be analyzed and interpreted. The complications and quality care to a particular patient can be assessed.

Disadvantages:
- Morbidity criteria to define MNM may be inaccurate
- Documentation unless of good quality, retrospective information might be inaccurate and difficult to use for ongoing audits.

Intervention-based criteria

Advantages: Simple to identify as based on the documents.

Disadvantages: As it is based on resources available, it may not be assessed uniformly. There may be variation of assessment eligibility criteria for intervention or ICU care.

Organ system dysfunction-based criteria

Advantages: It is similar to maternal death enquiries. It allows identification of critically ill women with a specific organ dysfunction.

Disadvantages: It is dependent on existence of resources for quality care, laboratory facilities, monitoring of critically ill women or women with organ dysfunction.

Maternal near miss is a retrospective event. From the theory of definition standpoint, a woman can only be recognized as a MNM, when she survives the severe complication in pregnancy, labor or postpartum 6 weeks. Hospitals with high- and moderate-resource settings, it is feasible to fulfill the criteria for assessment of maternal life-threatening conditions. Hospital with low-resource settings, as this is not feasible, periodic audits can be done.[2]

MATERNAL NEAR MISS CRITERIA (WHO)

A woman presenting with any of the following life-threatening condition and survived, is considered as a MNM case.[2]

Q. What are the specific defining criteria for MNM (SAMM)?
Ans.

Clinical criteria	
Acute cyanosis	Shock
Loss of consciousness (LC) lasting >12 hours	Uncontrollable fits/total paralysis
Gasping	Oliguria not responding to fluids or diuretics
LC and absence of pulse/heartbeat	Jaundice in pre-eclampsia
Respiratory rate > 40 breaths/min or < 6/min	Clotting failure (DIC)
Stroke	

Maternal near miss and maternal death

```
A                    B                      C
Women during   →   Complication(s)   →   Potentially
pregnancy,                                life-
childbirth                                threatening
or
postpartum
6 weeks
                                              │
                                              ▼
                                              F
                                         ┌─ Survival  →  Maternal
                  D              E       │               near miss
           Based on criteria → Outcome  ─┤
           1. Clinical                   │   G
           2. Intervention                └─ Death
           3. Organ system
              dysfunction
```
(Life-threatening conditions)

Laboratory-based criteria

Oxygen saturation < 90% for ≥ 60 minutes	pH < 7.1
PaO_2/FiO_2 <200 mm Hg	Lactate > 5
Serum creatinine ≥ 3.5 mg/dL	Acute thrombocytopenia (<50,000 platelets/cumm)
Serum bilirubin ≥ 6.0 mg/dL	Loss of consciousness and presence of glucose and katoacids in urine

Management-based criteria

Use of vasoactive drugs (dopamine, epinephrine)	Intubation ≥ 60 minutes not related to anesthesia
Hysterectomy following infection/hemorrhage	Dialysis for acute renal failure
Transfusion ≥ 5 units blood	Cardiopulmonary resuscitation

There is no gold standard criteria for defining SAMM specially where not all women give birth in a health facility or where women giving birth in a low-resource setting.

Q. What are the common life-threatening conditions in obstetrics?
Ans. Potentially life-threatening conditions commonly seen in obstetrics are:

Hypertensive disorders	Hemorrhagic disorders
Severe pre-eclampsia	Placenta previa
Eclampsia	Placental abruption
Hemolysis, Elevated Liver enzymes and Low Platelet count (HELLP) syndrome	Postpartum hemorrhage
Hypertension with complications (renal failure, encephalopathy)	Rupture uterus
	Ectopic pregnancy

Other systemic disorders	Management indicators
Pulmonary edema	Blood transfusion [> 5 units packed red blood cells (PRBCs)]
Sepsis	ICU admission
Shock	Central venous access
Respiratory failure	Hysterectomy
Uncontrolled seizures	Return to operating theater
Thrombocytopenia (<100,000 platelet/cumm)	Surgical intervention
	Prolonged hospital stay (> 7 days postpartum)
	Non-anesthetic intubation

Quality of obstetric care is assessed from the collection of data on MNMs together with maternal deaths. Reduction of mortality index (see below) would indicate improvement in the quality of emergency obstetric care.

Maternal near miss incidence ratio (MNM–IR) refers to the number of MNM cases per 1,000 live births (MNM–IR = MNM/1,000 LB).

Mortality index refers to the number of maternal deaths divided by the number of women with life-threatening conditions, expressed as a percentage. The higher the indexes, the more women with life-threatening conditions die (low quality of care).

Women with life-threatening condition (WLTC) refer to all women who either suffered as MNM and who died (WLTC = MNM+MD).

Maternal mortality is one of the worst performing health indicators in resource poor countries. In an effort to reduce maternal deaths, many countries are increasingly adopting policies to encourage births in institutions. Main purpose is to improve the identification of the areas of weakness or failure within the system. It is again important to assess the methods available in the institution for quality care. Therefore not only the deaths but also the care of a critically ill women need to be analyzed.

It is often not possible to analyze and identify the cause of actual maternal death where death occurred outside an institution, due to nonavailability of reliable documents.

A number of women with life-threatening conditions survive. This reflects the quality of emergency obstetric care. Indicators of MNM and maternal deaths can establish the quality of emergency obstetric care for comparisons between institutions and countries.

References

1. WHO. International Statistical Classification of Diseases and related health problems. Tenth revision (ICD-10), 10th edition. Geneva: Switzerland; 1992.
2. Say L, Pattinson R, Gülmezoglu AM. WHO systematic review of maternal morbidity and mortality: The prevalence of severe acute maternal morbidity (near miss). Reprod Health. 2004;1(1):3.

17 Cesarean Delivery on Maternal Request

Cesarean delivery on maternal request (CDMR) is defined when primary cesarean delivery (CD) is done electively before the onset of labor, on maternal request, without any maternal or fetal indications. Potential risks of CD are both to the mother and the neonate. Complications of subsequent pregnancies and delivery following prior cesarean section (CS) are also more. There are few potential short-term benefits of planned CD compared to vaginal delivery.

IMPORTANT ISSUES IN CESAREAN DELIVERY

- Cesarean delivery can save maternal and infant's lives.
- Cesarean section can cause significant complications and permanent disabilities or even death (in some settings).
- CD should ideally be undertaken when it is medically indicated.
- The ideal rates of CS is 10–15% (Table 17.1).
- CD rates >15% are not associated with further reduction in maternal and newborn mortality rates. However, currently WHO suggests no such fixed limit. CD maybe done as clinically indicated.
- Every effort should be made to provide CD to women in need, rather than striving to achieve specific rate—(WHO).
- The incidence of CD without medical or obstetric indications is increasing all over the World.
- A rising component of this is due to CD on maternal request.
- The magnitude of this problem is yet to quantify.
- We need to quantify the benefits and risks of CDMR versus planned vaginal delivery based on evidence.

Potential Benefits of CDMR (Maternal)	*Potential Risks of CDMR (Maternal)*
■ Decreased rate of postpartum hemorrhage (PPH)	■ Longer hospital stay
■ Lesser need of blood transfusion	■ Complications on subsequent pregnancy
■ Fewer surgical complications	■ Rupture uterus
■ Decreased urinary incontinence (weak-evidence quality)	■ Placental implantation problems
	■ Morbid adherent placenta
	■ Need for hysterectomy
	■ Thromboembolism

Table 17.1: Cesarean section rates—according to country

Country	Cesarean section rates
China	25.9
Brazil	45.9
US	30.3
Canada	26.3
Iran	41.9
Italy	38.2
Germany	27.8
India	31
UK	22.0
France	18.8
Australia	30.3
Switzerland	28.9
Chile	30.7
Argentina	35.2

Benefits of planned vaginal delivery

Maternal benefits	Neonatal benefits
▪ Short hospital stay	▪ Lower rate of respiratory morbidities
▪ Lower infection rates	▪ No risks of iatrogenic prematurity
▪ Less complications due to anesthesia	▪ Less admission to neonatal intensive care unit (NICU)
▪ Higher rates of breastfeeding	▪ Lower perinatal mortality
▪ Lower costs	

Risks of cesarean delivery on maternal request

Short-term risks	Long-term risks
▪ Longer hospital stay	▪ Rupture of uterus (scar rupture)
▪ Higher rates of infection	▪ Scar dehiscence
▪ Complications due to anesthesia	▪ Placenta previa
▪ Risks are more in the presence of medical disorders and increased BMI	▪ Placenta accreta, increta
▪ Higher costs	▪ Injury to bladder, bowel
	▪ Risks of peripartum hysterectomy
	▪ Risks of blood transfusion
	▪ Venous thromboembolism

Neonatal Outcomes

- Higher rates of **respiratory morbidities** when delivery is done on request, at <39 weeks
  - Transient tachypnea of the newborn (TTN)
  - Respiratory distress syndrome
  - Persistent pulmonary hypertension
- Other complications when delivery occurs preterm

  Respiratory morbidities:
  - Birth asphyxia
  - Hypoglycemia
  - Jaundice
  - Increased admission to in NICU.
  - Hypothermia
  - Sepsis
  - Encephalopathy

Because of these potential complications, cesarean delivery on maternal request should not be performed before gestational age of 39 weeks.

Other risk factors for CDMR must be reviewed. **Specific risk factors are**: Age (elderly), increased BMI and presence of any medical disorders, uncertain gestational age, reproductive plans and personal values.

Anxiety, fear of the unknown about labor process and delivery, prior poor obstetric outcomes, risk of trauma in delivery, may often aggravate the desire of CD. When the woman's main concern for the request of CD is the anxiety and fear, she need to be counseled with adequate information (Table 17.2). Prenatal classes for childbirth, education, emotional support in labor, presence of a labor companion of choice during delivery, provision of anesthesia when needed, to minimize pain may help her. However, maternal autonomy is to be respected.

Table 17.2: Risk of placenta accreta and hysterectomy by number of cesarean deliveries compared with the first cesarean delivery

Cesarean delivery	Placenta accreta [n (%)]	Odds ratio (95% CI)	Hysterectomy [n (%)]	Odds ratio (95% CI)
First*	15 (0.2)	-	40 (0.7)	-
Second	49 (0.3)	1.3 (0.7–2.3)	67 (0.4)	0.7 (0.4–0.97)
Third	36 (0.6)	2.4 (1.3–4.3)	57 (0.9)	1.4 (0.9–2.1)
Fourth	31 (2.1)	9.0 (4.8–16.7)	35 (2.4)	3.8 (2.4–6.0)
Fifth	6 (2.3)	9.8 (3.8–25.5)	9 (3.5)	5.6 (2.7–11.6)
Six or more	6 (6.7)	29.8 (11.3–78.7)	8 (9.0)	(6.9–33.5)

* Primary cesarean delivery; CI: Confidence interval.

Maternal Outcome Favor Neither Vaginal nor Cesarean Delivery

- Pelvic pain
- Sexual function
- PP depression, fistula
- Pelvic organ prolapse (POP)
- Anorectal dysfunction
- Maternal morbidity.

Weak-quality Evidence to Favor CDMR
- Urinary Incontinence
- Surgical and traumatic complications following planned vaginal delivery.

Neonatal Outcome Favor CDMR (Weak-quality Evidence)
Cesarean delivery causes reduction in:
- Fetal mortality
- Intracranial hemorrhage
- Brachial plexus injury.

These are based on weak quality evidence. Vaginal delivery is not associated with any such increase provided the vaginal delivery is done by a trained and skilled person.

There is no randomized controlled trial (RCT) that compared CDMR with singleton term pregnancy with vertex presentation.

National Institute of Health Consensus and State of the Science Conference on CDMR (18 member panel): March 2006:
- Risks and benefits of CDMR and peripheral vascular disease (PVD) does not provide the basis for a recommendation for either mode of delivery
- Approximate rate of CDMR: 4–18% (WHO)
- Patient's specific, cultural, societal, healthcare provider issues, ethical issues need to be considered.

Patients Specific Factors
- Age (elderly women may be considered for CD)
- Women desiring several children (these women need special counseling because of the long-term complications)
- Accuracy of GA
- Psychological/personality factor/ interpersonal violence/ traumatic delivery/depression } Medical indications
- Anxiety, fear.

Cultural and Societal Issue
Some cultures have rituals and customs for vaginal birth, other women may attribute more value to CD as the benefit. Throughout the world, there is rise in the rates of primary CS and decline in the rates of vaginal birth after CS (Fig. 17.1).

Any discussion of the relative benefits and risks of CDMR vs PVD, woman's cultural, personal view and her autonomy should be respected:
- Cesarean delivery is established as a safe alternative for **vaginal breech delivery** and also for **vaginal birth after cesarean delivery (VBAC).**
- These contribute to societal acceptance of cesarean birth as a safe method.
- Media also increase the concerns for vaginal birth. Such a shift in societal acceptance on safety, lead an increase in CDMR.

The unpredictability of timing of onset and the duration of labor, is a cause of concern for many women in the society.
- Each woman deserve individualized counseling, consistent with ethical principles and based on available scientific data, in the decision of CDMR. When a healthcare provider cannot support her request, the woman may be referred to another support provider.

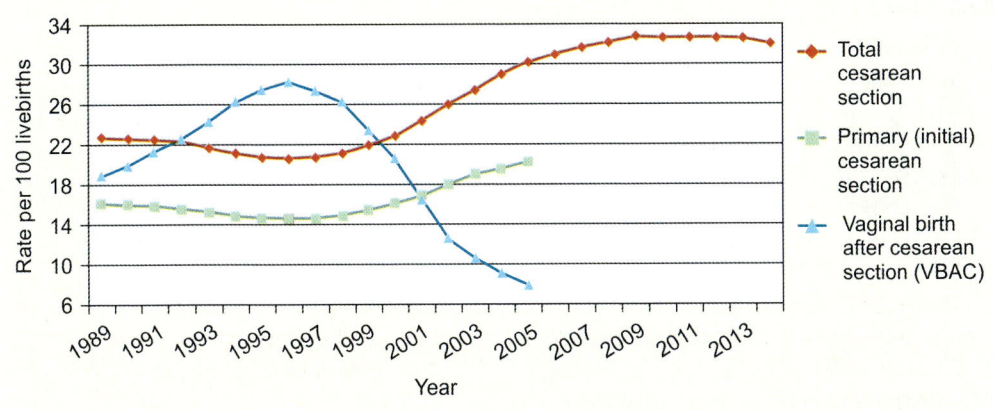

Fig. 17.1: Rates for total cesarean section, primary cesarean section and vaginal birth after cesarean (VBAC), United States, 1989–2014

Therefore, on balance of risks and benefits associated with CDMR the recommendations are **[WHO, The American Congress of Obstetricians and Gynecologists (ACOG)]**.
- In the absence of maternal and fetal indications for CS, a plan for vaginal delivery is safe, appropriate and should be recommended as it is the norm.
- Cases in which CS on maternal request is planned, the following are recommended:
  - Cesarean delivery should be performed at a gestational age >39 weeks.
  - It should not be motivated by unavailability of effective pain relief.
  - Women desiring for several children should be specifically counseled before accepting for CS on request. This is mainly due to the long-term complications of CD (see above).
  - Woman's cultural, personal view and her autonomy should be respected.
  - Further research is awaited for database studies and studies of modifiable factors for CDMR.

References

1. Silver RM, Landon MB, Rouse DJ, et al. Maternal morbidity associated with multiple repeat cesarean deliveries. National Institute of Child Health and Human Development Maternal–Fetal Medicine Units Network. Obstet Gynecol. 2006;107:1226-32.
2. Hannah MU, Whyte H, Hannah WJ, et al. Maternal outcomes at 2 years after planned cesarean section versus planned vaginal birth for breech presentation at term: the international randomized Term Breech Trial. Am J Obstet Gynecol. 2004;191:917-27.

18 Classification of Evidence Levels and Grades of Recommendations

CLASSIFICATION OF EVIDENCE LEVELS

1++	1+	1–	2++	2+	2–	3	4

- 1++ High quality meta-analysis, systematic reviews of randomized controlled trials (RCTs) or RCT with a very low bias
- 1+ Well-controlled meta-analysis, systematic reviews of RCTs or RCTs with a low risk of bias
- 1– Meta-analysis, systematic reviews of RCTs or RCTs with a high-risk of bias
- 2++ High-quality systematic reviews of case control or cohort studies or high-quality case control or cohort studies with a very low risk of confounding, bias or chance and a high probability that the relationship is causal
- 2+ Well-conducted case-control or cohort studies with a low-risk of confounding, bias or chance and a moderate probality that the relationship is causal
- 2– Case-control or cohort studies with a high-risk of confounding, bias or chance and a significant risk that the relationship is not causal
- 3 Nonanalytical studies, e.g. case reports, case series
- 4 Expert opinion.

GRADES OF RECOMMENDATIONS[1]

A	B	C	D

- **A** At least one meta-analysis, systematic review or RCT rated as 1++ and directly applicable to target population or a systematic review of RCTs or a body of evidence consisting principally of studies rated as 1+ directly applicable to target population and demonstrating overall consistence of results.
- **B** A body of evidence including studies rated as 2++ and directly applicable to target population and demonstrating overall consistency of results; or
Extrapolated evidence from studies rated as 1++ or 1+.
- **C** A body of evidence including studies rated as 2+ directly applicable to the target population and demonstrating overall consistency of results; or
Extrapolated evidence from studies rated as 2++.
- **D** Evidence level 3 or 4; or extrapolated evidence from studies rated as 2+.

GOOD PRACTICE POINT

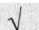

√   Recommended best practice-based on the clinical experience of the guideline developing group.

Reference

1. Royal College of Obstetricians and Gynecologists, London.

SECTION 4

Gynecology Discussion

Section Outline

- Ch. 19. Recurrent Miscarriage (First and Second Trimesters)
- Ch. 20. Tubal Ectopic Pregnancy
- Ch. 21. Cervical Insufficiency (Incompetence)
- Ch. 22. Heavy Menstrual Bleeding (HMB)
- Ch. 23. Urinary Incontinence
- Ch. 24. Polycystic Ovarian Syndrome
- Ch. 25. Male and Female Sterilization
- Ch. 26. Gestational Trophoblastic Disease
- Ch. 27. Carcinoma of the Endometrial (Early Stage Diseases)
- Ch. 28. Pregnancy of Unknown Location
- Ch. 29. Abnormal Uterine Bleeding
- Ch. 30. Endoscopy in Gynecology (Laparoscopic Surgery)
- Ch. 31. Robotic Surgery in Gynecology

19 Recurrent Miscarriage (First and Second Trimesters)

SINGLE BEST ANSWER (SBA) AND MULTIPLE CHOICE QUESTIONS (MCQs)

Q.1 Regarding etiology the epidemiological factors for miscarriage:
   a. Advanced maternal age
   b. Advanced paternal age
   c. Previous reproductive history
   d. Anesthetic gases for theater workers
   e. Exposure to video display terminal.

Ans. a. T b. T
   c. T d. F
   e. F

Q.2 Antiphospholipid antibody syndrome (APAS):
   a. It is an important cause of recurrent miscarriage
   b. Presence of antiphospholipid antibodies (APAbs) is a high risk factor
   c. Every woman with APA needs pharmacological intervention
   d. APAS inhibit trophoblast function and inhibition.

Ans. a. T b. F
   c. F d. T

Q.3 Anatomical factors for recurrent miscarriage:
   a. Overall prevalence of uterine anomalies in recurrent miscarriage population ranges between 2 and 38%
   b. Women with uterine malformations tend to miscarry more in the first trimester
   c. Cervical weakness is an independent risk factor in women with uterine malformations
   d. MRI scanning is an important tool in the confirmation of diagnosis.

Ans. a. T b. F
   c. F d. F

Q.4 Genetic factors for recurrent miscarriage:
   a. Overall prevalence is 2–5% in couples with recurrent miscarriage
   b. Most commonly is reciprocal or Robertsonian translocation
   c. Risk of miscarriage due to fetal aneuploidy increases with increasing number of pregnancy losses
   d. Risk of euploid pregnancy loss increases as the number of miscarriage increases.

Ans. a. T b. T
c. F d. T

Q.5 Immunological factors for recurrent miscarriage:
a. Human leukocyte antigen (HLA) incompatibility among couples is a known factor
b. Altered peripheral blood natural killer (NK) cells is an important factor
c. Uterine natural killer (uNK) cells are raised in these women
d. The response of T helper-1 (Th-1) cytokine is mounting in these women.

Ans. a. F b. F
c. F d. T

Q.6 Thrombophilia and recurrent miscarriage:
a. Thrombophilias are the known causes of systemic thrombosis
b. Activated protein C resistance is mainly due to factor V Leiden mutation
c. Thrombophilia may cause massive placental abruption
d. Hyperhomocysteinemia is not associated with adverse pregnancy outcome.

Ans. a. T b. T
c. T d. F

Q.7 Antiphospholipid antibody syndrome (APAS):
a. All women with recurrent miscarriage should be screened for APAbs
b. One clinical criteria is diagnostic
c. One laboratory criteria is confirmatory
d. Corticosteroid therapy improves the live birth rate.

Ans. a. T b. F
c. F d. F

One of the two clinical criteria in addition to at least one laboratory criteria must be present (*see* below).

Q.8 Management of an unexplained case of recurrent miscarriage should be done by:
a. Paternal cell immunization
b. Third party donor leukocyte infusion
c. Trophoblast membranes infusion
d. Immunoglobulin IV.

Ans. a. F b. F
c. F d. F

Q.9 Management of recurrent miscarriage due to endocrine factors:
a. Progesterone supplementation may be helpful
b. Human chorionic gonadotropin therapy is helpful
c. Insulin sensitizing agent (metformin and rosiglitazone) improve live birth rate
d. Suppression of high LH with GnRh agonist prepregnancy should be done.

Ans. a. T b. F
c. F d. F

MANAGEMENT ISSUES

Miscarriage is defined as the spontaneous loss of pregnancy before the fetus reaches the period of viability (24 weeks) (RCOG 2011). In Indian setup, we consider it 28 weeks.

Recurrent miscarriage is defined as the loss of three or more consecutive pregnancies. It is about 1% of all couples trying to conceive.

Q. **What are the important risk factors for recurrent miscarriage?**
Ans. A. **Advancing maternal age**
B. **Antiphospholipid syndrome**
C. **Genetic factors**
- Parental chromosomal factors
- Embryonic/fetal chromosomal abnormalities

D. **Anatomical factors**
- Congenital uterine malformations
- Cervical weakness (incompetence/insufficiency)

E. **Endocrine factors**
- Diabetes mellitus
- Thyroid dysfunction
- Polycystic ovarian syndrome (PCOS)
- Insulin resistance, hyperinsulinemia

F. **Immune factors**
G. **Infective agents: Bacterial vaginosis, genital tuberculosis**
H. **Inherited thrombophilias**
- Activated protein C resistance (factor V Leiden mutation)
- Antithrombin III
- Prothrombin gene mutation.

A. Advanced Maternal Age

It is associated with a reduction in both the number and quality of the remaining oocytes. Age-related risk of miscarriage is as follows:

Age 12–19 years = 13%
30–34 years = 15%
35–39 years = 25%
40–44 years = 51%
>45 years = 93%

Advanced paternal age has also been identified as a risk factor. Risk of miscarriage increases after each successive pregnancy loss.

Other environmental factors like smoking, excess caffeine and alcohol consumption increase the risk. Effects of anesthetic gases for theater workers are conflicting. Obesity is a factor for both sporadic and recurrent miscarriage.

B. Antiphospholipid Antibody Syndrome (APAS)

APAS is the most important treatable cause (15%) of recurrent miscarriage.[1] Antiphospholipid antibodies are:
- Lupus anticoagulant (LAC)
- Anticardiolipin antibodies (ACA)
- β_2 glycoprotein-1 (β_2 GP-1) antibodies.

Q. What are the mechanisms of pregnancy loss in association with antiphospholipid antibodies (APAS)?

Ans. The probable mechanisms are:
- Activation of complement pathway
- Release of local inflammatory mediators (cytokines, interleukins)
- Inhibitions of trophoblastic function and differentiation
- Thrombosis of uteroplacental vasculature.

However, the prevalence of APAS in low risk obstetric women is < 2%. Women with APAS having recurrent miscarriage, live birth rate without any pharmacological intervention has been reported only 10%.

APA syndrome and adverse pregnancy outcome:
- Consecutive miscarriage ≥ 3 before 10 weeks
- Fetal loss (morphologically normal) ≥ 1 beyond 10 weeks
- Preterm birth ≥ 1 before 34 weeks due to placental disease.

C. Genetic Factors

- ***Parental chromosomal rearrangements:*** Balanced structural chromosomal anomaly is present in about 2–5% of couples, most commonly a **balanced reciprocal** or **Robertsonian translocation**. This may result in live births with multiple congenital malformations and/or mental disability.
- ***Embryonic/fetal chromosomal abnormalities*** have been observed in about 30–57% of couples with recurrent miscarriage. Risk increases with advanced maternal age.

D. Anatomical Factors

Overall prevalence of uterine anomalies in recurrent miscarriage populations ranges between 2% and 38%. Second trimester miscarriage is commonly observed. This may be due to cervical incompetence and/or different types of uterine malformations (septate, bicornuate or unicornuate uterus).

Cervical incompetence: It is a known cause for second trimester miscarriage. Diagnosis is mainly clinical as the available objective tests have poor sensitivity and poor positive predictive value (*See* Dutta's Textbook of Obstetrics, 8th Edition, p. 197).

E. Endocrine Factors

Well-controlled diabetes mellitus and treated thyroid dysfunction do not have in any increased risk. Antithyroid antibodies have been linked to recurrent miscarriage. The increased risk of miscarriage in women with PCOS has been attributed to insulin resistance, hyperinsulinemia and hyperandrogenism.

F. Immune Factors

Natural killer cells present in peripheral blood and that present in the uterus is function differently. There is no relationship between uNK cell numbers and future pregnancy outcome. **HLA** incompatibility between couples or absence of maternal blocking antibodies is not considered as the cause of recurrent miscarriage.

Cytokines are immune molecules. Cytokine response may be either (1) Th-1 type or (2) Th-2 type. **Th-1 response** is the production of proinflammatory cytokines, [interleukin-2, interferon and tumor necrosis factor (TNF)]. On the other hand, **Th-2 response** is with production of anti-inflammatory cytokines (interleukins-4, 6 and 10).

Successful pregnancy might be the result of predominantly Th-2 cytokine response. On the other hand, women with recurrent miscarriage have a bias towards Th-1 cytokine response.

G. Infective Agents

TORCH and listeria infections are not associated with recurrent miscarriage. Therefore, routine screening for TORCH infection is not recommended. Bacterial vaginosis is a risk factor for second trimester miscarriage and preterm labor.

H. Inherited Thrombophilias

Thrombophilias are the disorders (acquired or inherited) of hemostatic mechanism that predisposes to intravascular thrombosis (British Committee for Standardization in Hematology 1990).

Factors for inherited thrombophilias

- Activated protein C resistance (factor V Leiden mutation)
- Antithrombin III
- Protein C } Deficiency
- Protein S
- Prothrombin gene mutation (PTG) 20210A
- Hyperhomocysteinemia.

Natural anticoagulants and their mechanism action

- **Activated protein C resistance:** It is most commonly due to factor V Leiden gene mutation. This makes factor V resistant to degradation by activated protein C (*see below*). As a result the unimpeded factor V predisposes to thrombosis due to increased generation of thrombin. Importantly, it is observed in 3–15% of European and 3% of African population but it has not been observed (till date) in the Asians.
- **Antithrombin III:** Inactivates factors IXa, Xa, XIa, XIIa and IIa. It inhibits thrombin generation. Homozygous antithrombin III deficiency is lethal and it is most thrombogenic. Risks of thrombosis varies between 3% and 40% depending upon whether the individual is heterozygous or homozygous.
- **β_2 glycoprotein-1:** It is a natural anticoagulant. It inhibits factor XII in the coagulation cascade. It is present with high concentration in the syncytiotrophoblasts. It helps implantation with increased vascularity of the endometrium. Damage to β_2 GP-1 with antibodies or complement activation results in intervillous space thrombosis and early pregnancy loss.
- **Prothrombin gene mutation 20210A:** It is observed in 2% of white population and it is uncommon in the Asians. Prothrombin gene mutation leads to excessive production of prothrombin. This is finally converted to thrombin. Pregnant women with prothrombin gene mutation run the higher risk of thromboembolism (3–15 times). Women who also inherit factor V Leiden mutation have the further higher risk of thromboembolism. Carriers of both the genes mutation should have lifelong anticoagulation therapy.

- **Hyperhomocysteinemia:** It results from deficiency of folic acid, vitamin B_6 and B_{12}. Folic acid acts as a cofactor in the methylation reaction of homocysteine to methionine. Hyperhomocysteinemia (C677T) is due to mutation of the enzyme 5, 10 methylenetetrahydrofolate reductase (MTHFR). It is an autosomal recessive disorder. Serum fasting level of homocysteine value ≥ 12 µmol/L is considered diagnostic. Hyperhomocysteinemia causes decreased activation of protein C. Therefore, it results in increased intravascular thrombosis and poor pregnancy outcome.

Besides this, hyperhomocysteinemia is associated with *increased risks of neural tube defects (NTD)*.

Thrombophilias and Adverse Pregnancy Outcome

- Recurrent fetal loss ≥ 10 weeks
- Severe IUGR (recurrent)
- Severe early onset pre-eclampsia
- Massive placental abruption
- Preterm labor.

Diagnosis of APA Syndrome

Clinical

- Unexplained thrombosis
- Unexplained fetal loss (≥ 1) at ≥ 10 weeks gestation
- Miscarriages (≥ 3) at ≤10 weeks gestation
- Preterm birth ≤ 34 weeks.

Laboratory

- Anticardiolipin antibodies (ACA)—IgG/IgM (99th percentile) at least two values 12 weeks apart
- Lupus anticoagulant (LAC)—detected twice 6 weeks apart (ACOG 2007).

Detection of APA syndrome is subject to considerable interlaboratory variation. It is mandatory that two tests must be positive at least 12 weeks apart for either LAC or ACA (IgG and/or IgM) above 99th percentile (40 g/L). There is also temporal fluctuation of APA titres in an individual woman. It may be positive transiently secondary to infections. Detection of LAC with dilute Russell's viper venom time test together with a platelet neutralization procedure is more sensitive and specific than either APTT test or the Kaolin clotting time test (RCOG 2011).

Definitive diagnosis of APA syndrome is made when atleast one of the clinical and one of the laboratory criteria are met.

Diagnosis of thrombophilias: There is a consensus on the diagnosis and treatment of antiphospholipid syndrome in pregnancy. But detection and management of inherited thrombophilias remained controversial.

Karyotyping and genetic factors: Cytogenetic analysis should be done with the products of conception of the third and subsequent consecutive miscarriage(s). Parental blood karyotyping of both the partners should be done for recurrent miscarriage where testing of products of conception report an unbalanced structural chromosomal abnormality. Risk of miscarriage as

a result of fetal aneuploidy decreases with an increasing number of pregnancy losses.[2] For any single miscarriage, sporadic fetal chromosome abnormality is most common. If the karyotype of the miscarriage pregnancy is abnormal, there is a better prognosis in the next pregnancy. Abnormal parental karyotype needs referral to a clinical geneticist.

Suspected uterine anomalies require investigations to confirm the diagnosis. These include pelvic ultrasound, hysterosalpingography, hysteroscopy, laparoscopy, sonohysterography or three-dimensional pelvic ultrasound (Fig. 19.1). The value of MRI in the diagnosis is yet to be determined.

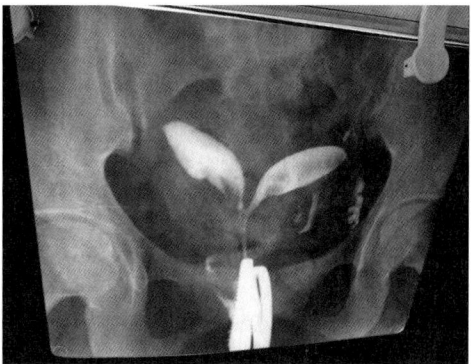

Fig. 19.1: Hysterosalpingography showing septate uterus (confirmed on hysteroscopy and laparoscopy). The woman suffered previous three miscarriages

MANAGEMENT OPTIONS FOR RECURRENT MISCARRIAGE

- **APAS:** Pregnant women with APA syndrome should be treated with low dose aspirin plus heparin to prevent further miscarriage. **Unfractionated heparin and low molecular weight heparin (LMWH) are equally safe and effective in the treatment of APA syndrome.**[3] **LMWH causes less thrombocytopenia and osteoporosis.** It is given once daily. This treatment combination improves live birth rate and significantly reduces the miscarriage rate by 54%. **Neither corticosteroid nor intravenous immunoglobulin therapy improve the live birth rate in women with recurrent miscarriage.** Women with recurrent first trimester miscarriage associated with inherited thrombophilia, role of heparin therapy is uncertain. **Heparin therapy during pregnancy may improve the live birth rate of women with second trimester miscarriage associated with inherited thrombophilia. The live birth rate of women with enoxaparin (LMWH) was 86% compared with 29% in women taking low dose aspirin alone**.
- **Immunotherapy:** Paternal cell immunization, third party donor leucocytes, trophoblast membranes and intravenous immunoglobulin in women with previous unexplained recurrent miscarriage do not improve the live birth rate. It increases maternal morbidity.
- **Infection:** Treatment of bacterial vaginosis with oral clindamycin reduces the risk of miscarriage and preterm birth.
- **Endocrine factors:** *Role of progesterone supplementation and/or hCG supplementation in prevention of recurrent miscarriage.*
  Progesterone is necessary for successful implantation and maintenance of pregnancy. This is explained due to its immunomodulatory actions. **Progesterone results in inducing a pregnancy protective shift from proinflammatory Th-1 cytokine response to a more favorable anti-inflammatory Th-2 cytokine response. Progesterone treatment reduces miscarriage.** The benefit of therapy with hCG in recurrent miscarriage is still in the context of randomized controlled trials (RCT).
- **Women with PCOS:** Increased miscarriage has been attributed to insulin resistance, hyperinsulinemia and hyperandrogenemia.

Metformin therapy during pregnancy is associated with reduction in miscarriage rate. However, there is no RCT to evaluate the role of metformin in women with recurrent miscarriage. Many uncontrolled studies have shown the benefits of metformin.

- **Anatomical factors:** Surgical correction of uterine anomalies improves pregnancy outcome. Compared to open uterine surgery, endoscopic surgery has got less complications. Hysteroscopic septum resection is effective in achieving successful pregnancy outcome. However, results of prospective RCT are awaited.

  Women with second trimester miscarriage due to cervical incompetence can be managed by ultrasound-indicated cerclage if cervical length is 25 mm or less (*See* Dutta's Textbook of Obstetrics, 8th Edition, p. 199).[4]

- **Unexplained recurrent miscarriage:** Women with unexplained recurrent miscarriage have an excellent prognosis for future pregnancy outcome (75%) without pharmacological intervention. Reassurance, support and tender loving cares are of value.

References

1. Pattison NS, Chamley LW, McKay EJ, et al. Antiphospholipid antibodies in pregnancy: Prevalence and clinical associations. Br J Obstet Gynaecol. 1993;100(10):909-13.
2. Ogasawara M, Aoki K, Okada S, et al. Embryonic karyotype of abortuses in relation to the number of previous miscarriages. Fertil Steril. 2000;73(2):300-4.
3. Empson M, Lassere M, Craig J, et al. Prevention of recurrent miscarriage for women with antiphospholipid antibody or lupus anticoagulant. Cochrane Database Syst Rev. 2005;(2):CD002859.
4. Konar H. Dutta Textbook of Obstetrics, 8th Edition, 2015. Jaypee Brothers and Medical Publishing, New Delhi p. 195.

20 Tubal Ectopic Pregnancy

Q.1 Regarding ectopic pregnancy:
   a. Laparoscopy should be done in all cases to confirm the diagnosis
   b. Laparoscopic salpingotomy increases the chance of subsequent intrauterine pregnancy
   c. Pregnancy of unknown location is a type of abdominal pregnancy
   d. Persistent ectopic and recurrent ectopic pregnancy are the same.

Ans. a. F b. F
       c. F d. F

Q.2 Tubal ectopic pregnancy can be managed by:
   a. Laparotomy once the patient is hemodynamically stable
   b. Laparoscopy when there is tubal rupture
   c. Medical method in all cases with unruptured state
   d. Observation alone occasionally.

Ans. a. F b. F
       c. F d. T

Women who are rhesus negative and nonimmune should be given anti-D immunoglobulin 50 mg IM who have an ectopic pregnancy.

MANAGEMENT ISSUES

When a patient with tubal ectopic pregnancy is hemodynamically unstable, it is mostly due to the rupture of tube resulting in massive intraperitoneal hemorrhage. Patient may be in hypovolemic shock. Hemoperitoneum can be diagnosed with transvaginal ultrasonography. Laparotomy should be done in such a patient as an emergent procedure with simultaneous resuscitation. It is indicated as the most expedient method to prevent further blood loss.

Laparoscopic surgery is preferable in the patient who is hemodynamically stable. This method has the advantage of shorter operation time, less intraoperative blood loss, shorter hospital stays and lesser need for analgesic drugs.

However, subsequent intrauterine pregnancy rate is similar in both the procedures, the risk of repeated ectopic pregnancy is lower in following laparoscopic procedure.

The actual surgical procedure on the tube includes salpingectomy or salpingotomy. The chance of subsequent intrauterine pregnancy appears to be the same following any of the procedure provided the contralateral tube is healthy.

When the laparoscopic conservative (salpingotomy) and radical treatment (salpingectomy) are compared, the chances of subsequent intrauterine pregnancy rates are similar but the risks of ectopic pregnancy rates are higher in the salpingotomy group. In the presence contralateral tubal disease, conservative tubal surgery (salpingotomy) is appropriate. This is done for the chance of future intrauterine pregnancy though the risk of ectopic pregnancy is increased. Therefore, the women must be counseled about the risk. Once understood, laparoscopic salpingotomy is the primary method of treatment when the contralateral tube is diseased and the women desires for future fertility. Otherwise, if salpingectomy is done, women needs *in vitro* fertilization.[1]

Irrespective of the type of surgery (laparotomy or laparoscopy), it is essential to follow-up the women when salpingotomy is done. Few patients need treatment for persistent trophoblastic activity (4–8%).

Medical Management of Tubal Ectopic Pregnancy

Estimation of serum human chorionic gonadotropin (hCG) and transvaginal ultrasonography can make the diagnosis of ectopic pregnancy confidently. Many women may not need the help of laparoscopy. However, the main reason for the use of laparoscopy is not only for the diagnosis but also for the purpose of therapy.

Therefore, medical therapy has got its place for selected woman.

Overall selection criteria of a patient for medical therapy includes:
- Unruptured tubal ectopic pregnancy (Fig. 20.1)
- Patient hemodynamically stable
- Serum hCG <3,000 IU/L
- Absence of fetal cardiac activity.

A variety of medical treatments are as effective as that of surgical treatment. Intramuscular methotrexate is commonly used. A single dose of 50 mg/m^2 is recommended. Serum hCG levels are checked on D_4 and D_7. There should be a fall in the level of serum hCG by more than 15%. Otherwise the women need further doses. About 14% of women require more than one dose. Another about 10% women will need surgical therapy in spite of medical therapy. Therefore, they should be counseled about the need of further therapy, follow-up and also the adverse effects of drug.

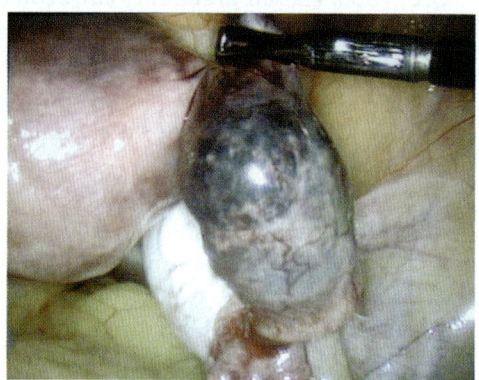

Fig. 20.1: Laparoscopy view of unruptured tubal ectopic pregnancy (right)

The adverse effects of the drug (methotrexate) are: (1) abdominal pain (75%), (2) stomatitis, (3) gastrointestinal upset, (4) conjunctivitis, (5) tubal rupture (7%).

Women should be advised to avoid sexual intercourse during the period of treatment. Similarly, forceful clinical pelvic examination should be avoided.

Pregnancy of unknown location is a situation when serum hCG level is positive but no pregnancy is visible neither within nor outside the uterus on transvaginal ultrasonography.

The level of serum hCG at which any viable intrauterine pregnancy will be visualized by transvaginal scan (TVS) is considered as the discriminatory zone. When serum hCG levels are <1,000 IU/L, no pregnancy is visible so as to define it as a pregnancy of unknown location. Levels of serum hCG between 1,000 IU/L and 2,000 IU/L have also been used as discriminatory levels.

Usually, 40–70% of such pregnancies resolve spontaneously with expectant management. Remainder of such cases were diagnosed subsequently as ectopic pregnancy (15–30%) and the rest were intrauterine that ended in miscarriage. However, these cases need follow-up with serum hCG levels until the levels are ≤ 20 IU/L. Woman needs to be counseled accordingly. About 20–30% women may need intervention.

Expectant Management for Unruptured Tubal Ectopic Pregnancy

The criteria for expectant management:
- Patient hemodynamically stable
- Woman without any symptoms
- Ultrasound diagnosis of unruptured tubal ectopic pregnancy
- Size of adnexal mass < 5 cm
- Initial value of serum hCG <1000 IU/L
- Follow-up hCG levels are falling (>15% in 24 hours)
- No evidence of rupture or blood in the POD.

PERSISTENT TROPHOBLASTS OR PERSISTENT ECTOPIC PREGNANCY

Persistent trophoblasts activity is observed in women treated with salpingotomy rather than following salpingectomy. This results in failure of serum hCG levels to fall as expected following initial treatment. Overall 10% women suffer from persistent trophoblastic activity. A single dose of methotrexate 50 mg/m^2 has been found to be effective.

Reference

1. Hajenius PJ, Mol F, Mol BW, et al. Interventions for tubal ectopic pregnancy. Cochrane Database Syst Rev. 2007;1:CD000324.

21 Cervical Insufficiency (Incompetence)

SINGLE BEST ANSWER (SBA) AND MULTIPLE CHOICE QUESTIONS (MCQs)

Q.1 Regarding cervical cerclage:
a. Use of perioperative tocolytics should be a routine
b. Perioperative antibiotic prophylaxis is a must
c. It should be under general anesthetic
d. Placement of two purse-string suture is better than a single suture
e. Shirodkar suture is much effective compared to McDonald's.

Ans. a. F b. F c. F d. F e. F

MANAGEMENT OPTIONS

No significant different results are obtained when tocolytic drugs are used or not during the perioperative phase. Similarly, there are no studies of perioperative antibiotic use in women undergoing cervical cerclage operation. Choice of anesthesia should be at the discretion of the anesthetic for any individual patient. Either of general or a regional anesthesia can be used. There is no study to support the placement of two sutures over one suture.

No significant differences of results in terms of fetal survival or major postoperative morbidity, had been observed between the two techniques (Shirodkar versus McDonald).

Midtrimester recurrent fetal loss and spontaneous preterm birth may be due to cervical incompetence (insufficiency). This is due to impaired anatomy and/or function of the cervix (internal os).

Etiological factors may be—uterine anomalies, cervical trauma (forceful dilatation of the internal os), conization, trachelectomy or vaginal operative delivery (forceps) through undilated cervix.

History suggestive of cervical incompetence are:
- Recurrent midtrimester fetal loss
- Painless cervical shortening and dilatation
- Painless expulsion of the products of conception
- Painless rupture of membranes.

Cervical Insufficiency (Incompetence)

Measures to prevent recurrent fetal loss due to cervical incompetence.
Cervical incompetence may be due to:
- Intrinsic weakness in the structure of the cervix
- Premature effacement and dilatation of the cervix.

Based on the etiology, measures are taken to provide a structural support to the weak cervix. This support, given by cerclage operation, maintains the cervical length and the endocervical mucous plug which is a mechanical barrier to ascending infection.[1]

Q. What are the different types of cervical cerclage operations?
Ans.
- History indicated cerclage
- Ultrasound indicated cerclage
- Rescue (emergency) cerclage.

History indicated cerclage: Cerclage is done based on woman's obstetric and gynecological history (discussed above). History indicated suture is performed prophylactically in an asymptomatic woman.

History indicated cerclage may be helpful to woman with previous two or more second trimester loss and/or preterm births.

Ultrasound indicated cerclage: Ultrasound indicated cerclage is done in cases with shortening of cervical length as seen on transvaginal sonography (TVS). This procedure is done electively (asymptomatic women).

Rescue (emergency) cerclage: Cervical cerclage is done in a case with premature cervical dilation and/or with herniation of fetal membranes in the vagina. Emergency cerclage usually done on the basis of patients' symptoms like vaginal discharge, bleeding or due to sensation of pelvic pressure. Often there are evidences of cervical effacements, dilatation and shortening of the cervix when the woman is examined by a speculum or by ultrasonography.

Q. What is the appropriate time for an elective cerclage procedure?
Ans. It is done electively at 14–16 weeks of gestation but may be done up to 24 weeks of gestation.

Q. What are the different routes and methods of cervical cerclage operation?
Ans. *Transvaginal (common)*
- **McDonald's operation:** A purse-string suture is placed at the cervicovaginal junction without dissecting the bladder.[2]
- **Shirodkar's operation:** Here, the similar type of purse-string suture is placed at the upper level of the cervix (level of internal os) after mobilization of the bladder.[3]
- **Wurm's operation:** Sutures are placed crosswise (from above-down and side-to-side) at or below the level of cervicovaginal junction. Purpose is to support the cervix and to retain the mucus plug.

Transabdominal: This procedure is performed via laparotomy or laparoscopy. Suture is placed at the level of cervicoisthmic junction (internal os). The mersilene tape is placed at the level of the isthmus, between the uterine wall and the uterine vessels.

Disadvantages of transabdominal procedure:
- Increased complications (injury to uterine vessels, ureter, bladder and hemorrhage), during the operation.
- Subsequent laparotomy for delivery or for removal of the tape when needed in pregnancy.

Q. What are the contraindications of cervical cerclage operation?
Ans.
- Presence of intrauterine infection (chorioamnionitis)
- Ruptured membranes (PPROM) before or during the operation
- Cervical dilatation > 4 cm
- Fetal compromise (malformation or death)
- Vaginal bleeding.

Q.2 Indications of cervical cerclage is (are):
a. Women with previous two or less second trimester fetal loss
b. Women with previous two or less preterm births
c. Women with cervical length >25 mm irrespective of history
d. Women with dilation of the internal os on ultrasound (funneling of the cervix)
e. Ultrasound indicated cerclage is not to be recommended in women with Müllerian anomalies.

Ans.
a. F   b. F
c. F   d. F
e. T

History indicated cerclage operation should be performed for women with recurrent (three or more) previous second trimester losses and/or preterm births. Three randomized controlled trials (RCTs) comparing history indicated cerclage with expectant management, showed no significant difference between the two groups in forms of fetal and neonatal outcome.

Women with a singleton pregnancy and no history of spontaneous midtrimester loss or preterm birth should not be considered for cervical cerclage operation, even if incidentally they are found to have short cervix (cervical length ≤ 25 mm) on ultrasonography.

Meta-analysis of four RCTs of cerclage versus expectant management in women with short cervix, reported no evidence of benefits of cerclage operation in women, who had no other risk factors for spontaneous preterm birth.[4]

The criteria to be fulfilled for performing cervical cerclage operation for a woman with singleton pregnancy are:
- History of spontaneous (≥ 2) midtrimester loss or preterm birth
- TVS surveillance revealed, cervical length ≤ 25 mm
- Funneling of the cervix (dilatation of the internal os) on TVS.

Women, found to have cervical length of ≤ 25 mm detected during serial sonographic examinations between 10+ and 21+ weeks of gestation, with history of spontaneous preterm birth/midtrimester loss, have reduced preterm birth and perinatal death with cervical cerclage.[5]

Therefore, women with a history of spontaneous second trimester loss or preterm delivery may be offered serial sonographic surveillance to detect cervical shortening. Women having cervical shortening, are benefited from ultrasound indicated cervical cerclage compared to a woman who has a long cervix.

Investigations to be done prior to insertion of cervical cerclage: First trimester ultrasound scan and screening for aneuploidy before insertion of cervical cerclage is recommended. This practice helps to ensure fetal viability and the absence of major or lethal fetal abnormality. It is a good practice to ensure an anomaly scan before a rescue cerclage.

Q.3 Regarding cervical cerclage:
   a. Progesterone supplementation following cerclage operation should be a routine
   b. Transvaginal cervical cerclage should be removed with the onset of labor
   c. Women with transabdominal cerclage, suture may be left in place if delivered by cesarean section
   d. Fetal fibronectin testing during the postcerclage period is very useful.

Ans. a. F   b. F
   c. T   d. F

A transcervical cerclage should be removed usually after 36 weeks of pregnancy. When the woman is in established preterm labor, the suture is to be removed immediately to avoid trauma to the cervix irrespective to the period of gestation. Fetal fibronectin testing in such a woman is not much informative because of its increased false-positive result. Women with transabdominal suture require delivery by cesarean section. In such a situation the suture may be left in place if further future pregnancy is desired. Routine use of progesterone supplementation following cerclage operation is restricted to clinical trials only. This is helpful in women with high risk of preterm delivery only.

References

1. Royal College of Obstetricians and Gynecologists: Clinical Governance. London: RCOG. 2006.
2. McDonad IA. Suture of the cervix for inevitable miscarriage. J Obstet Gynecol Br Emp. 1957;64(3):346-50.
3. Shirodkar VN. A new method of operative treatment for habitual abortion in the second trimester of pregnancy. Antiseptic. 1955;52:299-300.
4. Berghella V, Odibo AO, To MS, et al. Cerclage for short cervix on ultrasonography: Meta-analysis of trial using individual patient-level data. Obstet Gynecol. 2005;106(1):181-9.
5. Final report of the Medical Research Council/RCOG multicenter randomized trial of cervical cerclage. Br J Obstet Gynecol. 1993;100(6):516-23.

22
Heavy Menstrual Bleeding

For clinical purpose, **heavy menstrual bleeding (HMB) is defined as excessive menstrual blood loss which interferes with women's physical, emotional, social and material quality of life.** This can occur alone or in combination with other symptoms. Any intervention should aim to improve the quality of life measures.

HISTORY, EXAMINATION AND INVESTIGATIONS FOR HMB

History should cover the nature of bleeding, its duration, cycle interval, and related symptoms like pelvic pain, pelvic pressure, postcoital bleeding, metrorrhagia or any associated comorbidity.

Clinical examination and investigations should be through to reveal any structural (fibroid uterus) or any histological (endometrial carcinoma) abnormality.[1] However, if the history and physical examination suggests HMB without any structural or histological abnormality, treatment (pharmacotherapy) could be started without other investigations. **Usually, levonorgestrel-releasing intrauterine system (LNG-IUS)** is recommended. When history and clinical examination suggest any structural or histological abnormality, investigations are carried out.

Measurements of blood loss directly by alkali hematin or indirectly by 'pictorial blood loss chart' are not routinely recommended.[2]

Examination: Physical examination is done to exclude any structural abnormality (fibroid uterus) or any histological abnormality (atypical endometrial hyperplasia) (Figs 22.1A and B). Women with fibroid uterus that are palpable per abdomen and/or when the uterine length is ≥ 12 cm as measured by ultrasonography or hysteroscopy further investigations are carried out.

Investigations
- A full blood count (Hb%, TLC, DLC, PCV, blood film) should be done on all women with HMB.
- Thyroid hormone testing should be carried out when other signs and symptoms of thyroid disease are suggestive.
- Endometrial biopsy (EB) is taken with pipelle endometrial collection to exclude endometrial hyperplasia.
- Testing for blood coagulation disorders (von Willebrand's disease) should be done in women who have HMB since menarche or have personal or family history suggesting a coagulation disorder.

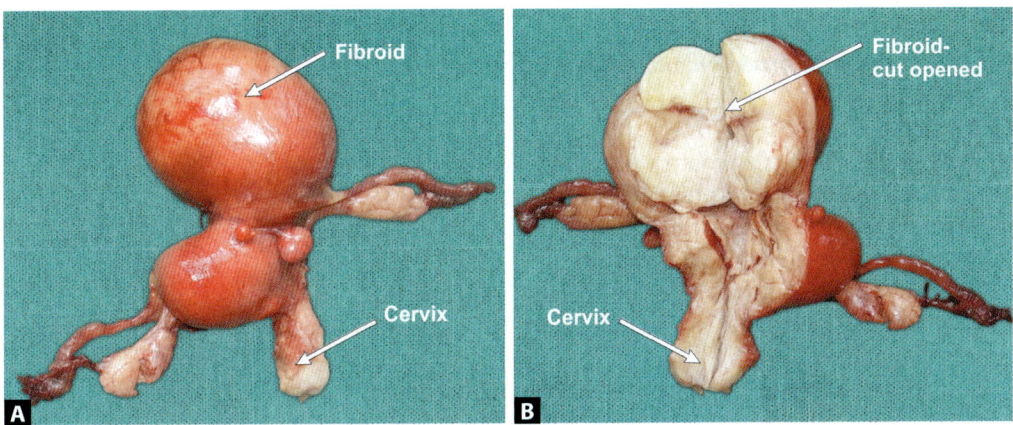

Figs 22.1A and B: Heavy menstrual bleeding (HMB) due to fibroid uterus

- Serum ferritin test is not a routine procedure.
- Female hormone (FSH, LH, estradiol) testing is not a routine procedure.

Indications for EB are:
- Women having persistent intermenstrual bleeding
- Women with age ≥ 45 years
- Women not responding to pharmacotherapy.

Indications of imaging study (USG) are:
- Uterus palpable per abdomen or feels bulky on clinical examination
- Vaginal examination reveals a pelvic mass of uncertain origin
- Women not responding to pharmacotherapy (treatment failure).

Special investigations are:
- **Ultrasound** is done as a first-line diagnostic tool to detect structural abnormality. Ultrasound should provide the information as regard the location, dimensions and number of fibroids.
- **Hysteroscopy** should be used when ultrasound result are inconclusive. Presence of uterine fibroids suggests appropriate treatment to control HMB (see below).
- **Saline infusion sonography (SIS)** is not recommended as first-line diagnostic tool.
- **Magnetic resonance imaging (MRI)** should not be used as a first-line diagnostic tool.
- **Dilatation and curettage (D and C)** is not recommended as a diagnostic tool.

PHARMACOTHERAPY FOR HEAVY MENSTRUAL BLEEDING

Q. What are the determinants of treatment?
Ans. Treatment options depend on the following factors:
- Presence or absence of uterine structural abnormality (fibroids)
- Presence or absence of histological abnormality (atypical endometrium)
- Women's desire for conception
- Women's desire to use contraception.

Treatment options are:

Pharmacotherapy is based on individual woman's need:
- LNG-IUS
- Tranexamic acid
- Nonsteroidal antiinflammatory drugs (NSAIDs)
- Combined oral contraceptives (COCs)
- Norethisterone 5 mg TID from D5–D26 of the menstrual cycle
- Injectable long-acting progestogens
- Gonadotropin-releasing hormone analog (GnRH analog):
- Women can have either tranexamic acid or NSAIDs when hormonal treatments cannot be recommended
- LNG-IUS takes some time (about 5–6 cycles) to give the therapeutic benefits
- Women with HMB and dysmenorrhea should be offered NSAIDs
- GnRH analog is considered in cases
  - Prior to surgery
  - In cases of having contraindications for surgery or uterine artery embolization (UAE)
  - HRT **add back** therapy should be recommended when GnRH, the analog therapy is continued for more than 6 months.
- Danazol should not be used routinely for the treatment of HMB
- Oral progesterone in the luteal phase only, should not be used in the treatment of HMB
- Ethamsylate should not be used for the treatment of HMB.

OPERATIVE TREATMENTS FOR HMB

Nonhysterectomy Surgery for HMB
- Endometrial Ablation
  Indications
  - When the bleeding is severe enough to affect the quality of life
  - Women does not want to conceive
  - Women with normal uterus or with small uterine fibroids (<3 cm in diameter)
  - Women with uterine size ≤ 10 weeks of pregnant uterus
  - Women should use effective contraception after endometrial ablation. Endometrial ablation techniques should be the **second generation ones** (see below).

  Second Generation Endometrial Ablation Methods
  - Impedance-controlled bipolar radiofrequency ablation. A metal fan-shaped device (fabric mesh) is used.
  - Fluid-filled thermal balloon endometrial ablation (TBEA). In this procedure, endometrial thinning is not needed. Therma choice III with silicon balloon at the tip is used.
  - Microwave endometrial ablation (MEA) is done in the postmenstrual phase.
  - Free-fluid thermal endometrial ablation.

  First generation ablation techniques like roller ball endometrial ablation and transcervical resection of endometrium (TCRE) are used when hysteroscopic myomectomy is needed at the same time.
- D and C should not be used as a therapeutic procedure.

Women with HMB due to fibroid uterus (>3 cm in diameter).

Treatment options are:
- Uterine artery embolization (UAE)
- MR-guided focused ultrasound (MRg FUS)
- Myomectomy
- Hysterectomy
  - **UAE:** It is an option for women, who want to retain their uterus and fertility.
  - **MRg FUS** is found to be effective. It induces coagulative necrosis in the myoma. It causes less pain compared to UAE. It is safe, effective and minimally invasive. Successful pregnancy following treatment has been observed.
  - **Myomectomy:** It is an option when preservation of uterus and childbearing function is desired.
  - **Indication of hysterectomy** for women with HMB are:
    - When other treatment options have failed or are contraindicated.
    - Women no longer wish to retain her uterus and fertility.
    - Women fully informed about the consequences of hysterectomy like sexual feelings, fertility, bladder function and the complications of the operation.

Route of hysterectomy (abdominal or vaginal) needs the following factors to consider:
- Size of the uterus and fibroids
- Mobility and descent of the uterus
- Size and space in vagina
- Previous surgery.

Place of Oophorectomy during Hysterectomy

- As a routine, oophorectomy during hysterectomy should not be done
- Women's informed consent must be there
- Women with family history of breast or ovarian cancer, need genetic counseling prior to a decision about oophorectomy
- Women with age ≥ 45 years
- Women with premenstrual tension syndrome
- Women should be counseled about the need of hormone replacement therapy (HRT), if oophorectomy is done during hysterectomy.

SIDE EFFECTS/COMPLICATIONS OF DIFFERENT TREATMENT OPTIONS FOR HMB

- **LNG–IUS:** Irregular uterine bleeding that may last for about 6 months; breast tenderness, acne or headache, amenorrhea and rarely uterine perforation at the time of insertion.
- **Tranexamic acid:** Indigestion, diarrhea, headache.
- **COCs:** Mood changes, headache, nausea, fluid retention, breast tenderness, deep vein thrombosis (DVT), stroke, heart attacks (*See* Dutta's Textbook of Gynecology, 7th Edition, p. 400, 402).
- **NSAIDs:** Indigestion, diarrhea, deterioration of asthma, peptic ulcer—may cause bleeding, peritonitis.

- **Oral progestogen:** Weight gain, bloating, breast tenderness, headache and acne, rarely depression.
- **Injectable progestogen:** Weight gain, irregular bleeding, amenorrhea, premenstrual-like syndrome (bloating, fluid retention, breast tenderness), temporary loss of bone mineral density. It is restored once the treatment is discontinued.
- **GnRH analog:** Menopausal like symptoms (hot flashes, increased sweating, vaginal dryness). Osteoporosis (trabecular bone) when used more than 6 months.
- **UAE:** Persistent vaginal discharge, post embolization syndrome (pain, nausea, vomiting and fever), need of additional surgery premature ovarian failure (women ≤ 40 years), hematoma, rarely hemorrhage, tissue necrosis and infection causing septicemia.
- **Myomectomy:** Hemorrhage; adhesion (causing pain and/or reduced fertility), need for further surgery, recurrence of fibroids, menorrhagia, HMB and infection.
- **Hysterectomy:** Hemorrhage, infection, intraoperative hemorrhage, damage to other organs (bladder, ureter), urinary dysfunction, incontinence, DVT and pulmonary embolism.
- **Oophorectomy during hysterectomy:** Postmenopausal (surgical menopause) like symptoms.

References

1. ACOG practice bulletin: Management of anovulatory bleeding. Int J Gynecol Obstet. 2001;72(3):263-71.
2. Heavy menstrual bleeding. [online] NICE guidelines—Gynaecological conditions. Available from "https://www.nice.org.uk/donotdo/measuring-menstrual-blood-loss-indirectly-pictorial-blood-loss-assessment-chart-is-not-routinely-recommended-for-heavy-menstrual-bleeding-hmb-whether-menstrual-blood-loss-is-a-problem-should-be" www.nice.org.uk. [Accessed January 2007].

23 Urinary Incontinence

Q.1 Assessment and investigations of a woman with urinary incontinence (UI):
a. Assessment of UI from history alone is often confusing
b. Urodynamic studies should be a routine for all women with UI
c. Multichannel filling and voiding cystometry are recommended before any surgical intervention for UI
d. Carrying out urodynamic studies before any initial treatment of UI improves outcome.

Ans. a. F b. F
c. T d. F

Q.2 Regarding the tests and management of UI:
a. Pad tests, Q-tip and Bonney tests are informative
b. Oxybutynin, darifenacin are used for women with overactive bladder (OAB)
c. Duloxetine is helpful for women with stress urinary incontinence (SUI)
d. Midurethral transobturator tape is recommended for OAB.

Ans. a. F b. T
c. F d. F

Urinary incontinence may affect physical, social and psychological wellbeing of the woman.
It is defined as the complaint of any involuntary leakage of urine (International Continence Society).

- **Stress urinary incontinence** is an involuntary leakage of urine on effort, exertion or on sneezing or coughing.
- **Urge urinary incontinence** is an involuntary urine leakage preceded immediately by urgency (a sudden compelling desire to urinate that is difficult to stop).
- **Mixed urinary incontinence** is an involuntary urine leakage associated with both urgency, exertion, efforts, sneezing or coughing.
- **Overactive bladder syndrome** is defined as an involuntary leakage of urine that occurs with or without urge incontinence as usually with frequency and nocturia.

Urinary incontinence (UI) is the involuntary leakage of urine. Woman with UI may be categorized symptomatically based on the history. History is sufficiently reliable to guide initial noninvasive treatment.

Bladder diaries for a period of 3 days, quantifying urinary frequency and incontinence episodes are reliable methods of assessment.

When a woman presents with clearly defined clinical diagnosis of pure SUI, multichannel cystometry is not routinely recommended.

CONSERVATIVE MANAGEMENT FOR SUI OR MIXED UI

- *Pelvic floor muscle exercise* (under supervision) for at least 3 months
- *Bladder training for a period of 6 weeks* for woman with urge or mixed UI
- *Medical management with antimuscarinic drugs*[1]
    - Oxybutynin tablet or transdermal patch
    - Darifenacin
    - Solifenacin
    - Tolterodine
    - Trospium.
- *Surgical management*
    - Woman with UI due to detrusor overactivity: Sacral nerve stimulation may be done
    - Retropubic midurethral tape procedure:
        - Macroporous tape made of polypropylene are recommended
        - Open colposuspension using rectus sheath (autologous sling) is an alternative procedure.

ASSESSMENT AND INVESTIGATIONS OF A WOMAN WITH UI

- Detailed *history-taking and physical examination* is done and the woman is categorized to any of the following groups:
    - Stress urinary incontinence
    - Urge urinary incontinence or overactive bladder
    - Mixed urinary incontinence

  Women having mixed symptoms should be treated with the predominant symptoms first.
- The relevant *predisposing and precipitating factors* should be taken care of simultaneously (e.g. cough, prolapsed uterus or obesity).
- *Urine analysis*
    - Routine urine analysis should be done. Urine dipstick test is done to detect the presence of blood, glucose, protein, leukocytes and nitrites.
    - Women with symptoms suggestive of urinary tract infection (UTI) (dipstick test positive for leukocytes and nitrites) should have midstream urine sent for culture and sensitivity. The woman should be treated with appropriate course of antibiotics.
- *Assessment of residual urine:* Women with symptoms suggestive of voiding dysfunction or recurrent UTI, should have postvoid residual volume measurement. It may be done with bladder sonography or catheterization.
- *Indications of referral to specialized unit*
    - Presence of hematuria (microscopic or visible)
    - Recurrent or resistant UTI
    - Presence of a pelvic mass
    - Associated neurological disease

- **Bladder diaries:** Minimum for 3 days covering both working and resting days
- **Pad testing:** Not done.
- **Urodynamic studies:**
  - Women having clearly defined clinical diagnosis of pure SUI, use of multichannel cystometry is not needed
  - Multichannel cystometry is not needed before starting conservative management. Urodynamic investigations in all cases of UI as routine before any initial treatment have not been found to improve outcome.
- **Indications of urodynamic studies are:**
  - Women having mixed urinary incontinence (both SUI and OAB)
  - Women with previous surgery for SUI or anterior compartment prolapse
  - Symptoms suggestive of voiding dysfunction.
- **Other tests of urethral competence are:**
  - The Q-tip and Bonney's tests are not recommended
  - Cystoscopy is not recommended in the initial assessment of women with pure SUI
  - Imaging (MRI, CT, X-ray) is not routinely needed. Ultrasound may be needed for the assessment of residual urine volume.

MANAGEMENT OF URINARY INCONTINENCE

Conservative management:
- Reducing intake of caffeine
- Modifying daily intake of fluid
- Obese women (BMI > 30 kg/m^2) should be advised to lose weight.

Treatment
Physical therapy: Supervised pelvic floor muscle exercise for 3 months period is advised. She is advised to perform pelvic floor muscle contraction, three times per day. Electrical stimulation or perineometry is not to be used as a routine.
Drug therapy: See above
Flavoxate, propantheline and imipramine should not be preferably used for the treatment of UI or OAB.
- **Desmopressin:** It may be used in women with UI or OAB with troublesome symptoms.
- Duloxetine is not given to women with a predominant stress UI.

Surgical Treatments for Overactive Bladder
- **Sacral nerve stimulation** is advised for women with UI due to detrusor overactivity when women are not responding to usual conservative management.
- **Augmentation cystoplasty** is done for women who have not responded with conservative management.
  Common complications are metabolic acidosis, mucus production, UTI and urinary retention.
- **Urinary diversion**
- **Injection of botulinum toxin** in the bladder wall.

Surgical Procedures for Stress Urinary Incontinence (SUI)
- Midurethral retropubic tape or tension-free vaginal tape[2] (TVT)
- Transobturator tape (TOT)

- Intramural bulking agents (glutaraldehyde cross-linked collagen) are used by injecting in the periurethral region
- Artificial urinary sphincter: When other surgical methods have failed
- Anterior colporrhaphy, needle suspensions, paravaginal defect repair and Marshall-Marchetti-Krantz procedure are not used for the treatment of stress UI.[3]

References

1. Nygaard IE, Kreder KJ. Pharmacologic therapy of lower urinary tract dysfunction. Clin Obstet Gynecol. 2004;47(1):83-92.
2. Basu M, Duckett J. A randomized trial of a retropubic tension-free vaginal tape versus a mini-sling for stress incontinence. BJOG. 2010;117(6):730-5.
3. Richter HE, Albo ME, Zyczynski HM, et al. Retropubic versus transobturator midurethral slings for stress incontinence. N Engl J Med. 2010;362(22):2066-76.

24 Polycystic Ovary Syndrome

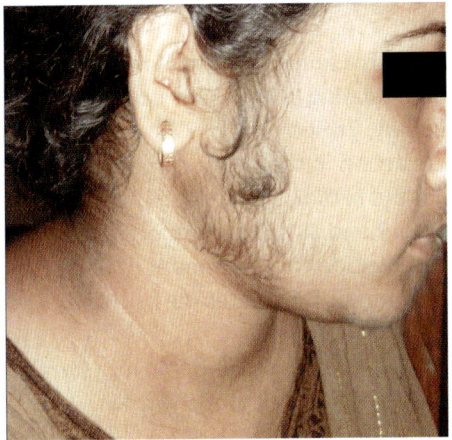

Fig. 24.1: Excess male type of facial hair and acanthosis nigricans in PCOS

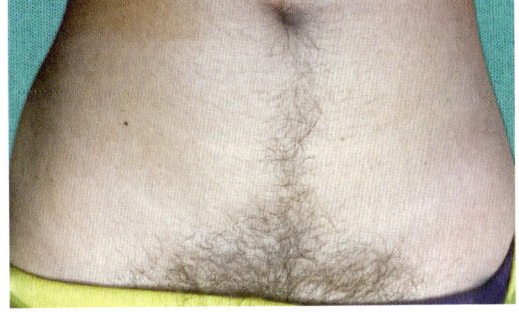

Fig. 24.2: 18-year-old girl showing male pattern of pubic hair distribution (male escutcheon)

Q. Metabolic abnormalities of women with polycystic ovarian syndrome (PCOS):
  a. Hyperandrogenemia is due to excess stimulation with follicle-stimulating hormone (FSH)
  b. Insulin resistance is observed in about 70–80% of women
  c. Obesity is included in the diagnosis of PCOS
  d. Slim PCOS women are more likely to develop type II diabetes.

Ans. a. F b. F
  c. F d. F

Metabolic Abnormalities in PCOS

Hyperandrogenism, insulin resistance, hyperinsulinemia, hypersecretion of luteinizing hormone (LH), hyperlipidemia, raised prolactin and lower levels of sex hormone binding globulin. Based on the metabolic abnormalities, the clinical features of PCOS are hirsutism, acne, alopecia, menstrual abnormalities, anovulatory infertility and obesity in about 40–50% of women (Figs 24.1 and 24.2). However, obesity is not a diagnostic criterion.[1] Ovarian hyperandrogenism is due to excess of LH (slim women) and insulin resistance (overweight women). Insulin resistance in women with PCOS is observed in 10–15% of slim and nearly 20–40% of obese women. Long-term risks of women with PCOS are development of type 2 diabetes, dyslipidemia, hypertension, cardiovascular disease, endometrial carcinoma and sleep apnea.

Q. Metabolic abnormalities in PCOS:
   a. Insulin resistance results in failure of all action of insulin
   b. Estimation of serum insulin level is a routine to treat the PCOS women
   c. Infertility in PCOS women is often due to poor quality of oocyte
   d. Glucose tolerance test should be done in women with positive family history only.

Ans. a. F b. F
         c. F d. F

Insulin Resistance in Women with PCOS

Insulin resistance is due to defect in receptor and postreceptor signaling. Insulin resistance and hyperinsulinemia are directly proportional. High-level of circulating insulin is the cause for excess androgen production (*See* Dutta's Textbook of Gynecology, 7th Edition, p. 378) and infertility due to anovulation. Insulin resistance exerts its adverse action in the ovary. Hyperinsulinemia contributes excess androgen production from the ovaries but in clinical practice it is not essential to measure the levels of insulin as a routine. On the other hand, it is more important to check for impaired glucose tolerance. Important screening test includes measurement of body mass index (BMI) and waist circumference. Fasting glucose ≥ 5.2 mmol/L indicates the risk of impaired glucose tolerance.

Asian women with BMI > 25 kg/m² (white women > 30 kg/m²), should undergo into standard 2 hours 75 g oral glucose tolerance test (OGTT) as they are the high-risk group women.

Polycystic Ovarian Syndrome and Metformin Therapy

Metabolic functions of metformin are:
- Inhibits hepatic glucose output
- Enhances insulin-mediated glucose utilization
- Decreases fatty acid oxidation
- Improves lipid profile by decreasing triglycerides, fatty acids, low-density lipoprotein (LDL) cholesterol and increases HDL cholesterol
- Does not stimulate insulin secretion
- Does not cause hypoglycemia
- Does not stimulate fetal pancreas to over secrete insulin
- Decreases intestinal absorption of glucose
- Appears to have direct effect on ovarian function
- Lowers serum androgen levels significantly
- Restores menstrual cyclicity
- Effective in achieving ovulation either alone or when combined with clomiphene citrate
- Cotreatment with metformin improves the response of exogenous gonadotropins or the results of assisted reproductive technology (ART) (IVF pregnancy)
- Appears to reduce body weight.

Q. Metformin therapy in PCOS:
   a. It enhances insulin secretion
   b. It is safe in pregnancy as it does not cross the placenta
   c. Once started should be continued in pregnancy
   d. Reduces the risk of significant ovarian hyperstimulation syndrome (OHSS).

Ans. a. F b. F
 c. F d. T

Dose schedule of metformin: 500–3,000 mg/day may be used. Commonly used dose regimens are 500 mg TID or 850 mg BID. Long-acting preparations are associated with less gastrointestinal side effects.

Metformin appears to be safe in pregnancy although it crosses the placenta. There is minimal effect on transplacental flux. However, it is advised to discontinue it, once pregnancy is diagnosed. There is no firm evidence that metformin reduces the risk of miscarriage.

Metformin is found to be less effective in those obese women with BMI ≥ 35 kg/m². Combined approach with lifestyle modifications and metformin therapy appear to be effective. Agents like metformin and thiazolidinediones (rosiglitazone, pioglitazone) improve symptoms and reproductive outcome in women with PCOS either by lowering insulin levels or improving insulin sensitivity at cellular level or both.[2,3]

Updated Cochrane review concluded that the benefit of therapy with metformin is limited. For young women with PCOS, lifestyle modifications (diet, exercise) remain the mainstay.[4]

Increased risk of miscarriage in women with recurrent miscarriage is attributed to hyperandrogenemia, insulin resistance and hyperinsulinemia. Uncontrolled studies have shown that use of metformin during pregnancy reduces the risk of miscarriage in women with recurrent miscarriage and PCOS. ***However, there is no randomized controlled trials to assess the role of metformin in women with recurrent miscarriage.***

Long-term Consequences of Polycystic Ovarian Syndrome

Q. What is the risk of developing gestational diabetes mellitus (GDM) in women with PCOS?

Ans. Women, who have been diagnosed with PCOS before pregnancy, should be screened for GDM.[5] Screening should be done at 24–28 weeks of gestation. Women who are overweight (BMI ≥ 25 kg/m²) and who are not overweight (BMI < 25 kg/m²) but with additional risk factors such as advanced age (> 40 years), personal or a family history of GDM should have 2 hours post 75 g glucose tolerance test is performed.

Q. What are the other long-term consequences of PCOS?

Ans. Women with PCOS have the risk of developing sleep apnea.

Q. What is the risk of developing cardiovascular disease (CVD) in women with PCOS?

Ans. Women with PCOS have the risks of developing CVD, besides the individual risk factors. Risk factors for CVD are obesity, family history of type II diabetes, dyslipidemia and hypertension.

Q. What are the risks of cancer in women with PCOS?

Ans. Women with PCOS suffering from oligo or amenorrhea, run the risk of developing endometrial hyperplasia and cancer. Women may be screened by transvaginal ultrasound in the absence of withdrawal bleeding. Women with thickened endometrium (>7 mm) or with a polyp should be considered for hysteroscopy and/or endometrial biopsy. Risks of ovarian or breast cancer are not associated.

Q. What are the strategies for reduction of risks?
Ans. Important issues are lifestyle modifications with exercises and weight control. First-line approach is diet, exercise and weight loss.[6]

Q. Could there be any place for pharmacological treatment?
Ans. Insulin-sensitizing agents are found helpful and safe.[7] But it is uncertain that the use of insulin-sensitizing agents confers any long-term benefit. Weight reduction itself is helpful to control hyperandrogenemia.

Q. What is the place of ovarian electrodiathermy (ovarian drilling)?
Ans. It is done in selected women with the problem of anovulation.

Q. What is the place of bariatric surgery for women with PCOS?
Ans. PCOS women with morbid obesity (BMI ≥ 40 kg/m^2 or ≥ 35 kg/m^2) with other high-risk factors are considered specially when standard management has failed to reduce weight.

References

1. Rotterdam ESHRE/ASRM-Sponsored PCOS consensus workshop group. Revised 2003 consensus on diagnostic criteria and long-term health risks related to polycystic ovary syndrome (PCOS). Hum Reprod. 2004;19(1):41-7.
2. Lord JM, Flight IH, Norman RJ. Insulin-sensitizing drugs (metformin, troglitazone, rosiglitazone, pioglitazone, D-chiro-inositol) for polycystic ovary syndrome. Cochrane Database Syst Rev. 2003;(2):CD003053.
3. Jakubowicz DJ, Iurno MJ, Jakubowiczs, et al. Effects of metformin on early pregnancy loss in the polycystic ovary syndrome. J Clin Endocrinol Metab. 2002;87(2):524-9.
4. Tang T, Glanville J, Hayden CJ, et al. Combined lifestyle modification and metformin in obese women with polycystic ovary syndrome (PCOS). A randomized, placebo-controlled, double-blind multicentre study. Hum Reprod. 2006;21(1):80-9.
5. Royal College of Obstetricians and Gynecologists. Diagnosis and Treatment of Gestational Diabetes. Scientific Impact Paper No. 23. London: RCOG; 2011.
6. Moran LJ, Hutchison SK, Norman RJ, et al. Lifestyle changes in women with polycystic ovary syndrome. Cochrane Database Syst Rev. 2011;(2):CD007506.
7. Gangale MF, Miele L, Lanzone A, et al. Long-term metformin treatment is able to reduce the prevalence of metabolic syndrome and its hepatic involvement in young hyperinsulinemic overweight patients with polycystic ovarian syndrome. Clin Endocrinol (Oxf). 2011;75(4):520-7.

25 Male and Female Sterilization

FEMALE STERILIZATION

Q.1 Regarding female sterilization:
  a. Laparoscopic method is quicker and should be done for all cases
  b. Filshie clip application is effective for postpartum sterilization
  c. Laparoscopic tubal occlusion should be done ideally by Filshie clip
  d. Lifetime risk of failure of tubal occlusion is estimated to be 1 in 200.

Ans. a. F; it is not suitable for all cases
  b. F; failure rate of Filshie clip application (postpartum) is high compared to Pomeroy procedure by minilaparotomy
  c. F; both Filshie clip or Falope rings (not only Filshie clip) should be the method of choice for laparoscopic tubal occlusion
  d. T.

Q.2 Regarding male sterilization (vasectomy):
  a. Compared to tubectomy, vasectomy has got more failure rates
  b. Vas division or occlusion by clips or by diathermy is equally effective
  c. It should be performed under local anesthetic whenever possible
  d. Following vasectomy men should use effective contraception until azoospermic.

Ans. a. F; vasectomy has got less failure rates (1 in 2,000) compared to tubectomy
  b. F; clips has got unacceptably high failure rates and should not be used. Division along with fascial interposition or diathermy should be done
  c. T.
  d. T; azoospermia is to be checked by semen analysis after 16 weeks postvasectomy or after 20 ejaculations, till then men should use some form of contraceptive.

Q.3 Tubal occlusion for female sterilization:
  a. Diathermy can be used as a primary method
  b. Hysteroscopic method is very effective
  c. Laparoscopic tubal sterilization needs general anesthesia
  d. Tubal occlusion can be done any time during the menstrual cycle.

Ans. a. F; diathermy cause more tubal damage, increases the risk of ectopic pregnancy and is more difficult to reverse if needed

b. F; effectiveness of this procedure is under evaluation
c. F; this procedure can be done under local anesthesia as an alternative to general anesthesia. It should be performed as a day care
d. F; it can be done so, provided the women have used an effective method of contraception up to the day of operation (see discussion below).

Case Selection

Q. Criteria to be fulfilled before regarding case selection for female sterilization:

Ans.
- Self-declaration by the client is accepted
- Client must be married (including ever married)
- Client's age is > 22 years but < 45 years
- The couple should have at least two children and the last child of age >1 year, unless sterilization is medically indicated
- Clients or their spouses/partners have not undergone sterilization in the past
- Client must be in a sound state of mind
- Mentally ill client must be certified by a psychiatrist and a statement should be given by the legal guardian/spouse regarding client's abnormal state of mind.

MALE AND FEMALE STERILIZATION

Management Options

Couple when requesting for sterilization, both the methods of vasectomy and tubectomy (tubal occlusion) should be discussed. Couple counseling and advice should cover details of information about the individual procedure.

Discussion about the other alternative long-term reversible methods of contraception [levonorgestrel-releasing intrauterine system (LNG-IUS) implants] with advantages, disadvantages and failure rates, should be made. Counseling must be done with up-to-date knowledge and it should be recorded.

Other Long-term Reversible Methods of Contraception

LNG-IUS, subdermal implants and copper intrauterine devices (IUDs) can work for 3–10 years depending upon the method. Some of these methods are as effective as tubal occlusion at the same time they have the benefit of reversibility. The cumulative rates of failure are as follows: Cu-T 380A at 12 years is 1.9/100 women; LNG-IUS is 1.1/100 after 5 years of typical use. These rates are comparable with tubal occlusion at the same time they have the benefit of reversibility. Currently, it is said that women should continue contraceptive use (once started) until up to a period of 2 years after menopause, if aged ≤ 50 years or one year if over 50 years (FPA-2001).

Tubal Sterilization (Occlusion)

Laparoscopic method of tubal occlusion is quicker. Compared to minilaparotomy, it has less morbidity. But surgeon need to be trained with this method. Postpartum sterilization procedure should be done by **modified Pomeroy's method**. Compared to laparoscopic method (Filshie clip or Falope ring) (Figs 25.2A and B), modified Pomeroy's methods has got lower failure rates.

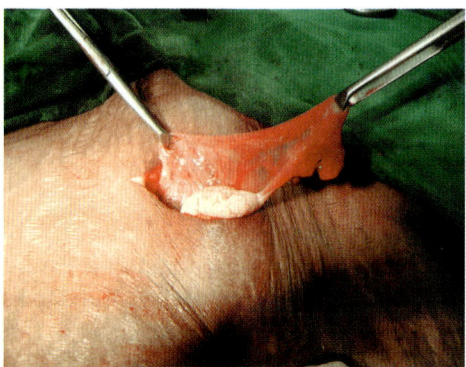

Fig. 25.1: Female sterilization (Pomeroy's method)

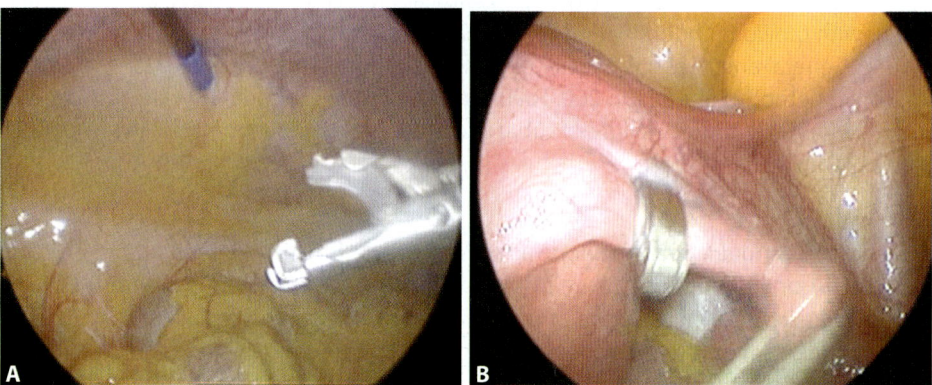

Figs 25.2A and B: Laparoscopic method of female sterilization (using Filshie clip). **A.** Filshie clip loaded applicator, **B.** Filshie clip is applied over the Fallopian tube

Minilaparotomy is the method of approach for an interval sterilization, though any effective surgical or mechanical method can be used.

Modified Pomeroy technique is the most widely used ligation technique. Absorbable sutures (chromic catgut) are used (Fig. 25.1). A loop of the tube is made near the mid portion (ampulla). The base of the loop is tied with chromic catgut suture. Finally, the loop is resected off (*See* Dutta's Textbook of Gynecology, 7th Edition, p. 408). Once the suture material is absorbed (10–14 days), the ends of the tubes fall apart. The chance of fistula formation is also less. However, the procedure removes 3–4 cm of the tube. The chance of reversal of the procedure is less compared to laparoscopic tubal occlusion method (Filshie).

Madlener technique: The tube loop is made. The base of the loop is crushed with a clamp or forceps. The base is then ligated with nonabsorbable suture material. This method has high failure rate.

Kroener technique: The entire fimbrial end of the tube is excised and removed. It is practically impossible to reverse the method.

Uchida technique (*See* Dutta's Textbook of Gynecology, 7th Edition, p. 408): This method is technically more difficult. It has high success rate but chances of reversibility are very low.

Laparoscopic Method of Tubal Sterilization (Occlusion)

Diathermy should not be used as method of tubal occlusion.
Disadvantages are:
- More damage to the tube (with monopolar)
- Damage (burn) to other organs (bowel/bladder)
- Not easy to reverse
- Increased risk of subsequent ectopic pregnancy.

Hysteroscopic method of tubal occlusion is done by using 'Essure' (*See* Dutta's Textbook of Gynecology, 7th Edition, p. 416). This is a new method. It is found to have good success rates. But this method is still under evaluation.

Laparoscopic Method of Sterilization[1]

Any women opting for laparoscopic method of tubal occlusion should be informed about the chance of laparotomy, if there is any problem with laparoscopy. This is particularly in cases with obesity or with previous abdominal surgery. Laparoscopic tubal occlusion can be done with local anesthetic. General anesthesia is usually used and it is done on a day care basis. Failure rate of laparoscopic method is about 1 in 200. Failure rate of Filshie clip after 10 years is 2–3 per 1,000 procedure. Whenever there is failure of tubal occlusion (sterilization) method, the risk of ectopic pregnancy is high.

Timing of Tubal Occlusion

Tubal sterilization should ideally be done as an interval method (in between pregnancies). Tubal ligation (occlusion) when done in the postpartum or postabortal period, the risk of failure is increased. There is also increased rate of regret following these two periods.

Tubal occlusion should be done during the follicular phase of the menstrual cycle. The woman should be advised to use some contraceptive measures until the next menstrual cycle. On the other hand, if the woman has used any method of effective contraception up to the day of operation in that case tubal occlusion can be done anytime during the menstrual cycle. Routine curettage at the time of tubal occlusion to prevent a **luteal phase pregnancy**, is not recommended.

Laparoscopic tubal occlusion should be performed as a day care. Use of local anesthesia can be done. Occlusion of the tubes is done mechanically using either Filshie clip which is applied at right angle to the tube over the isthmic portion, at a place 1–2 cm from the cornu. The entire circumference of the tube must be encased.

Tubal occlusion by mechanical method (using clips or rings) is very painful compared to methods done with diathermy. This is due to local tissue necrosis and ischemia at the site of tubal occlusion. Topical instillation of local anesthesia (bupivacaine) to the fallopian tubes at the end of the procedure is effective to reduce the pain.

Failure of Tubal Sterilization

Despite the use of any best method or approach of tubal sterilization, failure is present. Cumulative 10 years failure rate after sterilization was found 16.6/1,000 procedures Collaborative Review of Sterilization (CREST) study.[2]

Q. *What are the various reasons for failure following tubal sterilization?*
Ans.
- Fistula tract development of the occluded portion of the tube

- Ends of the tube can reconnect spontaneously (recanalization)
- Tubes may be occluded incompletely (partially)
- There may be slippage of the occlusive device
- Application of the occlusive device over a wrong anatomical structure (round ligament)
- Failure of recognition of pregnancy that has already taken place *(luteal phase pregnancy).*

Luteal phase pregnancy is defined when conception occurs unknowingly in the same menstrual cycle in which the sterilization operation is performed. Luteal phase pregnancies are estimated to occur in about 2–3/1,000 interval procedures. Therefore, it is a must, before the operation, to exclude the possibility of a preexisting pregnancy. However, a negative pregnancy test does not exclude the possibility of a luteal phase pregnancy. Routine curettage at the time of tubal occlusion, to prevent luteal phase pregnancy, is not recommended.

Luteal phase ectopic pregnancy can be caused iatrogenically by occluding the tube before the blastocyst has passed the site of occlusion.

If the woman has a copper intrauterine contraceptive device (IUCD) or LNG-IUCD *in situ*, it should be removed at the next period.

Whenever any method of tubal occlusion fails, the resultant pregnancy may be an ectopic pregnancy. The overall incidence of ectopic pregnancy following tubal sterilization ranges from 4.3–76.0% depending upon the method used to occlude or destroy the tube. Tubal occlusion with bipolar diathermy has much higher (27 times higher) rate of ectopic pregnancy.

Concurrent Method of Sterilization

Sterilization can be performed concurrently with cesarean delivery, induced abortion or medical termination of pregnancy. *In India majority of female sterilization procedures are concurrently done in association with all the above procedures.* Women should be counseled adequately beforehand at least a week prior to any procedure. Otherwise the woman regret (3–10%). *In Indian set-up, regret is mainly due to the death of a child, particularly that of a male child. In developed countries, regret is mainly due to the desire of a child with a new partner.* Failure rate of sterilization following concurrent procedure is high compared to an interval procedure.

Long-term Risk of Tubal Occlusion

There have been a report of significant **abnormal uterine bleeding** among women who have undergone tubal sterilization compared with a nonsterilized control group. There have been a debate, Whether the **post-tubal sterilization syndrome exists or not?**

CREST study found the risk of hysterectomy to be higher among these women compared to general population. However, there is no evidence to suggest that tubal occlusion leads to the problems that necessitate hysterectomy. It may be possible that **alteration in ovarian blood supply by the occlusion method is the cause for abnormal uterine bleeding**.

VASECTOMY

Methods of Vasectomy

No scalpel vasectomy is the optimum method to perform. It was developed by Li Shun Quiang of China in 1991. This method has low complications. Only *division of the vas* is not an acceptable

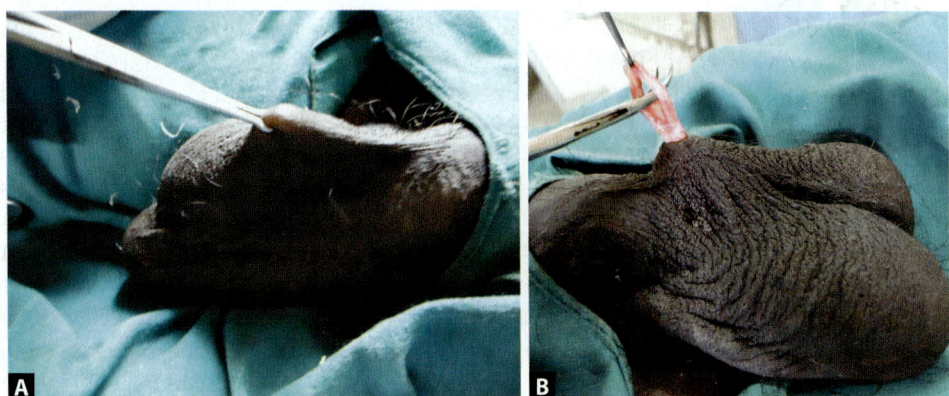

Figs 25.3A and B: No scalpel vasectomy: **A.** Holding the vas with ringed clamp; **B.** Dissection of the vas with forceps

technique because it results in failure. This method should be accompanied by *fascial interposition or diathermy* (*See* Dutta's Textbook of Gynecology, 7th Edition, p. 407).

Li's method takes less time. Complications are also low.

Common complications of vasectomy using scalpel method are: Injury to testicular blood vessels, bleeding, hematoma formation, infection and pain.

Methods of Vas Occlusion (Figs 25.3A and B)
- Ligation with absorbable (catgut) or nonabsorbable sutures (silk or cotton).
- Coagulation using monopolar or bipolar energy source. This method make reversal more difficult as damage to vas is much more.
- Application of clip.

Fascial interposition is done to reduce the risk of recanalization and the subsequent failure rates. Usually, a 2–3 cm segment of the vas is excised during the procedure. One end of the vas (usually the distal end) is allowed to fall back into the wound. The spermatic fascia is interposed over the defect so that the two ends are in different tissue planes. This makes the possibility of recanalization between the two ligated ends far less.

Fascial interposition makes no scalpel vasectomy much successful.

Application of clips and excision method has got high failure rate. Vasectomy is usually performed under local anesthetic and it is found safe.

Postvasectomy Considerations

Histological examination of the excised portions of vas is not routinely needed (unless when there is any doubt about their identity). Following vasectomy, men should use an effective contraception until azoospermia has been confirmed. This is to confirm the clearance of stored spermatozoa down the vasectomy site. Usually, semen analysis is done 16 weeks after vasectomy. Men should use other birth control methods for at least 20 ejaculations. ***Association for voluntary sterilization*** recommended at least 15 ejaculations or semen analysis 6 weeks after the procedure. By that time most men become sterile.

In a small group of men (2–3%), nonmotile sperm may be present in the postvasectomy period. Presence of ≤ 10,000 nonmotile sperm/mL, 7 month after vasectomy was not associated with any pregnancy report. In such a situation, men can be given, **special clearance** to stop contraception.

Failure of Vasectomy

Pregnancy can occur even several years after vasectomy. The rate may low as 1 in 2,000 after clearance has been given.

Vasectomy failure is defined as the presence of spermatozoa on semen analysis or presence of a pregnancy.

Causes of Vasectomy Failure

- Surgeon failure (operator)
- Method failure (technical failure)
- Unprotected intercourse soon after vasectomy while residual sperm is still stored in the reproductive tract
- Spontaneous recanalization of the vas
- Occlusion of a wrong structure instead of the vas, inadequate occlusion of the vas (loose tie), or congenital duplication of one or both vas (rare).

Risks of Vasectomy

- ***Prostate cancer:*** Population based study with systematic review found ***no association*** between vasectomy and prostate cancer.
- ***Testicular cancer***: ***No increased risk*** has been observed, based on contact and case control studies.
- ***Cardiovascular disease: No association*** has been observed between vasectomy and cardiovascular disease, atherosclerotic disease, hypertension, myocardial infarction or coronary artery disease.
- ***Chronic testicular pain*** may be observed months or years after vasectomy. The incidence of postvasectomy pain ranges from 12 to 52%.

References

1. Peterson HB, Xia Z, Hughes JM, The risk of pregnancy after tubal sterilization: findings from the US Collaborative Review of Sterilization. Am J Obstet Gynecol.1996;174(4):1161-8.
2. Hillis SD, Marchbanks PA, Tylor LR, Higher hysterectomy risk for sterilized than nonsterilized women: findings from the US Collaborative Review of Sterilization. The US Collaborative Review of Sterilization Working Group. Obstet Gynecol. 1998;91(2):241-6.

26. Gestational Trophoblastic Disease

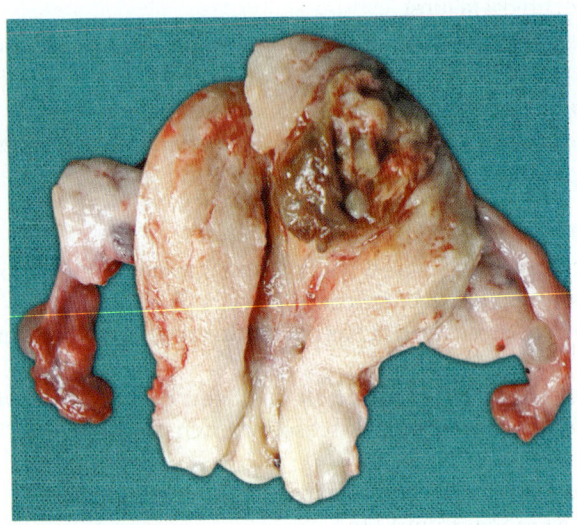

Fig. 26.1: Choriocarcinoma invading myometrium

Q. Regarding gestational trophoblastic neoplasia (GTN):
   a. Nearly 20–30% of patients with partial mole develop GTN following evacuation
   b. Metastatic tumor without established primary site with raised human chorionic gonadotropin (hCG) is diagnosed
   c. Decline in hCG level by >10% following chemotherapy indicates response
   d. Risk of recurrence is nearly 13% despite use of chemotherapy.

Ans. a. F b. T
 c. T d. T

Q. What is meant by gestational trophoblastic disease (GTD)?
Ans. GTD comprises a spectrum of neoplastic conditions derived from the placenta. GTN refers especially to those GTD cases with potential for tissue invasion and metastasis.

Q. How the diagnosis of GTN could be made following evacuation of hydatidiform mole?
Ans.
- Four or more values of plateaued hCG (±10%) over at least 3 weeks (days 1, 7, 14 and 21)
- Three or more values of rise in hCG (≥ 10%) over at least 2 weeks (days 1, 7 and 14)

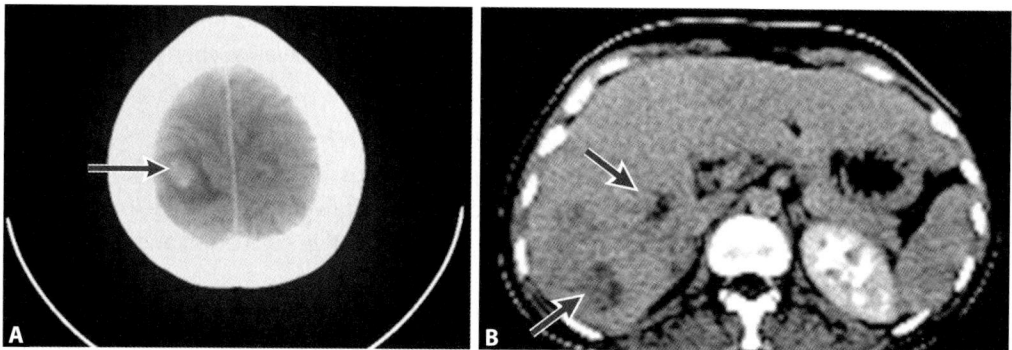

Figs 26.2A and B: Patient with choriocarcinoma, CT view showing: **A.** Brain metastasis, **B.** Multiple metastases in the liver

- Histologic diagnosis of choriocarcinoma, invasive mole or placental site trophoblastic tumor (PSTT)
- Metastatic tumor without established primary site with raised hCG.

Q. What percentage of women develops GTN following evacuation of a hydatidiform mole?

Ans. About 6–30% of patients develop GTN following evacuation of complete mole whereas, nearly 2–8% of patients develop GTN following evacuation of partial mole.

Q. How do you evaluate a case of GTN?

Ans.
- Complete general physical and pelvic examination
- Baseline hematologic parameters
- Baseline renal and hepatic functions
- Baseline hCG values
- Chest radiograph or computed tomography (CT) chest
- Brain magnetic resonance imaging (MRI) or CT scan (Figs 26.2A and B)
- CT or MRI scan of abdomen and pelvis.

Q. What is 'phantom' (false-positive) hCG? How this problem could be overcome?

Ans. Many patients after receiving chemotherapy or after surgery present with low level of hCG (200–300 mIU/mL).[1] This is due to interference with hCG immunometrics and sandwich assays caused by nonspecific heterophile antibodies in patient's serum. False-positive hCG assays will have markedly different values using different assay techniques. Heterophile antibodies are not excreted in the urine. Therefore, when serum hCG is detected in such a patient, a urine sample should be tested for hCG. Urinary hCG values would not be detected in a case with phantom GTN. This will avoid unnecessary chemotherapy for such a patient.

Q. What is 'real' low level hCG?

Ans. Persistent low levels of hCG in patients with GTN (< 500 mIU/mL) may be observed without any evidence of lesion. This is known as 'quiescent GTN' where hCG is not hyperglycosylated. These patients need follow-up for long-time. Risk of recurrence for such a patient is about 10%. Usually these patients respond well to chemotherapy in the event of recurrence.

Q. What factors have got prognostic importance for GTN?
Ans. Initially, World Health Organization (WHO) clinical classification (1980) and Federation of Gynecology and Obstetrics (FIGO) anatomic staging were considered. In 2000, FIGO revised its staging for GTN with uniformity for comparative evaluation and treatment in all the centers worldwide.
Adoption of current FIGO revised (2000) scoring system (*See* Dutta's Textbook of Gynecology, 7th Edition, p. 301) has categorized patients into low-risk (score: 0–6) and high-risk (score ≥ 7) groups. Low-risk group patients are treated initially single agent regimen. Patients with metastatic disease (score ≥ 7) are treated with multiagent chemotherapy.

Q. What hCG value should be considered for risk scoring?
Ans. It is important to note that the hCG level obtained immediately before starting treatment for GTN should be considered for **risk scoring**. The hCG level obtained at the time of evacuation is not to be used for this purpose. Current FIGO staging will help uniformity of patient evaluation and comparison of treatment results.

Q. How do you follow-up the women during and after chemotherapy for GTN?
Ans. Serum hCG level is monitored weekly during and after the chemotherapy:
- **Response:** Decline in hCG level by >10% following one cycle therapy.
- **Plateau:** Change ± 10% in hCG following one cycle therapy.
- **Resistance:** Rise > 10% in hCG following one cycle or plateau for two cycles of chemotherapy.
- **Remission:** Normal hCG values weekly for 3 consecutive weeks.
- **Maintenance** chemotherapy should be given for at least three more cycles after normalization of serum hCG values.

Q. How do you maintain the surveillance for remission after chemotherapy for GTN?
Ans.
- hCG values every 2 weeks for 3 months
- hCG values every month for 1 year
- hCG values every 6–12 months for lifelong (3–5 years at least).

Q. What is the risk of recurrence for women with high-risk disease after achieving initial remission?
Ans. In spite of using multiagent chemotherapy aggressively, nearly 13% of patients will develop recurrence.

Q. What would be your approach for management of such cases?
Ans. Even with intensive chemotherapy, patients may have recurrence following initial remission especially the women with high-risk disease.
Management options for such women are:
- Patient needs to be evaluated for metastasis.

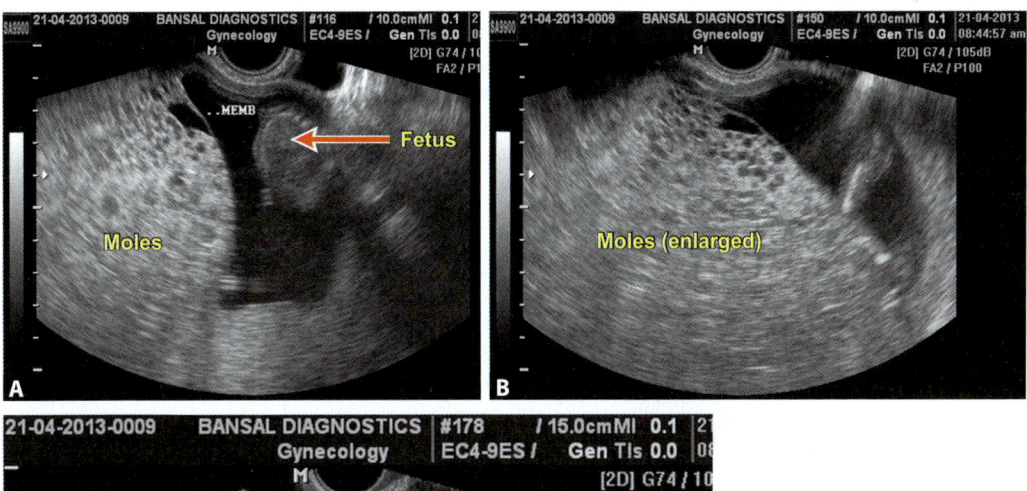
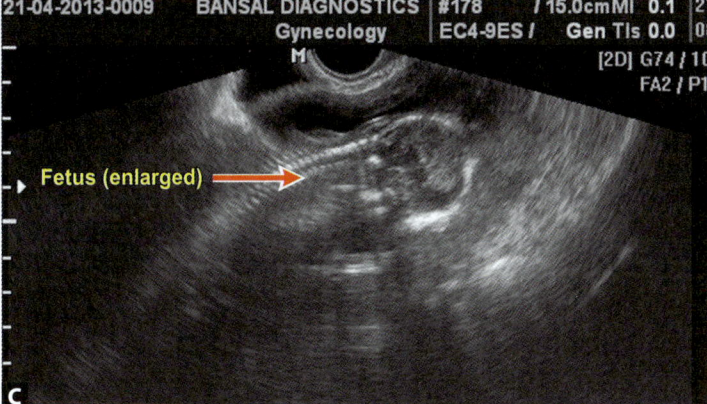

Figs 26.3A to C: Twin pregnancy: Coexistent molar pregnancy and a normal fetus

- Patient may be considered for alternative (EMA/CO, EMA-EP or MAC/CHAMOCA) chemotherapy regimens (*See* Dutta's Textbook of Gynecology, 7th Edition, p. 302).
- Patient may be considered for additional surgery (to extirpate drug resistant tissues, e.g. thoracotomy for lung wedge resection) or radiotherapy (for brain metastasis).

Twin pregnancy: Coexistent molar pregnancy and a normal fetus: Coexistent molar pregnancy with a normal fetus is relatively rare (1 in 22,000 to 1 in 1,00,000 pregnancies). Mrs R, a 34-year-old lady; P-0, G-4, A-3, L-0, conceived following IVF-ET. USG revealed the diagnosis (Figs 26.3A to C). Pregnancy ended in miscarriage at 18 weeks gestation due to the complication of excessive hemorrhage. Medical complications of such a twin pregnancy including hyperthyroidism, PIH and hemorrhage are increased. These patients have an increased risk of developing post molar GTN and metastatic disease.

Q. What is the reproductive outcome of a woman with GTN following remission of the disease?

Ans. Such a woman can have normal pregnancy and successful outcome in majority (79%). Risk of premature ovarian failure has been reported. However, risks of fetal congenital malformation are not increased at the risk of stillbirths may be high.

Q. What are the long-term health consequences of women treated for GTN?
Ans.
- Increased risk of second malignancy, especially following the use of multiagent chemotherapy with etoposide. Risks of developing myeloid leukemia and colon cancer are there.
- Early onsets of menopause and premature ovarian failure have been observed.

Reference

1. Hancock BW. hCG measurement in gestational trophoblastic neoplasia: a critical appraisal. J Reprod Med. 2006;51:859-60.

27 Carcinoma of the Endometrium (Early Stage Diseases)

FIGO STAGE I (2009)

***Stage I*:** Tumor confined to the corpus uteri
***Stage IA*:** No or invasion < 50% of the myometrium
***Stage IB*:** Invasion ≥ 50% of the myometrium (Fig. 27.1)
*Either grades I, II or III.
Positive peritoneal cytology has to be reported separately without changing the stage.
***Stage II**:** Tumor invades cervical stroma but does not extend beyond the uterus.
**Endocervical glandular involvement only is considered as stage I and no longer as stage II.

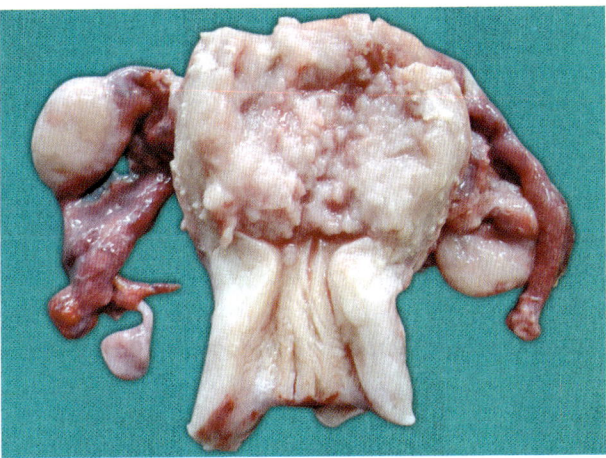

Fig. 27.1: Endometrial carcinoma diffuse type

FIGO GRADING SYSTEM (1989)

Grade I: <5% of the tumor shows a solid (nonsquamous or nonmorular) growth pattern.
Grade II: 6–50% of the tumor shows a solid (nonsquamous or nonmorular) growth pattern.
Grade III: >50% of the tumor shows a solid (nonsquamous or nonmorular) growth pattern.
Presence of any nuclear atypia increases the tumor grade by one.

Management Options

The current surgical management approach for a patient with endometrial cancer is:
(a) Laparotomy, (b) peritoneal cytology, (c) total hysterectomy and bilateral salpingo-oophorectomy and (d) surgical staging. Majority of women with endometrial carcinoma have endometrioid type of adenocarcinoma (80%) on histology. In women with non-endometrioid case, surgical steps are extended to include: (a) Omentectomy, (b) appendectomy and (c) peritoneal biopsies.

The place of lymphadenectomy (pelvic and para-aortic) is an important issue to detect extrauterine spread of the disease. This is essential as to formulate the postoperative management. Incorporation of lymphadenectomy in all patients of endometrial carcinoma is not universally accepted.[1] Two large prospective-randomized trials failed to show improved survival outcomes of the patients who underwent pelvic lymphadenectomy.[2,3] Patients with endometrioid type histology, grades 1 or 2 disease, tumor diameter < 2 cm and superficial myometrial invasion, did not have a lymphatic metastasis. There is no evidence of benefit in terms of overall survival or recurrence-free survival with pelvic lymphadenectomy in women with early endometrial cancer. Pelvic lymphadenectomy cannot be recommended as routine procedure for therapeutic purposes outside of clinical trials.[3]

Therefore, it was necessary to identify the group of patients in whom lymphadenectomy likely to improve survival outcome instead of increasing the risk of surgical complications and consequent morbidity.

The need to perform lymphadenectomy is based on the following factors:
- Histological type of the tumor
- Grade of the tumor
- Tumor size
- Depth of myometrial invasion as assessed during surgery
- Presence of extrauterine disease on exploration and biopsy.

Bilateral pelvic and para-aortic lymphadenectomy is performed in the presence of any of the following factors:
- Non-endometrioid type of endometrial cancer
- FIGO grade III tumor
- Tumor size > 2 cm
- Myometrial invasion >50%
- Evidence of extrauterine disease.

Differentiating features of type I and type II endometrial carcinoma

Features	Type I	Type II
Clinical		
High-risk factors	Unopposed estrogen	Age
Histology	Endometrioid	Non-endometrioid
Stage	Early I/II	Advanced III/IV
Differentiation	Well-differentiated	Poorly differentiated
Molecular		
HER2/neu overexpression	No	Yes
P-53 overexpression	No	Yes
K-Ras overexpression	Yes	No

Q. What is the significance of peritoneal cytology in the management of endometrial carcinoma?

Ans. FIGO (2009) recommends positive peritoneal cytology to be reported separately without changing the stage. It is not included in direct-staging procedure.
- Positive peritoneal cytology generally indicates spread of the disease.
- On the other hand in the essense of any evidence of extrauterine spread of disease or without any evidence of poor prognostic factor, positive peritoneal cytology has no significant impact in terms of disease recurrence and/or survival outcome of the patient.
- Positive peritoneal cytology along with presence of other known poor prognostic factor(s) worsens the survival outcome of the patient.

Postoperative radiotherapy in stage 1 endometrial carcinoma reduces locoregional recurrence but has no effect on overall survival. Radiotherapy increases treatment-related morbidity. Postoperative radiotherapy is not recommended in patients with stage 1 endometrial carcinoma below 60 years and patients with grade 2 tumors with superficial invasion.[4] However, patients with grade 3 tumors with a known propensity for deep myometrial invasion and lymph node metastasis may benefit from external beam radiotherapy.

Vaginal brachytherapy is better tolerated with high-dose rate (HDR) for women with endometrial cancer with high-risk of recurrence. Women with stage 1, grade 3 histology and invasion of lymphovascular space are the high-risk group. Women with these risk factors are benefitted with vaginal vault brachytherapy.[5]

FIGO STAGE II

Stage II: Tumor invades cervical stroma, but does not extend beyond the uterus.
Incidence of lymph node metastasis in stage II endometrial carcinoma is about 36%. However, reliable diagnosis of cervical involvement is difficult as endocervical curettage, has high false-positive and false-negative rates. Ultrasonography, hysteroscopy or MRI may be helpful. Therefore, risk of spread outside the pelvis to the para-aortic nodes, adnexal and upper abdomen is high in stage II disease.

Management options for endometrial carcinoma stage II disease are:
- **Radical hysterectomy, bilateral salpingo-oophorectomy, pelvic and para-aortic lymphadenectomy.**
  - ***Advantage:*** It provides accurate information as regard the spread of the disease.[6]
  - ***Disadvantage:*** The women with endometrial carcinoma are often (i) elderly, (ii) obese and (iii) suffer from some medical disorders. They are often not suitable for such an extensive surgical procedure. Operative morbidities are high.
- **Combined therapy**
  - ***Radiation therapy*** both external (pelvic) and intracavitary (cesium). This is followed after 6 weeks by ***total abdominal hysterectomy and bilateral salpingo-oophorectomy***. The results of the two above mentioned therapies are comparable.
  - ***Initial surgery:*** Exploratory laparotomy followed by extrafascial hysterectomy, bilateral salpingo-oophorectomy or modified radical hysterectomy with selected lymphadenectomy (clinically palpable nodes) is done. This is ***followed by pelvic or extended field external and intravaginal radiation*** depending upon the spread of the disease. Results reported are excellent.

References

1. Mariani A, Webb MJ, Keeney Gl, et al. Low-risk corpus cancer: Is lymphadenectomy or radiotherapy necessary? Am J Obstet Gynecol. 2000;182(6):1506-19.
2. Benedetti Panici P, Basil S, Maneschi F, et al. Systematic pelvic lymphadenectomy Vs no lymphadenectomy in early-stage endometrial carcinoma: randomized control trial. J Natl Cancer Inst. 2008;100(23):1707-16.
3. Kitchener H, Swart AM, Qian Q, et al. ASTEC study group. Efficacy of systematic pelvic lymphadenectomy in endometrial cancer (MRC ASTEC trial): A randomized study. Lancet. 2009;373:125-36.
4. Creutzberg CL, van Putten WL, Warlam-Rodenhuis CC, et al. Outcome of high-risk stage 1C, grade 3, compared with stage 1 endometrial carcinoma patients: The postoperative radiation therapy in endometrial carcinoma trial. J Clin Oncol. 2004;221234-41.
5. Mariani A, Dowdy SC, Keeney GL, et al. Predictors or vaginal relapse in stage I endometrial cancer. Gynecol Oncol. 2005;97(3):820-27.
6. Mariani A, Webb MJ, Keeney GL, et al. Role of wide/radical hysterectomy and pelvic lymph node dissection in endometrial cancer with cervical involvement. Gynecol Oncol. 2001;83:72-80.

28 Pregnancy of Unknown Location

Q. How do you define pregnancy of unknown location (PUL)?
Ans. The term PUL is used whenever there is no sign of either intra or extrauterine pregnancy or retained products of conception on transvaginal ultrasound despite positive pregnancy test.

Q. What is the current scenario about PUL?
Ans. The incidence of PUL is increasing. The reasons are:
- Initiation of early pregnancy assessment unit (EPAU)
- Early gestation scans
- Increased awareness.

Q. How do you assess a woman with the diagnosis of PUL?
Ans.
- Whenever a woman presents with a positive pregnancy test but no evidence of pregnancy on TVS, it is a case with PUL.
- **Clinical assessment and investigations are to be:**
    - Serum β-hCG estimation should be carried out
    - However, a positive serum β-hCG does not always indicate pregnancy
    - Molar pregnancy needs to be excluded
    - Possibility of heterotopic pregnancy is there
    - Combined TVS and serum β-hCG is more informative (PPV: 93.5–100%).

Q. How the diagnosis of PUL could be made?
Ans. Different investigative parameters either alone or in combination are done to make the diagnosis of PUL.
The different diagnostic methods are: Serum β-hCG estimation is to be done. The discriminatory zone of serum β-hCG is important. An intrauterine pregnancy (IUP) should be visible on ultrasound if serum β-hCG value ranges between 1,000 and 2,400 IU/L. However, the discriminatory levels of serum β-hCG are different in each unit. When the hCG levels are above the discriminatory zone and no intrauterine gestation sac is seen on **USG**, the ectopic pregnancy is the probability.[1]
Limitations of USG in early pregnancy are:
- Pregnancy site may not be visible in 8–31% of cases with early pregnancy scans
- The sonographer's experience is important. Even the sonographers in the early pregnancy assessment units may miss the diagnosis in 8–10 % of cases.

Q. What are the diagnostic criteria of ectopic pregnancy on USG?
Ans. Diagnosis of ectopic pregnancy:
- Identification of an extrauterine gestational sac
- Complex adnexal mass or
- Fluid collection rather than empty uterus on scan
- The combination of the above scan findings (PPV: 93.5–100% for diagnosing ectopic).

Q. Is there any added benefit of color Doppler sonography for the diagnosis of ectopic pregnancy?
Ans.
- Transvaginal color Doppler has not been shown to increase the detection rates of ectopic pregnancy, when compared with 2D ultrasound.
- It may be useful in showing enhanced trophoblastic blood flow.

Q. What is the place of serum progesterone estimation in the diagnosis of ectopic pregnancy?
Ans. Progesterone
- When serum progesterone levels are elevated, it indicates the viability of corpus luteum.
- Decreased levels of serum progesterone indicates failing pregnancy.
- Progesterone level < 25 nmol/L, associated with nonviable pregnancy (viable in 0.3%).
- Progesterone < 20 nmol/L predicts failing pregnancy (PPV > 95%).
- Levels > 25 nmol/L are associated with viable pregnancies.
- Levels > 60 nmol/L are strongly associated with IUP (2.6% ectopic).

Q. What is the relevance of β-hCG level estimation after 48 hours of interval?
Ans.
- hCG pattern after 48 hours—the value usually doubles (doubling time).
- Rise of hCG by 66%, predicts an IUP (PPV: 96.5%).[2,3]
- Fall of hCG by at least 15%, most likely suggests failing pregnancy.
- When the rise or fall in hCG is suboptimal, most likely the diagnosis is an ectopic one.

Q. What is the importance of endometrial study on USG in the diagnosis of ectopic pregnancy?
Ans. Trilaminar endometrium on USG: 94% specific for ectopic pregnancy but sensitivity is low (34%).

Q. What is the place of endometrial curettage in the diagnosis of PUL?
Ans. Curettage is done for the diagnosis, it helps by seeing the trophoblastic fronds, obtained on curettage. The trophoblastic tissues float on water when kept in a petri dish with water. However, it is not commonly done in India.
- It is not a usual practice in UK, although common in US.
- No clinical evidence of any added benefit.

Q. Is there any role of serum markers in the diagnosis of ectopic pregnancy?
Ans. Several tumor markers have been studied for this purpose. Nothing has been conclusively found to be helpful.
Important serum markers studied are:
- Serum CA 125
- VEGF
- Creatine kinase
- IL8-TNF

- PAPP-A
- PSPI, progesterone (PGN), leukemia inhibitory factor (LIF), GLY: VEGF, IL, TNF, HPL

Q. What is the place of MRI in the diagnosis of ectopic pregnancy?
Ans.
- MRI is highly (96%) sensitive. However, it is not commonly used.
- In 13–21% cases of ectopic pregnancy have an hCG rise similar to an IUP.

Q. What are the different outcomes of a case with PUL?
Ans. Clinical outcomes of PUL are:[4]
- Failing PUL (44–69%) and resolution
- Intrauterine pregnancy
- Ectopic pregnancy
- Persistent PUL.

Q. How do you define a case of persistent PUL?
Ans.
- Serum hCG levels fail to decline.
- There is no evidence of trophoblastic disease.
- Location of pregnancy cannot be identified.
- Usually hCG levels are low (<500 IU/L) and have reached to a plateau (2% of PUL).

Q. What are the benefits and the limitations of setting a high discriminatory level of hCG?
Ans.
- Setting high discriminatory level minimizes the risk of inappropriate intervention.
- On the other hand, it may delay the diagnosis of ectopic pregnancy by a few days.

Q. How do you manage a case of PUL?[5]
Ans.
- **Asymptomatic PUL** should be managed conservatively as none of the methods can predict the clinical outcome of PUL is 100% accurate.
- **Medical management** should be reserved for women with asymptomatic but persistent PUL.
- **Surgery** is indicated if the woman is symptomatic.

Q. How do you manage a case of asymptomatic PUL?
Ans. When no intrauterine or ectopic pregnancy or retained products of conception are seen on transvaginal sonography (TVS) and the woman is asymptomatic she can be managed conservatively.

Q. What are the benefits of the conservative management of PUL?
Ans. *Expectant management of PUL has the following benefits:*
- It has been shown to be safe.
- Reduces the need for unnecessary surgical intervention.
- Not associated with any serious adverse outcomes.
- **Limitations:** Unfortunately, multiple visits to EPAU are necessary before diagnosis can be made.

Association of Early Pregnancy Units guidelines 2007.

Q. Who are the women to be considered for medical management of PUL?
Ans. Medical management should be reserved for women with *asymptomatic but persistent PUL*.

Q. How medical management is done in such a case?
Ans. Medical management is recommended by EPAU.
Methotrexate, 50 mg/m^2, has been used successfully in persistent PUL (90% effective).

Q. What special care should be taken when a patient is under medical management with methotrexate?
Ans. Clinician's awareness is important to minimize any further complications.
The patients need to be observed closely. The following are the important observations:
- Abdominal pain between D3 and D7 in about 75% of women
- hCG levels may rise by D1–D4
- Risk of tubal rupture is about 7%
- Meantime for resolution is 35 days.

Immediate access to admission should be there, if needed for any complication.
Death has been observed in one case following such management (CEMACH, 2003–2005).

Q. What are the cases for surgical management of PUL?
Ans. When the woman is symptomatic or if an ectopic pregnancy is visualized, she should be considered for surgery. Method of surgery is by: Laparoscopy or laparotomy.

Q. Who are the modes of surgical management of PUL?
Ans. Laparoscopy or laparotomy should be undertaken without delay, if there are clinical signs suggestive of tubal rupture.

Q. How a patient with PUL under treatment should be followed up?
Ans. Follow-up is made with serum hCG estimation and ultrasound (TVS) examination. These are needed until the pregnancy is localized or intervention become necessary.

Q. What is the importance of estimating the levels of serum β-hCG?
Ans.
- When the fall or rise in hCG is suboptimal, ectopic pregnancy is the outcome.
- *hCG ratio*—hCG at 48 hours: hCG at 0 hours = < 0.87 (PPV: 96–99%), ectopic pregnancy is the possibility.
- However in 13–21% cases of ectopic pregnancy have an hCG rise similar to an IUP.
- hCG level above the discriminatory zone, with no intrauterine gestational sac on ultrasound, ectopic pregnancy is a possibility.

Q. What should be the management issues for a woman with the 'presumed' diagnosis of complete miscarriage having the diagnostic criteria of PUL?[6,7]
Ans.
- Management of such a women with 'presumed' complete miscarriage is to keep her under follow-up.
- Death had occurred, 3 weeks later due to ruptured tubal pregnancy (CEMACH, 2000–2002).

Often the patient passes a clot vaginally. This gives the impression of complete miscarriage showing an empty uterus on USG. The women should be under observation with monitoring by serum β-hCG and evaluation by USG. Risk of ectopic pregnancy for those women is still there.

Q. Is there any limitation of early laparoscopy in such a woman?
Ans. Laparoscopy has false-negative rate of 3–4% when done too early. It has false-positive rate of 5% because of retrograde uterine bleeding.

Q. What are the main areas of difficulties in the management of PUL and how it could be overcome?

Ans.
- Difficulties are mainly in the diagnosis.
  - **Discriminatory level** of β-hCG is varies in different laboratories. Different levels of each unit are mainly due to different hCG assay technique used in the laboratories.
    - High discriminatory values of serum β-hCG avoids many unnecessary intervention. However, it delays the diagnosis by 3–5 days.
    - Ultrasonographic diagnosis of early pregnancy may be missed by 8–10% cases even by an experienced sonographer working in an EPAU.

CEMACH: Confidential Enquiry into Maternal and Child Health
EPAU: Early pregnancy assessment unit
hCG: Human chorionic gonadotropin
TVS: Transvaginal sonography
USG: Ultrasonography
PPV: Positive predictive value
CA 125: Cancer antigen 125
VEGF: Vascular endothelial growth factor
IL-8: Interleukin-8
TNF: Tumor necrosis factor
PAPP-A: Pregnancy-associated plasma protein-A
HPL: Human placental lactogen
GLY: Glycodelin

References

1. Seeber BE, Sammel MD, Guo W, et al. Application of redefined human chorionic gonadotropin curves for the diagnosis of women at risk for ectopic pregnancy. Fertil Steril. 2006;86:454-9.
2. Barnhart KT, Sammel MD, Chung K, et al. Decline of serum human chorionic gonadotropin and spontaneous complete abortion: defining the normal curve. Obstet Gynecol. 2004;104:975-81.
3. Royal College of Obstetricians and Gynaecologists. The Management of Early Pregnancy Loss. Green-top Guideline no. 25. London: RCOG; 2006.
4. Kirk E, Condous G, Haider Z, et al. The practical application of a mathematical model to predict the outcome of pregnancies of unknown location. Ultrasound Obstet Gynecol. 2006;27:311-5d.
5. Association of Early Pregnancy Units. Guidelines 2007. [online] Available from www.earlypregnancy.org.uk/documents/AEPUGuidelines2007.pdf. [Accessed June, 2016].
6. Confidential Enquiry into Maternal and Child Health. Why Mothers Die 2000–2002. The Sixth Report of the Confidential Enquiries into Maternal Deaths in the United Kingdom. London: RCOG Press; 2004.
7. Lewis G (editor). Saving Mothers' Lives: Reviewing Maternal Deaths to Make Motherhood Safer—2003–2005. The Seventh Report on Confidential Enquiries into Maternal Deaths in the United Kingdom. London: CEMACH; 2007.

29 Abnormal Uterine Bleeding

Any menstrual flow outside the normal volume, duration, regularity or frequency is considered as abnormal uterine bleeding (AUB). Significant number of women (70%) in a gynecology clinic are seen due to AUB. In order to avoid the confusion of different terminology used, FIGO introduce this universally accepted nomenclature.[1] The acronym 'PALM-COEIN' is used (see below) to described AUB. AUB in an individual may be due to one or more than one causes. The nomenclature used terms such as menorrhagia, metrorrhagia or polymenorrhea are often inconsistent and confusing. This also makes investigation and management approach difficult. To avoid these difficulties newer classification system has been introduced by FIGO and approved by ACOG.[2]

CLASSIFICATION OF AUB (FIGO 2011)

Structural causes: PALM		*Nonstructural causes: COEIN*	
Polyp	AUB-**P**	**C**oagulopathy	AUB-**C**
Adenomyosis	AUB-**A**	**O**vulatory dysfunction	AUB-**O**
Leiomyoma (Fig. 29.1)	AUB-**L**	**E**ndometrial	AUB-**E**
Malignancy and hyperplasia	AUB-**M**	**I**atrogenic	AUB-**I**
		Not yet identified	AUB-**N**

Subclassification of Leiomyoma (AUB-L) (Figs 29.1 and 29.2)

Submucosal (SM)	0	Pedunculated intracavitary
	1	< 50% intramural
	2	≥ 50% intramural
Others (O)	3	100% intramural; contacts endometrium
	4	Intramural
	5	Subserosal ≥ 50% intramural
	6	Subserosal < 50% intramural
	7	Subserosal pedunculated
	8	Others (cervical, parasitic)
Hybrid (both endometrium and serosa)	2–4	Two numbers are listed separated by a hyphen. The **first** number refers to the relationship with endometrium and the **second** refers to that of serosa. Example: 2–4 = submucosal (≥ 50% intramural) and intramural.

Abnormal Uterine Bleeding 349

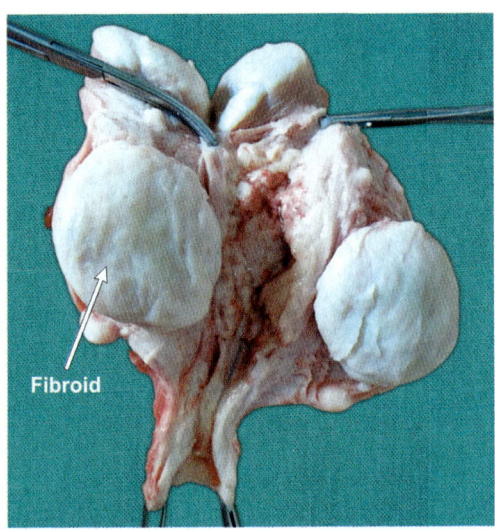

Fig. 29.1: AUB due to fibroid (leiomyoma) uterus (AUB-L)

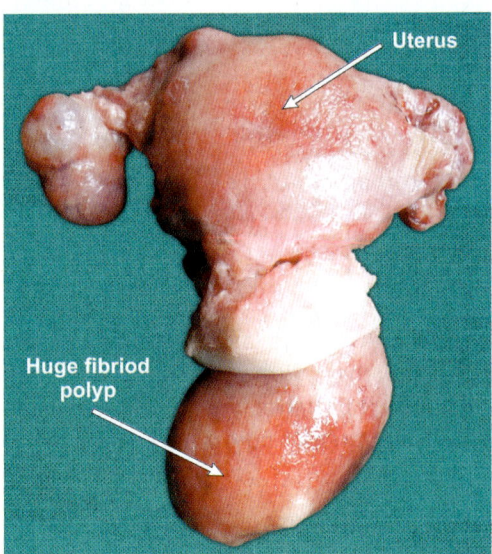

Fig. 29.2: AUB due to polyp (AUB-P)

Therefore, AUB includes a wide range of abnormalities (pelvic or systemic) that need to be investigated for diagnosis.

According to the new FIGO classification system of AUB, the 'PALM-COEIN' terminology used for expressing the pathology is as follows—AUB due to Polyp = AUB–***P*** (Fig. 29.3).
Similarly for the others: (1) AUB–***A*** (adenomyosis), (2) AUB–***L*** (leiomyoma), (3) AUB–***M*** (malignancy and hyperplasia), (4) AUB–***C*** (coagulopathy), (5) AUB–***O*** (ovulatory dysfunction), (6) AUB–***E*** (endometrial), (7) AUB–***I*** (iatrogenic) and (8) AUB–***N*** (not yet classified).

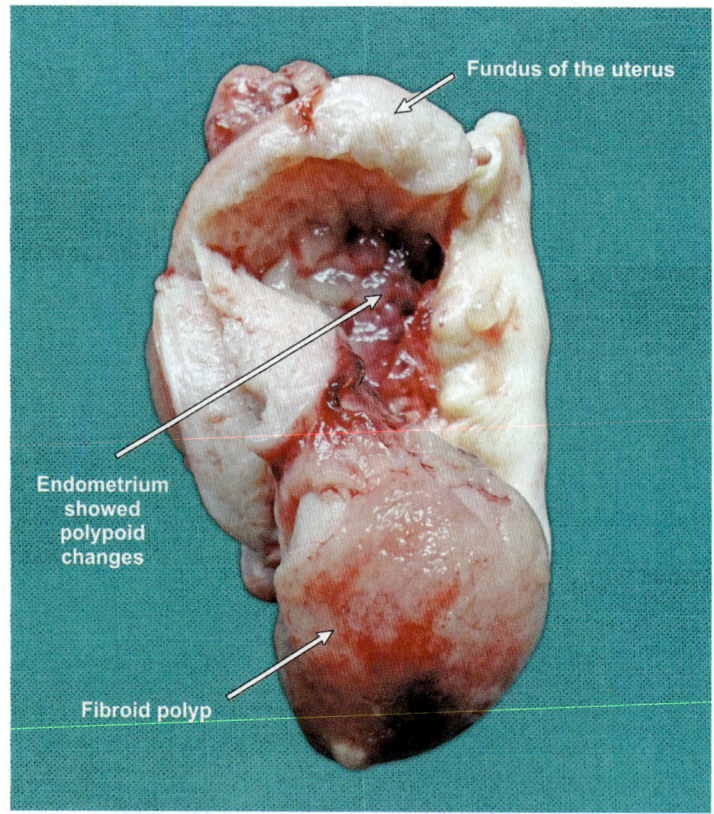

Fig. 29.3: Uterus is cut opened to show—a huge polyp protruding out of the cervical external os. Endometrium showed polypoid changes

Women with AUB may have one or more factors that may be responsible for the bleeding. The investigations should be comprehensive depending upon the available resources. However, it should be kept in mind that a mere presence of any abnormality may not be the contributory factor for AUB. Presence of a small subserous fibroid may not be the cause for AUB.

Notation

All the cases of AUB are evaluated in terms of presence or absence of each criterion. It is expressed as '**O**' if the criterion is absent; '**I**' if present and '**N**' if not yet assessed.

Once the investigations have been completed and the causes have been evaluated, the categorization of pathology and notation is done in a fashion for simpler understanding. For example, if a woman with AUB was found to have leiomyoma (type-1) and endometrial hyperplasia and no other abnormalities, the pathology would be categorized and notified as AUB $P_0 A_0 L_{1(SM)} E_1 - C_0 O_0 E_0 I_0 N_0$.

This notation may also be done in a simple form of categorization—AUB ($L_{(SM)}E$).

Example

$P_1 \quad A_0 \quad L_0 \quad M_0 - C_0 \quad O_0 \quad E_0 \quad I_0 \quad N_0$

In this case, endometrial polyp is the only cause of AUB and the rest are absent.

Diagnosis of Chronic AUB

It is made when a woman has suffered for a period of 3 months or more. In such a case, the following procedures are to be followed:

- **Structured history:** It is designed to determine: (a) Ovulatory function, (b) Fertility status, (c) Medical disorders, (d) Medications and (e) Thyroid function.
- **Physical examination:** Systemic and pelvic examination.
- **Investigations**
    - (i) Complete blood count (CBC), (ii) Hormone profile (thyroid function), (iii) Pap smear.
    - **Uterine evaluation**
        - Transvaginal sonography (TVS) → for any structural abnormality
        - Outpatient endometrial biopsy for women > 40 years age — To detect endometrial hyperplasia/atypia/carcinoma
        - Saline infusion sonography (SIS) is superior to TVS in detecting cavitary abnormalities
        - **Hysteroscopy and biopsy:** Hysteroscopy is highly accurate in diagnosing endometrial cancer
        - **Magnetic resonance imaging (MRI):** When needed (second-line test in cases like adenomyosis).

Differential Diagnosis of AUB (Age-based)

- **13–19 years**
    - **Anovulatory bleeding** due to dysregulation of hypothalamic-pituitary-ovarian axis.
    - **Coagulopathy** (laboratory tests needed are: CBC with platelets, PT and PTT).
    - **Irregular intake** of hormonal contraceptives (sexually active adolescents).
- **20–40 years**
    - Pregnancy complications
    - Uterine structural lesions (leiomyoma)
    - Anovulatory bleeding (PCOS)
    - Hormonal contraceptions
    - Endometrial hyperplasia.
- **41 years to menopause**
    - Anovulatory bleeding (declining ovarian function)
    - Cervical carcinoma (in developing countries)
    - Endometrial hyperplasia or carcinoma
    - Leiomyomas.
- **Management options:** Based on individual patient (*See* Manual of Obstetrics and Gynecology for the Postgraduates, p. 316).

References

1. Munro MG, Critchley HO, Broder MS, et al. FIGO classification system (PALM-COEIN) for causes of abnormal uterine bleeding in nongravid women of reproductive age. Int J Gynecol Obstet. 2011;113(1):3-13.
2. Committee on Practice Bulletins—Gynecology. Practice Bulletin no. 128: Diagnosis of abnormal uterine bleeding in reproductive–aged women. Obstet Gynecol. 2012;120(1):197-206.

30   Endoscopy in Gynecology (Laparoscopic Surgery)

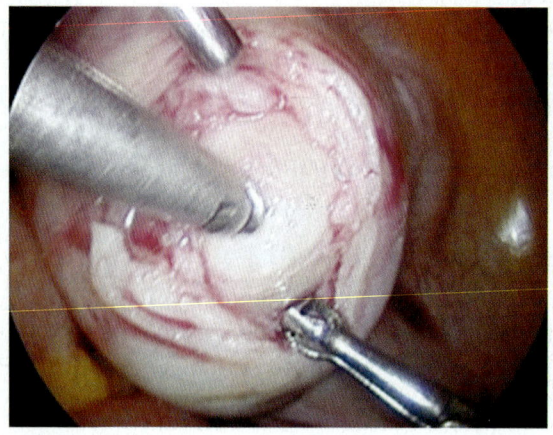

Fig. 30.1: Laparoscopic myomectomy. Enucleation of myoma is being done with a myoma screw

- **Q. Energy source used for hemostasis in endoscopy surgery are:**
  - a. Radio-frequency electricity is the most versatile method
  - b. Laser coagulation and cutting are the ideal one
  - c. Ultrasonic scalpel (harmonic) is the best
  - d. Stapling or knot tying is the better alternative.
- **Ans.** a. T   b. F
        c. F   d. F

- ***Radio-frequency electricity:*** It can be used either by monopolar or bipolar instrument. With optimum power settings tissues can be heated, desiccated and coagulated (Fig. 30.1). Ideally, the vessels should be compressed within the blades of a bipolar forceps and then the electrode is to be activated. This helps the vessel walls to seal by desiccation and coagulation when continuous low-voltage current is used (coaptive coagulation). ***In a bipolar forceps, when tissues between the blades are completely desiccated, there is no flow of electricity. This can reduce the problem of lateral thermal spread***. Automated generators are available that can stop pulse energy automatically. Laser and radio-frequency electrical sources of energy convert electromagnetic energy to mechanical energy, which is then turned into thermal energy.

High-current density energy, once delivered to tissues, the intracellular temperature rises >100°C and then intracellular water rapidly vaporizes. When this energy is **used in a linear fashion, tissue cutting effect is seen**. When radio-frequency energy with low-power density is used, effects such as desiccation and tissue coagulation are observed. **Monopolar** electrosurgical instruments with narrow ends generate high power density required to vaporize or cut tissues.

- *Laser energy:* It can be used to vaporize and cut tissues. KTP (potassium titanyl phosphate) and Nd:YAG lasers are used for cutting. CO_2 laser cannot be used effectively. KTP and Nd:YAG lasers, though much effective than CO_2 laser, have much higher risk of lateral thermal injury. Moreover, they are expensive.

- *Harmonic ultrasonic energy (harmonic scalpel):* It is a device used for coagulation and cutting of tissues. Electrical energy from the generator causes piezoelectric ceramics in the transducers (handpiece) to convert electrical energy into mechanical motion which is transferred to the blade extender. The ultrasonic wave is amplified as it travels down the blade tip, where it produces a maximum motion at 55,000 cycles/second. This results in simultaneous coagulation and cutting of tissues. No energy passes through the patient as opposed to that of electrosurgical instruments.

  Tissue effects with harmonic ultrasonic
  - **Coaptation** involves transfer of mechanical energy to tissues. The internal mechanical friction breaks the hydrogen bonds and causes protein denaturation. A sticky coagulum is formed that seals the vessels at temperature <100°C.
  - **Cavitation** occurs when the blade vibrates (50–100 microns). The cell water is vaporized and subsequently the cells rupture. There is minimum lateral thermal injury.

    This device reduces the need of frequent instrument change, as it coagulates and cuts the tissues simultaneously.

- *Hemostatic clips* can be applied with a specially designed clip applicator. Clips are generally used for vessels of 4 mm diameter or more. It is of special benefit, when a large vessel close to

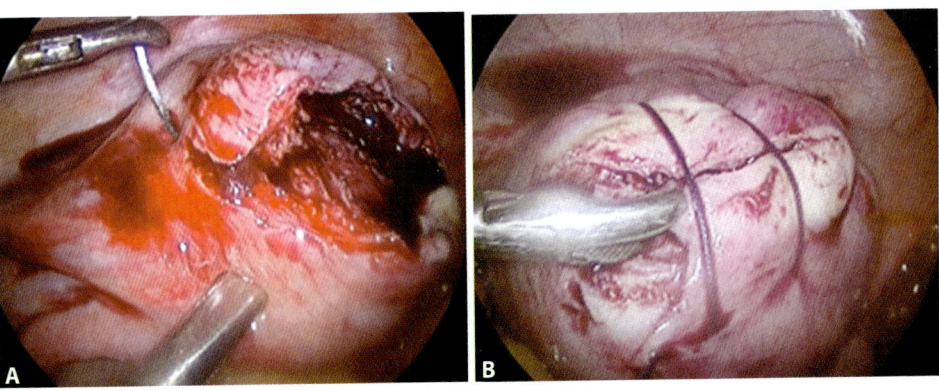

Figs 30.2A and B: A. Laparoscopic myomectomy; **B.** Myoma bed is being sutured
Courtesy: Dr P Kodtawala, Ahmedabad

an important structure (ureter) is to be ligated. Cost of stapling devices is high. Staplers cannot be used at all sites of bleeding, whereas electrodiathermy energy sources are of versatile use.

- ***Laparoscopic suturing:*** Intracorporeal suturing is done within the peritoneal cavity. This is similar to open surgery using the instruments. Extracorporeal knots are either (Figs 28.2A and B) pre-tied (endoloops) or created outside and then pushed inside the peritoneal cavity by knot pusher.

A surgeon needs to develop the skills with a number of combination methods of hemostasis to be used as and when required. There is no evidence that one device is best and safe in comparison to others.

31. Robotic Surgery in Gynecology

Q. Robotic surgery:
a. It is a facilitated laparoscopy having a computerized interface between patient and surgeon
b. From technologic point of view, robotic and laparoscopic surgery are the same
c. Robotic movements are intuitive
d. Learning curve for robotic surgery is long
e. Prior laparoscopic surgery skill is essential for robotic surgery.

Ans. a. T b. F
c. T d. F
e. F

Robotic technology facilitates the laparoscopic surgery with the use of a computer interface. Robotic technology enhances surgeon's ability with superior accuracy, dexterity, performance (suturing), shorter working times and reduces the number of complications compared to conventional laparoscopic surgery.[1]

TECHNOLOGY AND INSTRUMENTS USED IN ROBOTIC SURGERY

The surgeon controls the robotic arms with his two hands. Foot switches (five) to control are clutch, camera, focus, energy sources (monopolar and bipolar-cutting and coagulation).

Robotic technology: The surgeon sits at the console which is away from the patient. The assistant sits by the side of the patient. The stereoscopic view of robotic laparoscopy is different from laparoscopic image. Robotic system consists of a robotic column with robotic arms (Figs 31.1A to C) and a surgeon's console.

The robotic column has three or four robotic arms. The robotic arms work in a direction towards the robotic column. The robotic arms hold the robotic instruments with the robotic trocars (Figs 31.2A and B).

In gynecologic surgery, the robotic column placed between the patient's legs or lateral to the legs to get access to the vagina, rectum or urethra.

Docking: In robotic laparoscopic surgery docking is defined as the attachment of the robotic arms to the robotic trocars inserted in the patient. Mean docking time of about 3 minutes is observed and it is improved with progressive number of surgery.

Robotic laparoscopic surgery is especially useful in obese patients, surgery for gynecologic oncology—endometrial cancer, cervical cancer, retroperitoneal lymphadenectomy for advanced ovarian cancer and robotic pelvic exenteration operation.

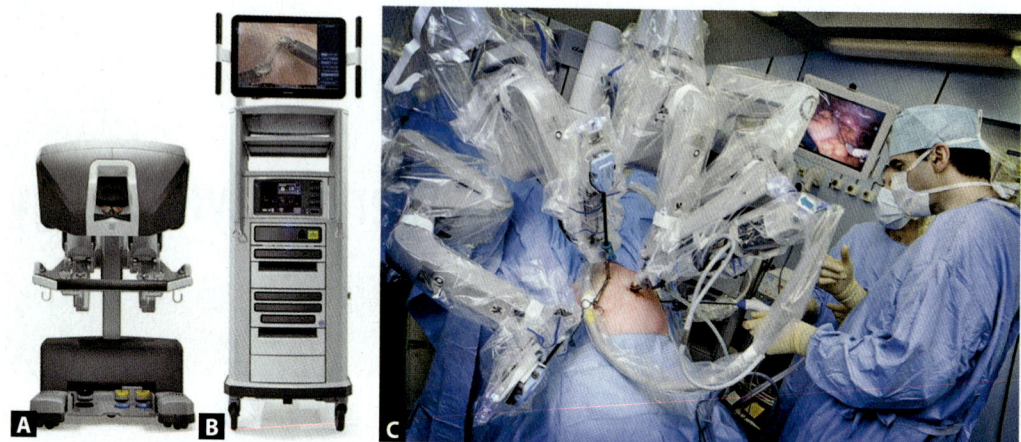

Figs 31.1A to C: A. Robotic console with foot pedals and the hand controls. Hand controls are used to manipulate the instruments and to move, rotate and focus the camera. The foot pedals are used to activate the energy sources and to move the camera, **B.** Telestration monitor, **C.** Robotic column: It is placed between the patient's legs while doing the pelvic surgery

Special advantages are: Operation time is similar compared to laparoscopic surgery, reduced blood loss, shorter hospital stay, higher number of lymph nodes removed and similar rate of postoperative complications. Tumor recurrence is not different compared to laparoscopic surgery.[1]

TECHNOLOGICAL AND OTHER ADVANTAGES OF ROBOTIC SURGERY

Advantages on the Part of the Surgeon

- **Surgeon** sits on the console, which is situated away from the operation site. He controls the robotic arms with hands and foot switches for camera and energy sources. Surgeon's arms and hands are in a comfortable position.
- **Docking** is the process of attaching the robotic arms to the robotic trocars inserted in the patient. One assistant sits with the patient in the theater. Assistant does the docking. The assistant is trained in robotics, so as to help the procedure (using vessel-sealing device, suction, irrigation) whenever needed.
- **Surgeon's morbidity** due to prolonged surgery (as observed in laparoscopy) is less.

Technological Advantages[2]

- Robotic image is stereoscopic (3D) which is different from laparoscopic view.
- Robotic movements are intuitive. The instrument tips are articulated such as to have seven degrees of movements. It mimics the movements of human wrist and fingers. So, any complex maneuver can be done within a limited space.[2]
- It helps suturing and intracorporeal knot tying with ease unlike that of laparoscopy.
- High precision and absence of tremor are of particular benefits in cases of ureteric anastomosis, fistula repair or retroperitoneal lymphadenectomy.

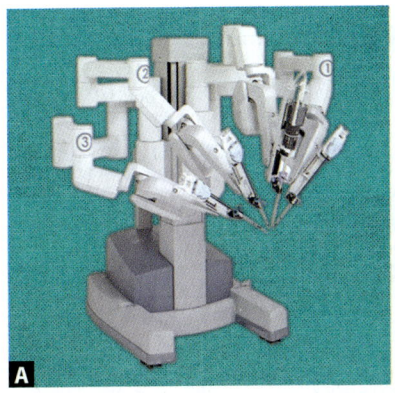 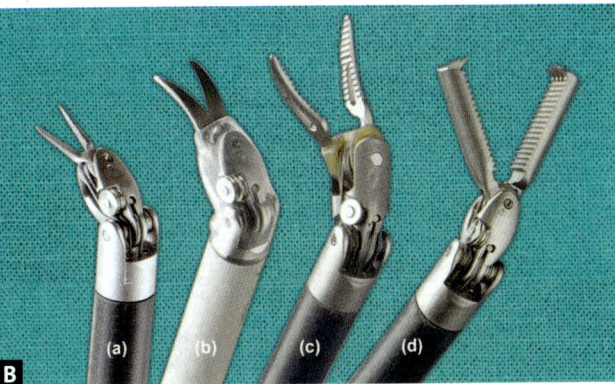

Figs 31.2A and B: A. Robotic column with robotic arms, **B.** Commonly used robotic instruments: (a) Maryland bipolar, (b) Hot shears, (c) Prograsp forceps (fenestrated), (d) Cobra grasper

The **third generation robotic system**, da Vinci Si model (2009), have a resident teaching console, where a trainee can learn robotic technology directly from the surgeon.
- Increased accuracy and enhanced dexterity are the distinct benefits compared to laparoscopic surgery.
- Robotic surgery has the benefits as the movements of the instrument tip are intuitive. In laparoscopic surgery, the movements are counter intuitive which is opposite to the movements of the surgeon's hands.
- Significant reduction in surgeon's morbidity and stress compared to laparoscopic surgery. In robotic surgery, the surgeon sits on a console whereas in laparoscopic surgery the surgeon stands in a strained position with hands and shoulders for a long time.

COMPLICATIONS OF ROBOTIC SURGERY

- Due to lack of tactile feedback, injury may occur to any organ unless done under visual control.
- Unwanted resistance due to collision of the robotic arms may occur.
- Prolonged pressure of the robotic arms on the patient's thighs or arms may cause injury.
- Sudden loss of pneumoperitoneum may result in pulling the instruments off the anterior abdominal wall. This is due to the fact that robotic trocars are fastened to the robotic arms and with that of robotic column.

DISADVANTAGES OF ROBOTIC SURGERY

- Robotic columns and its arms are heavy and risks of injury are there.
- Absence of tactile feedback.
- Repositioning of robotic column and arms when needed increases surgical time.
- Operating room must be spacious (6,000 sq feet or more) to accommodate equipments and the surgical team.
- The assistants must be versed with robotic surgery to comply with the required maneuvers, as the surgeon is away and sitting at the console.
- Cost (both initial or maintenance) is prohibitive for robotic programs.

LIMITATIONS OF LAPAROSCOPIC SURGERY

- Long-learning curve
- Long operative time
- Counterintuitive hand movements
- Limited degrees of instrument motion
- Ergonomic difficulty and there is tremor amplification.

OVERALL ADVANTAGES OF ROBOTIC SURGERY

- 3D visualization
- More accurate instrument movements
- Instrument movements mimics to complex hand movements
- Enhanced dexterity without tremor
- Faster suturing
- Shorter learning curve.

References

1. van der Schatte Olivier RH, Van't Hullenaar CD, Ruurda JP, et al. Ergonomics, user comfort, and performance in standard and robotic-assisted laparoscopic surgery. Surg Endosc. 2009;23(6):1365-71.
2. Pitter MC, Anderson P, Blissett A, et al. Robotic-assisted gynaecological surgery-establishing training criteria; minimizing operative time and blood loss. Int J Med Robot. 2008;4(2):114-20.

SECTION 5
Infertility and Assisted Reproductive Technology (ART)

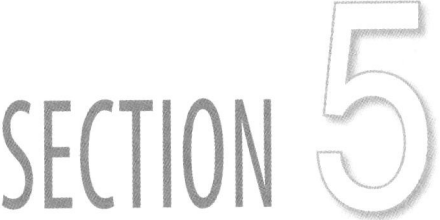

Section Outline

- Ch. 32. Current Concept in Physiology of Ovulation
- Ch. 33. Infertility Evaluation and Management
- Ch. 34. Female Infertility
- Ch. 35. Male Infertility
- Ch. 36. Assisted Reproductive Technology (ART)
- Ch. 37. Management Strategies for Low Responder Woman
- Ch. 38. Third Party Reproduction

32 Current Concept in Physiology of Ovulation

Q.1 Regarding folliculogenesis and ovulation:
a. Follicular development and differentiation takes about 85 days
b. Anti-Müllerian hormone (AMH) supports monofollicular development
c. First phase of follicular growth (60 days) is gonadotropin sensitive
d. Elevated and static level of estradiol is essential for ovulation
e. Menstrual cycle and ovulatory cycle are the same.

Ans.
a. T b. T
c. F d. F
e. F

GERM CELL MIGRATION AND POPULATION IN THE GONADS

Germ cells are endodermal in origin. The germ cells migrate from the yolk sac to the genital ridge along the dorsal mesentery between 30 days and 40 days. The germ cells undergo a number of rapid mitotic divisions and differentiate into oogonia. The number of oogonia reaches its maximum at 20th week numbering about **7 million**. The mitotic division gradually ceases and majority enter into the prophase of first meiotic division and are called ***primary oocytes***. These cells when surrounded by flattened granulosa cells, are called ***primordial follicles***. At birth, there is no more mitotic division and all the oogonia are replaced by primary oocytes. The estimated number of primary oocytes, at birth is about **2 million. At puberty**, some **400,000** primary oocytes are left behind, the rest become atretic. During the entire reproductive period, ***some 400*** are likely to ovulate. Germ cells degeneration start in intrauterine life and it continues throughout the childhood and the childbearing period. As a result, only few follicles with ova can be detected in menopausal women.

The phases of follicular growth, maturation and ovulation are discussed under the following heads.

Folliculogenesis:
- Follicular growth and maturation
- Emergence of dominant follicle (DF) and ovulation
- Follicular atresia
- Endocrine (estradiol) control of ovulation
- Difference in menstrual cycle and ovulatory cycle

- Events in ovulatory cycle
  - Endocrine
  - Biophysical.
- Events in nonovulatory cycle.

Follicular Growth and Atresia

Follicular growth and atresia is a continuous process, from intrauterine life to the age of menopause. This process is not interrupted by pregnancy, ovulation or by combined oral contraceptive therapy.

Initial recruitment, growth and development of primordial follicles are not under the control of any hormone (including gonadotropins). It is dependent upon a variety of factors that are produced locally (autocrine and paracrine mechanism). These are transforming growth factor β (TGF-β) subfamily of proteins, activins, inhibins, growth hormone and AMH.[1]

After a certain stage (>2 mm in size), the growth and differentiation of primordial follicles are under the control of follicle-stimulating hormone (FSH). Unless the follicles are rescued by FSH at this state, they undergo atresia. FSH also induces luteinizing hormone (LH) receptors on the granulosa cells of the DF.

Follicular Growth, Maturation and Emergence of Dominant Follicle

The cohort of growing follicles undergoes a process of development and differentiation which takes about 85 days and it spreads over 3 ovarian cycles. It is not clear as to how many and which of the primordial follicles amidst several thousands are recruited in a particular cycle. It is presumed that about 20 antral follicles (around 5–10 per ovary) proceed to develop in each cycle.

The cohort of follicles are recruited after puberty, as they become sensitive to gonadotropins. It is presumed that growth hormone (GH), insulin growth factor-I (IGF-I), androgen and also some other unknown growth factors play their role to make the follicles sensitive to gonadotropins. The cohort of follicles are recruited during last 20 days out of the total 85 days (3 ovarian cycles) of follicular growth and differentiation.

Each of these primordial follicles will compete for maturation under the influence of pituitary gonadotropins. Ultimately one will be successful for final maturation, leading to ovulation. The rest of the follicles will undergo the process of atresia beginning on D8.

Process of follicular growth and maturation: Primordial follicle → primary follicle → preantral follicle → antral follicle → preovulatory phase of Graafian follicle → final maturation and ovulation (Fig. 32.1).

Every 80 days cohort of follicles are recruited under the influence of GH, IGF-1 and androgens. Time interval from follicular recruitment, maturation, atresia or final phase of ovulation, is nearly

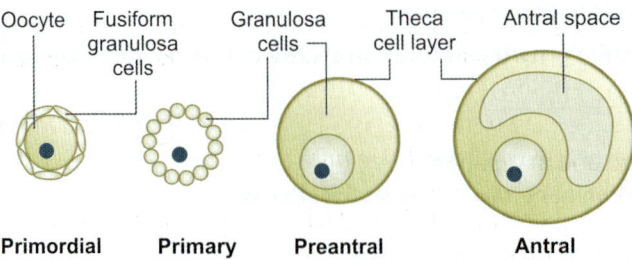

Fig. 32.1: Phases of follicular growth and maturation

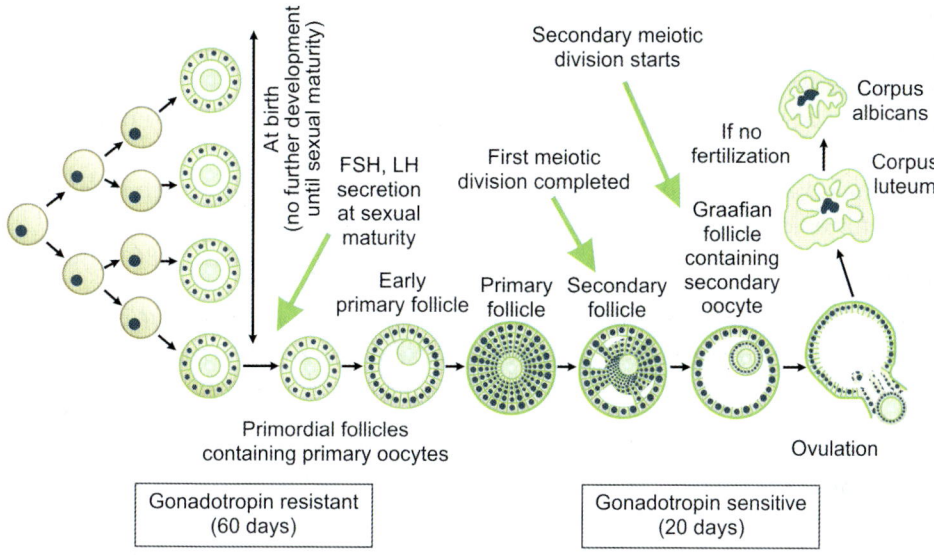

Fig. 32.2: Follicular growth-gonadotropin sensitivity-maturation and ovulation
Abbreviations: FSH—follicle-stimulating hormone, LH—luteinizing hormone

80 days. The entire process is divided into first phase of gonadotropin resistance (60 days) and second phase of gonadotropin sensitivity (20 days), coinciding with the late luteal phase of previous cycle (Fig. 32.2).

Role of AMH in follicular development: AMH inhibits initial recruitment of primordial follicles into the pool of growing follicles. It also decreases responsiveness of follicles to FSH. AMH plays an important role for monofollicular development and ovulation. It also prevents premature depletion of the follicular pool.

The probable mechanisms for monofollicular development and ovulation:
- All the primordial follicles that reach the preantral stage, produce AMH.
- AMH inhibits further growth of primordial follicles by decreasing the responsiveness of follicles to FSH.
- The growth of DF is however uninhibited as the DF has maximum number of FSH receptors, and it produces less AMH.
- Usually only one DF grows to maturity rest become atretic.

Endocrine Control of Ovulation

The primary endocrine control of ovulation is through estradiol (E2). Neither the pituitary nor the hypothalamus has the primary role, though estradiol is the outcome of hypothalamic-pituitary ovarian axis function.

The cyclicity of ovulation and menstruation depends upon the following sequence endocrine events where **estradiol (E2) plays the dominant role:**
- Estradiol level must decline in the late luteal phase.
- Estradiol level must rise in the midmenstrual or midfollicular phase.
- Follicular microenvironment must be E2 dominant (follicular androgens must be converted to estrogen with the help of enzyme aromatase).

As early as days 5–7, one follicle out of so many, becomes dominant and undergoes further maturation. The granulosa cells of the DF have the maximum number of FSH receptors. The rest of the follicles become atretic by D8.

The selection of DF depends primarily on FSH. However, the FSH action is modulated by autocrine and paracrine action of many other factors.

Basically the selection of dominant follicle is explained under the two categories of supports:
1. **Gonadotropic axis support:** FSH, LH, E2, inhibin, activin and AMH.
2. **Somatotropic axis support** is GH, IGF-I, sex hormone binding globulin (SHBG), insulin growth factor binding protein (IGFBP) and TGF-β.

Therefore, **when analyzed critically, the menstrual cycle and ovulatory (follicular growth, maturation, ovulation and atresia) cycle are not the same but are different to some extent.** This understanding is essential for the management of dysovulatory subfertility.

Menstrual Cycle and Ovulatory Cycle

- **Menstrual cycle:** Begins on D1 of the preceding cycle and ends on D1 of the subsequent cycle
- **Ovulatory cycle:** Begins on the late luteal phase (D21–D28) of the preceding menstrual cycle and ends in the early luteal period of the existing cycle.

The entire period of ovulatory cycle can be divided into five distinct phases:
1. Late luteal (postovulatory: D21–D28) phase
2. Early follicular phase (menstrual: D1–D4)
3. Midfollicular phase (D5–D6)
4. Late follicular phase (D7–D14)
5. Early luteal (D15–D21)

Important sequence of events in the late luteal phase are:
- Decline in E2 level
- Decline in inhibin level
- Rise in FSH level
- Recruitment of fresh follicles.

Endocrinological and Biophysical Events in the three Different Follicular Phases of an Ovulatory Cycle

Early follicular phase	
Endocrinologic events	**Biophysical events**
Adequate FSH level →	▪ Follicular growth
	▪ Proliferation of granulosa cells
	▪ Induction of receptors for FSH followed by LH
	▪ Aromatase activity
Optimum LH →	E2 synthesis and further follicular growth
Midfollicular phase	
▪ Rise in E2 levels	▪ Recruitment of dominant and co-dominant follicles
▪ Decline in FSH levels (negative feedback of rising E2)	▪ Induction of LH receptors in the granulosa cells of the dominant follicle by FSH
▪ Rise in LH levels than FSH	▪ Follicles become more LH responsive

Important events for selection of dominant follicle (in midfollicular phase) are:
- ***Estrogen dominant follicular microenvironment*** (privileged follicle).
- ***Induction of LH receptors*** in the granulosa cells of the DF. Luteinizing hormone receptor induction is essential for (i) midcycle LH surge to induce ovulation, (ii) luteinization of the granulosa cells to form corpus luteum[2] and (iii) secretion of progesterone.
- ***Rise in estradiol levels***—establishing negative feedback effect on FSH (suppression). This results in less competent follicles to undergo atresia. The additional events are:

Late follicular phase	
Endocrinologic events	**Biophysical events**
■ Peak and plateau levels of E2	■ Growth of dominant follicle(s)
■ Rise in LH level and its surge	■ Complication of oocyte meiosis
■ Further decline in FSH level	■ Ovulation
	■ Luteinization of granulosa cells
	■ Secretion of progesterone

Important Endocrinological Events in the Process of Ovulation
- There is induction of LH receptors in the DF by FSH.
- There is shift of dominant follicular control from FSH to LH since the midfollicular phase.
- LH in the late follicular phase causes follicular atresia other than the DF. This keeps multifollicular ovulation and multiple pregnancy under check. Multiple pregnancy is common after induction of ovulation.
- LH surge occurs when E2 level reaches a peak (100 pg/follicle) and is sustained for 48–50 hours.
- Peak level of LH should be 75–100 ng/mL.
- Duration of LH surge is about 24 hours. It has a crescendo → peak → decrescendo pattern.
- Progesterone within the follicle inhibits oocyte maturation inhibitory factor (OMIF). This event initiates release of the first polar body. Thus, the oocyte becomes haploid and fertilizable.
- Actual process of ovulation is induced by perifollicular leucocyte activation. The leads to matrix dissolution by production of specific enzyme including plasminogen activator. Absence of the enzyme leads to luteinized unruptured follicle syndrome.
- Rise in estradiol (E2) in follicular phase is controlled by FSH (early) and by LH (late follicular phase) → peak (D10–D11) levels (100 pg/mature follicle) → plateau level of E2 for 48 hours → positive feedback on pituitary LH → LH surge (any time within next 48 hours) → ovulation (within next 34–36 hours).
- The basic prerequisite in ovulatory cycle is the fluctuating levels of E2. If for any reason, the E2 levels become static, anovulation is the rule [as in polycystic ovarian syndrome (PCOS)].
- Attenuated LH surge may lead to ovulation with a dysmature egg. This egg is unsuitable for fertilization.
- Unscheduled LH surge (when the granulosa cells are not yet matured), leads to premature luteinization of granulosa cells and release of a 'progeric' egg. This egg is unsuitable for fertilization.
- Premature luteinization of granulosa cells leads to defective formation of corpus luteum. This makes the luteal phase defective.
- Androgenized follicular microenvironment leads to follicular atresia (as in PCOS).

Events in Nonovulatory Cycle

Static levels of estradiol → tonic stimulation of hypothalamus → release of tonic (levels) of luteinizing hormone-releasing hormone (LHRH) → more LH than FSH secretion → elevated but static levels estrogen (E2) → an ovulation (characteristic of PCOS).

Ovary, secreting the fluctuating level of estrogen (E2), is considered the band master of endocrine orchestra for a normal ovulatory cycle. When levels of E2 become static anovulation is the sequelae.

Events Leading to Failure of Ovulation

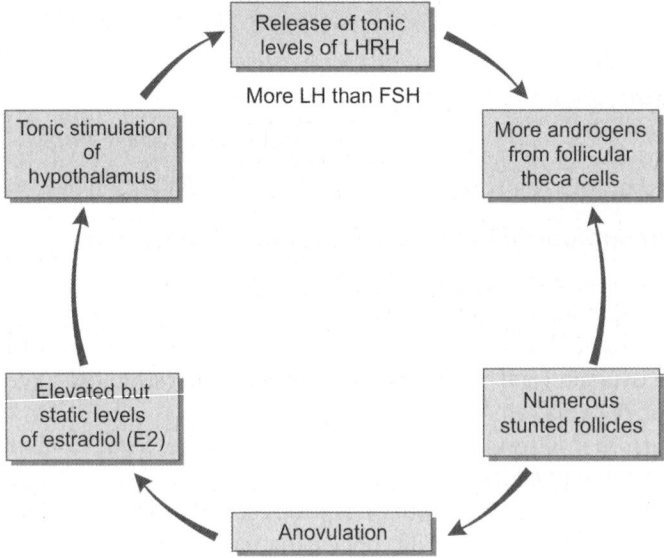

Abbreviations: LHRH—luteinizing hormone-releasing hormone, LH—luteinizing hormone, FSH—follicle-stimulating hormone

References

1. Demura R, Suzuki T, Tajima S, et al. Human plasma free activin and inhibin levels during the menstrual cycle. J Clin Endocrinol Metab. 1993;76(4):1080-2.
2. Anasti JN, Kalantaridou SN, Kimzey LM, et al. Human follicule fluid vascular endothelial growth factor concentrations are correlated with luteinization in spontaneously developing follicles. Hum Reprod. 1998;13(5):1144-7.

33. Infertility Evaluation and Management

INTRODUCTION

Infertility is a medical as well as social problem. Infertility does not cost life. But it perpetuates a devastating emotional and social trauma on the couple. Ultimately, it results in dissatisfaction, dejection and despair in the couple.

During the last two and a half decades, there has been a marked increase in the prevalence of infertility world over and so also in India. Overall incidence of infertility in India is 15–20%.

Broadly infertility can be classified under the following types

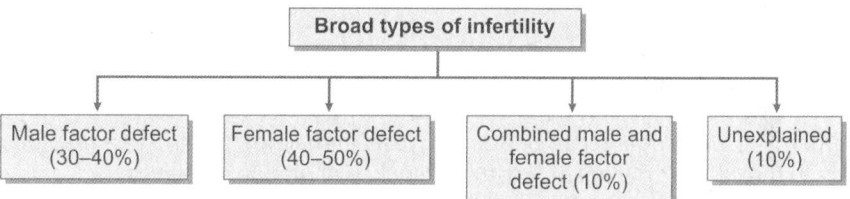

EVALUATION OF INFERTILE COUPLES

Basic Parameters for Evaluation of an Infertile Couple

- **Inspection:** Female partner: Obesity, hirsutism, acne → Polycystic ovarian syndrome (PCOS)
  Male partner: Scanty or absence of mustache and beard, presence of gynecomastia → Klinefelter's syndrome.
- **Interrogation**
  - Female partner
  - Male partner
  - Both the partners

  Female partner menstrual history
  - Amenorrhea
  - History of mumps, sexually transmitted infections (STIs)
  - Oligomenorrhea

  Male sexual dysfunction
  - Loss of erection
  - History of orchitis, STIs
  - Loss of libido

- **Examination of both the partners**

  Female partner
  - General physical examination
  - Systemic examination
  - Pelvic examination

  Male partner
  General and systemic examination and examination of genitalia— penis, urethra, testis (volume), epididymis and the vas

- **Basic Investigations**
  - Semen analysis
  - Ovulation detection/confirmation
  - Assessment of
    - Tubal patency
    - Tuboperitoneal factors (endometriosis)
    - Ovarian reserve (if history suggests see Manual of Obstetrics and Gynecology for the Postgraduates p. 372).

Following clinical evaluation, all infertile couples are broadly categorized into three groups:

1. **Easily treatable conditions**
   - **Female partner:** Ovulation dysfunction, tough hymen, mild endometriosis
   - **Male partner:** ▪ Mild oligospermia ▪ Phimosis

2. **Not easily treatable conditions**
   - **Female partner**
     - Premature ovarian failure, pelvic adhesions due to tuberculosis
     - Advanced pelvic endometriosis, uterine synechiae
   - **Male partner**
     - Azoospermia
     - Asthenospermia/teratospermia.

   There may be **multiple defects** in one or both the partners. Examples are—seminal defect (male partner) with tubal block or adenomyosis (female partner). There may be multiple defects in the one partner again, e.g. tubal block with uterine synechiae.

3. **Unexplained infertility (See Manual of Obstetrics and Gynecology for the Postgraduates p. 379):** Couples having apparently no defect, in either partner, based on basic evaluation parameter, belong to the unexplained group of infertility. Prognosis of these couples is somewhat better as compared to other two groups mentioned before.[1] However, better prognosis is expected provided (a) age of the female partner <35 years, (b) duration of infertility is <7 years, and (c) menstrual cyclicity is regular.

   Women having regular cyclical periods seldom suffer from ovulatory dysfunction, whereas women having delayed periods or having oligoamenorrheic cycles, usually have anovulation or oligoovulation. This is the common presentation of woman having polycystic ovarian syndrome (PCOS). (See Manual of Obstetrics and Gynecology for the Postgraduates p. 323).

PATIENT CATEGORIZATION AND MANAGEMENT PROTOCOL

Five types of treatment options are available:
1. Medical
2. Surgical
3. Assisted reproductive technology (ART)
4. **Combination treatment:** (a) Surgical and medical, (b) surgical followed by ART, (c) medical followed by ART, and if nothing works
5. Adoption.

Medical treatment: Women with PCOS or with unexplained infertility may be benefitted with induction of ovulation (clomiphene citrate).

Surgical treatment: Surgery for improvement of infertility may be:
- ***Obligatory:*** As in cases with narrow introitus (Fenton's operation), uterine synechiae (hysteroscopic adhesiolysis), fibroid uterus where no other cause for infertility present (myomectomy—laparoscopy/laparotomy).
- ***Complementary:*** Laparoscopic ablation of endometriotic implants, ovarian drilling (LOD) or hysteroscopic septal resection.

Combination of therapy may improve the results of infertility.

Surgical (laparoscopic) and/or medical (long-acting GnRH-A) treatment of advanced endometriosis may be effective. Similarly, ART preceded by surgical or medical treatment is more rational for fertility restoration in advanced stages of endometriosis.[2]

Summary: Infertility management protocol should be outlined based on the cause(s). Judicious planning may help in achieving an acceptable outcome.

Management Options for Couples with Multiple Defects

Corrections of multiple defects are seldom successful. Prospect of achieving spontaneous pregnancy is remote in such a couple having multiple defects. The options available for them are:
- ART with or without gamete donation (*See* Manual of Obstetrics and Gynecology for the Postgraduates p. 388).
- Surrogacy or (*See* Manual of Obstetrics and Gynecology for the Postgraduates p. 400).
- Adoption.

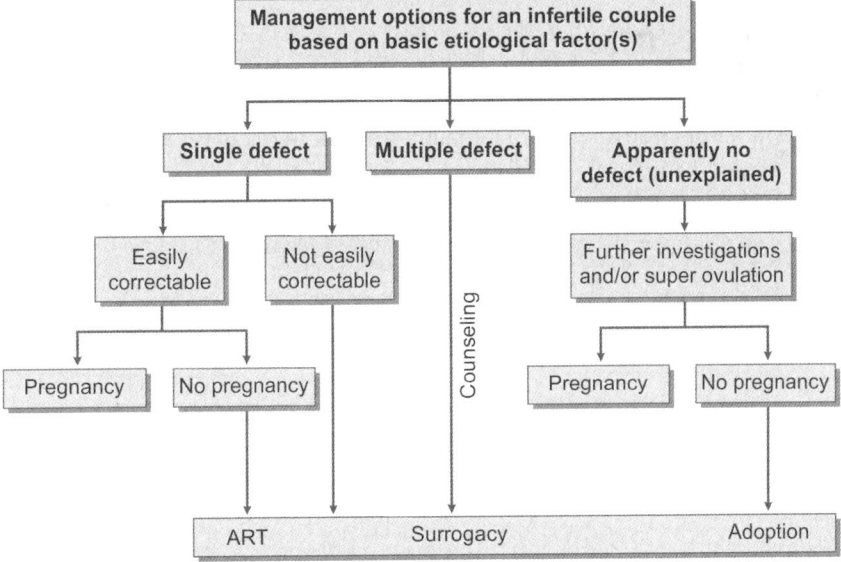

References

1. Practice Committee of the American Society for Reproductive Medicine. Effectiveness and treatment for unexplained infertility. Fertil Steril. 2006;86(5 Suppl 1):S111-4.
2. Jacobson TZ, Duffy JM, Barlow D, et al. Laparoscopic surgery for subfertility associated with endometriosis. Cochrane Database Syst Rev. 2010;1:CD001398.

34. Female Infertility

Q.1 *Regarding female infertility:*
  a. Antral follicle count >6 using TVS indicates adequate ovarian reserve
  b. High levels of AMH indicates poor ovarian reserve
  c. Abnormal endometrial perfusion may be a factor for unexplained infertility
  d. Premature LH surge results in poor quality of oocyte
  e. In ART cycle, younger the patient more the number (>3) of embryo to be transferred

Ans. a. T   b. F
         c. T   d. F
         e. F

OVULATORY DISORDERS

Nearly 30–40% of infertile women suffer from the problem of ovulatory dysfunction.
Ovulatory dysfunction may be due to: (a) failure to release (ovulate) an egg, or (b) inability to produce fully matured eggs.

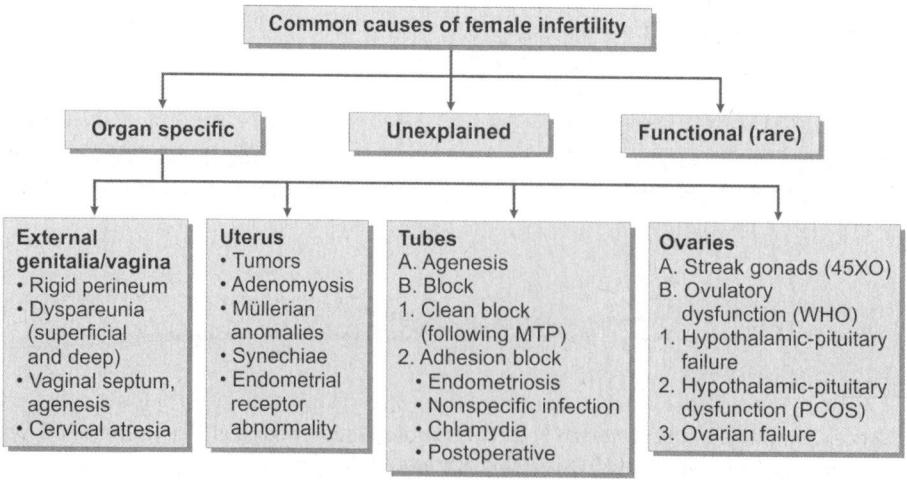

(*See* Dutta's Textbook of Gynecology, 7th Edition p. 188)

Classification of Ovulatory Disorders (WHO)
- Hypogonadotropic hypogonadism (hypothalamic-pituitary failure)
- Hypothalamic-pituitary dysfunction
- Hypergonadotropic hypogonadism—premature ovarian failure (POF).

Women need to be evaluated for the underlying pathology causing anovulation. Unless the underlying pathology is detected and corrected the main problem of ovulatory dysfunction could not be overcome even by therapy. The common underlying pathologies are:
- Thyroid dysfunction both (a) hypothyroidism, (b) hyperthyroidism
- Hyperprolactinemia
- Weight disorders: (a) Excessive weight loss, (b) Excessive weight gain (obesity)
- Polycystic ovarian syndrome (PCOS)
- Pituitary tumor
- Adrenal disease
- Galactorrhea.

Physiology of Ovarian Cycle in Menstruation and Ovulation

Principle events are
- ***Recruitment of a group of follicles:*** It takes about 85 days for a group of primordial follicles (15–20) to grow.
- ***Selection of dominant follicle:*** Out of so many follicles rescued by FSH, dominant follicle is the one that has the maximum number of FSH receptors and has the dominant estrogenic follicular micro-environment (high estradiol: androgen ratio).
- ***Ovulation:*** Sustained high level of estradiol along with LH surge principally triggers ovulation.
- ***Formation of corpus luteum:*** Once conception occurs, there is luteal-placental shift (8–10 weeks). Thereafter, secretion of progesterone continues from the placenta.

Fertile window: It is the 6 days interval ending on the day of ovulation (not after ovulation). Sperm survive up to 2–3 days in normal cervical mucus, but eggs survive for less than 24 hours. Generally a woman remains fertile between D10 and D17 of the menstrual cycle. Daily intercourse, during the window period, increases the probability of pregnancy.

Ovulatory disorders may be due to:
- Anovulation (complete absence of ovulation)
- Oligoovulation (infrequent ovulation).

Women having abnormal menstrual history (amenorrhea, oligomenorrhea, polymenorrhea or dysfunctional uterine bleeding) often suffer from ovulatory dysfunction. Successful treatment of ovulatory disorders depends on the correct identification of the underlying pathology for anovulation.

Management of Ovulatory Disorders

Hypogonadotropic Hypogonadism

(WHO Category–1)
This group of women is associated with (H-P failure) low level of serum FSH, LH and estradiol. Common causes of hypogonadotropic hypogonadism are: (a) Pituitary adenomas, (b) Craniopharyngioma and other factors like, (c) stress, anorexia, excessive exercise, extreme weight loss (BMI < 16 kg/m^2) or congenital hypothalamic failure—Kallmann syndrome.

Investigations
- Serum levels of FSH, LH, GnRH and serum estradiol are estimated.
- MRI study is done for the detection of central nervous system pathology.

Management issues: Single most important and effective treatment for this group of women with low BMI (<16 kg/m^2) is counseling and to encourage weight gain with good diet and nutrition.

Leptin is deficient in such women suffering from anorexia and exercise induced amenorrhea. Exogenous leptin restores ovulation in these women.[1]

Pulsatile GnRH every 60–90 minutes stimulates ovarian physiology for ovulation. Success rate of pulsatile GnRH therapy is high (90%). The added advantages are incidence of monofollicular development and the low subsequent risk of ovarian hyperstimulation syndrome (OHSS). The multiple pregnancy rates are also low. Exogenous gonadotropin (FSH and LH) can also be used for induction of ovulation as GnRH is not easily available.

Hypergonadotropic Hypogonadism (Premature Ovarian Insufficiency or Failure) (WHO Category-3)

Women's age and fertility: Age is an important determinant as fertility declines with advancing age. Many women are getting married in late 30s or early 40s. However, significant decline occurs in oocyte quality and quantity as the women enters late 30s, though it begins in early 30s. Primary ovarian insufficiency (failure) is the cessation of ovarian function prior to the age of 40 years. It is characterized by primary or secondary amenorrhea with elevated serum gonadotropin levels. However, ovarian failure is fortunately is a rare entity. Premature ovarian failure could be due to several reasons.

Causes of premature ovarian insufficiency (failure)
- Abnormal chromosomal pattern (45XO Turner, 47XXX) causing accelerated follicular atresia
- Pure gonadal dysgenesis
- Infections (HIV, mumps, tuberculosis)
- Iatrogenic: Radiation, chemotherapy, surgery (oophorectomy, excessive ovarian drilling)
- Metabolic: Galactosemia
- Autoimmune disorders (polyglandular autoimmune syndrome)
- However, 5–10% of women with POF achieve pregnancy and deliver successfully.

This indicates, women should be assessed for ovarian reserve before planning management.

ASSESSMENT OF OVARIAN RESERVE

Ovarian reserve tests are to assess the quantity as well as the quality of primordial follicles present in the women's ovary. These tests are done to determine how the ovaries will respond to therapy (ovulation induction). In other words, it is the assessment of the reproductive potential of the woman.

The tests are:
- **Estimation of basal level of serum FSH** on D3 and again on D10 following clomiphene citrate challenge test (CCCT): 100 mg orally each day from D5–D9: values >10 IU/L (more than 2SD) indicates poor ovarian reserve.
- **Basal (D3) serum estradiol level** > 70–80 pg/mL, poor ovarian reserve.
- **Serum inhibin B (D5):** Reduced inhibin B levels (less than 40 pg/mL) are observed in woman with advanced age.

- **Serum anti-Müllerian hormone (AMH):** Levels of serum AMH is a good predictor of ovarian stimulation response. Its level also comes with the direct proportion of antral follicle count (AFC). Levels of AMH (1 ng/mL) declines with age and with poor ovarian reserve. Levels of AMH can be measured any time in the menstrual cycle.

AMH: It is produced by the granulosa cells of the preantral small follicles. Serum levels of estradiol and inhibin B depend on pituitary FSH feedback mechanism. Level of AMH is not dependent on feedback mechanism. This is one of the reasons for which AMH is being considered as a better predictor of ovarian reserve compared to estradiol and inhibin B. Levels of AMH can be measured at anytime in the menstrual cycle. Therefore, understood that AMH is qualitative whereas AFC is a quantitative marker of ovarian reserve.

AFC is done by using TVS in early follicular phase in both the ovaries. AFC more than 7 (2–10 mm size) reflects adequate ovarian follicular reserve. AFC decreases with age. AFC reflects the primordial follicle pool in the ovary. AFC, less than 4 indicates poor ovarian reserve and there is poor response to ovarian stimulation (IVF).

Management Options for Ovarian Insufficiency
(WHO Category–3)
- **Chance of conception from autologous cycles is remote** though spontaneous recovery of ovarian function (5–10%) and pregnancy has been reported.
- **Pretreatment with high dose estrogen and progesterone** or gonadotropin releasing hormone agonist (GnRH agonist) followed by ovulation induction with clomiphene or exogenous gonadotropins.
- **Pretreatment with corticosteroids** followed by induction ovulation with exogenous gonadotropins.
- **Therapy with dehydroepiandrosterone (DHEA)**: 25 mg three times daily for 5–6 months is thought to increase oocyte pool and successful pregnancy.
- *In vitro fertilization (IVF)* is an option with autologous oocyte, whenever available.
- Women in this group have few follicles left, which are unresponsive to chronically elevated levels of FSH. The above mentioned treatment regimens suppress the elevated level of FSH. The follicles are then reactivated with induction of new receptors. These receptors then respond to stimulation protocols for folliculogenesis and ovulation.
- **IVF with donor's oocyte** may be an option.
- **IVF and embryo transfer.**
- **Adoption.**

Hypothalamic-pituitary Dysfunction
(WHO Category–2)
Hypothalamic-pituitary dysfunction: Polycystic ovarian syndrome (PCOS) is the most common cause of ovulatory dysfunction.

Diagnostic criteria of PCOS (Rotterdam ESHRE/ASRM-2004)[2]
- Oligo-ovulation or anovulation (clinically presenting as oligomenorrhea or amenorrhea)
- Hyperandrogenemia (clinical and/or biochemical)
- Polycystic ovarian changes (other etiologies of hyperandrogenism like androgen secreting tumors, congenital adrenal hyperplasia) are to be excluded.

Presence of any two of the three above mentioned conditions fulfill the diagnostic criteria of PCOS.

Emphasis is given on the **far reaching consequences** of PCOS in all ages.
Two significant long-term consequences are:
1. **Metabolic syndrome**
   ♦ Diabetes
   ♦ Dyslipidemia—mostly in insulin resistant PCOS women
   ♦ Hypertension (cardiovascular and coronary artery disease).
2. **Thrombophilic syndrome**
   ♦ Coronary artery disease
   ♦ Recurrent miscarriages.

Management Issues in PCOS (irrespective of age)
- Early detection and prevention
- Change in lifestyle
- Calorie restriction
- Weight reduction.

Weight loss is essential while intending for fertility improvement. Weight loss can be achieved by exercise, decreased calorie consumption and lifestyle modification. Weight loss can also be achieved by pharmacologic agents and/or by surgery.

Significant **biochemical abnormalities** observed in PCOS are: Hyperinsulinemia (insulin resistance), hyperandrogenemia, hyperprolactinemia, hyperglycemia, hyperlipidemia, hypersecretion of LH and low serum SHBG levels. **Management of women PCOS can be optimized under three groups**—mild, moderate and severe, depending on their clinical, biophysical and biochemical presentation.

Group A (mild): Usually, these women are nonobese (normal BMI) and nonhirsute. Often they have delayed menstrual cycle. USG reveals ovarian size either normal or slightly enlarged but there is no thecal hyperplasia.

Management options: These groups respond well with clomiphene citrate. Depending upon the other investigations, they may need adjuvant therapy like bromocriptine, eltroxin or dexamethasone.

Group B (moderate): These women present with features of mild hirsutism (excess androgen levels) and mild obesity. Often these women suffer from oligomenorrhea. On transvaginal sonography (TVS), these women presents with enlarged ovaries with peripherally arranged cysts with stromal hyperplasia.

Management options
- Women still respond well with clomiphene citrate.
- However, better option for them is clomiphene citrate combined with insulin sensitizing agents like.
- **Metformin (oral biguanide)**, 500 mg three times a day for a period of 3–6 months.
- **Rosiglitazone (thiazolidinediones):** Rarely used, as it is a category 'C' drug in pregnancy.

Metformin acts by several mechanisms (*See* Manual of Obstetrics and Gynecology for the Postgraduates, p. 234).

Evidences are still lacking to support the therapy of metformin alone for ovulation induction. Combination of therapy of clomiphene with metformin is commonly recommended. There is no randomized control trial yet to support the continuation of metformin in pregnancy in women with PCOS in order to prevent miscarriage. However, metformin unlike thiazolidinedione group (rosiglitazone) appears safe when used during pregnancy especially in women with gestational diabetes mellitus (GDM). It is particularly recommended in patients with glucose intolerance. Metformin in this group of women, has been shown to improve ovulation rate though clinical pregnancy rate remains same.

Group C (Severe): These women are typically obese (BMI >25), stocky build. They have the family history of diabetes mellitus, they often suffer from secondary amenorrhea. They also present with the features of HAIR–AN syndrome. HAIR–AN syndrome is characterized by—hyperandrogenemia, insulin resistance and acanthosis nigricans. Transvaginal ultrasonography reveals—typical PCOS changes and ovarian stromal hyperplasia.

Management: Besides the general management issues, the specific management options for induction of ovulation are:
- Insulin sensitizing agents
- Clomiphene citrate plus metformin
- Insulin sensitizing agent plus ovarian drilling
- Aromatase inhibitors (letrozole, anastrozole) off label use for induction of ovulation in clomiphene resistant women proved successful in 66–80%. Main concern with the use of letrozole is possible association of fetal congenital anomalies, though no such increased association has been observed when letrozole was compared with clomiphene citrate.[3] Physician should carry own responsibility when this drug is used (off label) with patient counseling.

Gonadotropin (hMG/FSH): Anovulatory PCOS women, who fail to ovulate with oral medications, may be considered for exogenous gonadotropins. Women need to be monitored carefully. Low initial dose of FSH are generally given. Ovulation triggering with hCG is given when one or two follicles are 16–18 mm diameter. A serum E2 level per mature follicle of 100–150 pg/mL is optimum for monitoring.[4]

Women with PCOS when treated with exogenous gonadotropin, run the high risk of multiple pregnancy (36%), OHSS (4.6%) and cycle cancellation (10%). These complications are due to high number of antral follicular development.

Sequential use of clomiphene or aromatase inhibitors and exogenous gonadotropins is an alternative to avoid the complications of gonadotropin use. Combined treatment of GnRH agonist for down regulation followed by exogenous gonadotropins (hMG/FSH) is an alternative. The regimen may overcome the problems of premature luteinization of ovarian follicle and inadequate luteal phases.[5] Women with PCOS may also require IVF.

Surgical treatment: Women with clomiphene resistant PCOS can be treated surgically by ovarian drilling. This surgical procedure reduces the ovarian androgen production and promotes ovulation. This procedure also minimizes the complications of exogenous gonadotropin therapy (multiple gestation and OHSS). Usually, laparoscopic drilling is done at 3–10 sites per ovary using electrodiathermy or laser. Results are similar to the use of exogenous gonadotropins. Cumulative ovulation rate within one year following laparoscopic ovarian drilling (LOD) is 52%. However, patients should be carefully selected for ovarian drilling.

Current Research and Management Options for Women with PCOS

Women who fail to respond with conventional management may be considered for other modes of therapy.
- Collection of immature oocytes using TVS
- *In vitro* maturation of these immature oocytes using an appropriate media
- Freezing the immature oocytes for future use.

Summary of Management Options for Women with PCOS

- ***First line management*** may be clomiphene citrate with or without adjuvant therapy insulin sensitizing agents.

- **Clomiphene resistant women** may be treated with exogenous gonadotropins with or without down regulation.
- **Surgical management:** LOD is an effective alternative in clomiphene citrate (CC) resistant cases. It is as effective as exogenous gonadotropins and has less complications compared to gonadotropins.
- **Collection of immature oocytes** for *in vitro* maturation and freezing for future use are the currently available options.

TUBAL FACTORS FOR INFERTILITY

Tubal factor is responsible for 25–40% of infertile women.
The common causes tubal blocks are:
- Pelvic infections (PID) due to (a) *C. trachomatis, N. gonorrhoea* (b) Tuberculosis, (c) Salpingitis isthmica nodosa. Risk of tubal block is as high as 75% after three episodes of PID
- Tubal polyps
- Mucus debris
- Pelvic endometriosis
- Previous tubal surgery or sterilization
- Tubal endometriosis.

Incidence and severity of pathology for tubal block rise with each episode of pelvic infection
Tuberculous salpingitis: Genital tuberculosis is almost always secondary to systemic tuberculosis. Common primary sites are lungs, lymph nodes, bones or gastrointestinal tract. Tubal affection of tuberculosis is almost 100%. Tubercular endosalpingitis (most common), interstitial salpingitis and perisalpingitis may occur (see Fig. 34.1). Diagnosis of genital TB could be made by investigations for detection of systemic TB (*See* Dutta's Textbook of Gynecology, 7th Edition, p. 115). Menstrual blood or endometrial tissue for TBPCR has got high sensitivity (85–95%). Tissue biopsy with endometrium or laparoscopically obtained peritoneal tubercles can be made. Genital TB has got poor reproductive outcome even following treatment. Failure of implantation and increased miscarriage rates are the consequences. Risks of ectopic pregnancy are high even if they conceive. Following successful chemotherapy, pregnancy can be achieved with the help of assisted reproductive technology (ART).

Tubal Patency Tests

Side and site of tubal block can be diagnosed by hysterosalpingography, laparoscopic chromopertubation, falloposcopy or with sonohysterosalpingography (less invasive).

Management Options for Tubal Factors for Infertility

In view of progressive success rate of ART, the place of tubal reconstructive surgery is gradually becoming less and less. However, there may be few situations where tubal reconstructive surgery may have a place.
Proximal tubal block is may be due to tubal mucosal adhesions, amorphous debris, cornual fibroid, fibrosis due to tuberculosis or mucosal polyp. It may be overcome with tubal cannulation under hysteroscopic guidance. A soft cannula is passed into the tubal ostia and a guidewire passed through contrast media (dye) is injected. Tubal patency (spillage of dye) could be seen simultaneously with laparoscopy. Successful pregnancy rate of proximal tubal cannulation is 20–40%.

 Midtubal block is mainly due to tubal sterilization. Regret is not uncommon in India due to accidental death of all the children or that of the male child. Reversal of tubal sterilization can

be done by laparotomy or by laparoscopy either by naked eye or by microsurgical procedures. Pregnancy rates following microsurgical procedure of tubal reconstructive surgery is around 60–80%. Risk of ectopic pregnancy is high (10%). The success of tubal reversal procedure depends on the following issues:
- Site of anastomosis—isthmic-isthmic or ample-ampullary—better prognosis
- Lesser the interval between tubal sterilization and reversal procedure better the outcome
- Final reconstructed tubal length > 4 cm gives better result
- Lesser the tubal damage (use of rings or clips), better the outcome
- No other pelvic pathology.

Distal tubal block: It may be due to infection, adhesion formation with PID, endometriosis or previous surgery. Young patient with mild adhesions, normal tubal mucosa, may be considered for reconstructive surgery. Different surgical procedures are done depending on an individual patient. Tubal surgery may be—salpingolysis, adhesiolysis, salpingostomy, fimbrioplasty or resection-anastomosis.

Advantages of tubal surgery
- One time procedure
- Couple may attempt conception every month without further intervention
- May conceive more than once with a single surgery
- Avoid the risks of IVF like OHSS, multiple pregnancy.

Disadvantages of tubal surgery
- Surgical complications like infection, bleeding, anesthesia
- Risk of ectopic pregnancy
- Success depends significantly on surgeon's expertize.

Summary of tubal surgery
- Tubal surgery may be considered in young women after previous tubal sterilization or in women with mild disease at the distal tubal segment.
- Tubal surgery may tried for proximal tubal block (hysteroscopic tubal cannulation and balloon tuboplasty). Nearly 80% of cases obstruction can be relieved.
- In women having genital tuberculosis, surgery should be withheld. IVF-ET may be employed following antitubercular therapy when endometrium becomes free from disease.
- Elderly women (age >37 years) with tubal pathology should be considered for IVF.
- Women with complicated tubal occlusive disease are considered for IVF.
- *Hydrosalpinx:* IVF better option (following tubal clipping or salpingectomy).

IVF VERSUS REVERSAL OF TUBAL STERILIZATION

Intrauterine pregnancy rates following reversal of sterilization range between 31% and 92%. This is particularly high in women that they had been sterilized with microsurgical techniques.

IVF was originally developed to overcome the tubal factors for infertility. The success rate of IVF and ET on an average is 30–35% per IVF cycle (*See* Manual of Obstetrics and Gynecology for the Postgraduates, p. 122). In a women with intrauterine pregnancy following reversal of tubal sterilization, the rates of miscarriage and multiple pregnancy are lower compared to IVF. Ectopic pregnancy rates after surgical reversal (2–10%) are not acceptable. Women with age over 40 years, reversal of sterilization achieves a good intrauterine pregnancy (40–70%). It is about 90% in age (<40), whereas, success with IVF decreases after that age with a live birth rate of per treatment cycle is low (5.4%). Tubal anastomosis has significantly higher cumulative pregnancy rates for women <37 years compared to IVF, but no significant difference over 37 years.

PERITONEAL FACTORS FOR INFERTILITY (FIG. 34.1)

Endometriosis: Infertility management in women with endometriosis is complex. The pathophysiology of infertility in a woman with pelvic endometriosis has been (*See* Dutta's Textbook of Gynecology, 7th Edition, p. 189, 250) observed due to multiple factors. It is mainly due to anatomic distortions, adhesions, associated endocrinopathy, presence of inflammatory mediators having gametotoxic effects or due to implantation failure.

Laparoscopy remains the gold standard for the diagnosis of endometriosis. It has the added benefit of therapy at the same time.

Management options: Determinant factors for the management are: (1) Age of the patient, (2) Stage of the disease (ASRM), (3) Severity of symptoms, (4) Results of previous therapy and (5) Location of the disease.

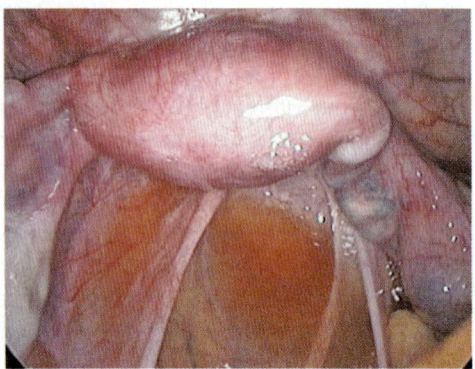

Fig. 34.1: Tuboperitoneal factors for infertility. A case of pelvic tuberculosis
Courtesy: Dr H Ray, Patna

Hormonal suppression of endometriosis has hardly any effect on the outcome of endometriosis related infertility.

Laparoscopy: Ablation of endometriotic implants, adhesiolysis in mild and minimal pelvic endometriosis can significantly improve pregnancy rates. Intrauterine insemination (IUI) with ovarian stimulation is effective to improve fertility in women with minimal to mild endometriosis. Laparoscopic treatment of moderate endometriosis including removal of endometrioma can improve fertility status.[6] Women may need ovulation induction with clomiphene citrate with or without exogenous gonadotropins. No randomized controlled trials or meta-analysis are available to support that surgical excision in cases with moderate to severe endometriosis, which enhances the pregnancy rates. However, majority of women with moderate to severe pelvic endometriosis are considered for IVF. Laparoscopic surgery is indicated prior to IVF as adhesions or endometrioma would interfere with oocyte retrieval.[7,8] IVF may be the option after laparoscopic surgery, as a first line therapy depending upon the individual woman. Controversy remains as regard the ovarian reserve following ovarian surgery for endometrioma. Most recent evidence suggests for direct IVF without prior surgery.

UTERINE FACTORS FOR INFERTILITY

Uterine factors may be associated with infertility in about 10–15% of cases. **The pathology responsible for infertility are**: Submucous fibroids, uterine synechiae, congenital uterine malformations (unicornuate uterus, uterine septum, bicornuate uterus or uterine agenesis) or uterine polyps.

Müllerian duct malformations may be responsible for infertility in about 10–37% of cases. These cases are often associated with urogenital malformations (40%). Müllerian malformations are also associated with recurrent early pregnancy loss.

Diagnosis of uterine cavity abnormalities can be made with hysteroscopy (gold standard), combined hysteroscopy and laparoscopy, hysterosalpingography, transvaginal ultrasonography,

(3D), sonohysterography or with magnetic resonance imaging (MRI). MRI is more informative compared to sonography for diagnosis of uterine malformations, fibroids and adenomyosis.

Management options: Surgical corrections improve obstetric outcome in few cases. Rudimentary horns are to be removed. Hysteroscopic metroplasty (septum resection) significantly improve the obstetric outcome.[9]

Submucosal myomas and interstitial myomas impair fertility due to several reasons (*See* Dutta's Textbook of Gynecology, 7th Edition, p. 225) and mainly due to distortion of the endometrial cavity and poor implantation. **Surgery**: Myomectomy (laparoscopic and/or hysteroscopic procedure) is recommended as a part of infertility treatment. Whether a myoma, not distorting the endometrial cavity, should be removed or not is not yet known.[10]

Uterine synechiae: Overzealous curettage damaging the basal layer of the endometrium results in uterine wall adhesion formation with subsequent development of fibrosis. Endometrial tuberculosis, myomectomy, cesarean section, all may have the similar effect and can cause intrauterine adhesions or Asherman's syndrome. Women usually give the history of surgical intervention. She usually presents with the problems of secondary amenorrhea, scanty period, secondary infertility or recurrent pregnancy loss. Diagnosis can be confirmed by hysterosalpingography or better with hysteroscopy. Intrauterine adhesions could be complete or partial.

Management: Adhesions could be released with hysteroscopic resection. Menstrual function and fertility status could be restored. Women suffering from synechiae due to endometrial tuberculosis usually have poor prognosis.

Postoperative management includes hormone therapy (estrogen and progesterone) for fresh endometrial growth. Combined therapy with hormones and placement of an IUCD to prevent re-adhesions may also be done. This therapy may be continued for 2–3 cycles.

UNEXPLAINED INFERTILITY

This group includes the couples in whom the basic infertility investigations have been completed and the reports revealed normal semen parameters, evidence of ovulation, patient fallopian tubes and there is no other obvious cause for infertility. Couples with unexplained infertility need counseling. They should be reassured that nearly 20% of such women will conceive in the next 12 months and over 50% in the next 36 months. **Nearly 10–20% of couples are diagnosed with unexplained infertility**.

Possible Explanations for Unexplained Infertility

- **Reduced endometrial vascularity:** Doppler ultrasound based studies have revealed that there is reduced and abnormal endometrial perfusion in women with unexplained infertility. However, no therapeutic approach has been made based on this observation as yet.
- **Unexplained male and female factors:** Sperm mitochondrial dysfunction, aberrant spindle formation or premature zona hardening are the areas thought to be responsible. However, these need further study.
- **Role of infection:** Subclinical endometrial infections have been thought for poor implantation. *Chlamydia trachomatis, M hominis, U urealyticum* infections may be associated. Prophylactic antibiotics (doxycycline 100 mg twice daily of 3–4 weeks) may be given to the couples with unexplained infertility. Prophylactic antimicrobial therapy is mostly given to couples before ART cycles.

- **Endometrial receptivity:** Besides reduced endometrial vascularity, endometrial receptivity including pinopode formation, biochemical expression of integrin and optimum endometrial genetic expression (HOXA genes) are thought to be inadequate in women with unexplained infertility.
- **Immunological:** Whether antisperm antibodies and other antibodies like antiphospholipid antibodies, antithyroid antibodies have any role, need further study. Till date no screening is recommended for this purpose.
- **Luteinized unruptured follicle (LUF) syndrome** is a known cause of infertility (20%) in women with unexplained infertility. In this condition, the follicle grows but undergoes luteinization before it ruptures and releases the oocyte. Mostly it can be diagnosed by transvaginal ultrasonography. These women should undergo IVF where follicles are aspirated. The oocytes are retrieved and fertilized *in vitro*.
- **Unexplained pelvic pathology:** Detection of undiagnosed pelvic endometriosis, adhesions may be made by laparoscopy. Whether the laparoscopic procedure has got any distinct advantage as a routine needs to be evaluated.

Management options for Unexplained Infertility

Young women are be counseled and advised for expectant management. However, some patients may need indepth investigations including laparoscopy. Women with unexplained infertility are treated stepwise as follows:
- With clomiphene citrate or letrozole (off label use) for 3–4 cycles
- Then exogeneous gonadotropins for 3–4 cycles
- Followed by IUI or ART (*See* Manual of Obstetrics and Gynecology for the Postgraduates, p. 389).

ART options for unexplained infertility include IVF and ICSI.

Baseline ovarian cyst: Baseline ultrasound scan is done on D2 or D3 of the cycle. Basal endometrium should be thin (< 4 mm) and the ovaries should be normal (without any cysts). Presence of functional ovarian cysts (> 2 cm) on baseline scan and baseline serum estradiol >80 pg/mL is associated with decreased pregnancy rate following ovulation induction with gonadotropins. Gonadotropin requirements are high. Embryo qualities are also poor.

Management: Pretreatment use of oral contraceptive prior to GnRH agonist cycle is associated with decreased rate of cyst formation.

Controlled ovarian stimulation (superovulation) is done to produce more than one egg for the purpose of either ART or non-ART cycles. This principle enhances the possibility of conception in women. Baseline USG scan is done on D2/D3 to assess the antral follicle count and to exclude the presence of any ovarian cysts. Clomiphene citrate and gonadotropins are started for induction of ovulation. In superovulation protocols, gonadotropins are started on D2/D3 of menses. The dose of gonadotropins are monitored each day until D6/D7 depending upon response. Thereafter, serum estradiol levels and TVS are done to monitor the ovarian response. Gonadotropin dose may need to be increased by 50–100 IU/day every 2–4 days until an optimum response is observed. Triggering of ovulation is done when at least two follicles of 17–18 mm diameter are seen and endometrial thickness is ≥ 8 mm. For non-ART cycles serum E2 and TVS are monitored. Cycle cancellation should be considered if serum E2 level of 1000–2500 pg/mL for 3 or more follicles of 16 mm or more, or ≥ 2 follicles of 16 mm size plus ≥ 2 follicles of 14 mm diameter or more are seen. **For ART (IVF) cycles ultrasound, monitoring alone of follicles are sufficient**.

Results: Pregnancy rates of unexplained infertility varies widely in studies. This may be due to heterogeneity in treatment protocols and also with patients' age. Overall pregnancy rates for

women with unexplained infertility with age < 40 years when grouped by treatment protocol are as follows:
- Clomiphene treatment protocol/IUI 10–12% per cycle
- Gonadotropins/IUI 15–20% per cycle
- IVF 30–35%.

Women with age ≥ 40 years should be offered IVF as a initial and early treatment option. ICSI may be a treatment option for these groups of women with unexplained infertility. ICSI improves fertilization rates. However, studies have shown no difference in pregnancy rates or live birth rate when treatment results of IVF and ICSI were compared. For management of women with unexplained infertility, optimum treatment options available are: Clomiphene/IUI for 3–4 cycles, failing which super ovulation regimen with IUI or they may be considered directly for IVF.

Luteal phase defect (LPD): During normal luteal phase adequate progesterone secretion by the corpus luteum is observed. This promotes adequate development of secretory endometrium for blastocyst implantation. *LPD is an inevitable phenomenon in all ART cycles.* Induction of ovulation using gonadotropins may cause LPD due to supraphysiological levels of estradiol along with GnRH agonist or antagonist therapy. LPD may cause implantation failure and is thought to account for 4% of infertility. Diagnosis of LPD is not based on uniform criteria. Low levels of midluteal serum progesterone (<5 ng/mL), endometrial histology >2 day out of phase or a shortened luteal phase <14 days are considered for the diagnosis.

Treatment for Luteal Phase Defect

Progesterone supplementation can be given via oral, intramuscular or vaginal route. Progesterone in a dose 25–50 mg daily IM is given. Micronized progesterone given orally has erratic absorption rate and decreased bioavailability. It is given best vaginally 200–600 mg daily. Vaginal and IM route has got similar effect. Progesterone therapy is begun 3–4 days following the hCG trigger or LH surge and it is continued for next 7–10 weeks, if pregnancy occurs. Role of progesterone therapy in a non-ART treatment cycle is not clear (Table 34.1).

Table 34.1: Patient categorization in terms of treatment outcomes

Parameters	Favorable	Unfavorable
Age	<37 years	>37 years
Duration of infertility	<7 years	>7 years
Type of defect	Single, treatable	Multiple, untreatable
Baseline FSH level	<10 mIU/mL	>10–12 mIU/mL
Basal antral follicle count	>6	<6
Pelvic adhesions/ chocolate cyst	Minimum or none	Dense
Uterine shape and size	Normal	Deformed/Distorted
Previous failed IVF	None	>3

References

1. Welt CK, Chan JL, Bullen J, et al. Recombinant human leptin in women with hypothalamic amenorrhea. N Engl J Med. 2004:351(10):987-97.

2. Rotterdam ESHRE/ASRM-Sponsored PCOS consensus workshop group. Revised 2003 consensus on diagnostic criteria and long-term health risks related to polycystic ovary syndrome (PCOS). Fertil Steril. 2004;81(1):19-25.
3. Tulandi T, Martin J, Al-Fadbli R, et al. Congenital malformations among 911 newborn conceived after infertility treatment with letrozole or clomiphene citrate. Fertil Steril. 2006;85(6):1761-5.
4. Kwan I, Bhattacharya S, Mc Neil A, et al. Monitoring of stimulated cycles in assisted reproduction (IVF and ICSI). Cochrane Database Syst Rev. 2008:(2);CD005289.
5. Lainas T, Zorzovilis J, Petsas G, et al. In a flexible antagonist protocol, earlier, criteria-based initiation of GnRH antagonist is associated with increased pregnancy rates in IVF. Hum Reprod. 2005;20(9):2426-33.
6. Vercellini P, Somigliana E, vigano P, et al. Surgery for endometriosis-associated infertility: A pragmatic approach. Human Reprod. 2009;24(2):254-69.
7. Giudice LC. Clinical Practice. Endometriosis. N Engl J Med. 2010;362(25):2389-98.
8. Jacobson TZ, Duffy JM, Barlow D, et al. Laparoscopic surgery for subfertility associated with endometriosis. Cochrane Database Syst Rev. 2010;1:CD001398.
9. Pritts EA, Parkar WH, Olive DL. Fibroids and infertility: An updated systematic review of the evidence. Fertil Steril. 2009;91(4):1215-23.
10. Sunkara SK, Khairy M, El-Toukhy T, et al. The effect of intramural fibroids without uterine cavity involvement on the outcome of IVF treatment: A systematic review and meta-analysis. Hum Reprod. 2010;25(2):418-29.

35. Male Infertility

Q.1 Regarding male infertility:
a. Leydig cells are the site of spermatogenesis
b. Varicocele repair improves male infertility
c. GnRH therapy is effective for an infertile male due to Kallmann's syndrome
d. Low volume and low levels of fructose in semen suggest vasal agenesis
e. Asthenospermia is an indication for intracytoplasmic sperm injection (ICSI).

Ans.
a. F
b. F
c. T
d. T
e. T

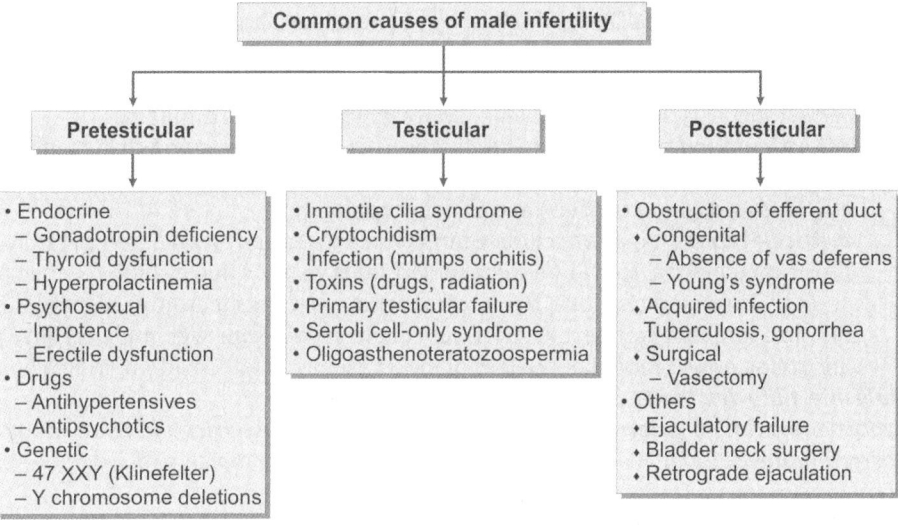

(See Dutta's Textbook of Gynecology, 7th Edition, p. 187)

MALE FACTORS FOR INFERTILITY

Male infertility may be due to:
- Defective spermatogenesis
- Obstruction in the efferent duct system

- Failure to deposit sperm in the vagina
- Errors in the seminal fluid analysis.

Male reproductive organs are: Testes, epididymis, vas deferens, prostate, seminal vesicles, ejaculatory duct, bulbourethral glands and urethra.

Two important cells in the testes are: Leydig cells and the **Sertoli cells**. Leydig cells produce androgens. Sertoli cells line the seminiferous tubules and, are the site of spermatogenesis. Luteinizing hormone (LH) stimulates leydig cells for the synthesis of testosterone. Follicle stimulating hormone (FSH) act on the Sertoli cells to stimulate spermatogenesis. It also stimulates Sertoli cells to produce androgen binding proteins (ABP) and inhibin-B. Spermatogenesis and sperm maturation need a high androgenic environment.

Spermatogenesis is controlled predominantly by the genes located on Y chromosome. Approximately, 75 days are required to complete the process of spermatogenesis (from spermatogonia stem cells to the mature sperm cells). Additional 12–20 days are needed for spermatozoa to travel the epididymis.

Basic semen analysis measures semen volume, sperm concentration, sperm motility and sperm morphology. WHO (2010) revised the normal values for semen analysis (*See* Dutta's Textbook of Gynecology, 7th Edition, p. 190).

MANAGEMENT OPTIONS FOR MALE INFERTILITY

- ***Medical treatment for male infertility*** (effective in few cases)
    - Infective causes (STIs)
    - Thyroid disorders
    - Endocrine causes (*See* Dutta's Textbook of Gynecology, 7th Edition, p. 187).
- ***Male infertility not due to azoospermia***
    - **Exogenous testosterone** should not be given for male subfertility because it decreases spermatogenesis due to negative feedback inhibition of the pituitary.
    - **Antioxidant food supplement:** Glutathione, carnitine and vitamin E do not affect semen parameters but administration of zinc and folic acid have been shown to be associated with improved sperm concentration and morphology.
    - **Varicocele repair:** It may affect male fertility due to rise in testicular temperature, reflux of toxic metabolites from left adrenal or left renal veins or due to high reactive oxygen species.[1] Treatment is done by surgical repair (varicocelectomy) or percutaneous embolization. It is not certain that varicocele repair improves male fertility status. Varicocelectomy is recommended in grade 3 cases associated with infertility.
- ***Male infertility due to azoospermia***
  Azoospermia classification and treatment (*See Manual of Obstetrics and Gynecology for the Postgraduates* p. 327): 1% of all men and 15–20% of infertile men are found to be suffering from azoospermia.
    - **Pretesticular azoospermia:** The important causes are hypogonadotropic hypogonadism. **Investigation to be done are:** Serum LH (↓), FSH (↓), testosterone (↓) levels. Pituitary imaging may be needed.
      Treatment options are: Pulsatile gonadotropin-releasing hormone (GnRH), Human chorionic gonadotropin (hCG) and exogenous gonadotropin therapy.
    - **Testicular azoospermia:** Important causes are (*See* Dutta's Textbook of Gynecology, 7th Edition, p. 187) genetic (Y chromosome deletions), infections (mumps), primary testicular failure, oligoasthenoteratozoospermia and developmental (cryptorchidism).

Management options
- In individuals having hypergonadotropic hypogonadism (raised levels of FSH and LH), testicular biopsy is not helpful. Donor sperm may be considered.
- Men having normal hormonal results—testicular biopsy may be done. If sperm is present in biopsy, ICSI is the option following retrieval of sperm by testicular sperm extraction (TESE) and percutaneous epididymal sperm aspiration (PESA).
- About 5–15% of infertile men suffer from chromosomal abnormalities. Prevalence is higher in (10–15%) in men suffering from azoospermia or severe oligospermia. **Common abnormalities are:** Klinefelter's syndrome (47 XXY), microdeletions of Y chromosome. These men need genetic counseling as the microdeletions can be transmitted to the male offspring following *in vitro* fertilization (IVF)/ICSI.

- **Post-testicular azoospermia:** Common causes are (*See* Dutta's Textbook of Gynecology, 7th Edition, p. 187) congenital absence of vas deferens (cystic fibrosis), obstruction due to infection (tuberculosis, gonorrhea) or vasectomy. About 40% of azoospermic men have obstructive pathology which again may be congenital bilateral absence of vas deferens (CBAVD) or infective etiology. Men with normal gonadotropin and testosterone level having low volume ejaculation should be tested for postejaculatory urine analysis.

Treatment: Men suffering from diabetes or past history of bladder neck or prostate surgery, suffer from the problem of retrograde ejaculation. Sperm received from neutralized urine of men can be processed for assisted reproductive technology (ART) or insemination. Men suffering from bilateral or unilateral vasal agenesis should have renal imaging as the association of renal agenesis is 10–25%. Men with CBAVD suffer seminal vesicle agenesis. So, they have low semen volume, low pH, and low fructose levels. Spermatogenesis is normal in such a male. About 75% of men with CBAVD have mutation of cystic fibrosis transmembrane regulator gene (CFTR). Men with CBAVD should have their female partner's carrier status tests done.[2]

Vasectomy reversal: It can be done successfully and subsequent pregnancy rate is about 80–100%. Microsurgical methods of vasovasostomy or vasoepididymostomy are effective. The time interval between vasectomy and reversal is an important determinant for success of surgery and pregnancy. Longer the interval, poorer is the result.

INFERTILITY AND INTRAUTERINE INSEMINATION (IUI)

Indications
- Oligospermia (mild)
- Asthenospermia (mild)
- Immune factor (male and female)
- Male factor (impotency, hypospadias)
- Hostile cervical mucus
- Unexplained infertility.

Intrauterine Insemination

About 0.3–0.5 mL of washed, processed and concentrated motile sperm (5–10 million) is pushed into the uterine cavity by transcervical catheterization. Patient should be in bed for about 15–20 minutes after the procedure. Pregnancy rates have been reported to be 10–11% per cycle and 40% after 4–6 cycle.

MALE INFERTILITY AND INTRACYTOPLASMIC SPERM INJECTION (ICSI)

Indications
- Severe oligospermia
- Asthenospermia, teratospermia
- Obstruction of efferent duct system (male)—obstructive azoospermia
- CBAVD
- Failure of IVF
- Unexplained infertility.

Methods of Sperm Recovery
- Microsurgical epididymal sperm aspiration (MESA)
- Percutaneous epididymal sperm aspiration
- Testicular sperm extraction
- Testicular sperm aspiration (TESA).

Fertilization rate of ICSI is about 70–80% and clinical pregnancy rate around 40%. Success rate of ICSI following sperm retrieval in obstructive azoospermia is 30–60%. Men with obstructive azoospermia need counseling as regard the transmission of genetic disorder to their offspring.

ICSI (Figs 35.1A to C): ICSI is associated with higher congenital anomaly risk (4.2%) when compared with conventional IVF (2–3%).[3]

Donor insemination: Men with azoospermia who do not desire ART, donor insemination is an effective alternative.

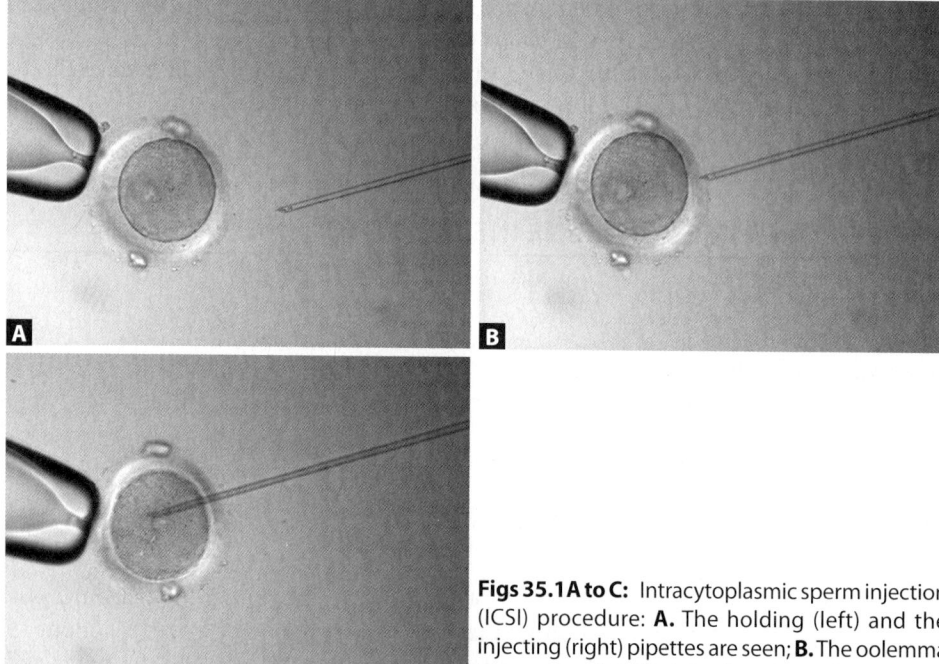

Figs 35.1A to C: Intracytoplasmic sperm injection (ICSI) procedure: **A.** The holding (left) and the injecting (right) pipettes are seen; **B.** The oolemma is penetrated; **C.** The injection pipette has reached nearly the center of the oocyte

References

1. Practice Committee of American Society for Reproductive Medicine. Report on varicocele and infertility. Fertil Steril. 2008;90(5 Suppl):S247-9.
2. Practice Committee of American Society for Reproductive Medicine in Collaboration with Society for Male Reproduction and Urology. Evaluation of the azoospermic male. Fertil Steril. 2008;90(5 Suppl):S74-7.
3. Practice Committee of American Society for Reproductive Medicine; Practice Committee of Society for ART. Genetic considerations related to ICSI. Fertil Steril. 2008;90(5 Suppl):S182-4.

36 Assisted Reproductive Technology (ART)

MCQs

Q.1 *Regarding gonadotropin stimulation for controlled ovarian stimulation (COS):*
   a. Gonadotropin stimulation could be done either using follicle-stimulating hormone (FSH) or human menopausal gonadotropin (HMG)
   b. Monitoring with serum estradiol levels with transvaginal ultrasound is essential in all assisted reproductive technology (ART) cycles
   c. Less aggressive stimulation increases cycle cancellation rates
   d. Pretreatment therapy with combined oral contraceptives (COCs) reduces pregnancy rates
   e. Supportive treatment in women with polycystic ovarian syndrome (PCOS) may prevent ovarian hyperstimulation syndrome (OHSS)

Ans.
   a. T   b. F
   c. F   d. F
   e. T

Q.2 *Use of gonadotropin-releasing hormone (GnRH) analogs and ART cycles:*
   a. GnRH agonists cause immediate down regulation
   b. GnRH agonists long protocols have better pregnancy rates
   c. GnRH antagonist use results of higher pregnancy rate
   d. Daily dose GnRH agonists have higher pregnancy rate
   e. GnRH analogs suppress premature luteinizing hormone (LH) surge

Ans.
   a. F   b. T
   c. F   d. T
   e. T

Q.3 *In ART cycles:*
   a. Blastocyst transfer has lower implantation failure
   b. Three embryo transfer is optimum in women age, < 35 years
   c. Embryo cryopreservation facilitates the multiple transfer cycles from single oocyte retrieval
   d. Overall success rates of fertility treatment following *in vitro* fertilization (IVF) and embryo transfer (ET) is 35%
   e. Live birth rate per cycle from donor oocyte depends on recipient's age

Ans. a. T b. F
c. T d. T
e. F

ART encompasses all the procedures that involve manipulation of gametes outside the body for the treatment of infertility. The procedures are exclusively carried out in tertiary care unit.

Most Frequently and Currently Practiced ARTs

- *In vitro* fertilization and embryo transfer (IVF-ET)
- Intracytoplasmic sperm injection (ICSI)
- Intrauterine insemination (IUI).

By strict criteria of definition, IUI is not included under the heading of ART, as the procedure does not involve in direct retrieval of oocytes from the ovaries. However, extracorporeal male gamete manipulation and superovulation of the female partner is involved in this procedure. Considering these issues, majority of the IVF clinics consider IUI as one of the technologies of assisted reproduction. **Other procedures of ART** are—gamete intrafallopian transfer (GIFT), zygote intrafallopian transfer (ZIFT), subzonal insemination (SUZI) and peritoneal oocyte and sperm transfer (POST).

Steps of Assisted Reproductive Technology

- Patient counseling and selection
- Pretreatment therapy with COCs to synchronize follicular growth and to prevent ovarian cysts
- Controlled ovarian stimulation
    - GnRH analog down regulation followed by gonadotropin stimulation
- Ovulation triggering with human chorionic gonadotropin (hCG) or GnRH agonist
- Oocyte retrieval (see Figs 36.1 and 36.2)
- Insemination (IVF or ICSI)
- *In vitro* embryo culture in nutrient media and incubation in CO_2 incubator
    - Embryo transfer (not more than 3) back into mother's uterus between D2 and D5 at the cleaving embryo (4–8 cell) stage or blastocyst stage
    - Cryopreservation of surplus embryos
- Luteal support mostly with micronized progesterone
- Serum βhCG estimation D14 postembryo transfer.

GnRH agonist: It has long half-life and increased receptor binding affinity. Initial 7 days of administration, GnRH agonist exerts a flare effect due to upregulation of GnRH receptors. This is followed by receptor desensitization resulting in fall in the level of gonadotropins (down regulation). Ultimately with prolonged use, GnRH agonist induces menopause-like state (low estradiol levels).

GnRH agonist are available either depot or daily use. Intramuscular/subcutaneous (IM/SC) or intranasal route can be used. The GnRH agonist protocols may be long or short. Long protocols may again be **long follicular or long luteal down regulation**.

In long luteal down-regulation protocol, GnRH agonist is started in the luteal phase, D21 of the previous cycle (*See* Dutta's Textbook of Gynecology, 7th Edition, p. 205). After 10–14 days of GnRH agonist therapy on D2 of subsequent menstrual cycle (whichever is earlier), a pelvic ultrasound and serum estradiol levels are done to confirm suppression. Thereafter, gonadotropin stimulation is begun. **Use of single-dose depot GnRH agonist is associated with higher gonadotropin (dose and duration) requirement and has lower pregnancy rates when compared with daily GnRH agonist formulation.**

GnRH antagonist (Cetrorelix, ganirelix) (*See* Dutta's Textbook of Gynecology, 7th Edition, Ch 32, p. 435): GnRH antagonists have no agonist action. Suppression to GnRH receptor and desensitization effect is immediate. There is immediate suppression of FSH and LH. GnRH antagonist is started on D4–D7 of stimulation in ART cycles. This schedule reduces the risks of premature LH surge. This also allows endogenous FSH-mediated follicular recruitments prior to GnRH suppression.

GnRH antagonists: Protocols may be fixed or flexible.
- ***Fixed protocol*** uses the antagonist on D4, D5, D6 or D7 of stimulation irrespective of follicular growth[1]
- ***Flexible protocol:*** Antagonist is used when the leading follicle has reached 12–16 mm or when serum estradiol level has reached above 600 pg/mL.

Till date, there is no randomized control trial to establish the superiority of one protocol over the other.[2] However, most of the centers have shifted to the antagonist protocol. ***Advantages are:*** (a) Shorter duration of therapy and (b) Simplicity of protocol.

Other protocols are flare, ultrashort, microdose and modified natural.

Comparison of GnRH agonists to GnRH antagonists

(*See* Dutta's Textbook of Gynecology, 7th Edition, Ch 32, p. 434)

Use of GnRH antagonist is associated with lower duration of stimulation, lower dose of gonadotropins and reduced rates of OHSS. According to 27 randomized controlled trials (RCTs), both the regimens have similar rates of production of good quality embryos.[3] However, clinical pregnancy rates are higher by 4.7% in agonist compared to antagonist cycles.[4]

What is early LH surge? How it causes premature follicular luteinization?

Due to high estradiol level in early follicular phase (as a consequence of gonadotropin stimulation), early LH surge occurs. GnRH agonist or antagonist is used to suppress it. Spontaneous ovulation prior to oocyte retrieval is observed in about 16% of nonsuppressed cycles. Premature LH surge occurs usually 5–7 days after starting follicular stimulation. Overall premature luteinization has been observed in 7–35% of cases. The possible mechanism of premature luteinization are: (a) Incomplete pituitary desensitization, (b) increased receptor sensitivity of granulosa cells to LH, (c) innate poor responder and (d) total amount of progesterone secreted from multiple follicles equals to the late follicular phase.

The main ***disadvantage of premature luteinization*** is endometrial advancement. Adverse effect on quality of oocyte or embryo has not been remarkably observed.

The different measures to overcome the problems of premature follicular luteinization are:
- Triggering ovulation at the appropriate time
- Using less aggressive stimulation protocols
- Cryopreservation of oocytes and embryos
- Use of antiprogesterone (mifepristone) at the time when hCG is given (less commonly used procedure).

Follicular growth and maturation: Initial growth of preantral and small antral follicles is independent of any hormone. Small antral follicles > 2 mm become responsive to FSH stimulation. The follicles become recruitable in the late luteal phase of the cycle. Preceding ovulation, FSH induces the receptors for LH on the granulosa cells once the antral follicle attains the size of 10 mm or more. At that state, LH can induce FSH-like actions on the granulosa cells (contrary to the 2-cell, 2-gonadotropin theory) and also stimulate the enzyme aromatase. Human menstrual cycles have two waves of follicular development. The **first wave** is the minor wave that occurs immediately after the ovulation in the preceding cycle. Once progesterone is available following ovulation, all the follicles, except the dominant one, undergo atresia. The subsequent wave is the **major wave** that occurs during the time of menstruation of the previous cycle. During this time, the dominant follicle is selected and other follicles are deprived of their growth. The follicle having the maximum number of FSH receptors and higher level of E2—androgen ratio in the follicular microenvironment is recruited as the dominant one. The dominant follicle is recruited by the cycle D6 or D7 which coincides with an estradiol rise that inhibits FSH.

Controlled ovarian stimulation (COS): Synchronous growth of dominant and codominant follicle(s) is achieved by gonadotropin stimulation. The main hormone in this process is the FSH. Most investigators suggest that the optimum number of retrieved oocytes in a given cycle is between 5 and 15. The optimal level of estradiol at the time of hCG administration is between 70 and 140 pg/mL per follicle. Estradiol monitoring *may not be that essential in the ART cycle*.[5] *Ultrasound monitoring alone may be adequate to maximize pregnancy and live birth rates.*[6]

Cycle cancellation in normal responders occurs in up to 6% of the cycles because of inadequate response. Cycle cancellation increases with advancing age and is decreased with ovarian reserve. It can be minimized by increasing the dose of gonadotropins. However, maximum upper limit of gonadotropin dose is 450 IU beyond which no benefit is observed.

Gonadotropin stimulation could be done either using FSH or with HMG: A systematic review of 14 RCTs found no significant differences between HMG and urinary FSH in rates per cycle pregnancy, multiple pregnancy, miscarriage, ovulation or hyperstimulation.[7] However, risk of OHSS was less with FSH compared to HMG. Similarly, no significant difference in the outcome was observed when urinary FSH was compared with recombinant FSH.[8]

However, recent studies have shown that HMG use is associated with higher androgen and lower progesterone levels on the day of hCG trigger for ovulation. This indicates a more favorable endocrine profile with HMG compared to FSH.[9]

Less aggressive stimulation reduces cycle cancellation rate: The problems of premature luteinization and lower pregnancy rates are encountered when more aggressive FSH stimulation protocols are used. **COCs given for 28 days prior to GnRH analogs, can give some benefits.** It helps in cycle regularity, synchronizes follicular development, prevents premature LH surge, reduces the incidence of ovarian cysts and hyperstimulation syndrome. More importantly, *it reduces the cycle cancellation*.

Therapy schedule of COCs for antagonist cycles: COS is to begin 2–5 days after stopping of COCs (irrespective of menses). For long agonist protocols, the agonist overlaps the last 5 days of COC pills followed by start of COS on D2 or D3 of withdrawal bleeding. **COCs pretreatment during GnRH agonist cycles is associated with higher pregnancy rates.**[10]

Supportive medications have been used with some benefits. Prophylactic antibiotics (doxycycline or azithromycin) are of help when subclinical infection is thought of. Glucocorticoids during peri-implantation period may improve pregnancy rates in women with autoimmune disease, assisted hatching or with advanced age. Metformin has been shown to prevent ovarian hyperstimulation (OHSS) in PCOS patients and is of benefit.

Growth and maturation of oocyte and ovulation (Figs 36.1A and B): In natural cycle, meiosis-I is completed just before ovulation. The oocyte will extrude the first polar body and the oocyte-cumulus complex will detach from the ovarian wall and ovulation will occur.

Ovulation triggering in ART: It is done when at least two follicles are 17–18 mm or larger in diameter (but <24 mm), with endometrial thickness 8 mm or more is observed. Recombinant hCG 250 µg SC or urinary hCG 10,000 IU is given. When there is the risks of OHSS, GnRH agonist can be given in place of hCG in antagonist protocol or recombinant LH can be given for hCG in agonist protocol.

Oocyte retrieval is performed by transvaginal ultrasound-guided needle aspiration. Each follicle is punctured and the follicular fluid is aspirated. In Kolkata, Institute of Reproductive Medicine protocol, intravenous conscious sedation is used. Prophylactic antibiotic (augmentin and metronidazole) is given. Oocyte retrieval is usually done 34–36 hours after the hCG injection. Luteal support (*See* Manual of Obstetrics and Gynecology for the Postgraduates, p. 121, 389) is started after embryo transfer.

In vitro fertilization insemination: 100,000–800,000 motile sperm/mL per oocyte is used. Processed sperm are incubated in media for 3–4 hours for sperm capacitation and acrosome reaction. Before insemination, retrieved oocytes are cultured in media.

Embryo culture: Assessment of embryo development is done after 15–20 hours of insemination or ICSI. Fertilization is characterized by the presence of two pronuclei and extrusion of second polar body. After another 24–30 hours, embryos are examined for cleavage. ***First embryo cleavage*** occurs about 21 hours after the fertilization, subsequent divisions occur every 12–15 hours up to the 8 cell stage on 3rd day of embryo development. Compaction to form the 16 cell morula occurs on 4th day of embryo development. Blastocyst formation with differentiation of inner cell mass and trophectoderm is completed on D5 or D6.

Blastocyst transfer is observed to have lower implantation failure, higher pregnancy rate and higher live birth rate (32–42%) than cleavage stage transfer.[11]

Embryo Morphology and Selection of Embryo for Transfer

Cleavage stage embryo with normal development is characterized by—early cleavage (2 cells) on D1, 4 cells on D2, and 8 cells on D3. ***About 10% or less number of blastomeres should have fragmentation***.

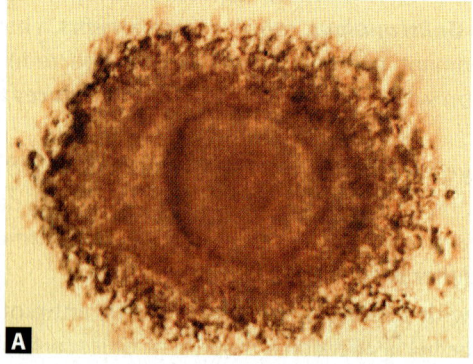 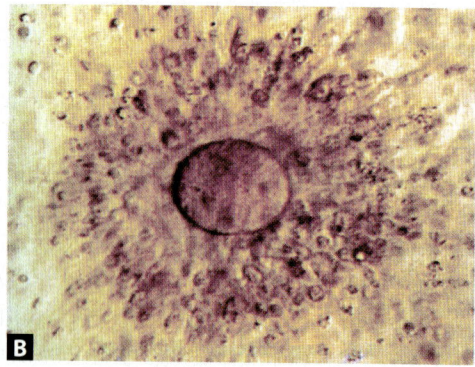

Figs 36.1A and B: A. *Very immature oocyte:* Tightly packed cumulus and corona, granular ooplasm, presence of germinal vesicle and absence of first polar body (FPB); **B. *Mature oocyte:*** Well-expanded cumulus, sun burst-like corona, clear ooplasm and FPB in perivitelline space (PVS)

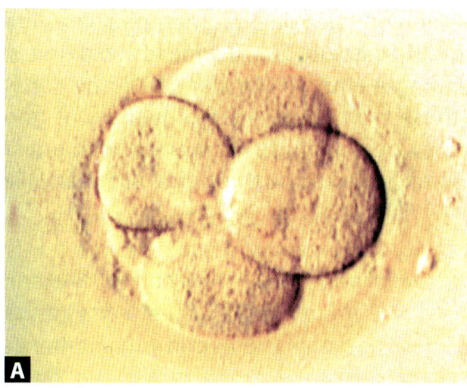
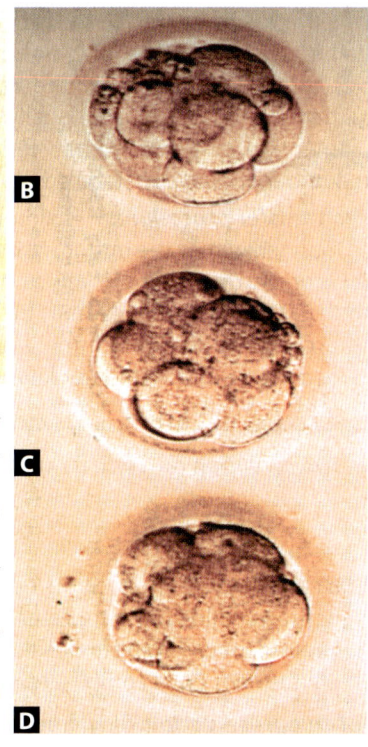

Figs 36.2A to D: Embryos are divided into four types depending upon the extent of fragmentation. **Type-A** is the best and **Type-D** is the worst.

Type-A: Minimal volume of fragmentation associated with one blastomere.

Type-B: Localized fragmentation mainly occupying the periphery of the blastomeres.

Type-C: Small fragmentation speckled in all the blastomeres over the embryo.

Type-D: Large volume of fragmentation in all the blastomeres.

The ***blastomere size*** should be regular and there should be no multinucleation. Scoring of blastocysts: ***Scale 1 (worst) to scale 6 (best)***, is done by Gardner and Schoolcraft. The trophectoderm in a grade 6 blastocyst has completely escaped or hatched from the zona. Similarly, the ***inner cell mass is graded from A to C*** depending upon tightness and cellularity (A is the best). Trophectoderm is graded from A to C based on cohesiveness and cellularity (A is the best) (Figs 36.2A to D).

Morphological Assessment of Embryo Quality

A good quality embryo is considered with the following morphological characters:
- All the blastomeres' size and shape should be almost equal
- Blastomeres should occupy almost whole of the space within the zona pellucida
- There should be no multinucleation
- The blastomeres should appear transparent with clear cytoplasm (less fragmentation).

Table 36.1: Number of embryo transfer [American Society for Reproductive Medicine (ASRM-2013)]

Age (years)	Embryo transfer
<35	1 (maximum 2)
35–37	2 (maximum 3)
38–40	3 (maximum 4)
41–42	5

Number of embryos to be transferred: It is not a uniform one. Current guidelines indicate 1–3 embryos to be transferred depending on age of the patient. This is done to avoid risks of multiple pregnancies and the complications thereof. Single embryo transfer should be considered for younger patients (age <35 years). Usually, these women have large quantity of good quality embryos. Otherwise, two embryo transfers may be optimum. For women with advanced age, maximum number of cleavage stage embryo transfer could be three (age >35 years) (Table 36.1).

Embryo transfer procedure: It is aimed to deliver the embryos transcervically, safely in an atraumatic manner, within the endometrial cavity for implantation. It is performed using a soft catheter. It is done to deposit the embryos at a level of about 0.5–1.0 cm below the uterine fundus. Transfer under ultrasound guidance may be helpful. Currently, multiple meta-analysis have shown Ultrasonography (USG)-guided ET improves clinical pregnancy rates and implantation rates. Most centers now do the ET under USG guidence.

Cryopreservation of Embryos/Oocytes

Embryo cryopreservation can be done at (a) pronuclear, (b) cleavage stage and also at (c) blastocyst stage.

Benefits

- Multiple transfer cycles from single oocyte retrieval
- Pregnancy rates following cryopreserved embryos are nearly similar or marginally less
- Fertility treatment can be optimized significantly
- Reduces treatment cycle complications, OHSS, and failure rates.

Methods of cryopreservation: Slow freezing or rapid freezing (or victification) are two methods. ***Slow freezing*** protocols take longer time and concentration of cryoprotectants is less. ***Victification*** uses high concentration of cryoprotectants for rapid cooling. It is less expensive and has higher postthaw embryo survival. Embryo thawing is done by brief exposure to air and warm water followed by rehydration. ***Pregnancy rates following frozen embryos are lower compared to fresh transfer cycles.***[12] This again may be due to embryo selection as best embryos are selected for fresh transfer.[13]

Endometrial preparation for frozen embryo transfer (FET): In natural cycle, no exogenous treatment is needed for the recipient. Transfer is timed to spontaneous ovulation.[14] Otherwise estradiol supplementation is started in early follicular phase and is continued for 13–15 days till endometrial thickness of 8 mm is obtained. Endometrial thickness is measured with transvaginal ultrasound. Progesterone supplementation begins 48–72 hours prior to transfer of cleavage state embryo. Blastocysts are thawed 5–6 days prior to transfer. GnRH agonists are sometimes used in medicated cycles to prevent premature LH surge, which may affect the endometrial maturation adversely.

Success rates of fertility treatment: Overall success rates are follows—clomiphene citrate (CC) and timed intercourse (TI): 3–17%; IUI, CC and IUI: 10–14%; Gonadotropins and IUI: 15–20% and IVF success: clinical pregnancy rate/cycle for age <35 years: 31–46%.[15]

Donor Oocyte

Indications of pregnancy from donor oocytes

- Woman with ovarian failure
- Poor ovarian response to stimulation
- Poor oocyte quality (as in advanced age)

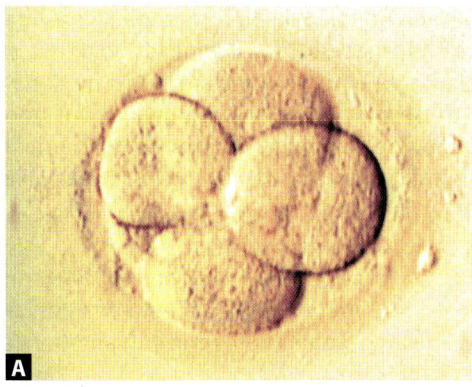
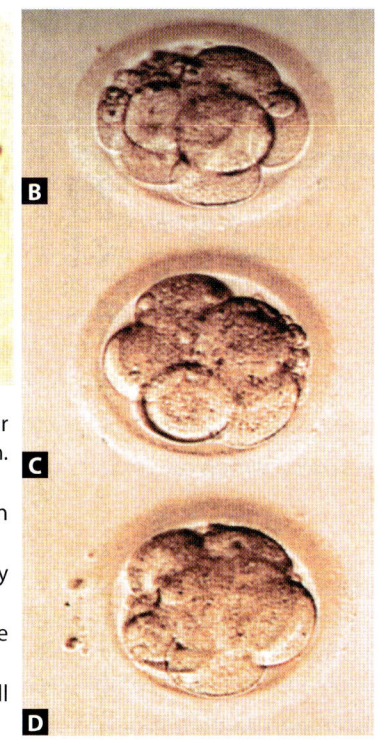

- Repeated failure of fertilization
- Failure of implantation after multiple ART
- Inherited genetic disorders.

Live birth rate per cycle of donor oocyte IVF are 50% regardless of the recipient's age. Oocyte recipient needs to undergo endometrial preparation (described above). At present, donor oocytes must be used to create embryos during the retrieval cycle (as oocyte freezing is considered experimental till date).

References

1. Devroey P, Aboulghar M, Garcia-Velasco J, et al. Improving the patient's experience of IVF/ICSI: A proposal for an ovarian stimulation protocol with GnRH antagonist co-treatment. Hum Reprod. 2009;24(4): 764-74.
2. Huirne JA, Homburg R, Lambalk CB. Are GnRH antagonists comparable to agonists for use in IVF? Hum Reprod. 2007;22(11):2805-13.
3. Reh A, Krey L, Noyes N. Are gonadotropin-releasing hormone agonist losing popularity? Current trends at a large fertility center. Fertil Steril. 2010;93(1):101-8.
4. Al-Inany HG, Abou-Setta AM, Aboulghar M, et al. Gonadotropin-releasing hormone antagonists for assisted conception: a Cochrane review. Reprod Biomed Online. 2007;14(5):640-9.
5. Lass A, UK Timing of hCG Group. Monitoring of IVF-ET cycles by ultrasound versus by ultrasound and hormonal levels:A prospective, multicenter, randomized study. Fertil Steril. 2003;80(1):80-5.
6. Kwan I, Bhattacharya S, McNeil A, et al. Monitoring of stimulated cycles in assisted reproduction (IVF and ICSI). Cochrane Database Syst Rev. 2008;(2):CD005289.
7. Nugent D, Vandekerckhove P, Hughes E, et al. Gonadotropin therapy for ovulation induction in subfertility associated with polycystic ovary syndrome. Cochrane Database Syst Rev. 2000;4:CD000410.
8. Smitz J, Andersen AN, Devroey P, et al. Endocrine profile in serum and follicular fluid differs after ovarian stimulation with HP-hMG or recombinant FSH in IVF patients. Hum Reprod. 2007;22(3):676-87.
9. Daya S. Follicle-stimulating hormone and human menopausal gonadotropin for ovarian stimulation in assisted reproductive cycles. Cochrane database Syst Rev. 2009;1.
10. Biljan MM, Mahutte NG, Dean N, et al. Effects of pretreatment with an oral contraceptive on the time required to achieve pituitary suppression with gonadotropin-releasing hormone analogs and subsequent implantation and pregnancy rates. Fertil Steril. 1998;70(6):1063-9.
11. Blake DA, Farquhar CM, Johnson N, et al. Cleavage stage versus blastocyst stage embryo transfer in assisted conception. Cochrane Database Syst Rev. 2007;4:CD002118.
12. Urman B, Balaban B, Yakin K. Impact of fresh-cycle variables on the implantation potential of cryopreserved thawed human embryos. Fertil Steril. 2007;87(2):310-5.
13. Wennerholm UB, Söderström-Anttila V, Bergh C, et al. Children born after cryopreservation of embryos of oocytes: a systematic review of outcome data. Hum Reprod. 2009;24(9):2158-72.
14. Glujovsky D, Pesce R, Fiszabjn G, et al. Endometrial preparation for women undergoing embryo transfer with frozen embryos or embryos derived from donor oocytes. Cochrane Database Syst Rev. 2010;(1):CD006359.
15. Centers for disease controls and prevention (2016). 2007 assisted reproductive technology success rates [online] CDC website. Available from http://www.cdc.gov/art/ART 2007/PDF/Complete.2007_ART.pdf.

37 Management Strategies for Low Responder Woman

The decline in female fecundity with age is well-documented. Spontaneous conception is low in women over the age of 45 years.[1] Deliveries after the age of 45 years are only 0.2%. It is documented that oocyte depletion accelerates after the age of 37 years. Moreover, ovarian response to stimulation in older women with low ovarian reserve is poor. This is due to the increased resistance of the ovaries to gonadotropin stimulation even with a high dose.

Factors for poor response of ovaries to gonadotropin stimulation:
- Age is an independent and significant determinant[2]
- Body weight
- Body mass index (BMI)
- Size and count of antral follicles (≥ 2–11 mm). A count of < 5 follicles of 2–5 mm diameter has been suggested as a poor responder
- Basal hormonal levels are also used to predict the response.

D3-FSH > 10 IU/mL; inhibin B (low), serum estradiol (high) and anti-Müllerian hormone (AMH), low—suggest poor response.

MANAGEMENT ISSUES

Gonadotropin stimulation for poor responders may produce more follicles when given 300–400 IU or even 600 IU of FSH per day.

Stimulation may done with fixed high dose FSH or with step down protocol depending upon the response.[3] Maximum dose of gonadotropin (FSH) used with the effective response is 450 IU/day.

GnRH agonists (GnRH-a) in the treatment of poor responders:
- **Long GnRH-a protocol:** Resulted in increased number of oocytes, improved clinical pregnancy rate per embryo transfer compared to conventional stimulation. Therefore, long GnRH-a protocol was found superior in terms of efficacy in low responder patients. However, in many patients with poor response, resulted in excessive ovarian suppression with GnRH-a. Consequently, hormonal stimulation was excessively prolonged with increased cost and duration of treatment. The ovarian unresponsiveness was very high.
- **Step down GnRH-a protocol:** Excessive ovarian dampening due to long GnRH-a made this protocol less popular. This supported the concept of a step down GnRH-a with the low dose (mini-dose) protocol. Mini-dose is found superior to standard agonist dose in terms of oocyte yield and cycle outcome.

- **GnRh-a 'stop' protocol:** Pituitary recovery and resumption of gonadotropin secretion following GnRH-a treatment usually takes up several weeks. Use of 'ultrashort protocol' was effective to suppress the endogenous LH secretion when GnRH-a (leuprolide acetate 0.1 mg/day from cycle day 21 reducing to 0.05 mg/day upon down regulation) was using to the stop protocol. The ultrashort protocol was stopped after 5 days. There was no premature LH surge. This forms the basis of 'stop protocol' or discontinuous GnRH protocol. This 'stop protocol' showed favorable results in terms of both cost effectiveness and clinical outcome.
- **Short GnRH-a protocol:** Patients who failed to multifollicular growth with long GnRH protocol were considered for a short protocol with short and ultrashort regimens. It had the advantages of the initial agonistic stimulatory effect of GnRH-a non-endogenous FSH and LH secretion which is also known as flare-up effects.

  Advantage is that it eliminates excessive ovarian suppression due to prolonged agonist use. Pituitary desensitization generally achieved within 5 days of treatment. Patients are protected from premature LH surge. This protocol was considered favorable for the poor responder woman.

  The limitations of the protocol was that its efficacy were not judged in prospective randomized controlled trials in comparison to standard long protocol. The live birth rate in flare-up group was found low (3.8%) when compared to the standard long protocol (25%).

  Adverse effects of flare-up protocol with GnRH-a was LH secretion and development of increase androgen levels in the follicular environment. This is detrimental to the process of folliculogenesis and meiosis leading to poor oocyte formation and reduced rate of fertilization and implantation. Early follicular use of GnRH-a (flare-up protocol) resulted in increased levels of LH, E2, androgens and progesterone compared to the mid luteal group of GnRH-a use.

  To improve the ill effects of flare-up GnRH-a use, the following measures could be taken:
  - Pretreatment use of oral contraceptive pills (OCPs)
  - Use of progestin (norethisterone) before the use of gonadotropin stimulation
  - Dose reduction of GnRH-a to minimize the flare (micro-dose flare).
- **GnRH antagonists in the treatment of poor responders:** Its use has an immediate effect (within 6 hours) of dose-related suppression of gonadotropin release and resulted in comparable therapeutic efficacy compared to agonists. GnRH antagonist is administered in the late follicular phase to suppress the LH surge.

  Other advantages are:
  - It avoids the 'flare-up' of LH
  - Shortens the overall treatment protocol
  - Reduces the risk of ovarian hyperstimulation syndrome (OHSS)
  - Reduces the menopausal side effects of the woman.

  The dose schedule may be fixed or flexible depending upon the response. In the beginning of controlled ovarian stimulation (COS), the pituitary is fully responsive to GnRH pulses. This allows more natural follicular recruitment without any inhibitory effect of GnRH-a.[4] This antagonist protocol for poor responders also permit the use clomiphene citrate (CC) with or without gonadotropin stimulation. Owing to the synergistic effect, the requirement of gonadotropin may be less and so also the concomitant cost. There is some modest improvement in oocyte retrieval, embryo transfer and clinical pregnancy rates.
- **Role of androgens:** Human follicular growth and development is regulated by different endocrine and paracrine factors that develop the favorable follicular microenvironment. Same

amount of androgens from theca cells are produced and this small amount contributes to the follicular environment.
Role of follicular androgens in folliculogenesis
- Reduces follicular apoptosis and responsiveness to gonadotropin
- Enhance the action of FSH for follicular growth and maturation

This concept encouraged the use of dehydroepiandrosterone (DHEA) for women with diminished ovarian reserve. The woman is given 75 mg of DHEA daily for an average of 4–5 months. With the concept of aromatase inhibitors were used to block the intraovarian androgen conversion to estrogens. Few studies support the beneficial effects of DHEA or aromatase inhibitors for women with diminished ovarian function. However, it needs authentication with prospective randomized control trials.

- **Role of human growth hormone (hGH):** Results are conflicting with the role of hGH when used in women with poor responders. Few studies showed improvements in follicular responsiveness and pregnancy rates.
- **Pre-treatment with oral contraceptive pills:** It is suggested that use of OCPs may increase the pregnancy rates of IVF specially in the poor responders.[5,6]
  The suggested mechanisms are:
  - Induction of estrogen receptors in the follicle and sensitization
  - Suppression effect on the pituitary with either alone or in combination with GnRH agonists
  - Improvement of local (intraovarian) growth factors
  - Changes in the endometrium.

  Cycle outcomes of gonadotropin stimulation with prior hypothalamic-pituitary suppression with OCP with or without GnRH-a were improved in terms of oocyte retrieval, embryo transfer, embryo quality and clinical pregnancy rates. However, more published data are needed to support the observation.
- **Low-dose aspirin:** It was used to improve follicular vascularity. However, available evidence does not support its use in the poor responder women undergoing IVF.

Aneuploidy screening: Women with advanced age produce oocytes with inadequate reserves of energy. Energy produced by mitochondrial DNA, is necessary for oocyte maturation, meiosis and process of disjunction. Mitochondrial dysfunction (due to related pathology), can lead to an increase in nondisjunction, abnormal chromatid separation and higher rates of oocyte apoptosis.[7] Because of this reason oocytes retrieved during ART procedures may be biochemically or chromosomally defective. Chromosome abnormalities are the important cause of embryo wastage. Preimplantation genetic screening (PGS) confirmed this association for women aged >35 years.

SUMMARY

- Treatment strategies for low responder or women with diminished ovarian reserve are difficult and at times frustrating.
- Development of any definitive treatment strategies is difficult as there is a paucity of any large-scale prospective randomized controlled trials (RCTs).
- High dose gonadotropins (300–450 IU of FSH daily) for women with diminished ovarian reserve or poor ovarian response are useful to yield a maximum number of oocytes.
- Long GnRH-a protocol—might be the protocol of choice when ovarian reserve is low and the response is poor. Mini-dose (low dose) agonist down regulation is found useful to increase ovarian responsiveness.

- Short (micro-dose) flare—GnRH-a protocol. It is found beneficial. Pretreatment of OCPs uses can prevent the adverse effects of LH and excess androgen secretion. OCP use prevents the high LH which is due to the endogenous gonadotropin flare-up effect.
- GnRH antagonists—results in immediate suppressive gonadotropins release. COS for follicular recruitment is done with the inhibitory effect of GnRH-a. Clomiphene citrate alone or combined with gonadotropins (synergistic effects) result in higher oocyte yield.
- Stop protocol: In some failed cases of long or short GnRH-a regimen, agonist administration can be withdrawn and gonadotropin stimulation is continued. No LH peak was observed and clinical outcomes were found favorable.
- ART treatment is recommended for women with declining years of fecundity. In addition to diminished ovarian reserve and poor response, other associated factors have been a challenge. Poor oocyte quality (aneuploid oocytes and embryos), uterine factors, women's psychological stress are also the hindrances.
- Use of donor oocyte has been considered the successful alternative.

References

1. Laufer N, Simon A, Samueloff A, et al. Successful spontaneous pregnancies in women older than 45 years. Fertil Steril. 2004;81(5):1328-32.
2. Chuang CC, Chen CD, Chao KH, et al. Age is a better predictor of pregnancy potential than basal FSH levels in women undergoing IVF. Fertil Steril. 2003;79(1):63-8.
3. Cedrin-Durnevin I, Bständig B, Herve F, et al. A comparative study of high fixed-dose and decremental-dose regimens of gonadotropins in a minidose GnRH-a flare protocol for poor responders. Fertil Steril. 2000;73(5):1055-6.
4. Craft I, Gorgy A, Hill J, et al. Will GnRH antagonists provide new hope for patient considered 'difficult responder' to GnRH-a protocols? Hum Reprod. 1999;14(12):2959-62.
5. al-Mizyen E, Sabatini L, Lower AM, et al. Does pretreatment with progesterone or OCPs in low responders followed by the GnRH-a flare protocol improve the outcome of IVF-ET? J Assist Reprod Genet. 2000;17(3):140-6.
6. Kovacs P, Barg PE, Witt BR. Hypothalamic-pituitary suppression with OCPs does not improve outcome in poor responder patients undergoing IVF-ET cycles. J Assist Reprod Genet. 2001;18(7):391-4.
7. May-Panloup P, Chretien MF, Jacques C, et al. Low oocyte mitochondrial DNA content in ovarian insufficiency. Hum Reprod. 2005;20(3):593-7.

38 Third Party Reproduction

When the ability to produce gamete(s) and to gestate a pregnancy is compromised, a third party reproductive option can be considered. This is done with the help of donor sperm, donor oocyte or donor embryos and a gestational carrier. Need of a gestational carrier may be due to several reasons.

SURROGACY

Surrogacy is the procedure where a woman (surrogate) receives gamete(s) or embryos and gestates (carries the pregnancy) on behalf of an intending mother. In surrogacy, there is an agreement between the third party (commissioning couple) and the woman (surrogate) that she (surrogate) will carry pregnancy with the objective of handing over the baby finally to the commissioning couple after delivery.[1]

Surrogacy could be of two forms:
1. ***Gestational surrogacy or full surrogacy or host surrogacy or IVF surrogacy:*** Gametes of the intended parents and/or donors are used for *in vitro* fertilization (IVF) and the embryos are transferred into the surrogate. The surrogate has no genetic link to the child.
2. ***Natural or straight or partial surrogacy:*** It involves intrauterine insemination (IUI) where either the intended father's or donor sperm is used for artificial insemination. The oocyte comes from the surrogate mother. The surrogate has a genetic link to the child.

Since 1980, surrogacy has gained acceptance gradually. Human Fertilization and Embryology Authority (HFEA) in 1984 branded surrogacy as ethically unacceptable.[2] British Medical Association (BMA) in 1996 accepted surrogacy as a reproductive option of last resort.[3] The legal issues surrounding surrogacy is mostly in relation to IVF legislation in India at the moment. The other forms of surrogacy are not well covered by law not only in India but also in many other countries of the world. Legally, surrogates are given reasonable financial support. However, commercialization of surrogacy is not permitted.

Human Fertilization and Embryology Act (2008), UK recommends:[4]
- The commissioning couple are married and are cohabitees and both are >18-year-old.
- The conception must be from placing the embryo, sperm or egg into the surrogate mother or by donor insemination. The egg or sperm must be from one member of the commissioning couple, thus providing a genetic link.
- The surrogate and the legal father (if not the commissioning father) must give consent for the parental order transfer within 6 weeks after delivery.

- Payment of the surrogate (other than medical, legal, maternity, travel cost, etc.) for expenses is decided by the court.

Counseling: In-depth counseling of all parties engaged in surrogacy arrangement is essential.[5] Medical and psychological risks of surrogacy must be explained and understood by both the parties. Potential psychological risk to the child must be considered and legal advice should be obtained.[6]

Specific Situations to Suggest Surrogacy
- Congenital absence of uterus: Mayer-Rokitansky-Küster-Hauser (MRKH) syndrome
- Women with surgically removed uterus (hysterectomy)
- Uterine shape has been distorted and deformed (fibroid or adenomyosis and Müllerian abnormalities)
- Uterine synechiae
- Renal and cardiac pathology
- Recurrent unexplained miscarriage
- Repeated IVF failure due to unknown causes.

Other extended indications are: Married woman seeking surrogacy for career plan.

Procedure of Gestational Surrogacy
- The procedure involves creation of an embryo by IVF.
- The embryo results from the union of gametes (sperm and egg) derived from the infertile couple.
- The infertile couple is the genetic or biological parents (commissioning couple).
- Surrogate mother (surrogate host) may be a friend or relative or she may be unknown to the commissioning couple.
- Endometrial preparation in the surrogate before embryo transfer is needed (*See* Manual of Obstetrics and Gynecology for the Postgraduates, Ch 36).
- This procedure is also known as ***IVF surrogacy*** or ***full surrogacy.***
- In India at the moment, there are few practical problems as well as legal considerations that need modifications. It is suggested that the agreement of surrogacy between the surrogate host and the commissioning couple should be signed in the presence of a lawyer. After all, the commissioning couple is the biological parents of the child.

In India Indian Council of Medical Research (ICMR), recommends:
- Assisted reproductive technology (ART) clinic would play no role in commercial surrogacy program.
- Surrogate must surrender all parental rights.
- Surrogate should have not more than five children in her life (including her own children).
- Procedures could be done only at ICMR recommended clinics.
- Birth certificate would have names of the genetic parents.

References
1. British Medical Association. Surrogacy: Ethical Considerations. Report of the Working Party on Human Infertility Services. London: BMA;1990.
2. Human Fertilization and Embryology Authority. (1984). Warnock Report. [online] Available from http://www.hfea.gov.uk/docs/Warnock_Report_of_the_Committee_of_Inquiry_into_Human_Fertilisation_and_Embryology_1984.pdf [Accessed June, 2016].

3. British Medical Association. Changing Conceptions of Motherhood. The Practice of surrogacy in Britain. Chichester: Wiley-Blackwell. London: BMA Publications;1996.
4. Parliament of the United Kingdom. (2008). Human Fertilization and Embryology Act 2008. [online] Available from http://www.legislation.gov.uk/ukpga/2008/22/pdfs/ukpga_20080022_en.pdf [Accessed June, 2016].
5. Jadva V, Murray C, Lycett E, et al. Surrogacy: The experiences of surrogate mothers. Hum Reprod. 2003;18(10):2196-204.
6. Committee on Ethics. ACOG committee opinion number 397, February 2008: surrogate motherhood. Obstet Gynecol. 2008;111(2 Pt 1):465-70.

SECTION 6
Maternal Medicine (Short Obstetric Reviews)

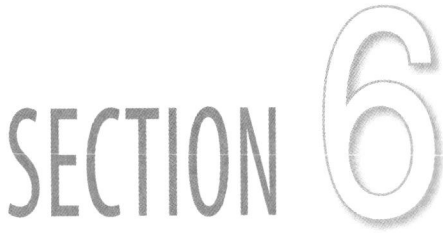

Section Outline

Ch. 39. Obstetric Case Presentation
Ch. 40. Anemia in Pregnancy
Ch. 41. Hemoglobinopathy
Ch. 42. Sickle Cell Disease in Pregnancy
Ch. 43. Thyroid Dysfunction in Pregnancy
Ch. 44. Heart Disease in Pregnancy
Ch. 45. Gestational Age and Cesarean Delivery
Ch. 46. Place of Thromboprophylaxis during Pregnancy
Ch. 47. External Cephalic Version
Ch. 48. Diminished Fetal Movements
Ch. 49. Transfusion in Obstetrics
Ch. 50. Obstetric Cholestasis
Ch. 51. Diabetic Nephropathy
Ch. 52. Renal Transplant
Ch. 53. Non Hemorrhagic Shock in Obstetrics

39 Obstetric Case Presentation

Mrs AT, 25-year-old homemaker with education of 4th standard, was admitted to the hospital on… She belonged to a family of low socioeconomic status. She was 4th gravida (G4: P0-A3-L0) at 33 weeks of gestation. Her chief complaints were progressive weakness and fatigue with occasional dyspnea for last 7–10 days. She did not have any history of vomiting, fever or bleeding neither from the vagina nor from any other site. She was earlier seen at a peripheral center where she had irregular supervision. She was immunized with tetanus toxoid and was on iron and folic acid supplementation therapy. Following admission she was investigated in this institute. Her details of hematological and other investigation reports were as recorded below:

- Hb% = 6.5 g/dL
- PCV = 32%
- MCV = 76 μ^3
- MCH = 25 pg (HbA2 >3.7%; HbF: 2%)
- Thyroid function tests: Normal
- Plasma glucose tests: Normal
- Routine urine analysis—within normal limit
- Serum iron = 80 µg/dL
- Serum ferritin = 106 µg/L
- Hb electrophoresis (HPLC) = β thalassemia minor
- MCHC = Normal
- Serum bilirubin: 1.5 mg/dL
- Liver function tests: Normal
- Stool for occult blood test: Negative

Fetal wellbeing assessment with USG revealed: Single live fetus with evidences of growth restriction. Liquor volume was reduced. She received two units of packed cell transfusion following the investigation. She was on folic acid therapy.

HISTORY

Obstetric history: She was G4 (P0-A3-L0). Her three previous pregnancies ended in miscarriage, two in the ***first trimester*** and the third in the early second trimester (14 weeks). She underwent ERPC following the last two miscarriages. She did not receive any transfusion during that period.

Menstrual history: She attended menarche at the age of 13 years. Her cycles were fairly normal and regular. Her LMP was… making her EDD on …… based on her LMP. She was at 33 weeks of gestation.

In the past, she did not suffer from any medical or surgical illness of significance. ***In the family,*** she was not aware of any member of her family to suffer from such illness or to receive regular transfusion.

Personal history: She had no history of using any habit forming drug. She also did not use any hormonal contraception.

EXAMINATION

With verbal consent and following evacuation of bladder.
General survey: She was alert, conscious and cooperative. She was with average build but her nutritional status was below average. She was 145 cm (4'10") tall, weighed 48 kg, with a BMI of 24. She had normal temperature; P-84 BPM, regular BP: 110/70 mm Hg. She looked pale, having mild pedal edema. Clinical examination did not reveal any jaundice, cyanosis, clubbing or koilonychia. Her oral hygiene was normal. There was neither any enlarged neck veins nor any palpable lymph node. Examination of thyroid and breasts were normal.
Systemic examination of cardiovascular, respiratory and CNS systems were normal.
Obstetric examination

- **Inspection:** Abdomen was found enlarged with an ovoid shape, from symphysis pubis to the junction of upper two-thirds and lower one-third of the line between umbilicus and xiphisternum. The umbilicus was everted, striae gravidarum and linea nigra were present. There was no scar mark. Hernial orifices were normal.
- **Palpation:** Superficial and deep palpation did not reveal any tenderness or any organomegaly. **Obstetric palpation:** Fundal height was approximately of 28–30 weeks size and the symphysis-fundal height measured 30 cm. Uterus was relaxed and non-tender. Palpation with the obstetric grips revealed: a single live fetus, longitudinal lie, cephalic presentation, head not engaged (three-fifths above the brim), back on the left hand side and limbs on the right. Liquor volume clinically appeared slightly less. On auscultation, FHS could be heard on the left spinoumbilical line with a rate of 147 bpm and was regular.

Pelvic examination of external genitalia were normal.
Speculum examination revealed that cervix was 2.5 cm long; os was closed; no discharge or leakage of liquor or bleeding was seen.

SUMMARY

A 25-year-old, 4th gravida (G4: P0-A3-L0) with previous three miscarriages, all in the first and early second trimester, was admitted at 33 weeks of gestation due to the gradually increasing symptoms of weakness, fatigue and occasional dyspnea. Her pregnancy was irregularly supervised in the first half. Her details of investigations revealed that she was suffering from inherited anemia of β thalassemia minor in nature. She received two units of packed cell transfusion following her admission.

On examination, she was moderately pale and had mild pedal edema. Her obstetric examination revealed: symphysis-fundal height of 30 cm, uterus was relaxed with a single live fetus longitudinal lie, cephalic presentation and the head was free and floating. On auscultation, FHS was 147 bpm and regular. There was associated growth restriction of the fetus and reduced liquor volume.

PROVISIONAL DIAGNOSIS

A lady, 25-year-old, G4 (P0-A3-L0) at 33 weeks of gestation complicated with inherited anemia (β thalassemia minor) and fetal growth restriction.
For case discussion (*See* Manual of Obstetrics and Gynecology for the Postgraduates, Ch 41, p. 412).

40. Anemia in Pregnancy

Anemia in pregnancy is the most common hematological disorder. In obstetrics, two causes are very common for anemia:
1. Iron deficiency
2. Hemorrhage in pregnancy [antepartum hemorrhage (APH), postpartum hemorrhage (PPH)].

Definition of anemia in pregnancy: Values of hemoglobin (Hb) or hematocrit (HCT) is less than 5th percentile of the values in a healthy reference population based on the stage of pregnancy [Centers for Disease Control and Prevention (CDC) 1998].

Accordingly, women with the following levels of Hb (g/dL) and HCT (%) are considered anemic (Tables 40.1 to 40.3).

Table 40.1: Levels of Hb and HCT to define anemia in pregnancy (CDC 1998)

	Pregnancy	Hemoglobin	Hematocrit
A	First trimester	< 11 g/dL	< 33%
B	Second trimester	< 10.5 g/dL	< 32%
C	Third trimester	< 11 g/dL	< 33%

Table 40.2: Classification of anemia in pregnancy

Acquired			Inherited
Deficiency of anemia			Thalassemia
• Iron	• Vitamin B_{12}	• Folic acid	
Hemorrhagic			Sickle cell anemia
• APH	• PPH	• Bleeding piles	
Anemia of chronic disease			Hereditary spherocytosis
• Renal	• Pulmonary Koch's		↓
			(Red cell membrane defect)
Hemolytic anemia			Metabolic disorders of red cell
• Malaria	• Drugs (nitrofurantoin)		G6PD deficiency
• Autoimmune			Pyruvate kinase deficiency
Aplastic anemia			
• Bone marrow aplasia	• Radiation		

Q. What is the significance of reticulocyte count?
Ans. Reticulocytes are normally < 2% of the red cells. Reticulocyte count gives a guide to the erythroid activity in the bone marrow.
- Increased reticulocyte count is seen in: (a) Following hemorrhage or hemolysis and (b) during the response to treatment with hematinic.
- Low reticulocyte count is seen in: (a) Bone marrow failure, (b) inappropriate response by the bone marrow and (c) deficiency of a hematinic.

Table 40.3: Classification of anemia by mean corpuscular volume (mcv)

Microcytic (MCV < 80 µ³)	Normocytic (MCV 80–100 µ³)	Macrocytic (MCV > 100 µ³)
■ Iron deficiency anemia ■ Thalassemias ■ Anemia of chronic disease	■ Hemorrhagic anemia ■ Hereditary spherocytosis ■ Autoimmune hemolytic anemia	■ Folic acid deficiency ■ Vitamin B_{12} deficiency ■ Liver disease ■ Drug induced (zidovudine)

Q. Enumerate the laboratory tests to diagnose iron deficiency anemia?
Ans.
- **Peripheral blood film:** Microcytic hypochromic anemia
- Low serum iron levels
- Raised total iron binding capacity
- Low serum ferritin levels.

Measurement of serum ferritin levels has the highest sensitivity and specificity for diagnosing iron deficiency anemia. Levels less than 10–15 mcg/L confirm iron deficiency anemia.

Q. What is the place of screening for anemia in pregnancy and routine iron supplementation?
Ans. Routine screening for anemia is recommended for all pregnant woman[1] (CDC 1998, 2002). Recommendation is also for universal iron supplementation to meet the increased iron demand in pregnancy except in few situations as with hemochromatosis.

Q. What is the rationale of universal iron supplementation in pregnancy?
Ans. Most women begin pregnancy with low iron store.[2] An average diet confers 15 mg of elemental iron per day. About 10% of ingested iron is absorbed. Total iron requirement during pregnancy is estimated to be approximately 1,000 mg. Using the criteria of diagnosis of anemia based on Hb (g/dL) and HCT (%) more than 50% of women throughout the world are anemic during pregnancy. About 75% of anemias that occur during pregnancy are secondary to iron deficiency. In adult women, most iron stores are in bone marrow, liver and spleen. If dietary iron intake is inadequate, absorption is poor from the gastrointestinal (GI) tract. **Moreover, if the pregnancies are too many and too frequent and delivery is complicated with hemorrhage, iron deficiency anemia is the eventuality.**

It is observed that nearly 80% of pregnant women have either low iron stores (100–500 mg) or no iron stores. Based on these data, it is wise to recommend iron supplementation to all pregnant women (Table 40.4).[3] They will improve maternal iron stores and are helpful for neonatal iron stores also.

Q. What are the food materials that enhances iron absorption?
Ans. Vitamin C, orange juice, grape fruit, strawberries, broccoli and peppers.

Q. What are the food materials that diminish iron absorption?

Ans. Dairy products, coffee, tea, pica (clay), antacids, soy products, spinach, GI disease (amebiasis) and proton pump inhibitors (PPI).

Table 40.4: Available iron supplements

Oral preparation (tablet)	Dose	Elemental iron
Ferrous sulfate	325 mg	65 mg
Ferrous fumarate	325 mg	106 mg
Ferrous gluconate	300 mg	34 mg
Parenteral		
Iron sucrose		20 mg elemental iron per mL: IV
Iron dextran		50 mg elemental iron per mL: IM/IV
Ferric gluconate		12.5 mg elemental iron per mL: IV

In practice, the diagnosis of iron deficiency anemia is often presumptive. It may be reasonable to start iron therapy empirically without first performing serum iron tests. Following iron supplementation to pregnant women with moderate iron deficiency, reticulocytosis may be observed after 7–10 days of iron therapy. This is followed by rise in Hb and HCT in subsequent weeks. Failure to response to iron therapy suggests incorrect diagnosis and should prompt to go for further investigations. Iron should be taken ideally 30 minutes before meals to allow maximum absorption. However, patient may develop dyspepsia and nausea with this schedule. Therefore, for compliance of therapy individual patient needs appropriate advise.

Q. What hematological investigations can differentiate the types of anemias?

Ans. Biochemical investigations for differentiation of anemia have been given in Table 40.5.

Table 40.5: Biochemical investigation

Investigations	Iron deficiency anemia	Thalassemia	Anemia of chronic disease
Serum iron	Decreased	Normal	Decreased
Total iron binding capacity	Increased	Normal	Decreased
Serum ferritin	Decreased	Normal	Increased

Q. When should parenteral iron be used in pregnant women?

Ans.
- Women who cannot tolerate oral iron.
- Women who will not take oral iron.
- Women with malabsorption syndrome.
- Women with severe iron deficiency anemia in later month of pregnancy.

Q. What are the different parenteral iron preparations used and what is the superiority of one over the other?

Ans. Iron sucrose complex given IV up to 100 mg. It may be given daily. Ten doses (1 g) can raise the levels of Hb and ferritin to the desired level. Iron sucrose have fewer allergic reactions compared to iron dextran (3.3 versus 8.7) and significantly lower fatality rate.

Oral versus intravenous sucrose for women with postpartum anemia showed significant rise in Hb levels on D5 and D14 when treated with IV sucrose therapy.[4] However by D40, there was no significant difference in Hb levels between the two groups. Thus, in most clinical situations oral preparations are appropriate and sufficient.

Iron dextran (50 mg/mL) can be given IM or IV. Intramuscular injections are painful. The preparation can cause anaphylaxis (1%). The reaction may be immediate or delayed.

Q. What is the role of erythropoietin for the treatment of anemia in pregnancy?

Ans. Role of erythropoietin in pregnant women with anemia have been studied in one randomized controlled trial. Hb level, reticulocytes count, HCT level was studied with the use of both parenteral iron and parenteral iron plus erythropoietin. All the parameters were found to be improved.[5] However, parenteral iron plus erythropoietin was associated with significantly shorter time to reach the targeted Hb level and other indices (reticulocyte count, HCT) levels within 2 weeks of treatment initiation. No difference in maternal and fetal safety was observed. However, no additional benefit was observed in the management of postpartum anemia with the use of erythropoietin and iron versus iron alone.

References

1. Recommendations to prevent and control iron deficiency in the United States. CDC. MMWR Recomm Rep. 1998;47(RR-3):1-29.
2. Scholl TO. Iron status during pregnancy: Setting the stage for mother and infant. Am J Clin Nutr. 2005;81(5):1218S-22S.
3. Pena-Rosas JP, Viteri FE. Effects of routine oral iron supplementation with or without folic acid for women during pregnancy. Cochrane Database Syst Rev. 2006;(3):CD004736.
4. Bhandal N, Russell R. Intravenous versus oral iron therapy for postpartum anemia. BJOG. 2006;113(11):1248-52.
5. Wågström E, Akesson A, Van Rooijen M, et al. Erythropoietin and intravenous iron therapy in postpartum anemia. Acta Obstet Gynecol Scand. 2007;86(8):957-62.

41. Hemoglobinopathy

Q. What is hemoglobinopathy?

Ans. Hemoglobinopathies are the inherited disorders of hemoglobin. Hemoglobin is composed of heme and four globin chains. When the abnormalities either in the quantity or in the quality of the globin chains are present in the hemoglobin molecule, the condition is known as **hemoglobinopathy**.

Q. What are the different types of hemoglobinopathies?

Ans. Hemoglobinopathies commonly are of two types:
1. **Qualitative abnormalities** of the globin chains may be there. This is due to substitution of amino acid in an alpha (α)-globin or in beta (β)-globin chain. This results in synthesis of an abnormal hemoglobin which can undergo sickling in certain situations.
2. Impaired (deficient) production of globin chains results in **quantitative imbalance** of globin chains in hemoglobin. The abnormality may affect the α-chain (α-thalassemia) or β-chain (β-thalassemia).

Q. What is the composition of adult hemoglobin?

Ans. In a normal adult:

Normal (%):	HbA ($\alpha_2 \beta_2$)	HbF ($\alpha_2 \gamma_2$)	HbA$_2$ ($\alpha_2 \delta_2$)
	96–98	0.5–0.8	1.5–3.7

Q. What type of hemoglobinopathy the woman presented in Chapter 39 belonged to?

Ans. The woman was diagnosed with a case of β-thalassemia minor. This was based on the investigations which was done in the hospital (Figs 41.1A and B).

Q. How the diagnosis of β-thalassemia trait is made?

Ans. The woman suffered due to mild to moderate anemia. Blood picture was of microcytic anemia. There was raised levels of HbA$_2$ ($\alpha_2 \delta_2$) more than 3.7% with normal or raised HbF ($\alpha_2 \gamma_2$) (2%). Serum iron either normal or raised and iron-binding capacity was normal. MCV and MCH were low but MCHC was normal.

Q. What is the reproductive outcome of such a patient with β-thalassemia in pregnancy?

Ans. Production in β-chain is directed by two genes. These genes are located (one copy each) on chromosome 11. More than 100 such gene mutations have been identified. In β-thalassemia minor, there is mutation of one gene. β-chain production is reduced by half. Excess of α-chains combines either with δ-chains producing HbA$_2$ ($\alpha_2 \delta_2$) or with

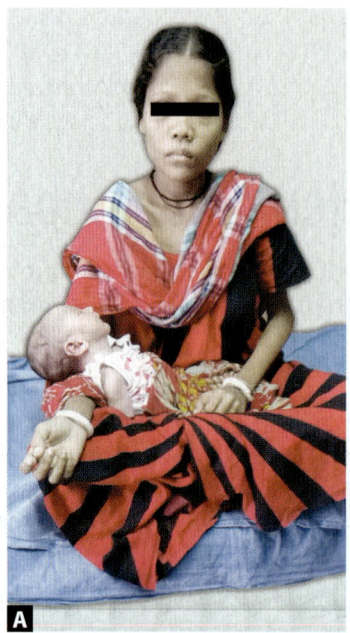 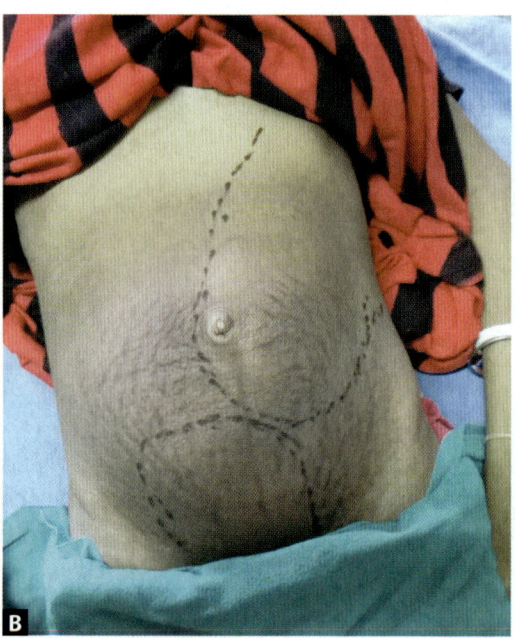

Figs 41.1A and B: A. 25-year-old woman with β-thalassemia minor in the postpartum period with her baby, **B.** The puerperal uterus and the hugely enlarged spleen is seen as outlined

gamma-chains ($\alpha_2 \gamma_2$). Pregnant woman with β-thalassemia minor usually tolerates pregnancy well. Thalassemia minor may coexist with sickle cell trait. In an individual with β-thalassemia major, both the genes are affected. Chance of survival for these subjects beyond teens is uncommon.

Q. What is the risk of transmission of the hemoglobinopathy to the baby?

Ans. Husband (partner) should be screened. When the husband of the woman is having β-thalassemia minor, the risk of the fetus being β-thalassemia major is 50%. Prenatal diagnosis could be done with chorionic villus sampling or amniocentesis.

Q. How do you manage such a woman in pregnancy?

Ans. The woman needs careful monitoring for her health as well as that of the fetus. Blood transfusion is required at a regular interval. Unnecessary iron loading should be avoided, oral and IV iron supplementations are generally contraindicated. Iron chelation therapy (desferrioxamine) is discontinued during pregnancy. Folic acid supplementation is given. Oral iron is given if ferritin level is low.

Q. What are the special risks for these women? How special care should be given?

Ans. Assessment of other organ function is needed. Iron overload is a problem for these women. For that reason, evaluation of functional status of heart, liver, thyroid and parathyroid glands and glucose testing should be done. Fetal well-being assessment should be done simultaneously. These patients need multidisciplinary team approach involving the hematologist and the fetomaternal medicine team involving obstetrician and the neonatologist.

Q. How do you manage the labor, delivery and puerperium?

Ans. Labor and delivery management are usual. However, some women may need additional care when there is any organ dysfunction (diabetes). Women may need blood transfusion if she is anemic. In the puerperium, she should be guarded against infection. Breastfeeding is not contraindicated.

Q. How the woman with β-thalassemia (major) behave?

Ans. Individuals with homozygous state of β-thalassemia (major) or Cooley's anemia are dependent on transfusion. Erythropoiesis is ineffective as there is no β-chain production. Usually, these individuals die of infections and cardiovascular complications in early life. They also suffer from infertility though successful pregnancies have been reported. These women who are transfusion-dependent often develop features of iron overload.

Q. What is the place of chelating agent in pregnancy?

Ans. Safety of chelating agent during pregnancy is unknown. There are reports of using chelating agents in the first trimester and successful pregnancy without any fetal malformations. Ideally, iron chelation is done before pregnancy. Chelating agent deferoxamine mesylate is commonly used.

Q. This patient (presented in Chapter 39) was given the replacement therapy with iron. How do you view the situation?

Ans. It is not common to see such a patient who is diagnosed to suffer from hemoglobinopathy late. She received oral iron therapy before the final diagnosis was made, for her problems of anemia. This is not uncommon again, as the deficiency (iron) anemia is the most common hematological disorder in our country. The suspicion is raised when the patient fails to respond to oral or parenteral iron therapy. Serum ferritin estimation is to be done to get the correct picture. These patients therefore carry risks of hepatic and cardiac hemosiderosis from iron overload. This is the reason that the patient with hemoglobinopathy should be screened for serum iron overload.

42 Sickle Cell Disease in Pregnancy

Q. What is the basic pathology in this disease?
Ans. It is caused by a point mutation in the β-globin gene on chromosome 11. This causes an amino acid change at position 6, changing valine to glutamic acid. This enhances the polymerization of hemoglobins in certain situations (hypoxia). There is increased cell rigidity and sickling. These sickled cells block the microcirculation. These sickled cells are not deformable and cannot squeeze through the microcirculation. Microvascular plugging causes local tissue hypoxia and infarction. Life span of sickle cells are 5–10 days compared to a normal RBCs of 120 days.

Gene mutation may be—homozygous (HbSS) or heterozygous (HbAS) (having 50–60% of HbA and 35–40% of HbS).

Q. What are the clinical manifestations of sickling phenomenon?
Ans.
- Vaso-occlusion in small vessels causing pain due to tissue infarcts (micro and macro) and organ damage
- Hemolytic crisis—anemia
- Others
  - Chest and girdle syndrome: Chest infections like pneumonia and avascular necrosis of femoral head
  - Renal dysfunction
  - Pulmonary hypertension
  - Cholelithiasis
  - Leg ulcers
  - Retinal disease
  - Neurologic (due to thrombotic events)—seizures.

Q. How these women become susceptible to different infections?
Ans. Recurrent episodes of sickling in the splenic circulation, results in splenic infarction. Most patients become hyposplenic at one age. They become susceptible to infections with encapsulated bacteria such as *Neisseria meningitidis, Streptococcus pneumoniae* and *Haemophilus influenzae*.

Q. How these women could be protected against such infections?
Ans. These women should be given penicillin prophylaxis. Erythromycin is the alternative for women who are allergic to penicillin. In addition, she should also be given pneumococcal vaccine, hepatitis B vaccine or influenza vaccine.

Q. How is the obstetric behavior of such women?
Ans. Obstetric complications are increased.
The complications are:
- Miscarriage
- Preterm labor
- Fetal growth restriction (FGR)
- Urinary tract infections (UTI)
- Pre-eclampsia
- Increased risks of painful crises
- Increased perinatal and maternal morbidity and mortality.

Q. How the offsprings are going to be affected when the mother is having sickle cell trait (HbAS)?
Ans. When the husband (partner) of the woman is also a sickle cell trait, there is 50% probability that the child will inherit the trait and 25% probability of inheriting the sickle cell disease (SCD).

Q. What is acute chest syndrome?
Ans. Acute chest syndrome (ACS) is a state of lung injury observed in association with SCD. It is different from the condition of pneumonia.
Pathology: ACS is the manifestations of lung injury caused by repeated episodes of embolism of fat from the bone marrow and also with the rigid sickled red cells. There is consolidation of lungs. The patient presents with cough, fever, pleuritic chest pain, leukocytosis and features of hypoxia.
Management: Resuscitative measures involve—blood transfusion, O_2 inhalation, bronchodilation and antibiotics. Patient may need intensive care management.

Q. What is the place of hydroxyurea in the management of SCD?
Ans. Hydroxyurea is a disease-modifying agent. It increases the levels of HbF, improves red cell hydration and decreases the rate of red cell polymerization of hemoglobins. Use of hydroxyurea reduces the episodes of sickle cell crises. However, hydroxyurea is not used in the pregnancy, though the risk of teratogenecity in human is unknown. Women on hydroxyurea should stop taking the medicine 3 months before conception.

Q. How these women should be managed in the antenatal clinic?
Ans.
- The woman is counseled with the information relevant with this disease (SCD).
- Antenatal care should cover a multidisciplinary team approach including obstetrician, hematologist, anesthetists, neonatologists and a skilled midwife.
- The woman need to be investigated for any chronic disease or end organ damage (renal and liver function tests, retinal screening, echocardiography for pulmonary hypertension and screening for iron overload). **Renal papillary necrosis and urinary tract infections are common**. Osteomyelitis is also observed.
- Folic acid (5 mg/day) supplementation is to be continued.
- Woman is advised to avoid certain factors that precipitate sickle cell crisis such as dehydration, sepsis, acidosis and extremes of temperature.
- Iron supplementation should be given when there are laboratory evidences of iron deficiency.
- Blood pressure measurement and urinalysis (including culture and sensitivity) should be done at each antenatal visit.

Q. Outline the intrapartum management of a woman with SCD.
Ans.
- Women with SCD are at high-risk. She should be delivered in a hospital and the availability of multidisciplinary team management is to be ensured.
  - Vaginal birth is preferred for the woman with SCD. Elective delivery may be done with induction of labor or elective cesarean section (if indicated) after 38+ (38 0/7) weeks of pregnancy.
  - Blood should be cross-matched for delivery or 'group and save' depending upon the case.
  - The precipitating factors for acute sickle cell crisis (dehydration, hypoxia, hypothermia, acidosis, sepsis) are to be avoided.
  - Fetal monitoring is to be done with continuous electronic fetal monitoring (EFM).
  - Regional anesthesia is preferred to general anesthesia during cesarean section.
  - O_2 saturation is maintained above 94% with pulse oximetry. Blood gas analysis may be needed when pO_2 level is <94%.

Patients with sickle cell anemia have increased amount of HbF. However, HbF is present in 0–20% of cells only. Cells containing little or no HbF become irreversibly sickled and are rapidly cleared from the system in the process of hemolysis.

Q. Outline in brief the postpartum management of a woman with SCD.
Ans.
- Women need to be managed with same degree of vigilance in the postpartum period. Risks of acute crisis and other complication (sepsis, ACS) are high.
  - Antithrombotic prophylaxis (LMWH) for 7 days following vaginal delivery and for 6 weeks following cesarean delivery is to be given.
  - Broad-spectrum antibiotics are to be given to prevent/control infections though routine antibiotic prophylaxis in labor is not supported.
  - Woman is advised for postpartum contraception.

Q. How to counsel the women for the use of contraceptions during the postpartum period?
Ans.
- Barrier methods of contraception are safe and effective in women with SCD. This method needs to be used correctly and consistently to minimize the failure rate.
  - Progestogen containing contraceptives
    - POP
    - LNG-IUS
    - Injectale (DMPA)
    - Implants (progestin)

    All are found safe and effective. Depot medroxyprogesterone acetate (DMPA) decreases painful crises more compared to other progestogens.
  - Estrogen containing contraceptives should be used as a second-line agent, concern is due to the risk venous thromboembolism.

Q. What is the place of prenatal diagnosis?
Ans. Women with SCD should have their husbands (partner) testing. When the partner is a carrier, woman needs to be counseled appropriately. Termination of pregnancy, if considered by the women for major hemoglobinopathy, it should be ideally done by 10 weeks of gestation.

Q. What is the place of blood transfusion in pregnancy?
Ans.
- Routine prophylactic transfusion is not recommended in pregnancy.
  - Hematocrit value is maintained >30% and HbA is about 50%.

- Exchange transfusion is indicated for women with ACS.
- Exchange transfusion increases the level of HbA.
- Women with anemia (hemoglobin <8 g/dL) should be given top up transfusion.

Q. How patient with acute painful crisis is managed?

Ans. Women having SCD with acute painful crisis should be managed in a hospital.
- Analgesia (pethidine to be avoided because of the risks of seizures). Analgesics are used depending upon the severity of pain. Commonly used analgesics are—paracetamol, NSAIDs (>12 weeks), dihydrocodeine or strong opiates like morphine.
- Fluids (IV) and oxygen inhalation.
- Thromboprophylaxis (low molecular weight heparin).
- Antibiotics—broad-spectrum when there is high clinical suspicion of infection.

Q. How the neonate should be screened?

Ans. Cord blood is sent to the laboratory for hemoglobinopathy screening. Maternal cell contamination is a possibility. Routine neonatal screening for sickle cell disorders is done in many countries (England).

Q. How the maternal and fetal risks are related with sickle cell hemoglobinopathy?

Ans. Sickling occurs in the homozygous condition (HbSS) or in compound heterozygous states (HbSC or HbS β-thalassemia, HbS D-Punjab). Sickle cell hemoglobinopathy with HbAS is essentially a benign condition. However, these individuals also need surveillance.

43. Thyroid Dysfunction in Pregnancy

Q. What are the physiological changes of the thyroid functions in pregnancy?
Ans. During pregnancy, the demand of thyroid hormones is increased. Thyroxin-binding globulin (TBG) level is raised due to raised levels of estrogens. Human chorionic gonadotropin (hCG) stimulates the thyroid gland and there is increased demand of iodine in pregnancy. Serum levels of maternal iodine falls due to increased renal clearance and transplacental shift to the fetus (Flowchart 43.1).

Daily requirement of iodine during pregnancy and lactation is about 200 mcg and 280 mcg, respectively. Fetal thyroid starts functioning between 10 and 14 weeks of gestation. At around 18 weeks, fetus starts secreting thyroid hormones.

Flowchart 43.1: Thyroid function tests in pregnancy and its interpretation

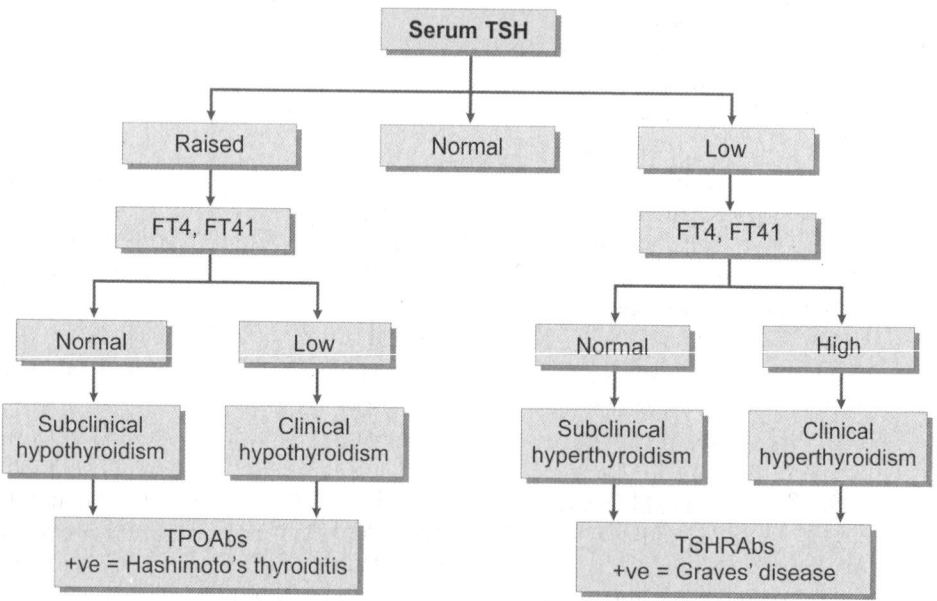

Q. What are the common causes of hyperthyroidism in pregnancy?
Ans.
- *Immune thyroiditis*
    - Graves' disease
    - Chronic thyroiditis

- **Non-immune thyroiditis**
  - Toxic nodule—solitary or multiple
- **Gestational hyperthyroidism**
  - Hyperemesis gravidarum
  - Gestational trophoblastic neoplasia (GTN)
  - Multiple pregnancy
- **Iatrogenic**
  - Excessive intake of thyroxin (overtreatment of hypothyroidism)
  - Iodine induced.

Q. **What are the important causes of hyperthyroidism in pregnancy?**

Ans. Autoimmune hyperthyroidism (Graves' disease) is the common cause of hyperthyroidism in pregnancy.

Q. **What are the important pathophysiological consideration with hyperthyroidism in pregnancy?**

Ans.
- **Maternal immunoglobulins (IgG):** Thyrotropin receptor autoantibodies (TSHRAbs), thyroid stimulating immunoglobulins (TSI) cross the placental barrier to reach the fetal circulation
- Maternal TSH does not cross the placenta but TRH crosses the placenta
- Maternal T4 crosses the placental barrier in the first half of pregnancy
- **Antithyroid drugs:** Methimazole, propylthiouracil (PTU), carbimazole (CZ), cross the placenta. These drugs may cause fetal goiter and hypothyroidism when given in high doses.

Gestational thyrotoxicosis
- Levels of FT4 and TT4 are raised (4–6 times the normal values).
- The women in early pregnancy (8–10 weeks) presents with nausea, vomiting, dehydration, ketonuria, mild palpitation, heat intolerance. In Graves' disease, these symptoms are preexistent to pregnancy.
- Features (biochemical and clinical) of hyperthyroidism subsides spontaneously by 20 weeks of gestation. Antithyroid drugs are rarely indicated.
- Serum levels of thyroid anti-TPO antibodies (TPOAbs) and TSHRAbs (markers of autoimmune disease) are absent. This is in contrast to Graves' disease where these antibodies are present.
- High levels of hCG molecules may have potent biologic activity as thyroid stimulators.
- Gestational hyperthyroidism usually does not affect the obstetric outcome adversely.
- Gestational thyrotoxicosis may recur in future pregnancies.
- Hyperthyroidism due to GTN usually subsides following evacuation of molar pregnancy as it eliminates the source of excretion of hCG. In some cases, treatment with β-adrenergic blocking drug (propranolol) is needed to control the adrenergic symptoms (palpitation, heart failure). Sodium iopanoate reduces the release of thyroid hormones and also block the peripheral conversion of T4 to T3. It can be used to control symptomatic hyperthyroidism.

HYPERTHYROIDISM IN PREGNANCY

Autoimmune hyperthyroidism (Graves' disease) is the common cause of hyperthyroidism in pregnancy.

Clinical diagnosis of thyrotoxicosis in pregnancy is difficult as many symptoms and signs are overlapped. The usual clinical presentation of hyperthyroidism are—palpitations, heat intolerance, tachycardia, goiter, proximal muscle weakness, orbitopathy, nervousness insomnia and weight loss despite increased appetite. Women may present with pre-eclampsia, eclampsia, systolic hypertension or small for gestational age (SGA) infants (Table 43.1).

Diagnosis is confirmed with thyroid function tests—a low or undetected TSH value in the presence of high values for FT4 or TT4 confirm the diagnosis of hyperthyroidism in pregnancy. Serum levels of TPOAbs (anti-microsomal antibodies) and TRAbs are elevated.

Table 43.1: Complications of hyperthyroidism in pregnancy

Maternal	Fetal	Neonatal
Pregnancy		
Miscarriage	Prematurity	Hyperthyroidism
Preterm labor	Fetal growth restriction (FGR)/SGA	
Pre-eclampsia	IUFD	Hypothyroidism
Eclampsia	Fetal hyper/hypothyroidism	Central hypothyroidism
Congestive cardiac failure	Craniosyntosis	
Placental abruption		
Postpartum		
Thyroid storm		

Management of Hyperthyroidism in Pregnancy

Principles of management are:[1]
- To prevent complications of the mother, fetus and the neonate.
- Monitoring the woman to maintain euthyroid state with an antithyroid drug (Table 43.2).

Table 43.2: Commonly used antithyroid drugs and their side effects

Drug	Dose	Side effects
▪ Propylthiouracil (PTU)	50–100 mg TDS	Polyarthritis, agranulocytosis, skin rash pruritus, hepatotoxicity, hepatitis, hepatic failure
▪ Methimazole (MM)	5–20 mg twice daily	Skin rash, pruritus, polyarthritis, embryopathy—aplasia cutis, hearing loss, facial abnormalities, developmental delay, choanal atresia

Considering the side effects of both the drugs, it is preferred to use PTU in the first trimester of pregnancy and thereafter, it is changed with MM (FDA and ATA).

Q. How the antenatal care is done and pregnancy is monitored?

Ans.
- The woman is seen at frequent interval (4 weeks) to assess clinical improvements.
  - Reduction of tachycardia, improvement of palpitation, nervousness, gain in weight and adequate fetal growth are essential.
  - Serum levels of FT4 and FT41 are maintained at the upper limit of normal.
  - Normalization of serum TSH suggests drug dose reduction.
  - Antithyroid drugs are maintained at the minimum level and an excess amount of antithyroid medications may cause fetal hypothyroidism and goiter.

- The need of antithyroid drugs decreases gradually after the second trimester. It is observed that about 40% of women remain euthyroid without any medications in the last few weeks.
- Drugs doses are to be monitored to avoid maternal (skin rash, hepatotoxicity) and fetal (hypothyroidism and goiter) side effects.
- Iodine (I^{131}) therapy is contraindicated in pregnancy as it induces fetal hypothyroidism.
- Iodine therapy is not done in pregnancy. Iodine crosses the placenta. Prolonged use of iodine may cause fetal goiter and hypothyroidism.
- Features of severe hyperthyroidism in pregnancy, labor or puerperium may be treated with β-adrenergic blocking drugs (propranolol).
- Surgery in pregnancy (subtotal thyroidectomy) may be done in selected cases.

Indications are few (a) Large goiter causing compression effects, (b) Cases where large amount of antithyroid drugs are needed (c) Woman found to be drug-resistant.

Postpartum management
- Use of antithyroid medication (in usual therapeutic doses) is not contraindicated for breastfeeding.
- The woman needs drug dose adjustment in the postpartum period.

Q. *What is the trimester-specific value of TSH and what is its importance?*

Ans. Table 43.3: Trimester-specific TSH reference ranges

Non-pregnancy	TSH reference range (mIU/L) 0.04–4.5
Pregnancy Trimester - 1st - 2nd - 3rd	TSH reference range (mIU/L) - 0.1–2.5 - 0.2–3.0 - 0.3–3.0

Importance: Using nonpregnant reference ranges, hypothyroid women could be misclassified during pregnancy as being euthyroid (TSH >2.5 but <4.0 mIU/L) (Table 43.3).

Trimester-specific reference ranges for TSH and T4 (total or free) should be done in each hospital antenatal setting.

Q. *What is thyroid storm and how it is managed?*

Ans. Thyroid storm is a clinical state with a severe form of thyrotoxicosis. The woman presents with hyperpyrexia (>103°F), tachycardia (pulse rate >140 bpm), nausea, vomiting, congestive cardiac failure and other neuropsychiatric symptoms. Confirmation is done with laboratory tests that reveal hyperthyroid changes (with raised FT4 values).

It is a life-threatening condition which needs immediate intervention. The patient needs management in an intensive care unit with a multidisciplinary team approach. Mortality is as high as 25%.

Management outlines are:
- ***Supportive care:*** Correction of dehydration, electrolyte imbalance, oxygenation and control of hyperpyrexia. Acetaminophen is commonly used.
- ***Control of infection*** (parenteral antibiotics) and management of congestive cardiac failure (digoxin therapy).
- ***Control of hyperadrenergic symptoms:*** Propranolol (β-adrenergic blocker) can be used.
- ***Control of hyperthyroid state*** with the antithyroid drug (MM or PTU) orally or through a nasogastric tube.

- **Corticosteroid (hydrocortisone IV)** is given to improve the clinical condition. It reduces the peripheral conversion of serum T4 to T3.
- **Lugol's iodine solution** 10–20 drops is given to block the synthesis of thyroid hormones.

FETAL AND NEONATAL THYROID DYSFUNCTION

Fetal hyperthyroidism: It is due to transplacental passage of high level of thyroid stimulating immunoglobulins (TSIs-IgG) that stimulates fetal T4 receptors to cause fetal hyperthyroidism. Fetal hyperthyroidism can be diagnosed with the features: (a) Fetal tachycardia (FHR >160 bpm), (b) FGR, (c) Oligohydramnios and (d) Development of fetal goiter as detected on ultrasonography. Cordocentesis can confirm the diagnosis.

Treatment is done with Antithyroid Drug to the Mother

Neonatal hyperthyroidism is commonly due to the transfer of maternal thyroid receptor antibodies to the fetus through placental barrier.

The fetus remained euthyroid as long as the mother received the antithyroid therapy during pregnancy. After delivery, the neonate develops hyperthyroidism as the protective effective of maternal antithyroid drug is absent. The neonate needs to be detected and managed for this problem urgently. The half-life of these immunoglobulins is short and the neonate becomes euthyroid soon.

Neonatal central hypothyroidism is observed in a neonate born to an untreated hyperthyroid mother. It is a phase of transient hypothyroidism due to the high level of T4 that reaches the fetal circulation through the placental barrier from the (untreated hyperthyroid) mother. This high level of maternal T4 in fetal circulation exerts a suppressive effect on fetal pituitary and hypothalamus. Diagnosis is made with the laboratory tests, low FT4 and low/normal TSH levels in the cord blood.

Treatment: Control of maternal hyperthyroidism.

UNIVERSAL VERSUS SELECTIVE SCREENING FOR THYROID DISEASE

Without evidence that identification and treatment of pregnant women with subclinical hypothyroidism improves maternal or infant outcomes, routine screening of subclinical hypothyroidism currently is not recommended (AACE, ATA-2011), (AES, ACOG-2007).

'It is reasonable to estimate serum TSH at the first obstetrical visit in those women of higher risk of thyroid dysfunction (ATA-2011)'.

INDICATIONS FOR THYROID TESTING IN PREGNANCY

- History of thyroid dysfunction or prior thyroid surgery
- Presence of thyroid symptoms or goiter
- Autoimmune disorder, type 1 DM
- Family history of thyroid dysfunction
- Use of amiodarone, lithium, iodinated radiologic contrast
- Unexplained infertility
- Geographic area with iodine deficiency
- Age >30 years
- TPOAb +ve
- BMI ≥40

In India, routine screening of pregnant woman for thyroid dysfunction should be considered to prevent adverse fetal and maternal outcome (FOGSI, ITS, ESI, API).[2]

HYPOTHYROIDISM IN PREGNANCY

Important Issues in the Management of Hypothyroidism in Pregnancy[3]

- Screening for the thyroid function in pregnancy—universal versus selective
- Management of subclinical hypothyroidism in pregnancy
- Management of hypothyroid women during pregnancy
- Isolated hypothyroxinemia.

    Q. What are the causes of primary hypothyroidism?
Ans.
- Insufficient dietary iodine
- Autoimmune thyroiditis (Hashimoto)
- Post-thyroid ablation (surgical I^{131} induced).

Case Summary

A 19-year-old girl was admitted to the medical ward for the problems of severe weakness, anorexia, abdominal pain and primary amenorrhea. She lost her interest to the environment. She stopped going to school.

On gynecological consultation and investigations, she was found to be severely hypothyroid, polycystic changes in the ovary. Her serum lipids and cholesterol levels were high. Sonography revealed cholesterol stones in the gallbladder. She was started thyroxin replacement therapy. She underwent cholecystectomy for the gallstones. She resumed her normal and regular menstruation. She returned back to her school. Her maintenance dose of levothyroxine was 150 mcg a day. This was her follow-up visit in GOPD six months during the treatment.

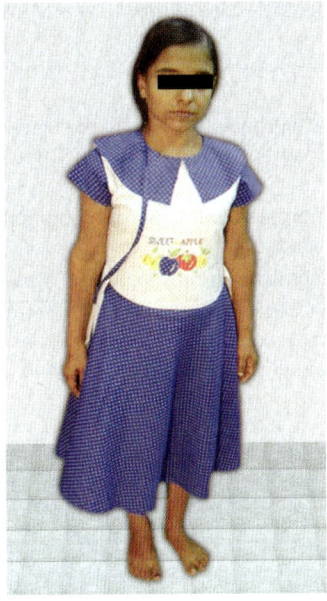

Fig. 43.1: Nineteen-year-old girl with hypothyroidism

    Q. What is postpartum thyroiditis (PPT)?
Ans. (Syn. postpartum thyroid dysfunction)[4]
- It is a transient thyroid dysfunction following delivery in euthyroid women.
- In majority of cases, it is due to Hashimoto thyroiditis.

- The best predictor of PPT is the presence of TPO antibodies regardless of its titer.
- However, it may develop in women with negative TPO antibodies also (1.7%).

Q. What is postpartum thyroid dysfunction (PTD)?
Ans.
- It is observed in 1.1–16.7% of all women
- Occurs around 8–16 weeks PP and lasts for 1–2 months
- Thyroid status may be ↑ or ↓ (transient or permanent)
- May be autoimmune or nonautoimmune form
- May be monophasic or biphasic
- There is increased association with type 1 DM (30%).

Q. How the diagnosis and the management of PTD is made?
Ans.
- Detection of serum anti-TPOAb, TgAb
- Estimate of serum TSH, FT4 levels
- May resolve spontaneously
- Blockers for symptomatic relief
- Medications for symptomatic cases only.

Q. What are the complications of hypothyroidism in pregnancy?
Ans. About 2% of pregnant women are hypothyroid.

Common complications in pregnancy are—miscarriage, pre-eclampsia, placental abruption, FGR, prematurity and stillbirths.

Others are: Mental slowness, decrease memory and psychomotor retardation.

References

1. Bahn RS, Burch HS, Cooper DS, et al. The Role of PTU in the Management of Graves's Disease in Adults: report of a meeting jointly sponsored by the American Thyroid Association and the FDA. Thyroid. 2009;19(7):673-4.
2. Clinical practice guidelines for management of thyroid dysfunction during pregnancy: Indian thyroid society and endocrine society of India.
3. American Thyroid Association Statement on Early Maternal Thyroidal Insufficiency: Recognition, Clinical Management and Research Directions. Thyroid. 2005;15(1):77-79.
4. Stagnaro-Green A, Abalovich M, Alexander E, et al. Guidelines of the American thyroid association for the diagnosis and management of thyroid disease during pregnancy and postpartum. Thyroid. 2011;21(10):1081-1125.

44

Heart Disease in Pregnancy

Q. Discuss the peripartum management of a woman with cardiac disease in pregnancy.

Ans.
- Management of such woman follows the standard obstetric care. **Additional care** specific to cardiac disease is to be provided also (Figs 44.1A and B).
- Majority of women **start labor spontaneously and deliver vaginally**. Babies are usually small.
- **Elective induction of labor** may be needed in few cases. This depends on the availability of multidisciplinary team members, to help the woman during the peripartum period.
- Monitoring of labor process, adequate pain control (epidural analgesia), O_2 inhalation (6 L/min), use of pulse oximetry, restricted fluid administration and use of cardiac monitor (ECG) are done.
- Avoidance for second stage stress (valsalva maneuver) and **to cut short the second stage** by forceps or ventouse.
- Management of third stage of labor—**oxytocin is preferred to ergometrine**.
- There is **circulatory overload** immediately following delivery due to autotransfusion from uteroplacental circulation. Aggressive diuresis (furosemide) therapy may be needed.
- When pharmacologic measures to treat pulmonary edema fail, noninvasive ventilation as biphasic positive airway pressure or intubation and **mechanical ventilation** are to be done.

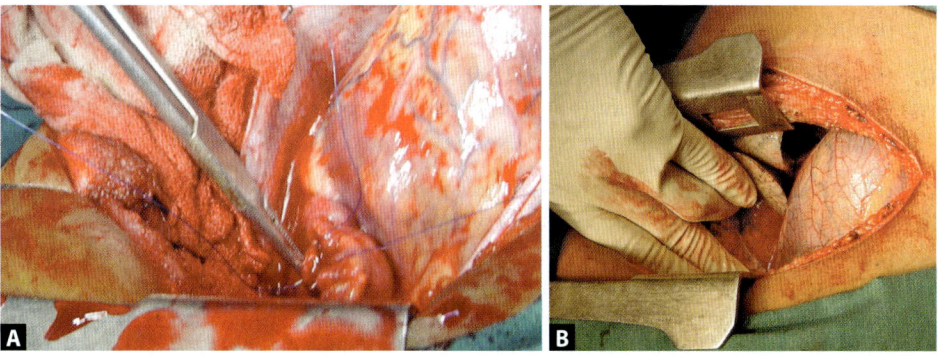

Figs 44.1A and B: Open heart surgery for mitral valve replacement in pregnancy (20 weeks of gestation), in a case with severe mitral stenosis

- **Patients on anticoagulation drug:** Administration of drug is to be stopped 4–6 hours before delivery or before induction of labor, cesarean delivery or regional anesthesia. PTT is allowed to normalize. Intravenous dose of UFH is stopped 4–6 hours before. LMWH is administered at the interval period of 24 hours. This interval reduces the risk of peripartum hemorrhage.

Q. How the problems of cardiac arrhythmias are managed?
Ans. Atrial arrhythmias, fibrillations will cause thromboembolic complications, pulmonary edema and deterioration of clinical situation.

Atrial arrhythmias are treated with digoxin and beta blockers. This will reduce the tachycardia. Anticoagulation therapy with heparin is to be started. Some patients may need direct current cardioversion. Anticoagulation therapy is useful to prevent thromboembolic stroke. Cardiologist should be involved.

Q. What are the different types of prosthetic heart valves?
Ans. Heart valves are of two types:
1. Mechanical heart valves (MHV) made of metal or carbon alloys
2. Bioprosthetic heart valves (BPV) derived from
   - Bovine or porcine tissue
   - Preserved human valves.

Q. What are the important differences between the two types of valves?
Ans. Differences are with two issues:
1. **Durability:** MHV work for 20–30 years whereas BPV work for 10–15 years. BPV undergo structural deterioration by 10–15 years.
2. **Thrombogenicity:** MHV are more thrombogenic and anticoagulation therapy has to be continued throughout the lifespan of the valve. BPV are less thrombogenic and anticoagulation therapy is not usually needed.

Anticoagulation therapy for patients with MHV: Warfarin vitamin K antagonist (VKA) is commonly used for thromboprophylaxis. Dose is maintained with a target INR of 2.0–3.0.
Other drugs used for anticoagulation: Unfractionated heparin or LMWH are commonly used. Both the drugs do not cross the placenta and have no fetotoxic effect. These drugs are used when VKA cannot be used. VKA (warfarin) is highly effective as an antithrombotic agent and to prevent thromboembolic complications (TEC). Warfarin when used in early pregnancy is associated with warfarin embryopathy.

Q. How the coumarin derivatives (VKA warfarin) act?
Ans. Warfarin depresses the synthesis of vitamin K-dependent clotting factors (factors II, VII, IX and X) in the liver. Warfarin crosses the placenta.

Q. What are the risks of warfarin use in pregnancy?
Ans. Warfarin embryopathy has been observed when it has been used in the first trimester of pregnancy.

These anomalies include—nasal bone hypoplasia, chondrodysplasia punctata, epiphyseal stipplings, limb or digital hypoplasia, microcephaly, cerebellar and cerebral atrophy, optic atrophy, cataracts, blindness, intraventricular hemorrhages, FGR and mental retardation. The risks of major birth defects with coumarin (warfarin) use, in the first trimester of pregnancy is 4.8% compared to 1.4% in controls. It is dose-dependent.

However, warfarin is an effective drug for thromboprophylaxis in pregnant women with MHV. Risk of TEC are doubled when warfarin is replaced with other agents.

Q. Discuss the role of LMWH and UFH in the management of pregnant woman with MHV.

Ans. Both the drugs LMWH and UFH can be used for this purpose. Both the drugs do not cross the placenta and are found safe to use in pregnancy even in the first trimester. LMWH is monitored with anti-Xa level of 1.0–1.5 IU/mL (peak levels drawn 3–4 hours after injection) and trough levels above 0.5 IU/mL. LMWH has got some advantages over by UFH. These are:
- Low risk for heparin-induced thrombocytopenia
- Low risk for osteoporosis
- Less risk for bleeding.

Q. What are the limitations of UFH and LMWH use in pregnancy?

Ans. Despite the use of UFH or LMWH with weight-adjusted doses, the risks of developing valve thrombosis is high (25%).

However, twice daily doses of LMWH is found superior compared to once daily dosing in pregnancy.

Q. What other agents can be used as antithrombotics?

Ans. Low dose aspirin (<100 mg/day) is used as an antiplatelet agent. It is used in pregnant woman with MHV concurrently with LMWH.

Q. What should be the optimum regimen for the use of antithrombotic agents in pregnant women?

Ans.
- Women need to be assessed for risk factors for developing valve thrombosis and the need of anticoagulation.
- Warfarin (VKA) is commonly used during the nonpregnant state and it is continued till pregnancy is confirmed (within 6 weeks).
- Warfarin (VKA) is changed to LMWH and close monitoring is maintained with anti-Xa levels. Peak levels (3–4 hours after injection) of 1.0–1.5 IU/mL and trough levels above 0.5 IU/mL are to be maintained. UFH can also be used instead of LMWH. Two or three doses a day may be given (SC). Monitoring is done by measuring APTT (twice the control).
- Warfarin may be restarted after 12 weeks and is continued till 36 weeks of pregnancy. INR is maintained at 2.0–3.5. Thereafter, LMWH or UFH is to be restarted and continued till 24 hours before the planned induction of labor or spontaneous onset of labor. This is done to reduce the risk of bleeding during the peripartum period.
- Postpartum anticoagulation is started with warfarin after 12–24 hours of delivery. Warfarin usually takes 2–5 days to reach the therapeutic levels of INR. During the gap period, LMWH or UFH may be used.

Q. How the risks of major hemorrhage could be minimized when the pregnant woman is on anticoagulation?

Ans.
- Inj. vitamin K with or without fresh frozen plasma (FFP) may be used to reverse the effect of warfarin.
- Dose adjustment (by delaying or withholding the drug with proper monitoring of serum parameters) can avoid the problem of major hemorrhage.

- Inj. protamine can reverse the effect of UFH completely but reverse the effect of LMWH partially.
- However, the management of cardiac disease in pregnancy needs the involvement of multidisciplinary team approach, including the cardiologist, anesthetist and the hematologist besides the obstetrician, neonatologist and the obstetric nurse.

Q. Should the woman breastfeed her baby when she is on warfarin (VKA) or UFH/LMWH?

Ans. Breastfeeding is not contraindicated in such a woman. The amount of secretion of these drugs in the breast milk is very low.

Q. How do you counsel a woman with heart disease for contraception during postpartum discharge?

Ans. Woman with cardiac disease needs contraceptive counseling as unplanned pregnancy may be life-threatening. Heart disease may be acquired (rheumatic) or congenital and each require special attention. Options of contraception include: (a) Barrier methods, (b) Hormonal contraception (oral and parenteral), (c) Intrauterine contraceptive devices (IUCDs) and (d) Sterilization.

Choice of contraceptive method depends on the maternal cardiac status, associated risk factors and the need of desired children.

Barrier methods are good, provided used correctly and consistently. Otherwise failure rate is high (up to 26 HWY). However, it can be used in conjunction with other method (progesterone only pill).

Contraceptives containing estrogen (COCs) preparation carry the risks of arterial and venous thrombosis. Hence, such contraceptives are generally avoided.

Progesterone only contraceptives are not contraindicated in women with cardiac disease; only limitations are irregular bleeding and slightly high failure rate compared to combined oral contraceptives (COCs).

The long-acting progesterone injectables (DMPA) are highly effective with very low-failure rates (0.3%). Irregular vaginal bleeding and/or formation of hematoma at the injection site is a problem for specially those women who are on anticoagulation therapy.

Intrauterine contraceptive devices (IUCDs) to consider are mainly of two types. Either of copper containing devices or LNG-IUS. IUCDs are very effective with a failure rate of 0.8 for CuT 380 and 0.1 for LNG 20. The fear with the use of these devices are the risks of bacterial endocarditis due to their predisposition to infection. However, WHO support their use in women with uncomplicated vulvular cardiac disease.

Sterilization: Women who has completed their families, are suitable for this method. However, women with complicated cardiac disease (severe pulmonary hypertension, left ventricular dysfunction, cardiomyopathy, NYHA class III and IV heart failure may also be considered for this permanent method of contraception.

Tubectomy or vasectomy needs to be discussed. Tubal ligation may be done by minilaparotomy under general anesthesia. Laparoscopic procedure of tubal ligation needs consideration of intraperitoneal CO_2 insufflations, raised intraperitoneal pressure and diaphragmatic elevation. Laparoscopic procedure should be done under general anesthesia as insufflations of the abdomen and pressure on the diaphragm is poorly tolerated under regional anesthesia. The risks are more in women with cyanotic heart disease and/or with pulmonary hypertension.

Vasectomy is a simple, safe and highly effective method. Complications of vasectomy, both short-term and long-term, are minimal.

45. Gestational Age and Cesarean Delivery

Q. What gestational age of pregnancy is considered the term pregnancy?
Ans. Conventionally, **term pregnancy** is considered the period extending from 3 weeks before and up to 2 weeks after the expected date of delivery.

Q. What was the purpose of defining the term pregnancy?
Ans. It was done with the expectation that perinatal outcomes of women delivered during this period were uniformly good.

Q. What are the current observations?
Ans. Term **pregnancy** is actually a long period of 5 weeks (37 0/7–41 6/7 weeks). Current research has shown that neonatal outcomes vary widely in terms of respiratory morbidity even when delivered within this wide range of 5 weeks of gestational age.

Q. What is the current recommendation in this issue?
Ans. The older definition 'term' has been replaced. It is currently designated as below.
Classification of term pregnancy (ACOG-2013)
- **Early term:** 37 0/7 weeks through 38 6/7 weeks
- **Full term:** 39 0/7 weeks through 40 6/7 weeks
- **Late term:** 41 0/7 week through 41 6/7 weeks
- **Postterm:** 42 0/7 weeks and beyond
- **Late preterm:** 34 0/7 weeks through 36 6/7 weeks.

Q. What is the significance of this work group recommendation (ACOG-2013)?
Ans. Uniform definitions of term are used to predict neonatal outcome more precisely and correctly. The new designations are to be used by all clinicians, researchers and data reporting systems.

Q. What is the clinical significance of using this new classification?
Ans. Currently, there is a growing trend of early delivery with an intention of improved neonatal and infant outcomes. Time of delivery often ranges from late preterm (34 0/6–36 0/7 weeks) to early term (37 0/7–38 6/7 weeks). Indications of such delivery may be medically indicated. In reality, it has been observed that morbidity and mortality rates are higher among the neonates and infants when delivered at early term period compared to those delivered by full term (39 0/7 weeks through 40 6/7 weeks) period of gestation.[1]

430 Manual of Obstetrics and Gynecology for the Postgraduates

Q. What are the morbidities associated with early term deliveries?

Ans.
- Respiratory distress syndrome (RDS)
- Transient tachypnea of the newborn (TTN)
- Birth asphyxia
- Ventilator use
- Hypoglycemia
- Pneumonia
- Respiratory failure
- Neonatal intensive care unit (NICU) admission (Fig. 45.1)
- Increased neonatal mortality.

Q. What are the overall risks of neonatal and infant morbidity and mortality when delivered at early term gestation?

Ans. The risks of adverse outcomes are greater for neonates delivered in early term (37 and 38 weeks of gestation). Respiratory failure rates [adjusted odds ratio (OR) 2.8; 95% confidence interval (CI) 2.0–3.9] and ventilation use (adjusted OR 2.8; 95% CI 2.3–3.4) were higher compared with infants delivered at 39 weeks of gestation.

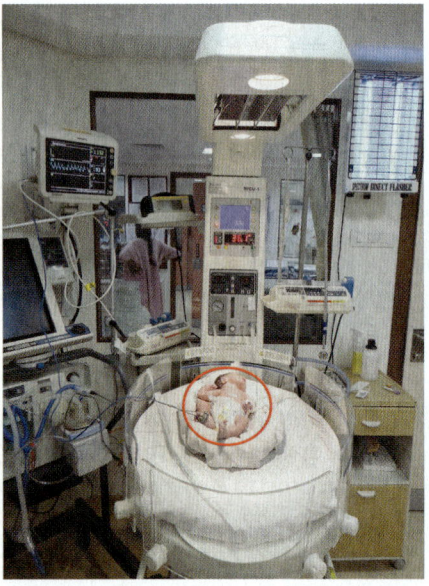

Fig. 45.1: Neonatal intensive care unit management of a preterm newborn weighing 1.1 kg.
Courtesy: Neonatal Care Unit—NRS Medical College and Hospital, Kolkata

Q. What would be the suggestions with these findings?

Ans. These findings suggest that scheduled cesarean delivery even a few days before 39 weeks of gestation should be avoided specially when it is not medically indicated.

Q. What is the difference in terms of mortality rate between the infants of the two groups?

Ans. Using 39 weeks of gestation as the reference group, the relative risk of neonatal mortality is 2.3 (95% CI: 2.1–2.6) at 37 weeks of gestation and 1.4 (95% CI: 1.3–1.5) at 38 weeks of gestation and 1.0 at 39 weeks of gestation.

Q. What are the different morbidities for the neonates when delivered late preterm or early term gestational age?

Ans. It is observed that respiratory morbidities are higher among neonates delivered during both the late preterm and early term periods when compared with neonates who are delivered at full term (39–40 weeks). It is also observed that non-respiratory morbidities are also increased in the first group compared to the full term neonates.

Q. What could be clinical guidelines in such a situation?

Ans. It appears that there may not be a clear universal approach to all category of women as regard the timing of cesarean delivery. However, for any non-medical reasons, early delivery before 39 weeks of gestation is not considered appropriate.[2]

Q. How the decision for timing of delivery is to be made?

Ans. Timing of delivery is an important decision to make. Maternal and newborn risks of the late preterm and early term delivery are to be balanced with the risk of further continuation of pregnancy. Decision has to be made in consideration with the available resources in the center. Moreover, such a late preterm or early term delivery should only be made for the benefit of the mother or the newborn or both. Therefore, decisions need to weigh the risks and benefits and must be individualized.[3,4]

Q. Should amniocentesis be done to determine the fetal lung maturation?
Ans. In a well-dated pregnancy, amniocentesis should not be used to guide the timing of delivery. The reasons are:
- When there is a clear indication of the late preterm or early term delivery for either maternal or newborn benefit, then delivery should be done, regardless of such maturity testing.
- Amniotic fluid indices for maturity do not suggest maturity in organ systems other than the lungs.

Q. Mention few situations in clinical practice that are medically indicated for late preterm and early term deliveries?
Ans. Examples (few) of medical scenarios (not all inclusive) commonly met in clinical practice are:
- Hypertensive disorders (pre-eclampsia, eclampsia)
- Placenta previa/placenta accreta
- Fetal growth restriction
- Prior cesarean delivery
- Diabetes with vascular disease
- Abruptio placenta
- Multiple pregnancy
- Oligohydramnios
- Alloimmunization of pregnancy with fetal affection
- Gestational diabetes with poor control

Q. What should therefore be the recommendation in the context of gestational age and cesarean delivery?
Ans. There are specific indications for delivery either late preterm or early term (before 39 weeks of gestation) that are medically indicated. This is mainly for the benefit of the mother or the newborn or for the both. However, in a clinical situation where the reason for cesarean delivery is for non-medical purpose, early term (before 39 weeks of gestation) is to be avoided.[5,6]

References

1. Hibbard JU, Wilkins I, Sun L, et al. Consortium on Safe Labor. Respiratory morbidity in late preterm births. JAMA. 2010;304(4):419-25.
2. Spong CY, Mercer BM, D'alton M, et al. Timing of indicated late preterm and early term birth. Obstet Gynecol. 2011;118(2 Pt 1):323-33.
3. Tita AT, Landon MB, Spong CY, et al. Timing of elective repeat cesarean delivery at term and neonatal outcomes. Eunice Kennedy Shriver NICHD Maternal-Fetal Medicine Units Network. N Engl J Med. 2009;360(2):111-20.
4. Reddy UM, Bettegowda VR, Dias T, et al. Term pregnancy: A period of heterogeneous risk for infant mortality. Obstet Gynecol. 2011;117(6):1279-87.
5. World Health Organization. International statistical classification of diseases and related health problems. 10th revision Vol 2, 2nd edn. Geneva: WHO; 2004.
6. Reddy UM, Ko CW, Raju TN, et al. Delivery indication at late preterm gestations and infant mortality rates in US. Pediatrics. 2009;124(1):234-40.

46 Place of Thromboprophylaxis during Pregnancy

Q. What are the indications of antithrombotic therapy in pregnancy?
Ans. Common indications are:
- To reduce the risk of thrombosis during pregnancy, labor and puerperium
- Pregnant women with prosthetic heart valves (See Manual of Obstetrics and Gynecology for the Postgraduates, p. 426).
- Women with thrombophilia
  - Inherited
  - Acquired
- Others
  - Systemic lupus erythematosus (SLE)
  - Women with obesity (BMI > 30 kg/m^2).

Q. Who are the women that need thromboprophylaxis in pregnancy?
Ans. Women with risk factors for venous thromboembolism (VTE) in pregnancy are considered for thromboprophylaxis.
  Risk factors are:
- **Previous thromboembolism**
- **Thrombophilia-inherited**
  - Antithrombin deficiency
  - Protein C deficiency
  - Protein S deficiency
  - Factor V Leiden
  - Prothrombin gene G20210A
  - Methylenetetrahydrofolate reductase (rare)
- **Antiphospholipid syndrome (acquired thrombophilia)**
  - Persistent lupus anticoagulant
  - Persistent anticardiolipin antibodies
  - β2 glycoprotein-1 antibodies
- **Medical comorbidities:** SLE, sickle cell disease, Nephrotic syndrome
  - Age >35 years
  - Obesity (BMI > 30 kg/m^2)
  - Multiparity ≥ 3
  - Smoking
  - Cesarean delivery, immobility, infection (postpartum).

Q. What are the different prophylactic measures against thrombosis and embolism during pregnancy and puerperium?

Ans.
- Women are encouraged to maintain mobility during labor and postpartum.
- Dehydration should be avoided.
- Considering thromboprophylaxis commonly used drugs are: Low molecular weight heparin (LMWH) and unfractionated heparin (UFH).
  Low molecular weight heparin (LMWH) is the drug of choice. LMWH is effective and safer than unfractionated heparin (UFH).
- Low dose aspirin may be used in some situation.
- Women with two or more persisting risk factors are considered for LMWH for 7 days following delivery.
- Women with three or more persistent risk factors (discussed above) should use graduated compression stockings.
- Thromboprophylaxis with LMWH for 7 days after delivery are considered for women with:
  - Obesity (BMI > 40 kg/m^2)
  - Emergency cesarean delivery (category 1, 2 or 3 *See* Manual of Obstetrics and Gynecology for the Postgraduates, p. 267).
  - Inherited or acquired thrombophilia.
- Women having LMWH antenatally should continue prophylactic doses of LMWH until 6 weeks postpartum.

Q. When to start antenatal thromboprophylaxis?
Ans. Thromboprophylaxis should be started antenatally as early as in pregnancy possible.

Q. How long should thromboprophylaxis to be continued by following delivery?
Ans. Woman with very high-risk for 6 weeks and woman with intermediate risk for 1 week.

Q. How the women are categorized for the risks of VTE?
Ans.

Risk category	Risk factors	Management outline
▪ **Very high**	▪ Previous VTE on long-term warfarin ▪ Antiphospholipid syndrome with previous VTE	▪ LMWH—antenatal + 6 weeks postpartum
▪ **High**	▪ Previous recurrent VTE ▪ Previous VTE + thrombophilia	▪ LMWH—antenatal + 6 weeks postpartum
▪ **Intermediate**	▪ Previous VTE + family history ▪ Previous single VTE with no risk factor at present	▪ LMWH—antenatal ± postpartum 7 days or 6 weeks depending upon the individual case

Q. What are the different LMWH used and what are the suggested doses?
Ans. Different LMWH need to adjust their doses according to the patient's weight. For weight adjusted doses (*See* Manual of Obstetrics and Gynecology for the Postgraduates, p. 240, 427).

47 External Cephalic Version

Areas of attention in writing review papers:
- Keywords of each question must be carefully noted.
- Not to write lists.
- A brief plan (with points) of answer for each question may be made in the beginning.
- Difficult question may be attempted with a clinical approach with an imagination of a patient management.
- Correct and concise answer begets marks. Too much writing is not encouraged.

Women with uncomplicated breech presentation should be offered external cephalic version (ECV) discuss.

Term **breech trial** (2000) revealed perinatal mortality and morbidity 1.6% in elective cesarean group and 5.0% in planned vaginal breech delivery group (RR 0.33, p < 0.001). Considering perinatal mortality alone, the respective rate for cesarean and vaginal delivery were 0.3% and 1.3% (RR 0.23, < 0.01). Similar rate for neonatal morbidity alone were 1.4% versus 3.8% (RR 0.36; p < 0.0003).[1]

Based on the review of current studies, it is considered that the route of delivery for term singleton breech, except in very rare circumstances, should be cesarean. **ECV** is the maneuver where fetal lie is changed to make it a cephalic presentation. Once it is successful, vaginal delivery of the fetus as vertex reduces all the risks of perinatal deaths and neonatal morbidity, compared to vaginal breech delivery. This also reduces the increased risks arising out of cesarean delivery.

With this knowledge, it is recommended that obstetricians should offer and perform ECV whenever possible (ACOG 2006).[2] ECV after 36 weeks should be attempted in the labor ward. Ultrasonography should be done to assess the fetal position, liquor volume and fetal heart rate (FHR).

Use of tocolytics and regional anesthesia (epidural/spinal) has been shown to increase the success rate of ECV. This is mainly due to significant abdominal wall relaxation with use of tocolytics and/or regional anesthesia. However, whether tocolytics should be used as a routine or selective is not known. Most centers prefer to use terbutaline 0.2 mg subcutaneously to increase the success rate of ECV. Use of regional anesthesia is not supported universally due to its lack of evidence (ACOG 2000). **ECV should be done at term pregnancy**.

The reasons for doing ECV at term are:
- Early ECV (32–36 weeks) associated with higher success rate (80%) but spontaneous reversion to breech presentation is also high (46%).
- Many breech fetuses would have been converted spontaneously to vertex had nothing been done.

- Any significant complication if arises, following ECV, immediate delivery by cesarean could be done as ECV is performed at term.

ECV has been found safe in a selected case. The reported complications are transient alteration in FHR pattern (5.07%), placental abruption (0.12%), vaginal bleeding (0.47%), emergency cesarean selection (0.43%) and low perinatal mortality (0.16%).[3] ECV should be done by trained professionals.[4]

Important predictors of failed version are:
- Engaged breech
- When fetal head palpation is difficult (maternal obesity)
- Irritable uterus.

Success rate of ECV was 0% when all the three factors were present and it was 94% when none was present. High success rate for ECV was observed with: (a) Parous women, (b) Adequate amniotic fluid, (c) Nonengaged breech and (d) Use of tocolytics.

Reduced success has been observed in:
- Engaged breech
- Anteriorly located placenta
- Fetal spine anterior or posterior
- Woman in labor
- Obesity.

Case need to be selected for considering ECV. Following are the contraindications of ECV:
- Fetopelvic disproportion
- APH, known uterine malformations
- Scarred uterus
- Fetal major malformations
- Maternal medical complications (severe PIH).

However, it has been observed that successful ECV does not reduce the cesarean rate completely, compared to a woman with spontaneous vertex presentation.[5] The intrapartum cesarean delivery rate even after successful ECV is twice the rate seen in spontaneous cephalic presentation. Success rate of ECV for a well-selected case is on an average of 60%.

References

1. Hannah ME, Hannah WJ, Hewson SA, et al. Planned cesarean section versus planned vaginal birth for breech presentation at term: A randomized multicentre trial. Lancet. 2000;356(9239):1375-83.
2. ACOG Committee on Obstetric Practice. ACOG Committee Opinion No. 340. Mode of term singleton breech delivery. Obstet Gynecol. 2006;108(1):235-7.
3. Collaris RJ, Oei SG. External cephalic version: A safe procedure? A systematic review of version-related risks. Acta Obstet Gynecol Scand. 2004;83(6):511-8.
4. Royal College of Obstetricians and Gynaecologists. The management of breech presentation: Guideline No 20, 2001.
5. Chan LY, Tang JL, Tsoi KF, et al. Intrapartum cesarean delivery after successful ECV; a meta-analysis. Obstet Gynecol. 2004;104(1):155-60.

48. Diminished Fetal Movements

Q. What factors influence the woman's perception about fetal movements?

Ans. **Maternal situation (positions):** Woman perceives most fetal movements while lying down compared to when sitting. Less movements are perceived when she is in standing position.

Maternal concentration toward fetal movements in a quiet surrounding is helpful (high) to perceive more movements compared to when she is busy or cannot concentrate to the movements of the fetus.

Placental position: Mother perceives less movement when placenta is localized to the anterior uterine wall.

Fetal situations:
- Fetal malformations (CNS, musculoskeletal systems) are associated with diminished fetal movements and have reduced perception by the mother. However, anencephalic fetus has been associated with more fetal movements.
- Fetal position—mothers perceive less fetal movements when fetal back is in anterior position.

Others
- Increased fetal movements have been observed by women following meals.
- Administration of corticosteroids for fetal pulmonary maturity has been observed to cause decrease in fetal movements.

Q. How the maternal perception of fetal movements are correlated with actual fetal movements?

Ans. Mother usually perceives fetal movements that are lasting more than 7 seconds. Fetal movements may be discrete kick, flutter, swish or roll. Maternal perception of fetal movements and the actual fetal movements detected on ultrasound showed a variation ranging from 45–88%. Maternal perception of fetal movements are more when she is on bed and concentrates her mind toward fetal movements.

Several other factors affect maternal perception of fetal movements. Important maternal factors are: Maternal activity, parity, obesity, medications and psychological factors including anxiety. Movement alarm signal is less than 3 movements in 1 hour or no movements in 12 hours time. Inability to count to 10 movements in a 12 hours period, known as **Cardiff count to 10** is also considered as an alarm signal.

Q. What is the significance of DFMC in relation to fetal wellbeing?

Ans. Maternal perception of fetal movements is regarded as the manifestation of a healthy fetus.[1] Principally, it is the increased state of maternal awareness and vigilance to the fetus with the perception to the fetal movements. Movement alarm signal (Sadovsky and Yeffe, 1974) is when there is < 3 movements in 1 hour. Cardiff count to 10 (Pearson and Weaver, 1976) warning is when there is < 10 movements in a 12 hours period. It has been suggested, reduced or absent FM, may be a warning sign of impending fetal death.

Most women (55%) had stillbirth perceived reduction or loss in fetal movements prior to the event. A significant reduction or sudden alteration in fetal movements is a potentially important clinical sign. However, several factors may alter maternal perception specially maternal anxiety. However, several studies have shown that maternal perception of RFM had a strong correlation with stillbirth.[2]

Q. At what period of gestation, a mother may be advised for DFMC and how she should report?

Ans. Mother may notice for FM counts after 28 weeks of gestation. She should be advised to follow her baby's movement patterns. When she perceives diminished or absent fetal movements, she should report to the physician in care. Failure to perceive 10 or more discrete movements in 2 hours period is considered to be reported to the physician concern.[3]

Q. What should be the management approach for a woman who presents with diminished or absent fetal movement?

Ans. Management approach includes detailed history-taking through clinical examination of the woman with auscultation of the fetal heart sound (FHS). Pinard stethoscope or usual stethoscope can be used. Ideally, a hand Doppler device will be of much use. Purpose is to exclude fetal death. Clinical examination is done to detect any risk factors, such as hypertension, FGR, SGA, placental insufficiency and congenital malformations.[4]

When there is a presence of FHS on auscultation and the woman has no risk factors, she can be reassured. She advised for follow-up antenatal visit with a next date. She should maintain the kick chart.

On other hand, if FHS could not be confirmed she should be referred for immediate ultrasound scan assessment for fetal cardiac activity.

Q. What should be the next course of management when fetal viability has been confirmed?

Ans. Depending upon the clinical assessment, as ultrasound scan fetal biometry determination is to be done. CTG would be the next course to exclude any fetal compromise.[5] It is initially done over a period of 20 minutes. **Four parameters of CTG** are assessed (baseline fetal heart rate, baseline variability, accelerations and decelerations). Presence of acceleration coinciding with fetal movement indicates a healthy fetus. It has been observed that a stillbirth rates (corrected for lethal congenital anomalies) after a reactive or non-reactive CTG were 1.9 or 26 per 1,000 births, respectively (Fig. 48.1).

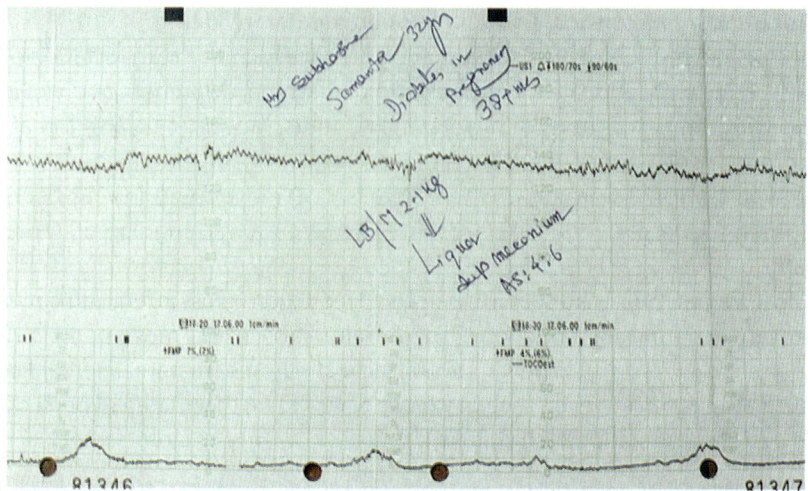

Fig. 48.1: Mrs S, 32-year-old lady, known diabetic, in labor at 38+ weeks of gestation with meconium stained liquor, CTG revealed: 1. Baseline FHR: 136 bpm; 2. Baseline variability: <= 5; 3. Acceleration: absent 4. Deceleration: absent. Trace pattern was: Pathological/category III. Cesarean delivery was done, baby boy was born weighing 2.1 kg with Apgar score: 4–6 and 10 at 0–5 and 10 minutes. Liquor was deeply meconium stained

Q. What would be the management plan when the woman complaints for RFM despite of normal CTG?

Ans. Ultrasound scan assessment should be performed as early as possible (preferably within 24 hours) in such a case. Fetal biometry should be done to detect FGR, SGA and the amniotic fluid volume. Fetal morphology should also be assessed at this time. During evaluation of this study, umbilical artery flow velocimetry could be done (Figs 48.2A and B). With the use of ultrasonography, there was significant reduction in all stillbirths from 3.0 to 2.0 per 1000 and from 4.2% to 2.4% of women presenting with RFM.

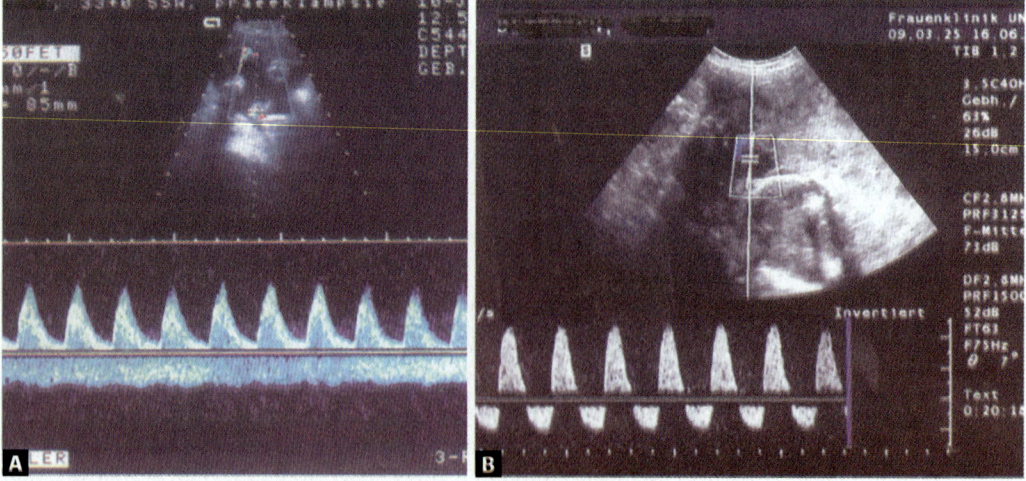

Figs 48.2A and B: A. Grossly reduced diastolic flow, **B.** Reversed diastolic flow is seen

Diminished Fetal Movements

Q. Could there be any role of fetal biophysical profile (BPP) as an investigation of RFM?

Ans. BPP may be used in a high-risk woman. It has good negative predictive value; that is fetal death is rare in women when BPP is normal.

Q. What should be the management approach for a woman with RFM when all investigations are normal?

Ans. The woman is explained with the investigation reports. She is reassured that in majority of cases (70%) following a single episode of RFM, the perinatal outcome is normal. However, the woman is advised to contact the physician in care if there are recurrent episodes of RFM.

Q. What should be the management approach when a woman presents with recurrent episodes of RFM?

Ans. She needs detail of assessment to detect any high-risk factor for fetal compromise. CTG and ultrasonography including Doppler studies may need to be done. Woman presenting with recurrent episodes of RFM has increased risk of poor perinatal outcome (Fig. 48.3).

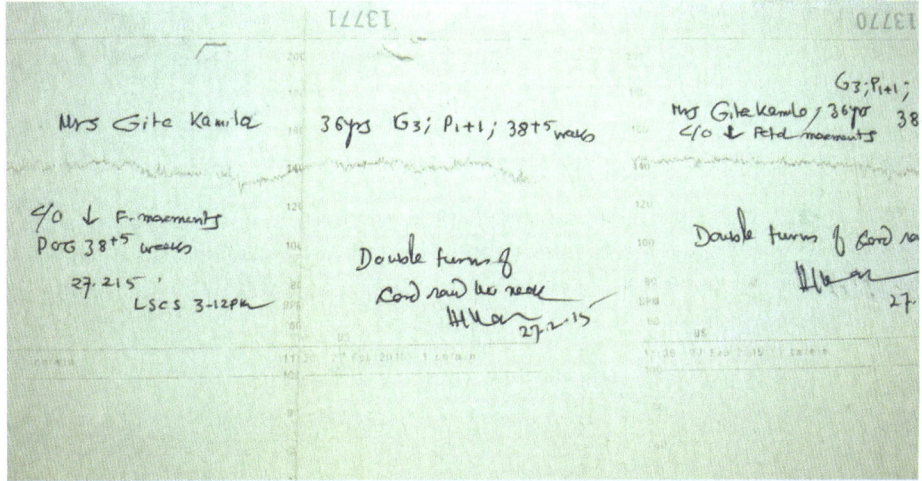

Fig. 48.3: Mrs G, 36-year-old woman, G2, P-1, A1, admitted with diminished fetal movements, at 38+5 weeks of gestation. CTG pattern was as shown: 1. Baseline FHR : 140; 2. Variability : ≤ 5; 3. Acceleration: absent; 4. Deceleration present. Trace pattern was: Pathological/category III. Emergency cesarean section was done for her. Double turns of tight cord round the neck was found

Q. What would be the definite management approach for such a woman?

Ans. Decision has to be made based on individual case analysis, period of gestation and presence of any high-risk factor. Based on these, induction of labor at term ≥ 37 0/7 weeks or late preterm ≥ 34 0/7 may be done. However, in all cases for early delivery (termination of pregnancy), center should have the facilities of special care neonatal unit. Betamethasone should be given to the mother when gestational age < 34 weeks.

References

1. Saastad E, Vangen S, Frøen JF. Suboptimal care in stillbirths—a retrospective audit study. Acta Obstet Gynecol Scand. 2007;86(4):444-50.
2. Freeman RK, Anderson G, Dorchester W. A prospective multi-institutional study of antepartum fetal heart monitoring. I. Risk of perinatal mortality and morbidity according to antepartum fetal heart rate test results. Am J Obstet Gynecol. 1982;143(7):771-7.
3. Pearson JF, Weaver JB. Fetal activity of fetal wellbeing: an evaluation. BMJ: 1976;1:1305.
4. Sadovsky E, Yaffe H, Polishuk W. Fetal movement monitoring in normal and pathologic pregnancy. Int J Gynecol Obstet. 1974;29(11):799-801.
5. Grivell RM, Alfirevic Z, Gyte GM, et al. Antenatal cardiotocography for fetal assessment. Cochrane Database Syst Rev. 2010;(1):CD007863. RCOG: Reduced fetal movement, Greentop Guidelines Feb 2011.

49. Transfusion in Obstetrics

Transfusion is the procedure that involves transfer of blood or blood components from one person (the donor) to another person (the recipient).

A blood transfusion can be a life-saving process. It is commonly done in:
- **Acute condition:** To replace the blood loss due to severe hemorrhage [major postpartum hemorrhage (PPH)].
- **Chronic condition:** Treatment of severe anemia (in pregnancy).

Oxygen carrying capacity is met for most nonpregnant women with a hemoglobin of 7g/dL, hematocrit (HCT) of around 21%. Adequate tissue perfusion is maintained. Transfusion is appropriate if there is associated active bleeding, surgery, chronic lung or cardiovascular disease. Each unit of transfused red blood cells (RBCs) will increase the Hb by approximately 1 g/dL.

Q. What are the principles of clinical transfusion practice?

Ans. Unnecessary transfusion could be avoided with the following measures:
- Early detection of anemia and its appropriate management
- Practice of good anesthetic and surgical management stopping/reducing the use of anticoagulants, antiplatelet agents before planned surgery
- Salvaging and reinfusing surgical blood losses
- Use of IV fluids replacement with crystalloids or colloids in cases with acute blood loss. This is done for volume replacement in a case with volume depletion
- Use of antifibrinolytic agents (tranexamic acid) to minimize blood loss.

Blood is a scarce and expensive resource, therefore, its use should be more rational.

Q. What is the whole blood?

Ans. Whole blood is the unseparated blood collected in an approved container with an anticoagulant preservative.

Q. What are the blood components?

Ans.
- Blood components are the constituents of blood, separated from the whole blood.

  Types of blood components are:
  - RBC concentrates or packed RBCs
  - Red blood cell suspension (RBCs + additive solution)
  - Plasma, fresh frozen plasma (FFP)
  - Platelets concentrates
  - Cryoprecipitate
  - Leukocyte depleted (filtered) red cells.

- Blood products are the plasma proteins prepared specifically as:
  - Albumin
  - Coagulation factors concentrates
  - Immunoglobulins.

Apheresis is a mechanical method of separating and collecting plasma or platelets directly from the donor.

Q. What are the different functions of anticoagulant and preservative solution in blood collection pack?

Ans.
- **Sodium citrate (C):** Binds with calcium ions and does not allow blood to clot
- **Phosphate (P):** Supports metabolism of red cells during storage
- **Dextrose (D):** Maintain red cell membrane to increase storage life
- **Adenine (A):** Provides energy.

Q. Discuss about whole blood transfusion in obstetrics:

Ans.
- Total volume in a bag: 550 mL, Hb: 12g/dL, hematocrit: 45%
- There are risks of all transfusion-transmissible infections

Storage: Between +2°C and +6°C

Indications:
- Red cell replacement in acute blood loss with hypovolemia
- Exchange transfusion
- Patients need red cell transfusions where red cell concentrates are not available

Contraindications: Risk of volume overload in patients with:
- Chronic anemia
- Incipient cardiac failure

Administration: Must be ABO, Rh compatible; Never add any medications.

Q. What are the major effects of storage on whole blood?

Ans.
- Fall in blood pH
- Rise in plasma K^+
- Progressive reduction in the red cell content of 2, 3-DPG, which may reduce the release of oxygen at tissue level
- Loss of all platelets function in whole blood within 48 hours of donation.

Reduction in factor VIII to 10–20% of normal within 48 hours of donation.

Q. Discuss about the PRBCs transfusion.

Ans.
- Virtually, all the plasma from the whole blood is removed
- **Volume:** 150–200 mL, Hb: 20 g/dL, Hct: 55–75%
- **Infection risk:** As for whole blood
- **Storage:** Between +2°C and +6°C
- **Indications:**
  - Replacement of red cells in anemic patients
  - Use with crystalloid replacement fluids or colloid solution in acute blood loss
- **Disadvantages:**
  - High PCV/Hematocrit with increased viscosity
  - White cells are a cause of febrile nonhemolytic transfusion reactions in some patients.

Q. What is the fresh frozen plasma (FFP) and what are its uses?

Ans.
- Plasma is separated from whole blood by centrifugation or by allowing the red cells to settle under gravity in a blood bank refrigerator.
- Fresh frozen plasma is used for the treatment of coagulation disorders (cases with deficient coagulation factors).
- FFP is frozen at −25°C or colder (FFP contains factors: II, V, VII, VIII, IX, X, XI).
- FFP can be stored for at least one year or longer.
- Volume: 200–250 mL.
- It contains multiple coagulation factors, including protein C and S, albumin and immunoglobulin.
- Plasma is not recommended as a replacement fluid to correct hypovolemia.
- Plasma carries the same risk like whole blood that of transfusion-transmissible infections.
- Plasma does not offer any additional clinical benefit over crystalloid or colloid fluids.
- Plasma is expensive; crystalloids or colloids replacement fluids are inexpensive.
- **Infection risk:** Very low-risk if treated with methylene blue or UV light.
- **Indications:**
  - Replacement of multiple coagulation factor deficiencies
  - Hemorrhage due to warfarin, DIC, HUS or in TTP.
- **Dosage:** 15 mL/kg
- **Administration:** ABO compatible, hypovolemia alone is not an indication.

Q. What is platelet concentrate and what are its uses?

Ans.
- Prepared from whole blood centrifugation or by plateletpheresis
- 40 mL contains 55×10^9: **Infection risk:** As in whole blood
- **Storage:** 20–24°C for up to 5 days
- **Indications:** Prevention of bleeding due to (a) Thrombocytopenia (b) Platelet dysfunction
- **Contraindications:** Not indicated in ITP, TTP, DIC. Thrombocytopenia associated with septicemia
- **Dosage:** 1 unit per 10 kg body weight
- **Platelet concentrate (PC):** D positive donor's PC should not be given to D negative child-bearing female
- Should be ABO compatible.

Q. What is cryoprecipitate and what are its uses?

Ans.
- Cryoprecipitate is prepared from fresh frozen plasma. It is rich in factors VIII, XIII, vWF and fibrinogen
- **Volume:** 20 mL
- **Infection risk:** As for plasma
- **Storage:** At −25°C or cooling for up to 1 year
- **Indications:**
  - Inherited deficiencies of
    - von Willebrand Factor
    - Factor VIII
    - Factor XIII
  - DIC
- **Administration:** Use ABO compatible products.

Q. What are the adverse reactions due to blood transfusion?
Ans.
- *Immunological*—alloimmunization and incompatibility
    - **Hemolytic reactions:** Immediate and/or delayed. It could be against red cells, leukocytes and/or platelets
    - **Nonhemolytic**—subfebrile reactions
        - Transfusion related lung injury (TRALI) due to anti-HLA antibodies
        - Urticarial reactions
        - Anaphylactic reactions
        - Graft versus host reaction
- **Infections**
    - **Viruses:** HAV, HBV, HCV, HIV, HHVB, CMV, HTLV-1
    - **Parasites:** Malaria, toxoplasma, trypanosomiasis
    - Bacteria
    - Others
- Circulatory failure due to overload
- Hypothermia
- Iron overload
- **Massive transfusion:** Bleeding, electrolyte imbalance (↑ K$^+$)
- Air embolism.

Q. How autologous blood could be used?
Ans.
- Collection and reinfusion of the patients own blood
    - Preoperative donation (Hb of 11 g/dL, Hct ≥ 34%), collection and storage of patient's own blood for the use in operation at a later date
    - Therapeutic dose of iron is given to build-up hemoglobin level.
      It may be done in cases with placenta previa where blood transfusion is often needed during the time of delivery.

Q. How intraoperative blood salvage could be done and used?
Ans.
- Collection of blood from the peritoneal cavity in a sterile method is done and reinfusion of shed blood is done to the same patient
    - A semicontinuous flow centrifugation device is done to wash the collected cells.

TRANSFUSION IN CLINICAL PRACTICE

- Woman in third trimester of pregnancy and Hb between 5.0 and 7.0 g/dL and in the presence of symptoms, blood transfusion should be given. It should preferably be PRBCs.
- Women listed for elective CS with the diagnosis of:
    - Placenta previa (antepartum hemorrhage)
    - Prior H/O PPH or prior cesarean delivery.
  All should have arrangement for transfusion ready.
- Hb between 8.0 and 10 g/dL: The following procedure should be done: (a) Blood grouping (ABO and Rh), crossmatching and (b) saving (at least one unit).

50 Obstetric Cholestasis

Obstetric cholestasis (OC) is the second most common cause of jaundice in pregnancy. The first is the viral hepatitis. In India, overall incidence is 1.2–1.5%. Hyperestrogenic conditions are the main cause though other factors like genetic (autosomal dominant) and familial (30–50%) are there. COCs intake is also associated with increased incidence. Geographically, commonly observed in South American Countries (Chile 12–22%). Cholestasis is mainly due to estrogen-induced disruption of the membrane transport mechanism in the hepatocytes and there is altered cholesterol, phospholipid ratio.

Diagnosis of OC is by one of exclusion. Details of history (family, COCs use, previous pregnancy, drug intake, pre-existing liver disease, alcohol abuse and of viral hepatitis) to be taken. Thorough clinical examination should be done. Jaundice is usually mild and bilirubin level is usually < 5 mg/dL. Woman often presents with itching specially at night. Liver function tests are done. Serum transaminases are elevated (2–4 fold). Bile acid levels are raised (10–100 fold). Ultrasonography (to exclude gallstones), serological test for hepatitis (HAV, HBV, HCV, CMV) and autoimmune liver diseases (anti-mitochondrial or anti-smooth muscle antibody) are done.

OC is associated with increased risks of IUFD, meconium-stained liquor, intrapartum fetal distress and neonatal bleeding diathesis (due to vitamin K deficiency). Risk of maternal hemorrhage (PPH) is also high due to decreased synthesis of vitamin K and the relative deficiencies of vitamin K dependent clothing factors (II, VII, IX, X).

Management issues: Treatment of OC with medication is not supported with evidence. Cholestyramine is effective for itching. It may cause steatorrhea and deficiency of fat-soluble vitamins. Ursodeoxycholic acid is found to be helpful. It reduces itching and improves liver functions. All women with OC should be given vitamin K. Water-soluble vitamin K (menadilol sodium phosphate) in doses of 5–10 mg daily is given. Neonates should be given vitamin K as in a routine. Women with raised levels of transaminases and bile acids should be counseled for planned delivery (induction of labor) after the 37 weeks of pregnancy. Intrapartum monitoring should be close to avoid the complications (discussed above). Third stage of labor is managed actively.

Obstetric cholestasis resolves spontaneously following delivery. LFTs should be done following 10 days of delivery to check the normalization of liver function. Woman need to be counseled as regard the risk of recurrence (50–60%) in subsequent pregnancy. She is advised to avoid COCs as it may alter liver the functions similar to pregnancy.

51
Diabetic Nephropathy

Q. How the severity of diabetes is classified?
Ans. Women with GDM or DM requiring insulin are designated by letters (B, C, D, F, R, T and H). Usually, such women have poor perinatal outcome compared to women whose diabetes is controlled by diet alone.

Q. What is diabetic nephropathy?
Ans. About 25–30% of women with IDDM develop nephropathy after a period of about 16 years. Nearly 10–20% of women with incipient diabetic nephropathy with microalbuminuria (30–299 mg/24 hours) turn to overt nephropathy (> 300 mg /24 hours of urinary albumin excretion). Such women run the risk of developing superimposed pre-eclampsia. The important biochemical parameter to predict perinatal outcome are:
- Proteinuria > 3g/24 hours
- Serum creatinine > 1.5 mg/dL (reduced creatinine clearance rate).

Q. How diabetic nephropathy could be managed?
Ans. The management of a diabetic woman with nephropathy needs control of hypertension to prevent further deterioration of kidney function. This is an addition to control the diabetes. Calcium channel blocking agents appear to be renoprotective and are not teratogenic. These drugs can be used in pregnancy. ACE inhibitors and angiotensin receptor blockers are contraindicated during pregnancy as they may result in fetal renal proximal tubular digenesis and oligohydramnios. Depending upon the level of creatinine clearance, woman with diabetic nephropathy may need renal transplantation.

Q. How retinopathy is related to diabetes?
Ans. Prevalence of retinal disease is directly related to the severity and duration of diabetes as well as with the age of onset. It usually develops over a period of 20 years. **Other factors are:**
- Levels of elevated HbA1C in first trimester
- Severity of hypertension.

Q. What are the pathological changes in the retina of a woman with diabetic retinopathy?
Ans. Class R diabetic women suffer with proliferative retinopathy with neovascularization and microaneurysms. These vessels may rupture and cause vitreous hemorrhage. With progress of pathology, there is retinal scaring and detachment. Ultimately, the patient suffers from loss of vision.

Q. How such women are managed?
Ans. Ideally, glycemic status should be maintained normal before the onset of conception. Hypertension need to be controlled. Laser photocoagulation is ideal for most women with proliferative retinopathy. Termination of pregnancy may be needed for women with florid retinal neovascularization and that is unresponsive to the therapy.

52. Renal Transplant

Q. Outline the management of a woman with renal transplant in pregnancy.

Ans. A woman with renal transplant in pregnancy need to be assessed for her health and for the wellbeing of the fetus. The following information suggests optimal maternal health status following transplant:
- No evidence of graft rejection for approximately 2 years of the post renal transplant
- Proteinuria either absent or minimal (≤ 299 mg/24 hours)
- Hypertension is either absent or well-controlled with antihypertensives
- Ultrasound examination of the kidney: Either normal or absence of any pelvicalyceal dilation
- Serum creatinine, < 125 µmol/L
- Immunosuppressive therapy: Lowest minimal dose (prednisolone ≤ 15 mg/day, azathioprine ≤ 2 mg/kg)

Pregnancy complications may be increased in some women. **Complications are:** Miscarriage, fetal growth restriction (FGR), preterm delivery, development of pre-eclampsia and also graft rejection (5%). The fetal and neonatal complications are infection, RDS, thrombocytopenia and adrenocortical insufficiency.

Management issues: Preconceptional counseling—woman should be managed carefully after transplant so that she is in a optimal state of health. She should be seen jointly by the nephrologists and the obstetricians.

Antenatal care: Assessment of renal function is to be done to detect any impairment of renal function.
- ***Mild impairment:*** Serum creatinine <125 µmol/L and well-controlled or absent hypertension.
- ***Moderate impairment:*** Serum creatinine 125–250 µmol/L and moderate hypertension.
- ***Severe impairment:*** Serum creatinine > 250 µmol/L and uncontrolled hypertension.

Fetal monitoring: Ultrasonography for fetal growth profile.
- Continued assessment of maternal health—anemia, serology for CMV, BP monitoring is continued. Serum creatinine assessment is maintained.
- Care during labor and delivery—close monitoring of maternal and fetal conditions are done.

- Cesarean section is done for obstetric indications only. Pelvic kidney is not an indication for cesarean delivery.

Postpartum care: Woman is counseled:
- To avoid breastfeeding (as the immunosuppressive drugs are excreted in the breast milk)
- Routine cervical cytology screening.

53 Non Hemorrhagic Shock in Obstetrics

Obstetric shock is not uncommon and is a life-threatening event. Commonly shock is classified into:
- Hemorrhagic shock
- Non hemorrhagic shock.
  Non hemorrhagic shock may be due to different reasons (see below).

Q. What are the cardinal events in maternal collapse?
Ans. Cardinal events are as follows:
- Maternal collapse is an acute event.
- It mainly involves the cardiac and respiratory system. } It may potentially lead to death.
- It involves the brain also.
- It may occur in pregnancy, labor or in the postpartum (6 weeks) period.

Q. What is severe acute maternal morbidity (SAMM)?
Ans. A woman who nearly died but survived a complication that occurred during pregnancy, childbirth or within 42 days of termination of pregnancy.

Q. What is the prevalence of SAMM?
Ans. Indian data is difficult to quote. However, in UK, it is 6 per 1,000 maternities, where maternal mortality rate (MMR) is 14 per 100,000 livebirths.

Q. What is the opinion of CEMACH report about the SAMM in UK?[1]
Ans. It is mainly due to:
- Poor resuscitation skills of the professionals working in the labor ward.
- However, death and disability may occur with best effort though.

Q. What are the common causes of obstetric shock (Fig. 53.1)?
Ans. Common causes of obstetric shock (Resuscitation Council, UK) are:

4Hs	4Ts	Others
- Hypovolemia - Hypoxia - Hypo/hyperkalemia (K$^+$) - Hypothermia	- Thromboembolism - Toxicity to drugs - Tamponade - Tension pneumothorax	- Eclampsia, severe pulmonary embolism (PE) - Epilepsy, seizures (other causes)

Non Hemorrhagic Shock in Obstetrics

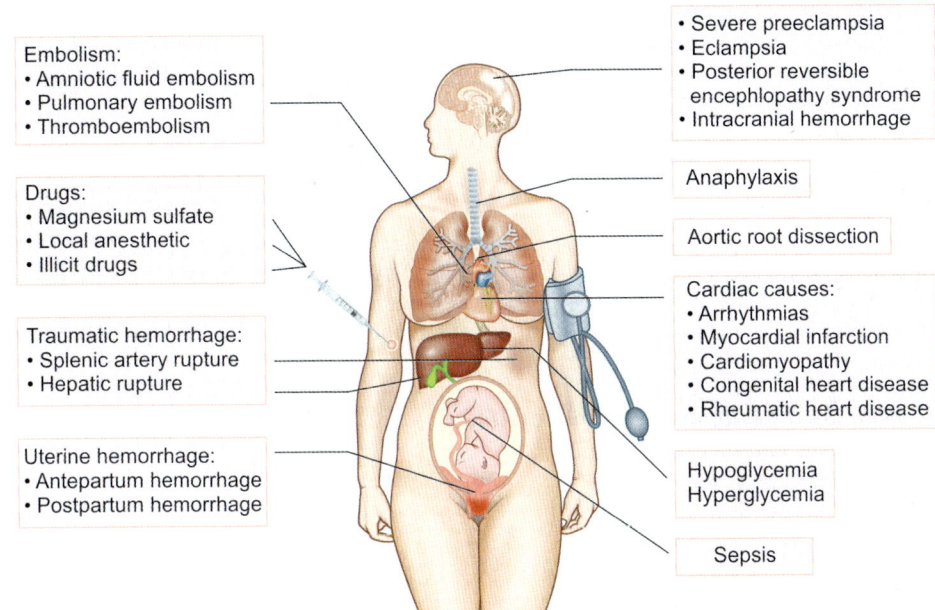

Fig. 53.1: Causes of obstetric shock

Q. Can a woman at risk of impending collapse be identified?[2]

Ans. Modified early obstetric warning score (MEOWS): Red alert features to identify a patient with impending collapse are:
- Heart rate > 100 bpm
- Respiratory rate > 21/min
- Temperature > 38°C
- Blood pressure:
  ◆ Systolic ≥ 160 mm Hg or < 90 mm Hg
  ◆ Diastolic ≥ 90 mm Hg.

A. AMNIOTIC FLUID EMBOLISM (AFE)

Q. What is the etiopathogenesis in AFE?

Ans. It is the entry of amniotic fluid in the maternal circulation at the time of delivery. It occurs through the minor breach in the placental membranes and tears in uterine veins. However, some amount of amniotic fluid enters the maternal circulation normally and it is innocuous. Fetal squames, trophoblasts are present.

An anaphylactoid reaction with complement activation has been considered as the underlying pathology. There is an activation of coagulation cascade (factor X) and the compliment pathways (↑serum: tryptase and histamine). In 60% of cases, coagulation failure is observed. There is dramatic onset of the clinical picture.

Q. What is overall scenario of AFE?[3,4]
Ans. Indian data is sparse. However, in UK, occurrence rate is 2/100,000 maternities.
- Maternal survival rate is 80% when prompt and effective measures are taken
- Neurological morbidity may be there
- Perinatal mortality is high (135/1,000 total birth).

Case Report 1

A multigravida, otherwise normal pregnancy was admitted at term because of pre-eclampsia. She was induced with prostaglandin E_2 (PGE_2) vaginally followed by a repeat dose by 4 hours. A rapid labor ensued which resulted in a vaginal delivery. She collapsed by an hour or so and within minutes she developed disseminated intravascular coagulation (DIC). She sustained cardiac arrest shortly afterwards from which she could not be resuscitated. Autopsy confirmed AFE (immunochemistry).

Q. What are the diagnostic criteria for AFE?
Ans. Diagnostic criteria for AFE are:
- Restlessness, numbness
- Agitation, tingling
- Seizures
- Cardiac arrest
- Dyspnea
- Hypotension
- Acute fetal compromise [fetal heart rate (FHR) abnormality].

Q. What are the risk factors for AFE?
Ans. Risk factors for AFE are:
- Increasing age
- Induction of labor (prostaglandins)
- Before delivery or at labor
- Cesarean delivery
- Multiparity
- Multiple pregnancy
- BMI ≥ 30 kg/m²
- Advanced pregnancy.

What are the Hemodynamic Abnormalities Associated with Amniotic Fluid Embolism?

It depends on the volume and the degree of meconium stained liquor in maternal circulation.
Pathology: Anaphylactoid reaction with complement activation.

Clinical Presentations with AFE

Dramatic onset of:
- Hypotension
- Acute respiratory distress syndrome
- Cyanosis
- Dyspnea
- Fetal distress.
- Pulmonary edema
- Cardiac arrest
- Coagulopathy
- Convulsions

CEMACH (Confidential Enquiry into Maternal and Child Health):[1,5] Sudden onset of breathlessness in a pregnant/postpartum woman (with exclusion of asthma), pulmonary embolism to be considered as the differential diagnosis.

Organ changes
- **Right ventricle:** Hugely dilated and akinetic
- **Left ventricle:** Contracted, cavity obliterated
- Profound hypoxia
- Coagulation failure.

Postmortem observation
- Fetal squamous cells
- Trophoblasts in the pulmonary artery
- Other debris.

Laboratory findings
- ↓Fibrinogen
- ↓ Platelets
- ↑ Fibrinogen degradation products (FDP).

Postmortem examination: Detection of cytokeratin positive hair in the lungs (immunochemistry).

Management of AFE
- Supportive therapy
    - Immediate resuscitation
    - Tracheal intubation for oxygenation, if not available—face mask
    - Cardiopulmonary resuscitation (CPR)
    - Inotropic support
- Correction of metabolic acidosis
- Blood/component therapy
- To combat coagulopathy
- Recombinant factor VIIa[2]
- Fresh frozen plasma, packed red blood cells
- Plasma exchange (hemofiltration for removal of amniotic fluid and cytokines)
- Emergency cesarean delivery.

B. CARDIAC DISEASE

Common causes of maternal collapse:
- Myocardial infarction, cardiac arrhythmias
- Aortic root dissection
- Congenital and rheumatic heart disease.
- Cardiomyopathy
- Infective endocarditis

C. SEPSIS (TABLE 53.1 AND FIG. 53.2)

Table 53.1: Common features of genital sepsis (CEMACH)

Symptoms	Signs
Fever	Tachycardia
Vomiting	Tachypnea
Diarrhea	Pyrexia
Abdomen pain	↑ WBC count
Skin rash (*Streptococci*)	↑ CRP
Vaginal discharge	

Temperature may not be present always.

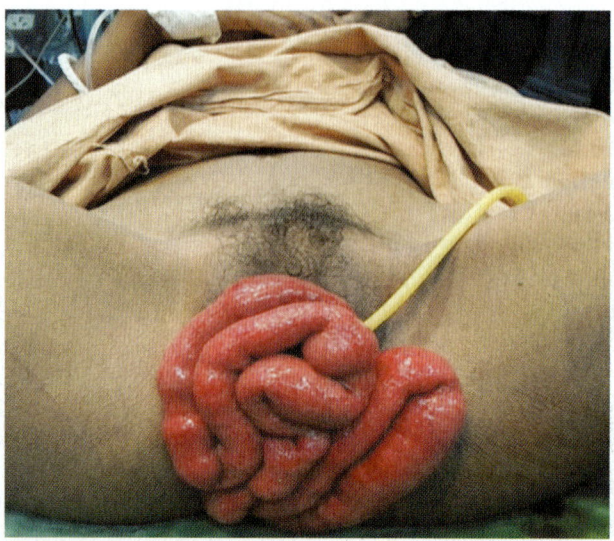

Fig. 53.2: Case of unsafe abortion. Loops of small intestine are seen outside the vagina. Small intestine loops were pulled down following perforation of the uterus during evacuation. The patient had the history of previous cesarean delivery (see the abdominal scar)

Sepsis Resuscitation Bundle (CEMACH)[6,7,8]

- To send blood for culture prior to antibiotic therapy.
- To start broad-spectrum antibiotics before the culture report is available. (*See* Manual of Obstetrics and Gynecology for the Postgraduates, p. 490)
- When hypotension persists, and/or serum lactate is > 4 mmol/L:
    - To start IV infusion with crystalloids or colloids.
    - Vasopressor (norepinephrine) and/or an inotrope (dobutamine) is used to maintain the mean arterial pressure ≥ 65 mm Hg.
- To measure serum lactate: Serum lactate > 4 mmol/L suggests metabolic acidosis.
- Surgical removal of the source of infection should be done when indicated.
- To maintain the central venous pressure: ≥ 8 mm Hg.
- Steroids may be given. Blood transfusion is needed when the hemoglobin level is < 7g/dL.
- Management with multidisciplinary team approach (MDTA).

D. SUDDEN UNEXPLAINED DEATH IN EPILEPSY (SUDEP)

E. SEVERE PRE-ECLAMPSIA AND ECLAMPSIA

Case Report 2

Mrs D, 23-year-old PGR, referred from a SDH with severe PE (BP 180/120) at 34 weeks of gestation → received MgSO$_4$ and labetalol before transfer → BP stabilized → induction of labor was done with PGE$_2$ → spontaneous vaginal delivery → immediate postpartum unconsciousness and hypotension → MDTA → resuscitation → MRI → massive cerebral edema, hemorrhage → infarction → bilateral occipitoparietal lobes → HDU → ITU → SAMM → slow recovery → survived → she improved slowly from the residual disability.

Severe Pre-eclampsia (MRI Brain) (Figs 53.3A and B) (*See* Manual of Obstetrics and Gynecology for the Postgraduates, p. 4)

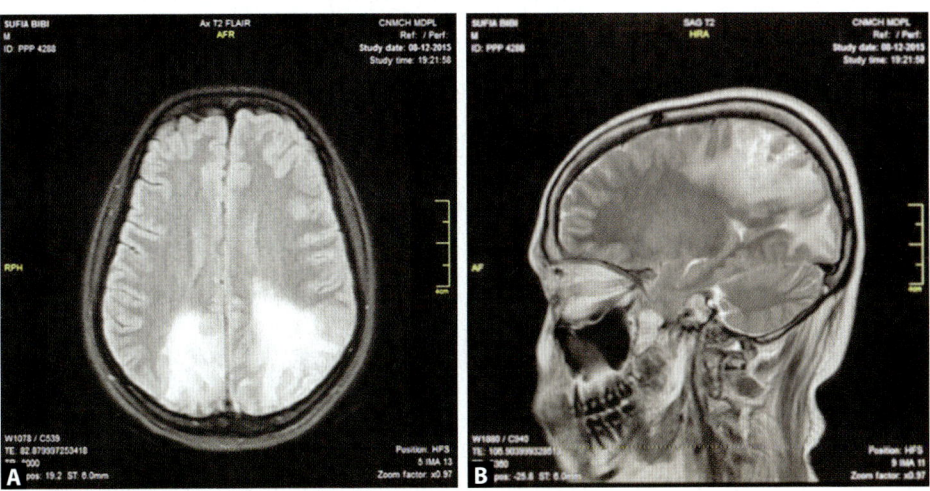

Figs 53.3A and B: MRI Brain: **A.** Axial view, T_2; **B.** Sagittal view, T_1. There is massive areas of cerebral edema and infarction in the bilateral occiput and parietal lobes

Case Report 3

19-year-old primigravida, referred from a SD hospital. She was in labor with severe hypertension. She received tab nicardia on transfer. On admission, BP was 160/120. She was given $MgSO_4$, soon thereafter, she developed convulsions.[9] Within an hour, she was delivered by low forceps. She developed sudden cardiac arrest and she collapsed. There was no PPH. She was resuscitated: Chest compression, tracheal intubation and ventilation IV, infusion, adrenaline, dobutamine in HDU (Fig. 53.4). She recovered completely following 31 hours of intensive care management.

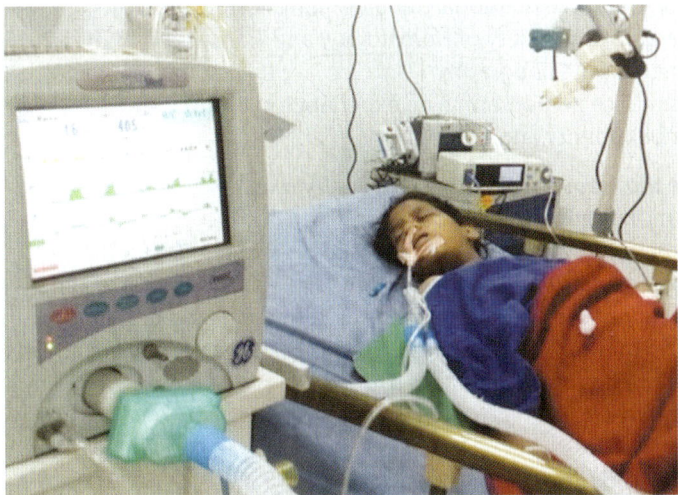

Fig. 53.4: A 19-year-old woman in the intensive care management (the same patient as described above). She developed sudden cardiac arrest immediately following delivery

F. VENOUS THROMBOEMBOLISM (VTE)

Venous thromboembolism and thromboprophylaxis based on risk categorization.

Risk factors evaluation	Risk category
▪ Age >35 years ▪ Obesity ▪ Multiparity	▪ Low-risk
▪ Medical comorbidities (heart disease) ▪ Operative delivery	▪ Intermediate-risk
▪ History of VTE ▪ Thrombophilia	▪ High-risk

Clinical Presentation
- Pleuritic chest pain
- Hypotension
- Tachycardia
- ECG changes
- Tachypnea
- Atelectasis
- Pulse rates: arrhythmias
- Friction rub
- Loss of vascular markings
- Alveolar-arterial O_2 tension > 20 mm Hg
- 70–80% occlusion: circulatory collapse
- Saddle embolism: echocardiography.

Diagnosis of VTE
- Computed tomographic pulmonary angiography (CTPA): (ACOG)
- Perfusion scan [British Society of Hematology and Transfusion (BSHT)-2013]
- Ventilation perfusion: scintigraphy
- Magnetic resonance angiography: no experience in pregnancy
- Intravascular pulmonary angiography.

> **Q. What are the measures in thromboprophylaxis?**
> **Ans.**
> - Early mobilization is encouraged
> - Compression stockings are to be used
> - Low molecular weight heparin (LMWH) is commonly started and is effective
> - Unfractionated heparin therapy is preferred in few cases
> - Heparin therapy may be continued in the antenatal and /or in the postpartum period
> - Hydration has to be maintained.
>
> **Management**
> - Thrombolysis
> - **UFH:** IV → SC (dose adjustment)
>   - Bolus IV: 70–100 U/kg
>   - Continuous IV 1,000 U/hour (15–20 U/kg/hour)

- Monitoring: aPTT: 1.5–2.5
  - Prophylactic LMWH
  - Warfarin
- Inhibitor to thrombin (dabigatran)
- Factor Xa—rivaroxaban.

Vena Cava Filters
Before surgery [cesarean section (CS)]: To stop anticoagulation due to the risks of:
- Life-threatening hemorrhage
- Hematoma formation.

To prevent these complications, vena cava filters can be placed in:
- Jugular or femoral vein
  These filters may be—retrievable.

Embolectomy
- Experience in pregnancy is limited
- Risks are both to the mother and the fetus (risks of stillbirth are: 20–40%).

Perimortem CS
- Decision for perimortem CS is difficult
- Reports are often poor gloomy
  - China: 90%
  - Canada: 25%
  - UK (CEMACH): 20%
- Perinatal mortality (PNM): 80%.

G. DRUG TOXICITY

Q. What are the conditions related to drug toxicity or drug overdose to cause sudden maternal collapse?

Ans.
- ***Magnesium sulfate*** toxicity especially in presence of renal impairment.
- ***Local anesthetics*** accidental intravenous injection
  - **Clinical presentation:** Patient presents with light-headedness, circumoral paresthesia, twitching of muscles, convulsions, circulatory collapse and loss of consciousness.
  - Cardiovascular collapse.
- ***Total spinal block or high spinal or epidural block*** may manifest with sudden circulatory collapse.
  - **Management:** Magnesium sulfate toxicity is managed by injection of calcium gluconate 10 mL (10%) IV slowly.
  - **Local anesthetic agents:** Injection is to be stopped immediately. ***Lipid rescue***, is recommended.

  Intralipid 20% (lipid emulsion) is given as IV bolus injection. Intralipid IV bolus, 20% 1.5 mL/kg over 1 minute followed by an IV infusion of intralipid 20% at 0.25 mL/kg /min is maintained. CPR should be maintained throughout the process until adequate circulation is established.

H. ANAPHYLAXIS

Causative factors are to be removed. A (Airway), B (Breathing)[10,11] and C (Circulation) resuscitation approach is maintained. Adrenaline is given by ***intramuscular injection*** in a dose of 500 mcg (0.5 mL) of 1:1,000. It may be repeated after 5 minutes, if needed. Adjuvant therapy with hydrocortisone 200 mg, slow IV may be given.

AORTOCAVAL COMPRESSION IN PREGNANCY

- It reduces (↓) cardiac output
- It causes supine hypotension
- Reduces efficacy of chest compression during CPR due to mechanical factors (gravid uterus, changes in pulmonary function)
- Intubation is difficult due to laryngeal edema
- Mendelson syndrome may occur due to the incompetence of the lower esophageal sphincter
- ***Physiological changes in pregnancy results in significant changes in all the body systems.***
  There is increase in plasma volume (40–50%), cardiac output (40%), pulse rate 10–15 beats/minute and placental blood flow (10% of cardiac output). There is decrease in systemic vascular resistance and venous return (due to pressure of the gravid uterus on the inferior vena cava). In the ***respiratory system***, respiratory rate (slight increase) and the tissue oxygen consumption is increased (20%). There is decrease in residual capacity (25%) and arterial pCO_2. The resultant effects of these changes are dilutional anemia, potential for rapid and massive hemorrhage when any hemorrhage occurs, rapid development of hypoxia and risk of developing acidosis more rapidly. There is decreased gastrointestinal motility, relaxation of the lower esophageal sphincter and splinting effects on the diaphragm due to the gravid uterus. At times, endotracheal intubation becomes difficult due to laryngeal edema (*See* Dutta's Textbook of Obstetrics, 8th Edition, p. 58). Mechanical position of the uterus and increased weight gain in pregnancy make the effort of CPR and ventilation more difficult.

Q. *Outline the optimal management of a case of maternal collapse:*
Ans. *Resuscitation Council (UK) Guidelines (A = Airway, B = Breathing, C = Circulation)*
- **Left lateral tilt—15°.**
- **MDTA in management is to be done.** (*See* Manual of Obstetrics and Gynecology for the Postgraduates, Ch 14, p. 277).

Q. *What is the place of perimortem CS? When, where, and how?*
Ans. *See* Manual of Obstetrics and Gynecology for the Postgraduates, Ch 14, p. 277.[12,13]

CLINICAL GOVERNANCE IN THE MANAGEMENT OF NON HEMORRHAGIC SHOCK IN OBSTETRICS

Debriefing: The family members and all the staff involved in the management, need debriefing. It reduces the post traumatic stress and depression. It is a holistic approach and must be done by an competent professional.

Documentation: Accurate documentation of all cases of maternal collapse is essential to avoid potential medicolegal consequences. Poor documentation or lack of documentation is a major deficiency that may create medicolegal problems.

Training in the management of non hemorrhagic shock in obstetrics: All maternity staff should have annual formal training in generic life support and management of maternal collapse. Life support training and drill reduces maternal morbidity and mortality.

References

1. Lewis G. The Confidential Enquiry into Maternal and Child Health (CEMACH). Saving Mothers' Lives: reviewing maternal deaths to make motherhood safer 2003–2005, The Seventh Report on Confidential Enquiries into Maternal Deaths in the United Kingdom. London: CEMACH. 2007.
2. Prosper SC, Goudge CS, Lupo VR, et al. Recombinant factor VIIa to successfully manage DIC from AFE. Obstet Gynecol. 2007;109(2 Pt2):524-5.
3. Knaus WA, Zimmerman JE, Wagner DP, et al. APACHE-acute physiology and chronic health evaluation: a physiologically based classification system. Crit Care Med. 1981;9(8):591-7.
4. Knight M, Tuffnell D, Brocklehurst P, et al. UK Obstetric Surveillance System. Incidence and risk factors for amniotic fluid embolism. Obstet Gynecol. 2010;115(5):910-7.
5. Royal College of Obstetricians and Gynecologists. Clinical Governance Advice No. 1c: Development of RCOG Green-top Guidelines: Producing a Clinical Practice Guideline. London: RCOG. 2006.
6. Tufnell DJ. United Kingdom amniotic fluid embolism register. BJOG. 2005;112(12):1625-9.
7. Working Group of the Resuscitation Council (UK). Emergency treatment of anaphylactic reactions. Guidelines for healthcare providers. London: Resuscitation Council (UK); 2008.
8. National Institute for Health and Clinical Excellence. NICE clinical guideline 50: Acutely ill patients in hospital. Recognition of response to acute illness in adults in hospital. London: NICE; 2007.
9. Royal College of Obstetricians and Gynecologists. Green-top Guideline No. 10(A): The Management of Severe Pre-eclampsia/Eclampsia. London: RCOG; 2006.
10. Rees GA, Willis BA. Resuscitation in late pregnancy. Anesthesia. 1988;43(5):347-9.
11. Howell C, Grady K, Cox C, editors. Managing Obstetric Emergencies and Trauma – the MOET Course Manual. 2nd edition. London: RCOG Press; 2007.
12. Harper NJ, Dixon T, Dugué P, et al. Working Party of the Association of Anesthetists of Great Britain and Ireland. Suspected anaphylactic reactions associated with anesthesia. Anesthesia. 2009;64(2):199-211.
13. Katz V, Balderston K, DeFreest M. Perimortem cesarean delivery: Were our assumptions correct? Am J Obstet Gynecol. 2005;192(6):1916-20.

SECTION 7

Short Reviews in Gynecology

Section Outline

Ch. 54. Place of Prophylactic Salpingectomy or Salpingo-oophorectomy in Current Gynecologic Practice
Ch. 55. Endometrial Carcinoma
Ch. 56. Bariatric Surgery in Gynecology and Obstetrics
Ch. 57. Fertility Conserving Options for Women with Gynecologic Malignancies
Ch. 58. Fertility Conserving Options for Women with Cervical Cancer
Ch. 59. Fertility Conserving Options for Women with Endometrial Cancer
Ch. 60. Advances in Contraception
Ch. 61. Interventional Radiology in Obstetrics and Gynecology
Ch. 62. Surgical Site Infection
Ch. 63. Abnormal Uterine Bleeding: Investigations and Management Issues
Ch. 64. Subfertility and Pelvic Endometriosis
Ch. 65. Medical Methods of Termination of Pregnancy

54. Place of Prophylactic Salpingectomy or Salpingo-oophorectomy in Current Gynecologic Practice

TYPES OF OVARIAN CARCINOMAS

Nearly 80% of all ovarian cancers are epithelial in origin. Epithelial ovarian cancers (EOCs) are the important cause of death from gynecological malignancy. Of all the epithelial ovarian neoplasms the important subtypes are: (a) Serous: 68%, (b) Clear cell: 13%, (c) Endometroid: 9% and (d) Mucinous: 3%.

Serous adenocarcinomas are further divided into:
- Type 1 or low grade (LGSOC)
- Type 2 or high grade (HGSOC)

Most deaths are from HGSOC (20 times higher than LGSOC). The life time risk of developing EOC is 1 in 70 (1.4%) by 75 years of age. Of the several high risk factors for EOC, the important ones are: (a) Advanced age and (b) Family history.[1]

Q. What is the risk with family history of ovarian cancer?

Ans. Nearly 5–10% of all ovarian cancers are associated with inherited genetic abnormality. Mutation in BRCA1, BRCA2, genes (most common) and mutations in mismatch repair genes (MLH1, MSH2 and MSH6) are associated. High rate (100%) of p53 mutations are associated with HGSOC.

The inherited ovarian cancers are commonly observed in young women. They are often bilateral and are high grade serous in type.

Q. What is the current concept in the pathogenesis ovarian carcinoma?

Ans. Nonuterine pelvic high grade serious carcinomas are currently considered as secondary to distal fallopian tube carcinomas. Other supportive hypotheses for ovarian carcinogenesis are:

- **Incessant ovulation theory (Fatallah-1971):** Repeated ovulatory trauma to the ovarian surface epithelium is a promoting factor causing error in cell replication. Women having repeated ovulations (ovulation inductions) with gonadotropins (gonadotropin hypothesis) are at increased risk of EOC. On the other hand women with COCs (suppression of ovulation) are at lower risk.
- **Hormonal hypothesis:** Excess androgen stimulation of ovarian surface epithelium increases the risk, whereas progesterone stimulation is protective to ovarian carcinogenesis.
- Distal tubal intraepithelial carcinoma (DTIC) as the origin (see below).

Q. **How the high grade serous ovarian cancers are etiologically related to distal tubal intraepithelial carcinoma (TIC)?**

Ans. Currently, there are several evidences to support that distal fallopian tube is the primary site of HGSOC.[1,2] The possibility is that fallopian tube is involved early in the disease process of the HGSOCs.

- Adult epithelial stem cells are essential for cell repair through clonal growth of cells and self-renewal. These process make the cells susceptible to DNA damage and subsequent development of cancers.
- The amount of such stem like epithelial cells are almost double in the distal fallopian tube compared to the proximal end of the tube. With this, the distal fallopian tube initiates the neoplastic transformation. Locally elevated levels of inflammatory cytokines in the distal fallopian tube also promote the process of malignant transformation.
- However presence of coexisting intraepithelial carcinoma is a prerequisite for the diagnosis of primary tubal carcinoma.
- Incorporation of Müllerian epithelium into the ovary.
  The mechanisms of incorporation of Müllerian epithelium into the ovary:
  - Exfoliation of tubal mucosal cells over the ovarian surface results in formation of endosalpingiosis, cortical inclusions or endometriosis. This may occur with formation of adhesions/contact of the tube with the ovary.[2]
  - Müllerian cells undergoing metaplastic change over the ovarian surface epithelium.
  - Molecular abnormality is the other pathway of ovarian carcinogenesis. At the molecular level, different mutations are observed for both the cases of LGSOC and HGSOC. Important one are: BRCA1, BRCA2, KRAS, BRAF, HER2 and p53.
- The incorporated cells on the ovarian surface, may give rise to neoplastic changes. The common tumors are serous tumors (either benign, borderline, low grade serous adenocarcinomas, endometrioid or clear cell tumors). Development of high grade serous ovarian cancers are rare with the mechanism of surface implantation.

There may be malignant transformation of the distal tubal mucosa through p53 mutations (p53 signatures). This may be the other pathway in the development of tubal intraepithelial carcinoma (TIC) lesions. These TIC cells may spread locally in the tubal wall, ex-foliate on the surface of the ovary, in the peritoneal cavity (peritoneal serous adenocarcinoma) or there may be a combination of these. Based on these evidences the association of the fallopian tube and HGSOC are considered as indisputable.

Q. **How high grade serous ovarian cancers (HGSOC) differ from that of low grade serous ovarian cancers (LGSOC)?**

Ans. These two cancers (HGSOC and LGSOC) differ at molecular level also besides their response to therapy and in terms of five year survival rate (Table 54.1).

Table 54.1: Difference between high grade serous ovarian cancers (HGSOC) and low grade serous ovarian cancers (LGSOC)

LGSOC	HGSOC
■ Associated gene mutations of KRAS or BRAF are observed in about 75% of cases. ■ HER2 mutations are also observed. ■ There is no mutation with p53 gene.	■ Extremely high rate of p53 mutations (almost 100%) ■ BRCA mutations (BRCA1 and BRCA2) ■ Absence of KRAS, BRAF or HER2 mutations.

Intense over expression of p53 is known as ***p53 signatures***. Serous tubal intraepithelial carcinoma (STIC) lesions are the precursors of HGSOC. There has been a link between STIC and HGSOC.[3]

There is a significant impact in clinical outcomes and response to chemotherapy in this group of HGSOC. HGSOC are a separate histological subgroup based on molecular pathology. The overall 5-year survival rate of ovarian carcinoma is 43%.

Q. How the risk of ovarian carcinoma be reduced?
Ans. High risk women having BRCA mutation:[4]
- Bilateral salpingo-oophorectomy provides the maximum reduction of risk for ovarian carcinoma (100%).
- It also reduces the risk of breast carcinoma (50%).
- Bilateral salpingectomy with delayed oophorectomy may be an alternative cost effective strategy for women with BRCA mutation carriers.[5]
- Ongoing epidemiological studies are likely to add strength to the current transitional research evidence to and change surgical practice.[6,7]

Prophylactic (opportunistic) bilateral salpingectomy in low risk women (without BRCA mutation) who have completed their families, should be carefully considered with conservation of ovaries at the time of gynecological surgery. This gives the benefit of risk reduction in one hand and at the same time it protects the woman from the disadvantages of surgical menopause.

Q. What is the current evidence in this field?
Ans. Evidence in human subjects are lacking. Trials in mice it is positive. But arguments is, 'if we wait until we have evidence before we offer the operation then, we will never generate evidence'.[8]

References

1. National Cancer Institute. Surveillance, Epidemiology, and End Results Program (SEER) Stat Fact Sheets: Ovary Cancer. [online] Available from [http://seer.cancer.gov/statfacts/html/ovary.html]. [Accessed June, 2016].
2. Seidman JD, Sherman ME, Bell KA, et al. Salpingitis, salpingoliths, and serous tumors of the ovaries: Is there a connection? Int J Gynecol Pathol. 2002;21(2):101-7.
3. Karst AM, Drapkin R. Ovarian cancer pathogenesis: a model in evolution. J Oncol. 2010;2010:932371.
4. Liu J, Cristea MC, Frankel P, et al. Clinical characteristics and outcomes of BRCA-associated ovarian cancer: genotype and survival. Cancer Genet. 2012;205:34-41.
5. Crump CP, Drapkin R, Miron A, et al. The distal fallopian tube: a new model for pelvic serous carcinogenesis. Curr Opin Obestet Gynecol. 2007;19:3-9.
6. Royal Australian and New Zealand. College of Obstetricians and Gynecologists. Managing the adnexae at the time of hysterectomy for benign gynecological disease. College Statement C-Gyn 25. Melbourne, Australia: RANZCOG; 2012.
7. Society of Gynecologic Oncology (2013). SGO Clinical Practice Statement: Salpingectomy for Ovarian Cancer Prevention. Chicago: SCOG. [online] Available from [https://www.sgo.org/clinicalpractice/guidelines/sgo-clinical-practice-statement-salpingectomy-for-ovarian-cancerprevention] [Accessed June, 2016].
8. Narod SA. Salpingectomy to prevent Ovarian Cancer. A concurrent series. Curr Oncol. 2013;20:145-7.

55 Endometrial Carcinoma

Q. Discuss the place of vaginal hysterectomy in a case with endometrial carcinoma (EC).

Ans. Vaginal hysterectomy is an alternative option for the management of EC in some selected cases only. Such cases are:
- Stage I disease with well-differentiated tumor
- Without any extrauterine spread of disease. It is considered as the simplest and least morbid approach compared to abdominal hysterectomy. Treatment outcomes are similar to other methods of clinical stage I EC. This is specially helpful in obese and in patients with poor surgical risks.

Limitations of vaginal hysterectomy:
- Exploration of the intraperitoneal cavity is not possible.
- To procure peritoneal cytological washings, it is not helpful.
- May pose increased difficulty in oophorectomy procedure at times.
- Lymph node sampling to assess the spread of disease is not possible.

Q. What is the place of minimally invasive surgery in the management of endometrial cancer (EC)?

Ans. Minimally invasive surgery (MIS) in the management of EC is considered effective and is with comparable outcome to open surgery. Presently, it is considered as a standard care in the management of EC. It is useful for comprehensive surgical staging and appropriate risk stratification. This is again useful for correct treatment initiative.

MIS includes:
- Laparoscopic assisted vaginal hysterectomy (LAVH)
- Total laparoscopic hysterectomy (TLH)
- Robotic-assisted laparoscopic hysterectomy (RALH).

Surgical procedure is total hysterectomy, bilateral salpingo-oophorectomy with pelvic and para-aortic lymphadenectomy. This is the recognized mode of surgery.

Para-aortic node dissection up to the level of renal vein is recommended. MIS is used for transperitoneal and extraperitoneal assessment of nodes during hysterectomy. It may also be used at a later date to restage the disease when initial surgery was incomplete.

Robotic surgery has got additional benefits for obese women as it reduces the morbidity significantly. The overall benefits of LAVH/TLH or RALH are—reduced operative and postoperative complications, reduced hospital stay, improved recovery, fewer bowel adhesions and radiation-induced bowel injury. Robotic-assisted surgery has got all the benefits of laparoscopic surgery in terms of lymph node yield, shorter hospital stay, operative time and blood loss. However, it is pertinent that all gynecologic oncologists need to be trained with MIS to get the actual benefits.

Q. Discuss the place of nodal dissection in the management of EC.

Ans. *Assessment* of nodal status is the single most important factors to categorize a patient for risk stratification.[1] Postoperative adjuvant therapy is decided with the comprehensive staging report. Routine nodal dissection is the best method by which only few patients are selected for adjuvant therapy. Accurate staging can only minimize the risk of unnecessary irradiation. With this, many patients are benefitted with the use of vaginal cuff brachytherapy (VCB) instead of radiation.

Risks: However, nodal dissection is not a complete risk-free procedure.

The known hazards are: Increased blood loss, increased operating time, vascular injury, injury to the genitofemoral nerve with subsequent development of paresthesia to the medial side of thighs, lymphocyte formation, ileus and lymphedema. The overall surgical complication of lymphadenectomy is above 20%. The major complication is about 6%. However, place of nodal dissection for EC is debated and controversy exists.[2] The postoperative radiation therapy in endometrial cancer (PORTEC) trial and a study in the treatment of endometrial cancer (ASTEC) could not establish any clear benefit of pelvic lymphadenectomy.[3] ASTEC members concluded nodal dissection could not be recommended as a routine procedure for therapeutic purposes.[3,4]

Surgical staging is considered the most accurate way to determine the extent of disease spread. Selective use of nodal dissection was done to balance the benefit of detecting unrecognized disease against the cost, morbidity and the use of adjuvant therapy. The overall risks and benefits of lymphadenectomy are to weigh against the risks, cost and morbidity of adjuvant chemo and/or radiation therapy.

Intraoperative gross inspection of the uterus guides the surgeon for the need of nodal dissection. Visual inspection correlated with microscopic assessment in 85% of cases. However, myometrial invasion may be more extensive microscopically than is evident with the clinical inspection. Considering all the above facts, **routine nodal dissection is considered.**

There are two principal nodal basins that drain the uterus.

1. **Pelvic lymph nodes:** The lower and the middle portion of the uterus drain to the following pelvic nodes. External iliac, hypogastric, obturator and common iliac nodes.
2. **Para-aortic node:** The corpus and the fundus drain into the para-aortic nodes. The nodes are bilateral, lymphadenectomy should be thorough and not sampling only. Isolated positive para-aortic nodes with negative pelvic nodes are uncommon[5] and are found in only 2% cases.

   Patients with positive pelvic and/or para-aortic nodes are treated with complete node resection followed by adjuvant (radiation and/or chemotherapy) therapy. This resulted in superior (100% for pelvic and 75% for para-aortic) 5-year survival outcomes. In the absence of nodal disease, the recurrence risk is low and 5-year survival outcome is high either with no radiation or with VCB only.[6]

References

1. Creasman WT, Morrow CP, Bundy BN, et al. Surgical pathologic spread patterns of endometrial cancer. A Gynecologic Oncology Group Study. Cancer. 1987;60(8 Suppl):2035-41.
2. Seamon LG, Fowler JM, Cohn DE. Lymphadenectomy for endometrial cancer: The controversy. Gynecol Oncol. 2010;117(1):6-8.
3. Creutzberg CL, van Putten WL, Koper PC, et al. Surgery and postoperative radiotherapy versus surgery alone for patients with stage 1 endometrial carcinoma: Multicenter randomized trial. PORTEC Study Group. Postoperative Radiation Therapy in Endometrial Carcinoma. Lancet. 2000;355(9213):1404-11.
4. ASTEC study group, Kitchener H, Swart AM, et al. Efficacy of systematic pelvic lymphadenectomy in endometrial cancer (MRC ASTEC trial): A randomized study. Lancet. 2009;373(9658):125-36.
5. Abu-Rustum NR, Gomez JD, Alektiar KM, et al. The incidence of isolated para-aortic nodal metastasis in surgically staged endometrial cancer patients with negative pelvic lymph nodes. Gynecol Oncol. 2009;115(2):236-8.
6. Onda T, Yoshikawa H, Mizutani K, et al. Treatment of node-positive endometrial cancer with complete node dissection, chemotherapy and radiation therapy. Br J Cancer. 1997;75(12):1836-41.

56. Bariatric Surgery in Gynecology and Obstetrics

Q. What is the relevance of this problem and the importance of pregnancy management for such patients?

Ans. Obesity is a growing problem in the developed world and also in many other countries including India. Obesity poses problems in achieving pregnancy, its successful continuation also causes problems in labor and puerperium. Operative interventions, weight reduction or bariatric surgery is becoming the common procedure to overcome this situation. Pregnancy following surgery may face nutritional and many surgical complications. These complications may affect the pregnancy outcome adversely. It is essential that obstetricians should be aware of these procedures, the need of counseling and management of women who undergo the bariatric surgery and conceive subsequently.

Q. What is the magnitude of the problem of obesity?

Ans. Most centers consider BMI = weight in kg/(height in meters)^2 is equal 30 or more is obesity. With this cut off value the prevalence of obesity in US has been reported to range between 16% and 50%.[1,2] Obesity is an epidemic in US as one study revealed 66% adults were either overweight or obese. Women, with a pregnancy BMI > 30 or a pregnancy weight more than 200 pounds, have been used to stratify risk during pregnancy. In India, exact data is difficult to quote, but the BMI values of > 25 and > 30 are considered overweight and obese, respectively. Overall prevalence of obesity in India is 16% (ICMR 2013–2014).[3]

Q. Discuss the different complications of obesity in pregnancy:

Ans. *See* Manual of Obstetrics and Gynecology for the Postgraduates, p. 238.

Q. Discuss the different fetal and neonatal effects of obesity in pregnancy:

Ans. *See* Manual of Obstetrics and Gynecology for the Postgraduates, p. 238.

Q. Mention the different modes of management for obesity in pregnancy:

Ans.
- **Nonsurgical methods** are initially done. These includes: dietetic restriction, exercise, behavioral changes and pharmacotherapy. Patients with BMI < 40, are usually considered for nonsurgical method of management.
- **Surgical method (bariatric surgery):** Considered for women with BMI ≥ 40, woman with associated comorbidities (hypertension, ischemic heart disease) are considered for bariatric surgery even if BMI is < 40.
  Bariatric surgery has been started since 1960s.

Q. How much is the success of bariatric surgery?
Ans. Bariatric surgery is a highly effective therapy especially for women with morbid obesity. Bariatric surgery significantly improves the obesity and the associated comorbidities. It improves the quality of life also.[3]

Q. What is the principle of bariatric surgery in the management of obesity?
Ans. The objective is to reduce the body weight. It can be done in two ways:
1. Restriction and
2. A combined method of restrictive and malabsorptive operations.

Q. What is the type of operation commonly done these days?
Ans. The combined method is commonly done. It is the Roux-en-Y gastric bypass procedure. An adjustable gastric banding (restrictive) and Roux-en-Y gastric bypass (malabsorptive) is done.

The proximal stomach is separated from the remaining part of the stomach with staples. In banding procedure, a fluid-filled band is placed around the stomach close to the fundus. This reduces the volume of the functional stomach. These methods could be performed by laparoscopy or laparotomy. Many other techniques like biliopancreatic diversion (malabsorptive) or jejunoileal bypass (malabsorptive) were used.

Q. What is the place of bariatric surgery at present?
Ans. Presently increasing numbers of bariatric surgical procedures are performed in each year. The majority of the procedures are done in women (80%) of which about 50% are done for women of reproductive age (with the mean age of 40 years). Interestingly bariatric surgery is also being done in adolescents with morbid obesity.

Q. What is the effect of surgery on future fertility and obesity?
Ans. Bariatric surgery is most effective for morbid obesity and to improve the quality of life. There is significant improvement of reproductive behavior of women with obesity. Improvement of PCOS, hyperinsulinemia, hyperandrogenemia, obesity, irregular menses are there. Improvement of fertility is also observed.[4,5] However, bariatric surgery should not be recommended as a treatment of infertility. Due to the effects of compromised absorption (malabsorptive surgery), the patient may develop nutritional deficiencies (vitamin and minerals).

Unintended pregnancies are high in these women as the absorption of combined oral contraceptive is low.

Q. What are the effects of surgery on health in their subsequent pregnancies?
Ans. Weight reduction either by medical or surgical method has got significant impact on women's health to improve the maternal comorbidities especially diabetes and hypertension and the quality of life. One systematic review of pregnancy after bariatric surgery described decreased rates of gestational diabetes and pre-eclampsia. However, late complications of bariatric surgery like intestinal obstruction, gastrointestinal hemorrhage, have been observed during pregnancy.

Q. What are the effects of bariatric surgery on perinatal outcome?
Ans. Bariatric surgery is not associated with increased perinatal death. Congenital abnormalities are not increased. Macrosomia (birth weight > 4 kg) was less. Babies of lower mean birth weights or small gestational age were observed, especially after Roux-en-Y gastric bypass.[4,6,7]

Q. What should be contraceptive counseling in the patients following bariatric surgery?

Ans. Pregnancy rates following bariatric surgery are improved significantly. There is an increased risk of combined oral contraceptive failure after bariatric surgery. These women should therefore be counseled for nonoral administration of hormonal contraception. Woman is advised not to become pregnant within 12–24 months of bariatric surgery till the full weight loss is achieved. Woman needs closed monitoring as regard maternal weight gain, nutritional status and fetal growth.

Q. What is the concern for nutritional status during pregnancy in a woman who has undergone bariatric surgery?

Ans.
- The woman may suffer from nutritional deficiencies especially after malabsorptive surgery (Roux-en-Y gastric bypass).
- The common deficiencies are protein, iron, vitamin B_{12}, folate, vitamin D and calcium.
- The woman needs evaluation for these micronutrients at the start of pregnancy. Investigations including complete hemogram, serum ferritin, calcium and vitamin D at each trimester of pregnancy are to be done.
- Oral supplementation has to be continued. If there is no improvement based on laboratory data, parenteral route supplementation should be done. Consultation with a nutritionist should be done.
- Folic acid supplementation (0.4 mg/day) may be increased to prevent birth defects. Whereas vitamin A should be limited to 5,000 IU/day during pregnancy to reduce the risk of birth defects.
- Postpartum monitoring should also be continued especially for the women who are breastfeeding.
- Women having restrictive surgical procedures (adjustable gastric banding procedure) may be allowed more oral intake by adjusting the band (by removing the fluid from the band). This 'active band management' procedure is found to improve woman's nutritional status.

Q. What are the special care during the antenatal period for women who had undergone bariatric surgery?

Ans.
- Complications of bariatric surgery should be diagnosed early. These may be anastomotic leak, bowel obstructions band erosion, internal hernias, band migration and abdominal pain.
- Dumping syndrome can occur after gastric bypass procedures. It is due to fluid shifts from the intravascular compartment into the bowel lumen following ingestion of high glycemic carbohydrates.
  Symptoms: Abdominal cramps, bloating, nausea, vomiting, diarrhea, hypoglycemia (due to hyperinsulinemia), tachycardia and palpitations. Women with dumping syndrome should avoid 50/75 g oral glucose screening test in pregnancy.
- The absorptive surface of the intestine is decreased. Extended release preparations are avoided instead oral solution and rapid release preparations are used. Drugs like NSAIDs are to be avoided to minimize gastric ulcerations.

Q. What special management issues are to be maintained during labor and delivery for women who underwent bariatric surgery?

Ans.
- Women that they remained obese even after bariatric surgery, should be managed similar to that of an obese women (*See* Manual of Obstetrics and Gynecology for the Postgraduates, Ch 7)
- Cesarean delivery rates are higher after bariatric surgery (up to 62%). However, bariatric surgery itself should not be considered an indication for cesarean delivery. Otherwise, bariatric surgery itself should not alter the course of management during labor and delivery from a normal woman.

References

1. Ogden CL, Carroll MD, Curtin LR, et al. Prevalence of overweight and obesity in the United States, 1999-2004. JAMA. 2006;295(13):1549-55.
2. Ehrenberg HM, Dierker L, Milluzzi C, et al. Prevalence of maternal obesity in an urban center. Am J Obstet Gynecol. 2002;187(5):1189-93.
3. Pradeepa R, Anjana RM, Joshi SR, et al. Prevalence of generalized & abdominal obesity in urban & rural India—the ICMR-INDIAB study (Phase-I) [ICMR-INDIAB-3]. Indian J Med Res. 2015;142(2):139-50.
4. National Center for Health Statistics. Health, United States, 2007 With Chartbook on Trends in the Health of Americans. Hyattsville; 2007.
5. Colquitt J, Clegg A, Loveman E, et al. Surgery for morbid obesity. Cochrane Database Syst Rev. 2005;(4):CD003641.
6. Maggard MA, Yermilov I, Li Z, et al. Pregnancy and fertility following bariatric surgery: a systematic review. JAMA. 2008;300(19):2286-96.
7. Patel JA, Patel NA, Thomas RL, et al. Pregnancy outcomes after laparoscopic Roux-en-Y gastric bypass. Surg Obes Relat Dis. 2008;4(1):39-45.

57. Fertility Conserving Options for Women with Gynecologic Malignancies

Q. What is the clinical relevance of this subject in context of current gynecologic practice?

Ans. Gynecologic malignancies are commonly diagnosed in elderly and postmenopausal women. However, no age is immune to any malignancy. When such a malignancy is diagnosed in a premenopausal woman fertility conservation is a major concern. Standard treatment of such malignancies ends in sterility. There are now few options for fertility conservation for such women who are diagnosed with a gynecologic malignancy before they are married or child bearing is completed.[1]

Q. What is the prevalence of such gynecologic malignancies?

Ans.
- Ovarian cancer
  - For women < 20 years   0.7–1.4 per 100,000 women
  - For women 20–49 years   1.6–16.6 per 100,000 women
- For cervical cancer
  - For women 20–49 years   1.5–14.9 per 100,000 women
- Endometrial cancer

MALIGNANT OVARIAN TUMOR

Q. What is the significance of fertility conservation in malignant ovarian tumors?

Ans. Ovarian malignancy is most lethal and 5-year survival rate of ovarian malignancy in spite of all modalities of treatment remained the same for last four decades. Most patients are in advanced stage except few (39%) that are diagnosed in stage IA. Presently, there is delay in women's child bearing. Therefore, it is important to have the fertility conservation options that are safe and available.

Q. What are different options for fertility conservation in a young woman with ovarian malignancy?

Ans. Options available are:
- **Surgery:** Conservation of the uninvolved ovary while doing surgery to the pathological one.
- **Medical**
  - Assisted reproductive technology
  - Surrogacy.

Q. How the woman with gynecologic malignancy should be counseled for available fertility conservation options?

Ans.
- Oncologist should keep in mind that the desire to have a biological child is strong in most couples.
- Before cancer therapy, oncologists should address the possibility of infertility in women with reproductive age.
- Options for third-party reproduction should be given.
- Oncologists should discuss the issues of limitations, as regard to nonavailability of accurate data to predict for any individual.

Q. What are the different options available for fertility preservation with the help of ARTs?

Ans. Options available are:
- **Before treatment:** Embryo cryopreservation following harvesting eggs, IVF and embryo freezing. This procedure is standardized now.
- **Oocyte cryopreservation:** Harvesting and freezing unfertilized eggs. This procedure is still investigational.
- **Ovarian tissue cryopreservation:** Freezing healthy ovarian tissues and reimplantation later on. This procedure is investigational.[2]
- **Gonadal shielding during radiotherapy:** It is done to reduce the radiation dose and damage to the gonads. This procedure is standardized.
- **Ovarian transposition (oophoropexy):** It is the surgical repositioning of the ovary (ies) away from the field of radiation. This procedure is standardized.
- Ovarian suppression with GnRH (agonist/antagonist) for conservation of ovarian tissue during therapy.
- Conservative ovarian surgery like ovarian cystectomy or preserving healthy contralateral ovary.

Q. What are the criteria for selecting a woman with ovarian malignancy for fertility conserving surgery?

Ans. These are the selected women who may be considered following counseling only:
- Epithelial ovarian cancers with stage IA and may be stage IB
- Borderline tumor of the ovary
- Malignant ovarian germ cell tumor (stage I)
- Sex cord stromal tumors (stage I).

Surgery in stage I, grade I and possibly grade 2 ovarian cancer does not significantly compromise survival and allows future fertility.

However, it is important that removal of the preserved ovary may be considered after pregnancy(ies) is over, to reduce the risk of recurrence.

Q. How the staging of ovarian cancer is made?

Ans. Ovarian cancer is staged following surgical and pathological procedures. These include laparotomy and findings on exploration and histopathological reports.
Surgical (exploratory laparotomy) procedures include:
- Peritoneal fluid cytology
- Multiple peritoneal biopsy
- Biopsy of any suspicions area
- Retroperitoneal lymph node sampling

- Pelvic and para-aortic node sampling
- Infracolic omentectomy

It is important that tumor should be removed intact without any cyst rupture or intraperitoneal spread of the disease.

Q. How to assess the involvement of the contralateral ovary?

Ans. Contralateral ovary may be involved even it looks clinically normal. Confirmation of involvement may be done only following biopsy that may be with wedge-resection or tissue biopsy only. However, such methods are unreliable. Risks of microscopic involvement for a normal looking contralateral ovary is 2.5% only. It is virtually absent when the stage of the disease is IA.

Q. What should be the surgical approach in a young woman with unilateral and stage I (grade 1) ovarian cancer?

Ans. Unilateral salpingo-oophorectomy with preservation of the contralateral healthy ovary and the uterus is now considered the appropriate surgical treatment.[3]

Q. What is the effect of adjuvant chemotherapy on fertility outcome after conservative surgery?

Ans. Actual situation is unclear and it is different with different chemotherapeutic agents.
- Alkylating agents (cyclophosphamide) may cause menstrual abnormalities and even premature ovarian failure (high risk).
- Methotrexate, 5-FU and vincristine cause less ovarian dysfunction (low risk).
- Taxanes, oxaliplatin are of unknown risks.
- Pubertal ovary has been found to be more resistant to the adverse effects of chemotherapy. However, successful pregnancy has been reported even following combined chemotherapy.

Q. What are the important issues that the oncologists should know and accordingly counsel the patients?

Ans.
- Oncologists should be familiar with the fertility sparing management options for a young woman with ovarian malignancy.
- Women must be counseled with the options available, limitations, eligibility criteria and importantly the risks and the benefits of such a procedure.
- Multidisciplinary team approach (oncologists, reproductive endocrinologists and perinatologists) should be there.
- It is difficult to predict outcome for anyone individual woman as there is nonavailability of accurate data that are based on large number of controlled studies.

References

1. Heintz AP, Odicino F, Maisonneuve P, et al. Carcinoma of the ovary. FIGO 26th Annual Report on the Results of Treatment in Gynecological Cancer. Int J Gynaecol Obstet. 2006;95(1):S161-92.
2. Meirow D, Levron J, Eldar-Geva T, et al. Pregnancy after transplantation of cryopreserved ovarian tissue in a patient after chemotherapy. N Engl Jr Med. 2005;353(3):318-21.
3. Ayhan A, Celik H, Taskiran C, et al. Oncologic and reproductive outcome after fertility-saving surgery in ovarian cancer. Eur J Gynecol Oncol. 2003;24(3-4):223-32.

58 Fertility Conserving Options for Women with Cervical Cancer

Cervical cancer is treated in majority by hysterectomy (simple or radical and/or pelvic radiation). Unfortunately, this treatment results in sterility. The surgical options available for fertility conservation are:
- Excisional procedures on the cervix—(a) cervical amputation, (b) conization.
- Other extensive procedures are—(a) radical abdominal trachelectomy (RAT), (b) radical vaginal trachelectomy (RVT).

Q. Who are the women that may be considered for excisional procedures?
Ans.
- Women with stage IA1 (< 3 mm stromal invasion, microinvasive carcinoma)
- Without any lymphovascular space involvement (LVSI)
- There should be negative endocervical curettings and the cone margin (following excision) should be free of disease.

Q. What is the place of ovarian transposition for a woman with cervical cancer?
Ans. It is done to reduce the risk of radiation injury to the ovaries, in the event that the woman needs radiation therapy following treatment of cervical cancer.

Q. How and at what place ovarian transposition could be done?
Ans. Ovarian transposition could be done either laparoscopically (commonly) or by laparotomy. Ovaries are transposed to a position away from the pelvis, in the paracolic gutters below the lower pole of the kidneys.

Q. What are the suggested eligibility criteria for ovarian transposition?
Ans.
- Any gynecologic malignancy that needs pelvic radiation therapy where ovarian function is to be preserved.
- Patient's age < 40 years seeking fertility conservation.
- Cancer confined to the cervix only.
- No evidence of LVSI.
- Extent of tumor spread has been assessed and excluded by pelvic magnetic resonance imaging (MRI).

Q. What is radical vaginal trachelectomy (RVT)?
Ans. RVT was originally performed by Daniel Dargent in 1987. RVT has two-step procedure:
1. A laparoscopic pelvic (with or without para-aortic) lymph adenectomy is done.
2. Trachelectomy is done via vaginal route.

Principle steps of vaginal trachelectomy are:
- A rim of 1–2 cm of vagina is delineated and a vaginal incision is made.
- Posterior colpotomy is performed.
- Paravesical and pararectal spaces are developed.
- Uterosacral ligaments are transected.
- The bladder pillars are transected mobilizing the ureters.
- Descending cervical branch of the uterine artery is ligated.
- The cervix is amputated keeping 1 cm of cervix attached to the body of the uterus.
- A permanent cerclage is placed at the remaining cervical stroma.
- The vaginal margin is sutured to cervical stroma without occluding the new external os.

The cervical tissue is sent for frozen section biopsy for examination of the resected margin. RVT is abandoned and a radical hysterectomy is done if the resected margin is found positive.

Q. What are the eligibility criteria for RVT?

Ans.
- Histologically confirmed cervical cancer—squamous cell carcinoma, adenosquamous carcinoma or adenocarcinoma. Neuroendocrine tumors of cervix are not considered for RVT.
- Women desirous to preserve fertility and ready for regular follow-up.
- Stage of the disease: FIGO stages IA1 (without LVSI), IA2 or IB1.
- Size of the lesions < 2 cm.
- No evidence of distant metastatsis on preoperative assessment using MRI.
- Adequate cervical length (≥2 cm).
- No evidence of lymph node metastasis.

Q. What is the outcome of RVT?

Ans. Pregnancy has been documented after RVT.[1,2] However, risks of miscarriage, preterm labor are there. Recurrence risks (3.1%) have also been observed.

References

1. Shepherd JH, Mould T, Oram DH. Radial trachelectomy in early stage carcinoma of the cervix: outcome as judged by recurrence and fertility rates. BJOG. 2001;108(8):882-5.
2. Schlaerth JB, Spirtos NM, Schlaerth AC. Radical trachelectomy and pelvic lymphadenectomy with uterine preservation in the treatment of cervical cancer. Am J Obstet Gynecol. 2003;188(1):29-34.

59 Fertility Conserving Options for Women with Endometrial Cancer

Up to 35% of endometrial cancers are diagnosed in premenopausal women. Endometrial cancers are diagnosed even in women younger than 25 years of age less commonly though.

High-risk factors to develop endometrial cancer are: (a) Hyperestrogenism, (b) anovulation, (c) obesity, (d) dyslipidemia, (e) diabetes mellitus (carbohydrate intolerance) and (f) women with polycystic ovarian syndrome (PCOS).

Standard treatment of early stage endometrial cancer (See Manual of Obstetrics and Gynecology for the Postgraduates, p. 340) is total abdominal hysterectomy bilateral salpingo-oophorectomy (BSO), pelvic and para-aortic lymph node sampling. Few patients may need adjuvant therapy either radiotherapy and/or chemotherapy.

Q. Who are the women to be considered for fertility conservation options?
Ans. Women with:
- Stage I, grade I endometrioid adenocarcinoma limited to the endometrium
- Without any evidence of lymph vascular space involvement (LVSI)
- Without any evidence of extrauterine spread of the disease based on CT imaging
- No evidence of myometrial invasion based on MRI
- No evidence of a suspicious adnexal mass on CT or USG.

Q. What are the different parameters that should be reviewed as pretreatment evaluation of the woman?
Ans.
- Detailed history and physical examination and to look for any signs and symptoms of advanced or metastatic disease.
- Dilatation and curettage of the endometrium should be done.
- Hysteroscopy and endometrial sampling is considered for women who are considered for hysterectomy. It is extremely operator dependent.
- Contrast-enhanced MRI is most reliable, accurate and is comprehensive for assessment of women with endometrial carcinoma to assess myometrial invasion. MRI is superior to TVS and CT in assessing myometrial invasion.

Q. What are the fertility sparing treatment options available for endometrial carcinoma?
Ans. Preventive measures to be taken are:
- To stop any unopposed estrogens
- Other risk factors are to be taken care of; (i) weight reduction, (ii) glycemic control, etc.

- **Progestin therapy:** Medroxyprogesterone acetate (MPA) or LNG-IUD. MPA is given continuously 40 mg (orally) per oral a day or higher is recommended for 6–9 months.[1]

Q. How do you follow-up these women?

Ans.
- Office endometrial sampling is done at an interval of 10–12 weeks or sooner if necessary. Dilatation and curettage may be performed if endometrial sampling results are not informative.
- Women are followed up depending upon their response with endometrial histology.
  - **Complete regression:** Therapy may be continued or stopped and advised for fertility improvement therapy.
  - **Persistence of disease:** Therapy may be continued and repeat evaluation is to be done. Persistent disease may need hysterectomy.
  - **Progression of the disease:** Recommended for hysterectomy.

Indications of hysterectomy:
- Poor compliance of the women with medication and/or follow-up.
- Evidence of progression of the disease.
- Child bearing is completed.

Q. What is the outcome of fertility conservative management of a woman with endometrial carcinoma?

Ans. Experience of managing such patients are less as the total number of patients managed are less as yet. Pregnancy has been documented and live birth rate is 47%.[2]

References

1. Gotlieb W, Beiner ME, Shalmon B, et al. Outcome of fertility-sparing treatment with progestins in young patients with endometrial cancer. Obstet Gynecol. 2003;102(4):718-25.
2. Niwa K, Tagami K, Lian Z, et al. Outcome of fertility-preserving treatment in young women with endometrial carcinomas. BJOG. 2005;112(3):317-20.

60. Advances in Contraception

Q. What is the significance of knowing advances in contraception?
Ans. Advances in contraceptive research contribute greatly to better health and healthcare. Progressive research in this field has made contraceptive measures more safe and effective for all the ages of clients. It is also essential that the healthcare providers should also know 'what is new' so that they can communicate with the clients more effectively.

Q. How the service of the healthcare providers is important?
Ans. A holistic approach brings the well-informed clients together for good quality services. Contraceptive care providers need to be well-informed, skilled and competent to communicate the clients sympathetically and should also deal the complication if any develops.

INTRAUTERINE CONTRACEPTIVE DEVICES (IUCDs)

Q. What are the new directions for the use of IUCDs (IUDs)?
Ans. The modern IUDs (CuT380 A, Multiload 375 and LNG-IUD) are safe, effective and quickly reversible. They can be used for long-term contraception. They are also cost-effective. CuT380 A is supplied free of cost by the Government of India through family planning program. CuT380 A can be used for ≥10 years, and Multiload 375 and LNG-IUD for 5 years each. They can be used to delay pregnancy or even to end child bearing (Figs 60.1A to C).

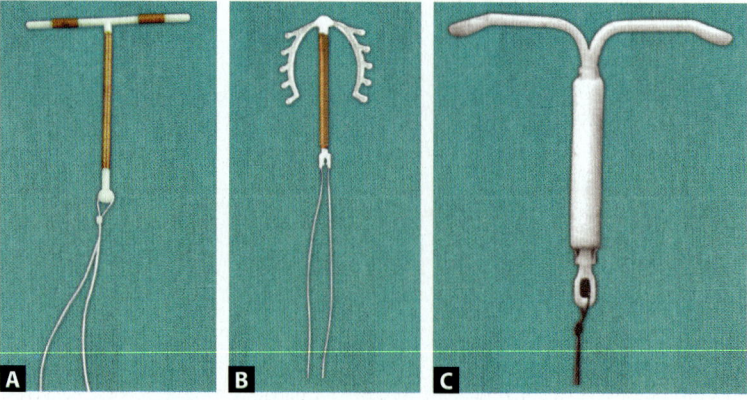

Figs 60.1A to C: A. CuT380 A; **B.** Multiload 375; **C.** LNG-IUD

- Effectiveness of IUDs is similar to that of female sterilization.
- **Failure rate:** LNG-IUD: 1 in 1,000 women; CuT380 A: 3–8 in 1,000 women.

Q. What are the other advantages of using IUDs?

Ans.
- In reality most women can use IUDs safely and effectively
- Including women who are breastfeeding
- Other advantages are:
  Women can use IUDs:
  - Without any tests for sexually transmitted infections (STIs), including human immunodeficiency virus (HIV)
  - Without any blood tests or laboratory tests
  - Without cervical cancer screening
  - Without breast examination.

Q. What is the current guidance to the use of IUDs in women with STIs?

Ans.
- Women who are at risk of HIV or are infected with HIV can safely use IUDs.
- Women having gonorrhea and chlamydia or purulent cervicitis are not recommended for the use of IUDs.

Q. What are advances in contraception as regard to the use of IUDs?

Ans.
- Refusing women IUDs in the absence of laboratory tests for STIs, blood tests, would deny benefits to a great majority of women.
- There is no significant increase in infertility associated with IUD use, which has been observed.
- About 72–96% women conceived within a year after the removal of IUDs.

Q. What is the medical eligibility criteria for contraceptive use?

Ans. According to WHO, categories for temporary methods are described in Table 60.1.

Table 60.1: The medical eligibility criteria for contraceptive use

Category	With clinical judgement	With limited clinical judgement
1.	Use method in any circumstances	Yes (use the method)
2.	Generally use method	Yes (use the method)
3.	Method is not usually recommended unless other more appropriate methods are available or acceptable	No
4.	Method not to be used	Do not use the method

Q. What is the current guidance to IUD users having HIV (Medical eligibility criteria category 2 and 3; WHO 2008)?

Ans.
- A woman with HIV (not AIDS) can have Cu-IUDs or hormonal IUD inserted.
- A woman having AIDS on highly active antiretroviral therapy (HAART) and is clinically well can have IUD inserted.
- IUD insertion is not recommended for women with AIDS and not on HAART (WHO category 3).
- However in all the situations the woman must be urged to use condoms along with IUD.

Q. Compared to the worldwide use of IUDs, which country has the maximum use of IUDs?
Ans. Most IUD users are in China (60%), thereafter eastern Europe and central Asia (11%) and other Asia (12%).

Q. What is the place of immediate postpartum insertion of IUCD (PPIUCD)?
Ans. Immediate postpartum insertion of IUCDs is safe. It can be inserted as:
- **Post placental:** Immediately following delivery of the placenta (following vaginal or cesarean delivery).
- **Early postpartum** (<48 hours) before the woman leaves the hospital following childbirth.

Q. What is the importance of PPIUCD?
Ans. Postpartum insertion of IUCD is encouraged in India as a measure of population control. Risk of unplanned and unintended pregnancy is high during the period following completion of exclusive breastfeeding. Majority of women resume menstruation, ovulation and sexual activity during this period. As such in India, unmet need of contraception in the postpartum period is still there. Currently, the rate of institutional delivery has increased significantly. While in hospital postpartum women have opportunity to use it without coming to the hospital for the second time. At that time the family planning, health workers have easy access to these women for counseling during the antenatal as well as postpartum period. PPIUCD is proved to be safe, effective and convenient for long-term use.

Q. What is the concern with breastfeeding in woman with HIV?
Ans.
- Risks of mother-to-child transmission (MTCT) for HIV infection with breastfeeding is 30%.
- Lactational amenorrhea may be an option for contraception in women with HIV.
- Exclusive breastfeeding carries lower risk of HIV transmission (MTCT) as compared to mixed feeding.
- Exclusive breastfeeding is the preferred feeding option for HIV exposed infants up to < 6 months of age (National guidelines 2011).
- Exclusive replacement feeding should be done only when AFASS criteria is fulfilled (A: Affordable, F: Feasible, A: Acceptable, S: Sustainable, S: Safe).
- Mother is counseled and helped to make her own choice regarding the use of exclusive breastfeeding or exclusive replacement feeding.

COMBINED ORAL CONTRACEPTIVES (COCs)

Q. What is the current guidance for the missed pills while the woman is on COCs or the pill?
Ans. **A.** When there is missing of one or two active pills (between days 1 and 21)

Take the missed pill as soon as you remember → Take the next pill usual → Keep taking active pills usual

B. However, there are special rule for special cases (situations).

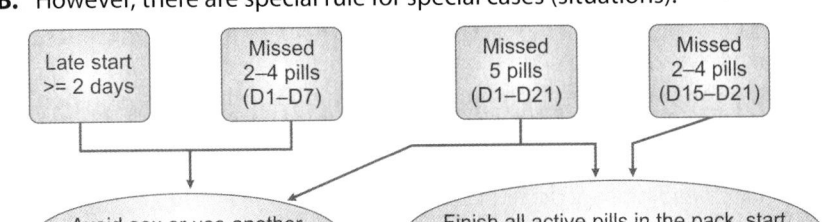

C. With 28 pills pack missed any of the last 7 (inactive) pills.

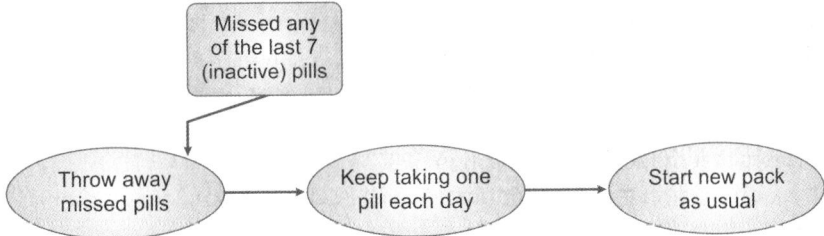

Q. What are the risks of missed pills and pregnancy?
Ans. Women who are late starter and/or missed pill in the third week, run the higher risks of failure and pregnancy. This is due to speeded development and growth of follicles resulting in ovulation and pregnancy. There are some women who are biologically active in this response.

Q. What about the ultra dose pills and shortening the hormone free interval?
Ans. Ultra dose pills contain ethinyl estradiol (EE) 15 µg and gestodene 60 µg. It is quiet effective but have more risks of break through bleeding. Withdrawal bleeds are more.
   Shortening the hormone free interval is done using hormone pills for 24 days and nonhormone pills for 4 days. This reduces the amount of withdrawal bleeding both in the amount and duration.

Q. Does the woman need to have menstruation to start the pill?
Ans. Woman can start the pill at any time when it is certain that she is not pregnant.

Q. Who are the women suitable for COCs?
Ans. Nearly all healthy women are found safe and suitable for COCs irrespective of marital status or parity.

Q. What examination she needs to have before using COCs?
Ans. Women who are clinically fit and otherwise healthy, can begin COCs:
- Without a pelvic examination
- Without any routine blood or laboratory tests
- Without cervical cancer screening
- Without breast examination.

Q. What are the extended and continuous use of COCs?
Ans. Taking the pills for 12 weeks without a pause followed by 1 week of no pills (break) is the **extended use** of pills. Whereas taking the pills without a break at all is called **continuous use**.

Q. What are the advantages and disadvantages of extended or continuous use of the pills?
Ans. Advantages
- Women have vaginal bleeding only for four times a year or no bleeding at all.
- Reduce the problems of premenstrual tension syndrome, dysmenorrhea, heavy bleeding and mood changes.

Disadvantages
- Irregular bleeding may occur initially
- More pills need to be used.

Q. How the pill effectiveness is affected?
Ans. Drug interactions are the important areas that often alter the pill effectiveness.
- **Drugs that reduces pill effectiveness are:** Rifampicin, griseofulvin, barbiturates, ritonavir and topiramate.
- **Anticonvulsants:** Carbamazepine, phenytoin, primidone.

The drugs induce hepatic enzymes to cause enhancement in metabolic degradation of pills.
- Drugs that reduces the absorption of EE.
    - **Broad-spectrum antibiotics:** Ampicillin, ciprofloxacin, doxycycline.
    - **Others:** Fluconazole, ofloxacin, tetracycline, triazole.

Q. How she can avoid the failure rate in such a situation?
Ans. She is to be counseled:
- If these drugs are for short-term use she can use a back-up method along with COCs.
- When these drugs are used for long-term, she may use a different method (progestin injectables, CuT380 A or LNG-IUD).

Q. What is the guidance regarding the hormonal contraception for the women with HIV?
Ans. The main concerns are:
- Risks of acquiring HIV
- Progression of disease
- HIV transmission
- Adverse interaction with HAART.

Current situation and guidance is as below:
- Regarding acquisition—no additional risk has been observed.
- Regarding progression of the disease, mixed observation has been mentioned.
- Risks of infectivity, evidence is limited and conflicting. So more study results are awaited.
- Drug interactions with HAART [nucleoside reverse transcriptase inhibitors (NRTIs), nonnucleoside reverse transcriptase inhibitors (NNRTIs)] do not reduce the efficacy of Depo-Provera® (DMPA).

IMPLANTS

Q. Discuss about the implants used as the next generation?
Ans. The implants of the next generation are:

- One rod system: IMPLANON® (etonogestrel 68 mg) (Fig. 60.2)
- Two rod system:
  - JADELLE® (Levonorgestrel) (Fig. 60.3)
  - Sino-implant (Zarin)
- Six-capsules (Norplant)
- These implants are safe, highly effective and quickly reversible
- Duration of use is 3–5 years
- Ease of insertion (1–2 min) and removal (2–3 min).

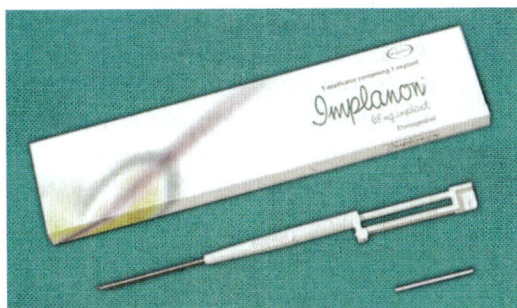

Fig. 60.2: IMPLANON® implant

Q. What are the special issues with the use of the new generation of implants?

Ans. The new generation implants are safe and suitable for nearly all women including adolescents and breastfeeding (> 6 weeks) and women with anemia.
- Implants are more effective than injectables and pills. Effectiveness is comparable to sterilization.
- Women with implants can be almost certain not to get any unintended pregnancy for up to 3–5 years.
- Women with HIV, AIDS on antiretroviral (ARV) therapy can safely use implants.
- Women with HIV, AIDS should be urged to use condoms also.
- Provision should be there to ensure routine, regular follow-up and reliable removal services.

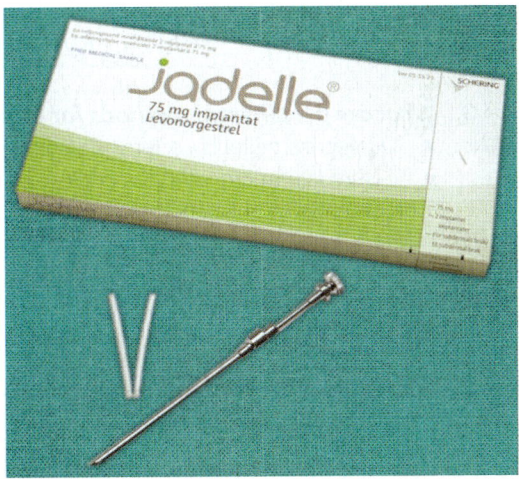

Fig. 60.3: JADELLE® implant

Progestin only contraception (PGN only injectables): Depot medroxyprogesterone acetate (DMPA) and norethisterone enanthate (NET-EN) each contains hormone progesterone (PGN) and no estrogen (EGN). DMPA is widely used.

Q. What is new about DMPA?

Ans.
- DMPA reinjection schedule is unchanged but the grace period or the extended period has been permitted for the late clients (WHO-2008).
  Schedule injection is at 3 months interval and grace period of 4 weeks has been added.
- Average delay in pregnancy is there for 7 months, since the last injection.

Q. What is the effect on bone mineral density (BMD) with the use of DMPA?

Ans. There is slight decrease in BMD with its use but it is reversible. Decreased BMD should not limit its use.

Q. Is there any contraindication of its use?
Ans. Contraindications are very few:
- Breastfeeding < 6 weeks of birth
- Severe high BP (systolic ≥ 160 mm Hg or diastolic ≥ 100 mm Hg)
- Ischemic heart disease
- History of prior stroke
- Arterial cardiovascular disease
- Severe liver disease, breast cancer.

Q. What is the place of PGN-only injectables for women with HIV?
Ans.
- Women with HIV or AIDS on ARV can safely use PGN-only injectable.
- They should use condoms also.

TRANSCERVICAL STERILIZATION

Q. What are the different methods for transcervical sterilization?
Ans.
- Quinacrine pellet is a sclerosing agent used to block the tubes. Failure rate is 2–3/100 WY.
- Essure is a microcoil (spring-like). It is used hysteroscopically and placed within the cornual end of the fallopian tube.

VASECTOMY

(*See Manual of Obstetrics and Gynecology for the Postgraduates, p. 332, Figs 25.3A and B*)

Q. What is the current scenario of vasectomy as a permanent method of male contraception?
Ans. It is a very effective method but neglected and under utilized due to misconceptions.

Q. What are the advantages of vasectomy over tubectomy?
Ans. Advantages of vasectomy are:
- It is a quicker method
- Safe
- Cheaper and
- Associated with faster recovery and above all it is a highly effective method (failure rate is 0.2 per 100 couples). It needs 3 months delay or 20 ejaculations to become effective.

Q. What is the over all prevalence rate of vasectomy throughout the globe?
Ans. It is performed in Bhutan (13.6%), Australia/New Zealand (11.8%), China (6.7%) and India (1.0%).

Q. Is there any health risk associated with vasectomy?
Ans. Generally-there is nothing such.
- Does not cause impotence
- No increased risk of testicular cancer
- No increased risk of cardiovascular disease
- Risk of prostate cancer is likely to be noncausative.

61 Interventional Radiology in Obstetrics and Gynecology

Interventional radiology is currently being carried out in the management of many areas in obstetrics and gynecology. Embolotherapy can obviate the need of many major operations like myomectomy or hysterectomy.

PLACE OF INTERVENTIONAL RADIOLOGY IN OBSTETRICS

- **Uterine artery embolization (UAE)** in the management of postpartum hemorrhage (PPH) (primary and secondary) is an effective intervention. It is an alternative to hysterectomy. In many hospitals, it is now routinely used in the management of PPH where resources and expertize permit. **Cases of PPH due to atonicity,** following cesarean section are effectively managed with UAE.
- Cases with placenta previa and accreta where placenta is morbidly adherent to the uterine wall, often bleeds profusely following delivery either vaginal or cesarean section. Such problems are commonly faced in cases with prior cesarean delivery. Care plans could be organized in such cases for doing UAE procedure electively just prior to the operation.
- UAE is considered as the most effective management for hemorrhage caused by uterine vascular malformations (uterine artery malformation, arteriovenous malformation or aneurysm formation). These women suffer from profuse secondary PPH. Diagnosis of such vascular malformations is often difficult. Doppler study may be helpful in few situations. Uterine vascular angiography is the gold standard in the diagnosis. UAE is the most effective management to control the abnormal bleeding in these cases.

Benefits of UAE: Besides the therapeutic benefit of control of hemorrhage, preservation of the uterus and the fertility are the other important benefits. The overall success rate of UAE is 90–95%. Pregnancies have been reported following UAE for treatment of PPH.

UAE in gynecology: UAE has been done in cases with fibroid uterus. It reduces the size, vascularity and problems of bleeding and pressure effects of the tumor. However, complications are also reported. Other uses of selective UAE in gynecology are: (a) To control hemorrhage after abdominal and vaginal hysterectomy, (b) hemorrhage from cervical cancer, (c) hemorrhage from abdominal pregnancy and (d) retroperioneal hemorrhage.

Procedure: Both the uterine arteries are selectively catheterized through the femoral artery under fluoroscopic guidance. Polyvinyl alcohol particles are used to embolize the vessels. This method is simple. It is done by a skilled interventional radiologist under local anesthesia.

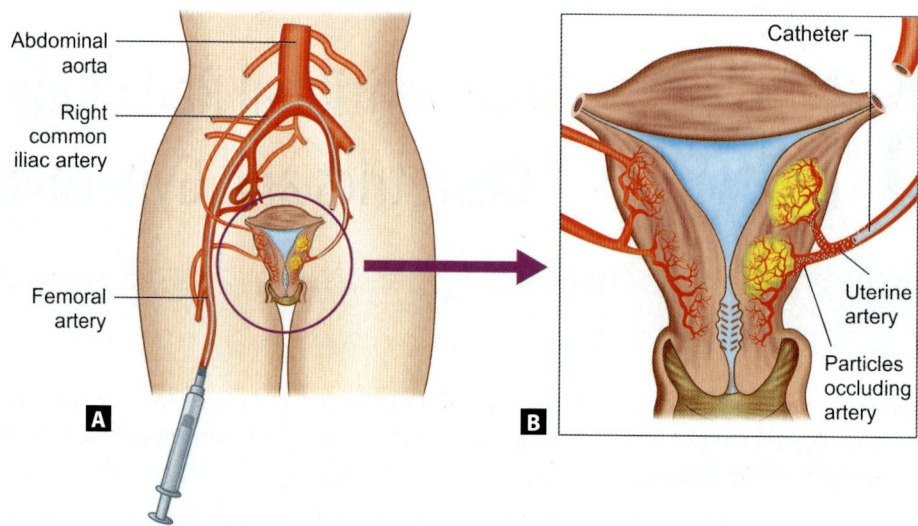

Figs 61.1A and B: Uterine artery embolization. **A.** Pelvic angiography is done through femoral artery catheterization, **B.** Uterine artery embolization is done through the catheter

Contraindications of UAE are: (a) Pregnancy, (b) active pelvic infection, (c) allergy to contrast media, (d) desire for future pregnancy, (e) undiagnosed pelvic mass and (f) pedunculated myoma.
Overall success rate of UAE: 96–98% (Figs 61.1A and B).
Benefits are: Improvement of menorrhagia, reduction in volume and size of fibroids (60%), conservation of uterus.
Common complications of UAE are low-grade fever, pain, pelvic infection, injury to femoral and iliac arteries and ischemia of buttock. Other complications following treatment of uterine fibroids are: abdominal pain, fever, vaginal discharge, nausea, vomiting, amenorrhea, sepsis (<1%) and ovarian failure (<5%). Future pregnancy complications are: miscarriage, preterm delivery, fetal growth restriction (FGR), PPH and increased risk of cesarean delivery. However, regarding future fertility and pregnancy following UAE, more studies are needed.

62 Surgical Site Infection

Postoperative surgical site infections (SSIs) are the important cause of patient mortality and prolonged hospital stay. This increases hospital cost. Some patients have increased risk factors for SSI.

Risk Factors for Surgical Site Infection (SSI)

- Pre-existing anemia
- Older age
- Excess operative blood loss
- Prolonged operative time (> 3.5 hours)
- Placement of foreign body (drain, catheter)
- Obesity
- Smoking
- Immunocompromised individual
- Preoperative HbAIC >7 % or
- Capillary blood glucose >200 mg/dL
- Presence of systemic disease.

Classification of Surgical Site Infection (Mangram–1999, Modified)[1]

A. ***Superficial incisional***
   - Involves superficial tissues only
   - Develops within 30 days of operation
   - Clinical features
     - Purulent discharge with positive bacteria in culture
     - Pain, tenderness, redness.

B. ***Deep incisional***
   - Involve abdominal wall muscles and fascia
   - Develops within 30 days of operation
   - Clinical features
     - Purulent discharge from deep tissues, not from organ/space component
     - Temperature ≥38°C, localized pain, tenderness
     - Detection of abscess by reoperation or radiology.

C. *Organ/space involvement*
- Develops within 30 days of operation
- Bacteria recovered from the fluid/tissue in that organ/space
- Purulent discharge through drain/stab wound from the organ/space.

Management: Details of history-taking and clinical examination is done. Investigations are organized including wound and/or vaginal swab. Broad-spectrum antimicrobials (piperacillin-tazobactum or imipenem-cilastatin) are started till the culture reports are available. Anaerobic coverage is done with metronidazole or clindamycin. Surgical intervention (laparotomy, drainage of abscess/hematoma) may be needed.

Interventions for Preventions of Surgical Site Infection (SSI)

A. Preoperative
- To reduce HbA1c levels to <7% before operation
- Improvement of nutritional status and level of hemoglobin
- To control any preoperative infections (respiratory/urinary tract).

B. Perioperative
- Removal/clipping of hair
- Thorough antiseptic scrub of hands, forearms of the surgical team members
- Preparation of the skin around the operative site with antiseptic agents (povidone iodine/chlorhexidine)
- Use of prophylactic antibiotics.

C. Intraoperative
- To reduce dead space
- To follow standard principles of asepsis
- Use of surgical drains (selective)
- Use of antibiotics (prophylactic/therapeutic as needed)
- To maintain intraoperative normothermia.[2]

D. Postoperative
- To maintain plasma glucose < 200 mg/dL on postoperative day-1 or day-2
- To monitor wound healing and early detection of SSI.

References

1. Mangram AJ, Horan TC, Pearson ML, et al. Guideline for prevention of surgical site infection, 1999. Hospital Infection Control Practices Advisory Committee. Infect Control Hosp Epidemiol. 1999;20(4):250-78.
2. Kurz A, Sessler DI, Lenhardt R. Perioperative normothermia to reduce the incidence of surgical-wound infection and shorten hospitalization. Study of wound infection and temperature group. N Engl J Med.1996;334:1209-15.

63. Abnormal Uterine Bleeding: Investigations and Management Issues

Q. What are the common causes of abnormal uterine bleeding (AUB)?

Ans. Neoplasm (fibroid, polyps, cancers), hormonal therapy, trauma, infection, coagulopathies and pregnancy complications (See Manual of Obstetrics and Gynecology for the Postgraduates, p. 348) are the common causes of AUB.

Q. What is the prevalence of AUB?

Ans. Overall prevalence in the women of reproductive age is 10–30%. It is as high as 50% in the premenopausal age group.

Q. How to assess the severity of AUB?

Ans. There are several methods in practice to assess the severity of uterine bleeding.
- Estimation of blood hemoglobin (usually < 12 g/dL)
- Hematocrit level
- Estimation of hematin (spectrophotometrically) not commonly done
- Pictorial blood assessment chart (PBAC): By assessment of pads soaked—lightly, moderately or completely
- Measurement of clots (> 1 cm)
- Pad changing with time (frequency):
    - Scoring system has been introduced with scores 1, 5, 20
    - Similarly measurement score: 1–20
    - Total score >100 points suggests menorrhagia.

Q. How saline infusion sonography (SIS) is correlated with transvaginal sonography (TVS)?

Ans. Saline infusion sonography is more helpful to detect the uterine intracavity pathology like polyps, submucous fibroid and blood clots. With these advantages SIS is found superior to TVS.

Q. What are the contraindications of SIS?

Ans.
- Pregnancy
- Pelvic inflammatory diseases
- Unexplained abdominal tenderness.

Q. What are the disadvantages of SIS?

Ans. Performance of SIS is cycle dependent. Thickened endometrium in the second half of the cycle may cause difficulty in diagnosis. The risk of false-positive diagnosis is more. SIS is good for the detection of focal lesion. Difficulty is there when the lesion is diffuse. Moreover difficulties are faced in cases where there is cervical stenosis and in postmenopausal women.

Q. How do you correlate AUB with different clinical scenarios?
Ans. The different clinical situations manifested with AUB are:

- Obesity
- Polycystic ovary syndrome (PCOS)
- Thyroid dysfunction
- Infections (chlamydia)
- Coagulopathies [idiopathic thrombocytopenic purpura (ITP), thrombocytopenia, leukemia, Von-Willebrand disease]
- Cervical ectopy
- Cervical pathology
- Enlarged uterus:
  - Fibroid
  - Adenomyosis
- Endometrial carcinoma
- Uterine sarcoma
- Adnexal pathology
  - Tubo-ovarian mass
  - Fallopian tube cancer

Q. What are the causes of uterine arteriovenous (AV) malformations?
Ans. Exact cause is not well understood. Common observations are: trauma (difficult cesarean delivery), cancer [cancer cervix, endometrium or gestational trophoblastic neoplasia (GTN)] or congenital.

Q. How do the women with AV malformations present?
Ans. Women may present with irregular or intermittent bleeding. Bleeding may at times be heavy and life-threatening.

Q. How the diagnosis of AV malformations could be made?
Ans. *Exclusion* of other causes for AUB is essential: (a) TVS may show hypoechoic tubular structure, and with, (b) color Doppler study: reverse blood flow is observed. However (c) contrast-enhanced computed tomography (CECT), (d) magnetic resonance imaging (MRI) may be used when needed, (e) angiography is considered as the gold standard for the diagnosis.

Q. How AV malformation could be treated?
Ans.
- Hysterectomy may be considered for women who have completed their family.
  - Uterine artery embolization is an option where facilities are available (*See* Manual of Obstetrics and Gynecology for the Postgraduates, p. 28).

Q. What is procedure of UAE?
Ans. *See* Manual of Obstetrics and Gynecology for the Postgraduates, p. 28.

Q. What are the contraindications of UAE?
Ans.
- Pregnancy
- Acute pelvic infection
- Endometrial hyperplasia

- Genital tract cancer
- Postmenopausal women
- Women desiring to presence fertility
- Intrauterine contraceptive device (IUCD) in place
- Larger or distorted endometrial cavity.

Q. What are the complications of UAE?
Ans.
- Nausea, vomiting
- Malaise, fever
- Infection
- Ovarian failure (rare).

Q. Outline your approach for management of a woman with AUB.
Ans. Details of history-taking and physical examination are done:
- Pregnancy is to be excluded [serum, beta-human chorionic gonadotropin (β-hCG), ultrasonography (USG)]
- **Hematological parameters:**
    - Complete blood count (CBC), platelets, thyroid-stimulating hormone (TSH)
    - Coagulation studies [partial thromboplastin time (PTT), prothrombin time (PT)], prolactin
- **Infections:** Chlamydia, others sexually transmitted infections (STIs)
- Cervical cytology (Pap smear)
- Ultrasonography (Flowchart 63.1).

Flowchart 63.1: Evaluation of cavity, myometrium and endometrium through transvaginal sonography

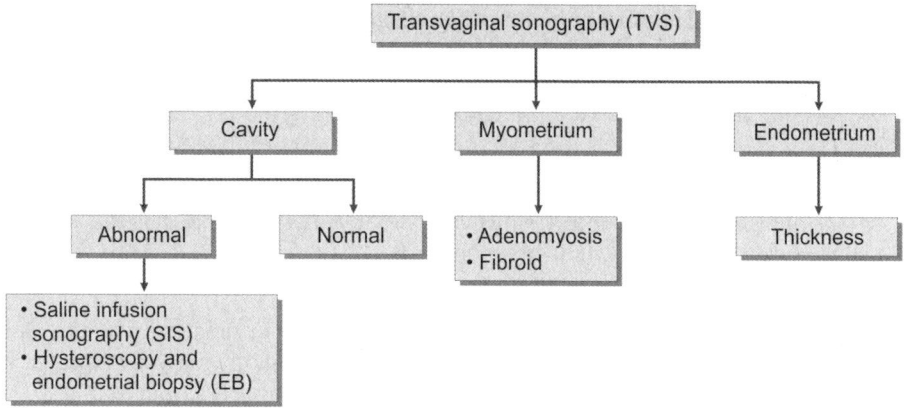

- **Endometrial thickness on TVS[1]**
    - Thickness 3.4 ± 1.2 mm mostly (postmenopausal atrophic endometrium)
    - Thickness 9.7 ± 2.5 mm (commonly endometrial hyperplasia)
    - Thickness 18.2 ± 6.2 mm (endometrial cancer).

Endometrial thickness > 4 mm requires additional evaluation with SIS, hysteroscopy, EB [American Congress of Obstetricians and Gynecologists (ACOG) 2009].

SIS is simple, minimally invasive sonographic procedure to evaluate endometrium, myometrium and the endometrial cavity.

Q. What are the iatrogenic causes of AUB?
Ans.
- IUCD (CuT380 A)
- Mirena
- Combined oral contraceptive (COC) (breakthrough bleeding)
- Progestin-only pill (POP)
- Hormone replacement therapy (HRT) (discontinuation)
- Tamoxifen.

Q. How does IUCD cause AUB?
Ans. Initiation of subclinical inflammatory changes in the endometrium. There is release of prostaglandins, thromboxanes, and increase in local leukocyte population. All these results in increased endometrial vascularity, thrombosis and infraction.

Q. How tamoxifen is associated with AUB?
Ans. Tamoxifen is a selective estrogen receptor modulator. It is commonly used in the management of breast carcinoma following surgery. Tamoxifen is an estrogen receptor antagonist in the breast tissue as well as an agonist in the endometrium. Prolonged use results in endometrial hyperplasia and carcinoma. Women with tamoxifen therapy need to be screened for endometrial abnormalities.

Q. What are the advantages of USG in the management of AUB?
Ans. Ultrasonography is considered as the first-line tool in the management of AUB. USG either transabdominal sonography (TAS) or TVS can detect any anatomical abnormality located in the myometrium or endometrium or with other pathologies like fibroid uterus, adenomyosis or submucous polyps. However, limitations are: high false-negative rate due to focal uterine cavity pathology. In such a situation, hysteroscopy or SIS is performed.

Q. What are the limitations of pipelle endometrial sampling?
Ans.
- Collected sample may be inadequate.
- False-negative rate for detection of endometrial cancer is 0.91%.
- False-negative rate due to local pathology is high.

Q. How do you evaluate the place of TVS versus SIS in the management of AUB?
Ans. Both the procedure have similar diagnostic accuracy. But limitations for the both are due to lack of histological diagnosis. However, operative hysteroscopy has the advantage of taking endometrial biopsy (EB) when desired.

Q. What are the advantages of hysteroscopy?
Ans. Hysteroscopy (3-5 mm diameter) may be considered as a primary tool in the diagnosis of uterine polyps, submucous fibroid. Operative hysteroscopy may be helpful as biopsy could be done simultaneously when endometrial carcinoma is suspected.

Q. What are the limitations of hysteroscopy?
Ans. It is an invasive procedure and is expensive. Difficulties may be faced due to cervical stenosis and in postmenopausal women. Complications may occur due to uterine perforation, spread of infection in the peritoneal cavity or peritoneal spillage of cancer cells in a case with endometrial carcinoma.

Q. What are the different structural abnormalities?
Ans.
- Endometrial polyps
- Adenomyosis
- Cervical ectopy
- Infections—chlamydia, other STIs

- Leiomyoma
- Hypertrophic myometrium
- Arteriovenous malformation (fistulous communications).

Q. What are the different systemic diseases that may cause AUB?

Ans.
- Severe renal dysfunction
- Liver disease
- Thyroid dysfunctions
    - Hypothyroidism
    - Hyperthyroidism (5%)
- Coagulopathy.

Q. What are the underlying basic pathology of AUB where the woman suffers with such a systemic disease?

Ans.
A. **Renal dysfunction** is accompanied by endocrine disturbances. This causes hypoestrogenism and this ultimately leads to amenorrhea and infertility.

B. **Liver disease:** There is often association of hypothalamic-pituitary ovarian dysfunction as in a case with renal dysfunction. Liver dysfunction is associated with high level of serum estradiol. This causes low levels of serum follicle-stimulating hormone (FSH) and luteinizing hormone (LH). Hemostatic dysfunction have also been observed in such cases.

C. **Thyroid dysfunction:** Hyperthyroidism often presents with amenorrhea or hypomenorrhea and menorrhagia in about 5% of cases. Hypothyroidism presents with menorrhagia. Women with hypothyroidism suffers from anovulation, amenorrhea and anovulatory dysfunctional uterine bleeding (DUB). Some woman also suffers from decreased coagulation factors to cause AUB. Treatment of hyperthyroidism corrects the AUB abnormalities.

D. **Coagulopathy:** AUB in women with coagulopathy is due to:
- Deficient platelet number (thrombocytopenia)
- Dysfunction of platelets (thrombasthenia)
- Defects in platelet plug stabilization
- Deficient clotting factors (factors VIII, IX disorder)
- Disorder of Von Willebrand factor (VWF).

Q. What are the different options for operative management of AUB?

Ans. Selection of cases is important. The management options are:
- **Dilatation and curettage:** Intractable cases when medical management has failed (ACOG). Endometrium can be tested for histological diagnosis.
- Endometrial ablation or resection
- Indications are:
    - Women with failed medical treatment
    - Women not desirous to preserve menstrual or reproductive function
    - Women with normal uterine size (< 10 weeks pregnant size)
    - Fibroid uterus but fibroids < 3 cm in diameter
    - Where longer surgical time is to be avoided.
- Myomectomy (*See* Manual of Obstetrics and Gynecology for the Postgraduates, p. 317, 379)
- Uterine artery embolization
- Hysterectomy.

Q. What is the overall success rate of endometrial ablation or resection?
Ans. Overall success rate is 70–80%. About 30–40% women become amenorrheic and another 50% get significant decrease in blood loss. But 10% women need repeat procedures or hysterectomy.

Q. How one should organize the investigations for the management of a case with AUB?
Ans. There is no such clear sequence of events. However, investigations should preferably be simple, less invasive with less discomfort and with much information. Considering all these TVS appears the logical first step. It can differentiate the pathologies that are focal, diffuse or located in the endometrial cavity, endometrium itself or in the myometrium. Once anatomical localization is made, subsequent investigations are carried out as follows:
- Endometrial hyperplasia → EB (Pipelle)
- Focal lesion: ♦ Hyteroscopy ♦ SIS } → Biopsy

Endometrial thickness: 3.4 ± 1.2 mm → Atropic endometrium (postmenopausal)
9.7 ± 2.5 mm → Hyperplasia
18.2 ± 6.2 mm → Endometrial cancer

Q. Describe the management options for DUB?
Ans. *Acute bleeding:* Premarin 25 mg IV 4 hourly 3 doses.
→ Then tablet 2.5 mg 6 hourly till bleeding stops.
Chronic cases: Inhibitor of cyclooxygenase (COX-1 and COX-2).
Reduces blood loss by 90%.
Progestogens
- Medroxyprogesterone acetate
- Norethisterone

Levonorgestrel-intrauterine system (LNG-IUS) reduces blood loss by 70–90%.
Danazol/gestrinone: 17α-isoxazole derivative of testosterone. Reduces serum estradiol levels and increases androgen levels. There is amenorrhea. It is the second-line drug of choice.
- ***Tranexamic acid:*** It is an antifibrinolytic agent. It is contraindicated in patients with risks of thrombosis.
- ***Ethamsylate:*** It is used as a hemostatic. It is not so effective.

Surgery
- Dilatation and curettage; cases with severe bleeding and refractory to medical management
- Uterine artery embolization in selective cases (*See* Manual of Obstetrics and Gynecology for the Postgraduates, p. 317, 487)
- Endometrial ablation/resection
- Hysterectomy in a selected case.

Reference
1. Granberg S, Wikland M, Karlsson B, et al. Endometrial thickness as measured by endovaginal ultrasonography for identifying endometrial abnormality. Am J Obstet Gynecol. 1991;164(1 Pt 1):47-52.

64. Subfertility and Pelvic Endometriosis

Discuss the management issues of subfertility in association with pelvic endometriosis:
- Approximately 40–60% of women in the reproductive age suffer from the problem of subfertility in association with pelvic endometriosis. Often they remain asymptomatic. Laparoscopic pelvic evaluation is the **gold standard** to detect pelvic endometriosis even if they are without any symptoms. Laparoscopy is helpful to stage the disease [allergic fungal sinusitis (AFS)] also.
- Arguments are there both in favor and against this association.[1] However, majority support the concept of causal relationship between the presence of endometriosis and subfertility.
- Women with pelvic endometriosis have reduced fecundity rate when compared to a woman with normal pelvis. Reduced monthly fecundity rate is observed for such women even after husband's sperm insemination compared to a woman with normal pelvis. This is also the observation that there is reduced implantation rate per embryo transfer after *in vitro* fertilization (IVF) in women with pelvic endometriosis.
- **The reasons for the association of subfertility are:[2]**
    - **Ovarian dysfunction:** (a) Defective folliculogenesis, (b) anovulation, (c) luteal phase defect (LPD), (d) hyperprolactinemia and (e) poor oocyte maturation.
    - **Tubal dysfunction:** (a) Pelvic adhesions, tubal obstruction (moderate to severe endometriosis) and (b) distorsion of normal tube and ovarian relationship.
    - **Others:** (a) Dyspareunia, (b) altered immunity and (c) subclinical peritoneal inflammation.

    Endometriosis is a progressive disease. Treatment of endometriosis is justified regardless of the symptoms because in 30–60% of women it progresses within a year.[3]

    However, association of subfertility and minimal or mild endometriosis is not well-established. Management of infertile women with minimal to mild endometriosis is therefore controversial.

    Current evidence suggests that **medical treatment** has no benefit over no treatment in terms of crude pregnancy rate.

    Association between endometriosis and subfertility is established especially in women with moderate to advanced stage disease.

    Laparoscopic surgical management (excision of endometriotic deposits, ovarian cystectomy for endometriomas, deep rectovaginal septum endometriosis, restoration of normal pelvic anatomy and adhesiolysis) has got some advantages over medical management to improve pregnancy rate (44%). However, **role of surgery in minimal to mild endometriosis is yet to be established**.

    Addition of **postoperative medical therapy** has not been observed with improved pregnancy outcome. Chance of spontaneous pregnancy is high during the first 6–12 months after conservative surgery alone.

Intrauterine insemination (husband)**, along with controlled ovarian stimulation **(superovulation) is found to improve pregnancy rate in women with mild to moderate disease.

IVF is an effective method to achieve pregnancy, irrespective of the stage of the disease. IVF may be considered following surgical treatment of endometriosis.[4]

References

1. D' Hooghe TM, Debrock S, Hill JA, et al. Endometriosis and subfertility: is the relationship resolved? Semin Reprod Med. 2003;21(2):243-54.
2. Kennedy S, Bergqvist A, Chapron C, et al. ESHRE guideline for the diagnosis and treatment of endometriosis. Hum Reprod. 2005;20(10):2698-704.
3. Dutta DC, Konar H. Endometriosis and adenomyosis. In: Konar H (ed). Textbook of Gynecology, 7th edition. New Delhi, India: Jaypee Brothers Medical Publishers; 2016. p. 248-59.
4. Feinberg EC, Levens ED, DeCherney AH. Infertility surgery is dead: Only the obituary remains? Fertil Steril. 2008;89(1):232-6.

65. Medical Methods of Termination of Pregnancy

Mrs CL, a 30-year-old woman, presents in the clinic for her unplanned third pregnancy that occurred due to failure of contraception. She had previous two spontaneous vaginal deliveries uneventfully. She is otherwise fit and healthy. She is now 8 weeks following the last USG report. She requests for medical methods for termination of pregnancy (TOP). Discuss the management issues.

Misoprostol is a synthetic prostaglandin analog. Currently, misoprostol is most commonly used for medical termination in the first as well as in the second trimesters of pregnancy. It ***stimulates myometrial receptors to cause strong myometrial contractions***. It also ***causes cervical softening and dilatation***. As a result, there is expulsion of the products of conception. In the first trimester, it may be used either alone or in combination with other drugs like mifepristone (600 mg) or methotrexate (50 mg/m^2). Standard drug regimen includes 600 mg mifepristone on day 1 followed by oral misoprostol 400 mg on day 3. Efficacy of this regimen is up to 95% when used with gestation ≤ 49 days. In 50% cases, expulsion occurs within 4–5 hours of misoprostol intake. Other evidence-based regimen had shown that **lower dose mifepristone** (200 mg) and **higher dose misoprostol** (800 mg vaginal or sublingual) increases the efficacy of abortion (95%) up to 63 days of pregnancy.

For **second trimester pregnancy termination** the commonly used regimen is misoprostol 400 μg intravaginally every 6 hours. ***Vaginal route misoprostol is more effective than oral administration***. When used in the second trimester, success rate of vaginal misoprostol is 86% within 24 hours.

Misoprostol has been highly effective and safe in many clinical trials for medical termination of pregnancy (MTP). It is acceptable and highly effective, and privacy is maintained.

The **common side effects** are: Vaginal bleeding, cramping abdominal pain and nausea. The woman should be counseled and explained of the side effects. She should be assured of medical help in case of any emergency. **Complications** of misoprostol induced abortion are rare (0.5%). Incomplete abortion occurs in 3% of cases. This can be managed by giving additional misoprostol or by suction curettage. Risk of endometritis is rare (0.09%). The maternal death rates remain 1 woman per 10,000 use.

Benefits of misoprostol compared to surgical methods: No risk of injury to cervix, uterine perforation, anesthetic reaction, hemorrhage, infection (endometritis), Asherman's syndrome, infertility, chronic PID or psychological problems.

Considering all the safety, efficacy and benefits, misoprostol has almost replaced the other methods for termination of pregnancy.

SECTION 8

Intrapartum Electronic Fetal Monitoring

Section Outline

Ch. 66. Fetal Response in Labor
Ch. 67. Fetal Heart Rate Patterns
Ch. 68. Fetal ECG
Ch. 69. Management of Nonreassuring Fetal Status (NRFS)

66
Fetal Response in Labor

Labor is a stressful event. The goal of intrapartum fetal monitoring (IFM) is to detect hypoxia in labor and to initiate management depending upon the severity of hypoxia. ***Severe hypoxia in labor when associated with metabolic acidosis can cause fetal organ damage or even fetal death.***

During labor, there are uterine contractions. In between contractions, the intraluminal pressure within the spiral artery (85 mm Hg) is higher than the intramyometrial pressure (10 mm Hg) and this maintains the uteroplacental blood flow. During peak uterine contractions myometrial pressure (120 mm Hg) exceeds the arterial pressure (90 mm Hg) causing temporary halting of O_2 delivery to the fetus through the placenta. Depending upon the intensity and duration of uterine contractions, fetal hypoxia may develop.

Fetus is under stress even during the course of a normal labor
The reasons are:
- Temporary halting of uteroplacental circulation during uterine contractions
- Fetal head compressions affecting the functions of the vital centers.

A healthy fetus can withstand the stress of labor within the physiological limits. But fetal distress may appear when the labor is abnormal or the fetus is already compromised. Therefore, there may be non-reassuring fetal status when labor events are abnormal to cause fetal hypoxia and acidemia.

Fetoplacental circulation: The deoxygenated fetal blood is transported via umbilical arteries to the placenta. After placental gas exchange, the oxygenated blood is transported back to the fetus via the umbilical vein. The most oxygenated blood is delivered to the cardiac muscle and the brain.

Grades of fetal hypoxia (oxygen deficiency): Hypoxemia is the initial phase of oxygen deficiency. There is fall in O_2 saturation in arterial blood. However, the cell and the organ functions remain intact.

During this phase of organ oxygen deprivation, fetus develops some defense mechanism for survival. It depends upon the severity of hypoxia.
- Fetal tissues try to extract more oxygen from blood.
- Fetus tries to reduce oxygen requirement by reducing non-essential activities (reduced fetal movements).
- Continued hypoxemia for days together leads to fetal growth restriction.
- With progressive severity of hypoxia—the defense mechanism becomes more forceful to maintain the energy balance.
- There is release of stress hormones—catecholamines and the corticosteroids. In the presence of reduced oxygen to the peripheral tissues, there is redistribution of blood flow. Anaerobic metabolism is initiated in the peripheral tissues.

- The fetus can manage the situation for several hours.
- Asphyxia as it develops ultimately, glycogen reserve in the heart and liver is used for energy production. Anaerobic metabolism sets in redistribution of blood becomes more pronounced. There is rise in the serum levels of K^+ and lactate (acidemia).
- When fetal defense mechanism reaches its final stage the system collapses. There is failure of all vital organs (heart, brain) functions.

Q. How is the fetal defense response during the phase of hypoxia?

Ans.
- **Full fetal defense:** As long as the fetus is healthy (low risk of asphyxial damage), fetal defense mechanisms are intact. In such a situation, the characteristic CTG and ECG signs of fetal distress are observed. The fetus is capable of responding to hypoxic stressfully.
  - **Reduced fetal defense:** With progressive severity of hypoxia, the situation becomes worse. The defense mechanisms are reduced. The fetal response is blunted due to progressively diminished reserve. The signs of distress may not be characteristic. The fetus is in a state of reduced compensation.
  - **Absent fetal defense:** There is high risk of asphyxial damage, fetal defense is lacking. The signs of fetal distress are uncharacteristic. The fetus is in decompensated state.

67. Fetal Heart Rate Patterns

FETAL HEART VARIABILITY

Normal variability suggests normal fetal cardiac response to an intact and active central nervous system (CNS). The differences in beat-to-beat in the fetal heart rate (FHR) are mainly with the control of sympathetic and parasympathetic nerve input. The parasympathetic (vagus) has the dominant control over the cardiac behavior. The earlier concept of short- and long-term variability has no significance in terms of fetal behavior (NICHD 1997).

Normal and increased variability indicates a healthy fetus. However, reduced variability may be due to several other reasons (see below), though fetal hypoxia and acidosis are the important ones. Severe hypoxia resulting in metabolic acidosis depresses the CNS. This is reflected with the reduced variability. Therefore, reduced variability must be interpreted with caution as several other factors need to be carefully analyzed including the clinical scenario (Fig. 67.1).

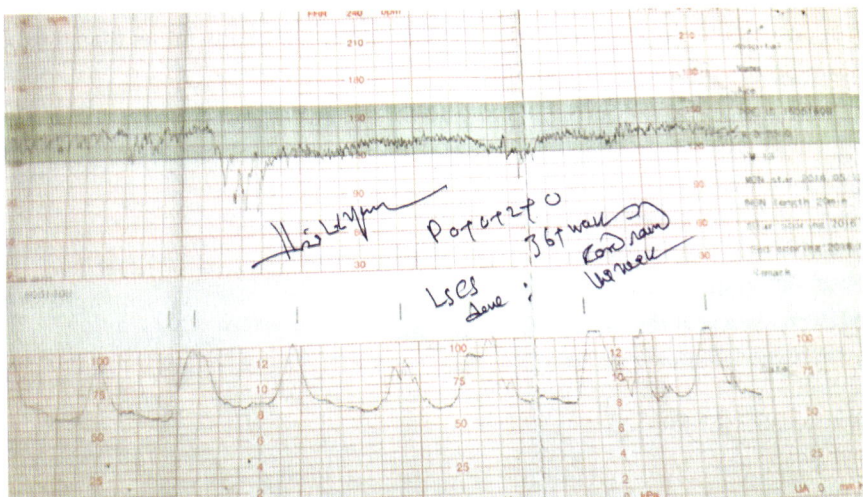

Fig. 67.1: 32-year-old lady (P0+0+2+0), at 36 weeks was in labor with meconium stained liquor. CTG revealed: 1) Baseline FHR: 130 bpm; 2) Baseline variability: ≤5; 3) Acceleration: absent; 4) Deceleration present. Trace pattern was: Pathological/category III. Cesarean delivery was done, baby girl was born, weighing 2.6 kg with Apgar score: 4–6 and 10 at 0–5 and 10 minutes time. Baby had tight cord round the neck

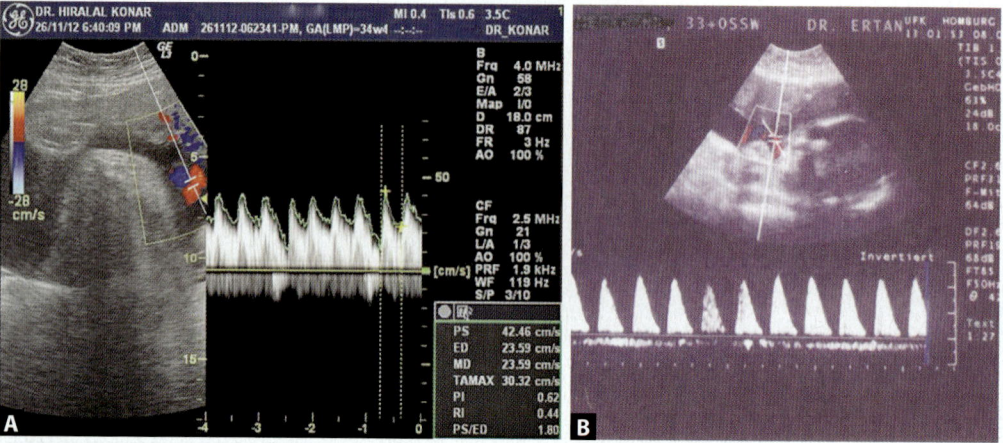

Figs 67.2A and B: A. Doppler evaluation of the umbilical artery. Pulse Doppler study revealed normal diastolic flow velocity waveform, **B.** Pulse Doppler showing absent diastolic flow velocity waveform

Cord compression results in compression of the umbilical vein first as it has a thin wall. There is fetal hypotension due to decreased blood flow return to the heart. There may be fetal tachycardia to maintain cardiac output. With progressive increase in compression effects, the arteries are occluded (Figs 67.2A and B). Cord blood flow interruption causes retention of CO_2 and cessation of O_2 delivery. With time, there is retention of CO_2 and fetus develops respiratory acidosis. With longer duration of cord compression, there is insufficient supply of oxygen and metabolic acidosis also develops. Thus, fetal acidosis due to cord compression is either respiratory or combined respiratory and metabolic.

The onset of variable deceleration is often abrupt and sharp. Variable deceleration is mainly a reflex response to the changes in pressure due to cord compression rather than hypoxia.

Pathophysiology of diminished variability

Hypoxia → stress response → acidosis → depressed brain function → reduced variability. Otherwise, normal variability indicates normal brain function and absence of severe hypoxia and acidosis.

Types of FHR variability
- **Absent:** No detectable amplitude of variability.
- **Minimal:** Amplitude detectable but < 5 bpm.
- **Marked:** Amplitude > 25 bpm.

Causes of decreased variability of FHR
- CNS depression: Hypoxia and acidosis
- Fetal sleep
- Fetal anomalies (CNS)
- Tachycardia
- Prematurity
- Fetal heart block (SLE)
- Drugs to mother
    - Pethidine, antihypertensives (β-blocker, methyldopa), tranquilizers, $MgSO_4$
    - General anesthesia.

Decelerations

Early deceleration: Fetal heart rate does not descend more than 30–40 beats/minute below the baseline. It is due to compression of the fetal head by the lower uterine segment or the cervix. They do not indicate fetal hypoxia.

Variable deceleration: It is due to the interruption of blood flow within the umbilical cord (umbilical cord compression). It is variable in size, shape, depth, duration and timing in relation to uterine contractions (Box 67.1).

Box 67.1: Classification of the severity of variable Decelerations (Kubli 1969)

Mild deceleration	Duration < 30 seconds and or depth not <80 bpm
Moderate deceleration	Depth < 80 bpm
Severe deceleration	Depth < 70 bpm and/or duration > 60 seconds

It is usually preceded and followed by accelerations. This is due to the reflex response of fetal systemic blood pressure changes. Variable decelerations may occur without fetal hypoxia.

Causes of variable deceleration: Cord compression due to (a) Oligohydramnios, (b) Nuchal cord (resulting in stretching of the cord with progressive head descent), (c) Cord abnormalities, e.g. short cord, true knots and (d) cord prolapse.

Late decelerations: In majority of the situations, the onset, nadir and the recovery of decelerations occur after the start, peak and end of the uterine contractions, respectively. FHR may go below the baseline by 30 to 40 bpm or more. Late decelerations are caused by uteroplacental insufficiency. There is slowing down of uteroplacental blood flow along with uterine contractions. The fetus becomes hypoxic when the placental insufficiency is sufficient enough to cause decreased tissue perfusion. Persistent hypoxia with severity causes fetal myocardial hypoxic damage. When the fetus becomes sufficiently hypoxic, metabolic acidosis develops.

Prolonged decelerations lasting 90–120 seconds or more are of severe and persistent in nature. Prolonged decelerations (due to severe hypoxia). Severity of hypoxia depends on the depth, duration, loss of variability during and after the deceleration.

Common causes are: Uterine hyperstimulation, hypotension and hypoperfusion following regional anesthesia, placental abruption, cord prolapse or eclamptic convulsions.

Accelerations

Accelerations are the transient increase in FHR lasing at least 15 seconds and rising ≥ 15 beats above the baseline. Acceleration lasting > 10 minutes are considered as the change in baseline. Presence of an acceleration indicates a healthy and well-oxygenated fetus. However, absence of acceleration does not always mean the fetus is hypoxic. Presence of spontaneous accelerations or accelerations induced by stimulation of fetal scalp or accelerations following other artificial stimulation measures indicates fetal pH > 7.20.

Sinusoidal patterns

Sinusoidal patterns are characterized by
- Stable baseline FHR (110 to 160 bpm with regular sine wave-like oscillations)
- Amplitude between 5 and 15 bpm

- Fixed or absent short-term variability
- Oscillations of sine wave above and below the baseline
- Absence of accelerations.

Sinusoidal patterns are seen in cases with fetal hypoxia and acidosis mostly due to fetal anemia. This pattern when seen following maternal narcotic therapy is called pseudosinusoidal pattern as the fetus is well-oxygenated and is nonanemic.

Q. *How the CTG traces are categorized?*
Ans. *Based on four features:*
    a. Baseline FHR
    b. Variability
    c. Decelerations
    d. Accelerations.

All the CTG traces are categorized into:
A. *According to RCOG and NICE:*
- Normal
- Suspicious
- Pathological.

B. *According to NICHD and AJOG:*
- *Category I*
- *Category II*
- *Category III:* (*See* Dutta's Textbook of Obstetrics, 8th Edition, p. 693, 694 and Manual of Obstetrics and Gynecology for the Postgraduates, p. 17).

68. Fetal ECG

Q. What are the limitations of cardiotocography (CTG)?
Ans. There are wide variations in CTG interpretation and also there is uncertainty about the clinical value of CTG. There is also lack of clarity in terminology, nomenclature and data-interpretation. It has been observed that CTG is good to identify a healthy fetus but unable to provide diagnostic information when there is fetal hypoxia.

Q. What is studied in fetal ECG?
Ans. ST segment analysis (STAN) of fetal ECG can reflect the function of the fetal myocardium during stress of labor. It is important to recognize that fetal heart and brain are equally sensitive or insensitive to oxygen deficiency. With this, myocardial behavior provides an indirect assessment of the condition of the fetal brain during labor (Fig. 68.1).

Q. What is the basic difference in recording of CTG and ECG?
Ans. CTG records the RR interval of the ECG. The STAN system combines RR interval measurements with the changes in the ST interval. The ratio between the amplitude of

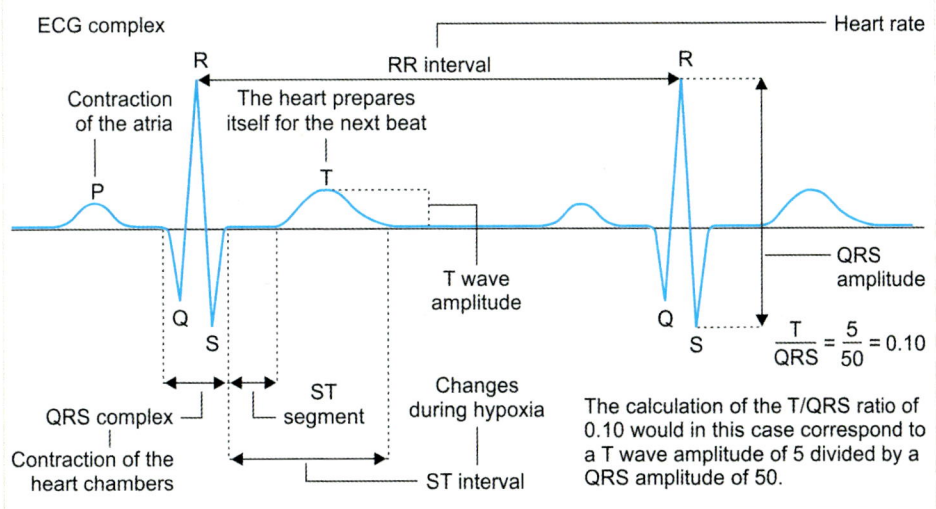

Fig. 68.1: Fetal ECG complex

the T wave and the QRS amplitude (the T/QRS ratio) gives an accurate measurement of the changes in T wave amplitude. In adult cardiology, ST analysis is done to assess myocardial insufficiency.

Generally, an average ECG waveform is created from 30 accepted ECG complexes. From this, an average ECG, a T/QRS calculation and ST segment analysis are done.

Q. What are the specific changes in the ECG during hypoxia?
Ans. During hypoxia, the myocardium adapts to the hypoxia situation. Glycogenolysis and anerobic metabolism are initiated. As the rate of glycogenolysis increases, the T wave amplitude rises. There may be biphasic patterns of the ST segments.

Q. How the ST changes are observed?
Ans. During the course of a normal labor, the fetus displays a fairly stable T/QRS ratio. There is no marked ST elevation and no biphasic STs. Absence of significant ST events indicates that the fetus is well control of the situation.

The change in ST segment or the T/QRS rise may be episodic (< 10 minutes) or it may be a baseline T/QRS rise. A baseline T/QRS rise indicates fetal response to hypoxia with anerobic metabolism.

Q. How STAN system is important in clinical management?
Ans. STAN system provides continuous information about the ability of the fetus to respond to the stress of labor.
However, the specific information should be used together with CTG.
- Generally, a normal reassuring (reactive) CTG indicates a healthy fetus in labor.
- In presence of CTG abnormality, ST waveform is analyzed to have more information about the severity of the stress.
- Based on the combined evaluation of CTG and ST analysis (ECG) clinical management action is developed.

Q. What are the main concerns with CTG?
Ans. A large number of fetuses show changes in the fetal heart rate without being asphyxiated. This has caused an increased rate of unnecessary intervention (cesarean delivery) and concern is the uncertainty about the clinical value of CTG.

Q. What are the benefits of fetal ECG (STAN) in intrapartum surveillance?
Ans. Compared to CTG alone, ST analysis is cost effective in terms of lowering the rate of fetal acidosis and reducing cesarean delivery, when used in term high-risk deliveries.

69 Management of Nonreassuring Fetal Status (NRFS)

FHR PATTERN AND INTERPRETATIONS (NICHD-2008, ACOG-2009)

Interpretations of fetal heart rate (FHR) patterns are difficult. Detection of fetal hypoxia, acidosis and correlation with neonatal hypoxia are often poor with the use of electronic fetal monitoring (EFM). However, according to NICHD (2008) FHR patterns are classified into three categories:
1. **Category I:** Reassuring pattern—fetus is normally oxygenated and baby is born with normal pH and Apgar score)
2. **Category II:** Nonreassuring fetal status (NFRS) (baby is more often normal)
3. **Category III:** NFRS and it is often associated with fetal acidosis. These fetuses need further evaluation.

MANAGEMENT OF NRFS (NICHD CATEGORIES II AND III)

The management of NRFS is to detect the cause of hypoxia or acidosis. The underlying pathology is to be detected and goal is to reverse the pathology whenever possible. Initial approaches are to organize the measures that help to deliver maximum oxygen to the fetus and improve the placental perfusion.

Medical Management (Noninvasive Measures)
- **Left lateral positioning** of the woman to avoid aortocaval compression. This is expected to improve cardiac return, cardiac output and ultimately uterine perfusion.
- **Oxygen administration** by face mask can improve oxygen delivery to the fetus through the placental circulation.
- **Maternal hydration** with IV fluids and to increase intravascular volume is to be done. Most women in labor are not allowed to drink fluids for the fear of surgical risks. Optimum hydration improves uteroplacental perfusion.
- To stop **oxytocin infusion** or to decrease it, when the FHR is nonreassuring pattern. It may be restarted once the reassuring pattern is established. However, the patient needs continued monitoring.
- **Tocolytic drugs** may be used when the contractions are excessive to cause NRFS or persistent decelerations. Commonly terbutaline 0.25 mg SC is used.
- **Amnioinfusion** is done in cases with oligohydramnios, premature rupture of membranes (PROM) and meconium stained liquor.

Advantages of amnioinfusion are:
- It increases the liquor volume
- Dilutes the meconium by increasing the liquor volume
- Minimizes fetal gasping (by reducing cord compression) effort.

Disadvantages of amnioinfusion are:
Evidences (Cochrane database 2010) do not support the benefits of reduced risk of meconium aspiration or any reduction in perinatal death following amnioinfusion.

Meconium: Passage of meconium is often due to hypoxia. Hypoxia causes increased vagal response in the fetus. It is manifested with excessive gut movements, relaxation of anal sphincter and passage of meconium. Passage of meconium may be in the absence of hypoxia again. But meconium is not only a potential sign of fetal hypoxia but also a toxin when the fetus aspirates it. Thick meconium indicates oligohydramnios. Oligohydramnios → cord compression → vagal response → increased gut motility → passage of meconium. Prolonged hypoxia leads to fetal gasping and aspiration of meconium.

Presence of reassuring FHR tracing in cases with meconium stained liquor can be managed expectantly. But presence of thick meconium, oligohydramnios and nonreassuring FHR pattern mandates urgent delivery.

EVALUATION AND MANAGEMENT OF A FETUS WITH NONREASSURING PATTERNS

- ***Fetal scalp pH:*** pH > 7.25—reassuring, pH between 7.20 and 7.25 is borderline and it needs to be repeated immediately and pH < 7.20 indicates fetal acidosis and urgent delivery.
- ***Fetal CTG*** (*See* Manual of Obstetrics and Gynecology for the Postgraduates, p. 227, 437, 509).
- ***Fetal ECG*** analysis, is done using computerized interpretations to detect changes in the ST segment. ST waveform changes indicate fetal metabolic acidosis.
  Fetal pulse oximetry initially was used to determine fetal oxyhemoglobin saturation in labor. But currently its accuracy in predicting fetal hypoxia has not been established.
- ***Computerized interpretation:*** Limitation of FHR monitoring using electronic modes (CTG and ECG) are due to lack of agreement in terminology and interpretation of records (FHR patterns). Intraobserver and interobserver variations are there. **The computer-based interpretation of FHR** patterns are found to be more accurate. This can predict fetal acidosis more accurately.

Interventions for NRFS (NICHD-2008)
Category I: Absence of hypoxia → no intervention.
Category III: Fetal metabolic acidosis → immediate evaluation and nonsurgical management → if no improvement → delivery (operative vaginal/cesarean delivery).
Category II: (a) Evaluation of fetal status, (b) Continued surveillance, (c) Re-evaluation including the clinical scenarios.

Management of this group is difficult. Some fetuses with category II may not have any hypoxia or acidosis. Whereas other fetuses may be hypoxic and/or acidotic.

Interpretation of the results of continued fetal surveillance is important. Moreover, integration of the fetal surveillance reports with the clinical scenario of the mother [pregnancy-induced hypertension (PIH)] and the fetus [fetal growth restriction (FGR)] should always be done. Time for intervention is a question of judgement with experience.

In the event of a persistent nonreassuring FHR, operative intervention is appropriate.

Unpredictability of NRFS is a known limitation and the medicological pressure of present day medical practice must be kept in mind.

Confusing pattern of EFM are those that does not fit into any one of the categories defined previously. Obstetrics emergencies like—abruptio placenta, cord prolapse, uterine scar dehiscence, persistent cord compression mandates expeditious delivery.

- **Operative interventions for NRFS: Interventions for nonreassuring fetal status**
   Indications
    - FHR pattern—persistently nonreassuring.
    - EFM, scalp blood pH, ST analysis can not assure that the fetus is nonacidotic.
    - When the fetus needs to be delivered expeditiously.

Category II: Majority (80%) of the laboring women belong to this group. EFM is most, reliable with category I (normal) and category III (acidotic). It is most unreliable when equivocal (category II).

Mode of operative delivery may be: (A) Operative vaginal delivery, (B) Cesarean section.

Decisions are made on the assessment of:
- Stage of labor process and the ease and safety of vaginal operative or instrumental delivery.
- Time interval (onset of NRFS to delivery) required to deliver the baby.
- Severity of fetal acidosis, clinician's skill and available resources (theater availability).

Delivery should preferably be done within 30 minutes of decision to deliver.

SECTION 9

Perinatal Medicine

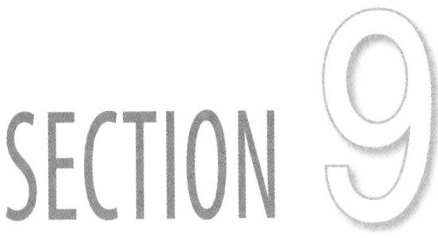

Section Outline

- Ch. 70. Immunization during Pregnancy and Breastfeeding
- Ch. 71. Noninvasive Prenatal Testing for Fetal Chromosomal Abnormality
- Ch. 72. Congenital Perinatal and Neonatal Infections
- Ch. 73. Congenital HIV Infection and AIDS
- Ch. 74. Varicella Zoster Virus (Chickenpox) Infection
- Ch. 75. Rubella in Pregnancy
- Ch. 76. Cytomegalovirus Infection in Pregnancy
- Ch. 77. Viral Hepatitis in Pregnancy
- Ch. 78. Listeriosis in Pregnancy
- Ch. 79. Toxoplasmosis in Pregnancy
- Ch. 80. Group B Streptococci Infection in Pregnancy

70 Immunization during Pregnancy and Breastfeeding

Q. What are the benefits of immunization in pregnancy and postpartum?
Ans. *Immunization in pregnancy*
- Protects the mother from infections
- Protects the fetus, neonate and the infant from infection. This is achieved through placental transfer of antibodies.

Vaccination during the postpartum period
- Protects the mother from vaccine preventable diseases. This also protects the infant indirectly by preventing maternal infection. Ideally women should have all vaccination covered before pregnancy.
- Breastfeeding protects the neonate/infant by supplying antibodies (secretory IgA).

Preconception clinic counseling is another area where immunization records are verified and updated.

However in our country, pregnancy gives us a scope for complete immunization for many women that they have missed it.

Guidelines for vaccination during pregnancy and breastfeeding (ACIP 2000).

Precaution for vaccination[1]

Conditions are:
- Risks of serious adverse reaction due to vaccination may be a problem.
- Ability of the vaccine to produce immunity may be compromised.
- Safety of vaccine given is unknown.
  In such situations, vaccination is deferred during pregnancy. However, vaccination may have to be considered when benefits outweigh the risks.
- **Contraindications:** When vaccination is known to cause serious maternal, fetal or neonatal adverse effects as based on evidence.
  No vaccine should be given when a contraindication is present.

Q. What are the different types of immunizations?
Ans. **A. *Active immunization:*** Depending upon the type of antigen used.
Vaccine may be—(a) Live or live attenuated; (b) killed or inactivated.
Live or live attenuated vaccines have the risks of fetal damage due to maternal viremia.
Killed or inactivated vaccines can be recommended in pregnancy.
Vaccines used are: Tetanus-diphtheria (TD) and influenza.

B. **Passive immunization:** Immunoglobulin therapy.
   Post exposure prophylaxis in cases:
Varicella zoster immune globulin (VZIG) is given to exposed nonimmune subject to reduce the morbidity. Similarly, it is given in cases with: hepatitis A and B, measles or tetanus.

Q. What are the differences between live and killed vaccines?
Ans.

Live vaccines	Killed vaccines
▪ Only a single booster dose is needed	▪ Multiple booster doses are needed
▪ Less stable	▪ More stable
▪ Humoral and cell-mediated immunity	▪ Mainly humoral immunity
▪ May revert to the virulent form	▪ Cannot revert to a virulent form
▪ Small dose needed	▪ Large dose needed

Q. Is breastfeeding a contraindication for vaccination?
Ans. Breastfeeding is not a contraindication for most of the available vaccines. Vaccinia (smallpox) virus is contraindicated as there is risk of transmission of vaccinia from mother to child through breast milk.

Q. What are the different vaccines recommended in pregnancy and breastfeeding?
Ans. Vaccines recommended in pregnancy are:[1]

Vaccine	Type
▪ Influenza	▪ Inactivated
▪ Pneumococcus	▪ Inactivated
▪ Meningococcus (polysaccharide)	▪ Inactivated
▪ Tetatus-diphtheria	▪ Inactivated

Q. What are the different vaccines that can be given with precaution?
Ans. Vaccines can be given with precaution are:
- Poliomyelitis (Salk) live attenuated—vaccine when needed for immediate protection.
- Yellow fever—live attenuated (when travel to a susceptible area is unavoidable).
- Rabies (live attenuated)
- Hepatitis A (inactivated)
- Hepatitis B (recombinant inactivated)
- Typhoid
- Pertussis (inactivated): It is given in combination with tetanus-diphtheria (TD) and
- Japanese encephalitis (inactivated).

Q. What are the vaccines contraindicated in pregnancy?
Ans. Live or live attenuated vaccines are contraindicated in pregnancy.
Vaccines that are contraindicated during pregnancy are:
- BCG vaccine
- Mumps vaccine
- Measles vaccine
- Rubella vaccine

- Varicella vaccine
- Human papillomavirus vaccine.
- Vaccinia vaccine

Q. What are the vaccines preferably to be avoided during pregnancy?

Ans. Inactivated polio vaccine (IPV), yellow fever and rabies vaccines under normal circumstances should be deferred. However, when the benefits outweigh the risks such as unavoidable travel during pregnancy to areas where risks of infection are high for yellow fever or post exposure prophylaxis after possible exposure for rabies, vaccines should be given. Generally, women should be advised not become pregnant within at least 1 month of vaccination.

Q. Are these varicella, and MMR vaccines contraindicated during breastfeeding?

Ans. The vaccines mentioned above, varicella, measles, mumps and rubella (MMR) can be used. Breastfeeding is not a contraindication or caution to vaccination for these two (varicella and MMR).

However, vaccinia (smallpox) is contraindicated both for pregnancy and breastfeeding.

Q. What are the risks when these vaccines are used in pregnancy inadvertently?

Ans. Inadvertent use of vaccinia virus during pregnancy and breastfeeding has been reported to cause fetal and neonatal infections. However, this is not the case for the other vaccine (varicella). No fetal or neonatal diseases have been reported till date with the use of the other vaccination. This is also not an indication for termination of pregnancy.

Ideally pregnancy should be avoided until 28 days after vaccination.

Q. What are the vaccines specially indicated in pregnancy?

Ans.
- Inactivated influenza vaccine
- Inactivated polio vaccine
- Tetanus toxoid.
- Pertussis (whooping cough) vaccine
- Diphtheria toxoid

Q. What are the vaccines recommended in pregnancy in certain situations?

Ans.
- Hepatitis A vaccine
- Meningococcus vaccine
- Rabies vaccine
- Yellow fever vaccine.
- Hepatitis B vaccine
- Pneumococcal vaccine
- Typhoid vaccine

Q. What is the current situation of human papillomavirus (HPV) vaccines for its use during pregnancy?

Ans. Currently, HPV vaccine is not recommended during pregnancy due to lack of its safety data. However, till date no adverse effect has been reported.

Q. Justifiable use of vaccines (when indicated): FDA category C

Ans.
- The following vaccines in the category C are: (a) Diphtheria, (b) Tetanus, (c) Hepatitis A, (d) Hepatitis B, (e) Influenza, (f) Immunoglobulin, (g) Inactivated polio vaccine, (h) Tuberculin test.
- The following vaccines are rarely justified.
  Live vaccines: (a) MMR, (b) Sabin polio vaccine (oral), (c) Varicella.

Q. What are the vaccines that can be used during breastfeeding?

Ans. The following vaccines are justified when indicated:

▪ HPV	▪ Hepatitis A	▪ Hepatitis B
▪ Influenza	▪ MMR	▪ Diphtheria
▪ Tetanus	▪ Varicella	▪ Pneumococcal
▪ Meningococcal	▪ Polio	▪ Rabies
▪ Typhoid	▪ Tuberculin PPD	▪ BCG

Yellow fever vaccine should be avoided unless the infant is in significant high risk of exposure.

MCQs

Q.1 Regarding immunization during pregnancy:
  a. Immunization is contraindicated during pregnancy.
  b. Active immunization during pregnancy is safe.
  c. All inactivated vaccines are to be avoided.
  d. Vaccination should ideally be done prior to pregnancy.
Ans. a. = F; b. = F; c. = F; d. = T

Q.2 Following vaccines are contraindicated during pregnancy:
  a. Pneumococcus
  b. Pertussis
  c. Varicella
  d. Yellow fever
  e. Japanese encephalitis.
Ans. a. = F; b. = F; c. = T; d. = F; e. = F

Q.3 Following vaccines are contraindicated both during pregnancy and breastfeeding:
  a. Varicella
  b. Measles, mumps and rubella
  c. Vaccinia (smallpox)
  d. Human papillomavirus
  e. Japanese encephalitis.
Ans. a. = F; b. = F; c. = T; d. = F; e. = F
  a and b. are contraindicated during pregnancy but not a contraindication or precaution during breastfeeding.
  d. It is not recommended during pregnancy due to lack of safety data but it can be used during breastfeeding.
  e. It can used during pregnancy with caution when travel to susceptible area is unavoidable. Its use during breastfeeding is with caution due to lack of safety data.

Reference

1. Advisory Committee on Immunization Practices Centers for Disease Control and Prevention (CDC). Guiding principles for development of ACIP recommendations for vaccination during pregnancy and breastfeeding. MMWR Morb Mortal Wkly Rep. 2008;57(21):580.

71 Noninvasive Prenatal Testing for Fetal Chromosomal Abnormality

Q. What is the clinical relevance of noninvasive prenatal testing?

Ans. Many biochemical analytes are used for screening of fetal chromosomal abnormality. Despite combined test procedures, the test accuracy is low. Invasive procedures for aneuploidy diagnosis include: chorionic villus sampling (CVS), amniocentesis or cordocentesis. Each of these diagnostic procedures has got a small but significant risk of pregnancy loss.

Improved testing with accuracy for fetal aneuploidy such as PCR, fluorescence *in situ* hybridization (FISH), microarray comparative genomic hybridization (CGH) and fetal whole genome sequencing using massively parallel sequencing (MPS) are found promising.

Cell-free fetal DNA (cffDNA) obtained from pregnant woman's plasma is a noninvasive testing. It offers a tremendous potential as a screening tool for fetal aneuploidy.

Q. What is the principle behind this test?

Ans. cffDNA can be detected in the maternal blood since the first trimester of pregnancy. Therefore, it is a reliable source of material for noninvasive method of prenatal testing.[1]

Q. What difficulties are faced for detection of cffDNA?

Ans. In maternal plasma cffDNA is mixed up with a large proportion of maternal cell-free DNA. This created confusion in identifying cffDNA.[2]

Q. How this was overcome?

Ans. Initially detection of paternally inherited fetal DNA sequences that are not present in mother (Y chromosome sequences with a male fetus) or rhesus D (RhD) sequences in women who are Rh-negative had been done.

Recent introduction of DNA sequencing technologies has allowed very precise relative quantification of DNA fragments. This can detect the extrachromosomal material for fetal trisomy within the maternal plasma DNA.

The newer technology of massive parallel sequencing (MPS) allows virtually all DNA molecules in the plasma sample to be analyzed.

Genotype of the fetus can be determined from maternal plasma by noninvasive prenatal testing (NIPT).[3,4]

Q. How testing of cffDNA is helpful?

Ans.
- cffDNA is thought to be derived primarily from the placenta.
- Circulating levels of cffDNA comprise about 3–13% of the total cell-free DNA in maternal plasma.

- cffDNA is cleared from the maternal blood within hours after the childbirth.
- cffDNA analysis is now clinically available for testing fetal aneuploidy with the help of MPS.
- Although cffDNA test is not a diagnostic test, it has high sensitivity and specificity.

Q. Could there be any possible source of error in testing?
Ans. The amount of cffDNA in maternal blood increases with gestational age. Blood samples taken too early in pregnancy may result in false-negative report.

Q. When should ideally the NIPT for aneuploidy be done?
Ans. Currently, it is suggested to do testing only when the fetal DNA percentage in maternal plasma is at least 4–5%. The commercially available aneuploidy tests based on MPS are generally done from 10 weeks of pregnancy. However, a pregnancy dating scan to establish the gestational age is required. Tests based on MPS are generally used for aneuploidy testing.

Q. What are the other reasons for the possible sources of error?
Ans.
- **Maternal obesity:** Increased maternal weight is associated with lower fetal DNA percentage in maternal blood.
- **Multiple pregnancies:**
  - *Monochorionic twins (monozygotic)*
    - Both the fetuses will be affected or unaffected.
    - The amount of cffDNA is almost double compared to a singleton pregnancy. Hence, the testing for aneuploidy will be more effective.
  - *Dichorionic twins:* Shotgun sequencing-based approaches are done. It is dependent upon the availability of sufficient DNA from each fetus to yield a valid test result. Because of several reasons, the use of NIPT in twin pregnancies is still at a very early stage of development.
- **Placental mosaicism:** The source of cffDNA is the placenta. 'Confined placental mosaicism' has been observed from the results of CVS where abnormal cell lines are present in the placenta but not in the fetus. This is observed in approximately 1% of CVS procedures. This necessitates an invasive procedures for confirmation, before the decision for pregnancy termination is made.
- **Maternal conditions:** Maternal chromosomal abnormalities including mosaicism or malignant disease may be the rare cause of discordant reports.

Q. What is the current status of cffDNA testing when compared with the existing current procedures (karyotyping/microarray)?
Ans.
- Invasive procedures (CVS, amniocentesis) and karyotyping provide information about all the 46 chromosomes. Invasive procedures carry the risks also.
  In NIPT, DNA sequencing should also target all the 46 chromosomes.
- It is not yet resolved whether tests for chromosome 21 with PCR or FISH alone or combined with karyotyping is accurate. Microarray CGH and shotgun massively parallel sequencing (MPS) use of all DNA molecules are coming up with more information. However, each method has its own advantages and disadvantages.

Q. Who are the women, they should be offered NIPT?
Ans. Currently, it is not recommended as a part of routine prenatal testing. Moreover, it is not recommended to low-risk women. It is also not recommended to women with multiple gestations.[5]

Q. What would be the pretest counseling for a woman about the NIPT results?
Ans.
- Woman following a negative cffDNA test result should be counseled that the test result does not ensure an unaffected pregnancy (ACOG 2012).
- A woman with a positive test result should be referred for genetic counseling and should be offered invasive prenatal diagnosis for confirmation of test results (ACOG 2012).

Q. What is MPS (MPGS)?
Ans. It is a newer DNA sequencing technology known as **massively parallel genomic sequencing (MPGS)** which is a highly sensitive assay to quantify millions of DNA fragments from maternal plasma (biological samples) in a span of days. MPGS can detect accurately trisomy 13, trisomy 18 and trisomy 21 as early as the 10th week of pregnancy.[6]

The test results are available approximately 1 week after the maternal sample is taken.

Q. How much accuracy the test carries?
Ans. This test has high sensitivity and specificity. So far reported (several large studies), detection rates for fetal trisomy 13, trisomy 18 and trisomy 21 are of greater than 98% with a very low false-positive rates (<0.5%). cffDNA testing appears to be the most effective screening test for aneuploidy in high-risk women.

Q. What are the prerequisites before offering a woman with NIPT?
Ans.
- A baseline ultrasound examination to confirm—viability, gestational dating, singleton gestation and to rule out fetal structural anomalies.
- Referral for genetic counseling when test results are positive (see above).
- Discussion with the woman when the test results are negative (see above).

Q. Mention the indication for cffDNA testing (ACOG 2012)?
Ans.
- Maternal age ≥35 years at delivery
- Fetal USG findings suggesting an increased risk of aneuploidy
- History of a prior pregnancy with trisomy
- Positive test result for aneuploidy, including first trimester, sequential or integrated screen or a quadruple screen
- Parenteral balanced Robertsonian translocation with increased risk of fetal trisomy 13 or trisomy 21.[7,8]

Q. What other conditions the cffDNA testing could be used besides detecting chromosomal abnormality?
Ans.
- Fetal RhD typing to determine fetal blood group status from maternal blood. This is essential while managing a woman (RhD negative) for the problem of hemolytic disease of the fetus and newborn (HDFN) or with Rh alloimmunization problem.[3,9]
- Fetal sex identification in the management of X-linked disorders or single gene disorders.

Q. What is the opinion of cffDNA testing in the foreseeable future?
Ans.
- It appears that the need for prenatal cytogenetic procedures will gradually go down.
- Invasive procedures of prenatal diagnosis will be done in fewer cases.
- Prenatal genetic testing will gradually shift from cytogenetics to molecular genetics.
- Ultrasound scanning will be used for detecting nonchromosomal fetal anomalies.
- Fewer biochemical tests may be required.
- MPGS which uses a highly sensitive assay can quantity millions of DNA fragments in biological samples within few days. It can accurately detect trisomy 13, trisomy 18 and trisomy 21.[10]

References

1. Lo YM, Corbetta N, Chamberlain PF, et al. Presence of fetal DNA in maternal plasma and serum. Lancet. 1997;350(9076):485-7.
2. Lo YM, Zhang J, Leung TN, et al. Rapid clearance of fetal DNA from maternal plasma. Am J Hum Genet. 1999;64(1):218-24.
3. Illanes S, Soothill P. Management of red cell alloimmunization in pregnancy: the non-invasive monitoring of the disease. Prenat Diagn. 2010;30(7):668-73.
4. Devaney SA, Palomaki GE, Scott JA, et al. Noninvasive fetal sex determination using cell-free fetal DNA: a systematic review and meta-analysis. JAMA. 2011;306(6):627-36.
5. Guo X, Bayliss P, Damewood M, et al. A noninvasive test to determine paternity in pregnancy. N Engl J Med. 2012;366(18):1743-5.
6. Canick JA, Palomaki GE, Kloza EM, et al. The impact of maternal plasma DNA fetal fraction on next generation sequencing tests for common fetal aneuploidies. Prenat Diagn. 2013;33(7):667-74.
7. Stumm M, Entezami M, Trunk N, et al. Noninvasive prenatal detection of chromosomal aneuploidies using different next generation sequencing strategies and algorithms. Prenat Diagn. 2012;32:569-77.
8. RCOG. Noninvasive prenatal testing for chromosomal abnormality using maternal plasma DNA. Scientific Impact Paper No. 15. 2014.
9. American College of Obstetricians and Gynecologists Committee on Genetics. Committee Opinion No. 545: noninvasive prenatal testing for fetal aneuploidy. Obstet Gynecol. 2012;120(6):1532-4.
10. Palomaki GE, Deciu C, Kloza EM, et al. DNA sequencing of maternal plasma reliably identifies trisomy 18 and trisomy 13 as well as Down syndrome: an International Collaborative Study. Genet Med. 2012;14:296-305.

72. Congenital Perinatal and Neonatal Infections

Maternal and perinatal infections are the common complications during the peripartum period. It is an important cause of mortality and morbidity both for the neonates and the mother.

Q. What is understood by congenital perinatal and neonatal infections?

Ans. **Perinatal period**—extends from 24 weeks (in India 28 weeks) of gestation up to 6 completed days of the birth of the baby.

Neonatal period—extends from birth to 27 completed days. It may again be subdivided in early neonatal period (since birth to 6 completed days) and late neonatal period (from 7th day to 27th completed days).

There is considerable overlap between congenital perinatal and neonatal infections. Such infection account for about 5% of all stillbirth and 10.1% of all neonatal deaths.

Q. What are the different types of congenital infections?

Ans. Common congenital perinatal infections are given in Table 72.1.

Table 72.1: Congenital infections

Virus	Sexually transmitted infections	Bacterial and others
Rubella	Chlamydia	Group B streptococci (GBS)
Human immunodeficiency virus (HIV)	Gonorrhea	*Escherichia coli*
Cytomegalovirus (CMV)	Syphilis	Toxoplasma
Varicella zoster virus (VZV)		Listeria monocytogenes
Hepatitis viruses (HAV, HBV, HCV, HDV)		Malaria
Measles		
Parvovirus		
Influenza virus		

Q. What are the implications of congenital perinatal infections?

Ans. Some of infections are more serious in pregnancy than in the nonpregnant state specially due to vertical transmission. This results in significant perinatal morbidity and mortality.

Q. What are different modes of transmission of congenital perinatal and neonatal infections?

Ans. ■ Across the placenta: HIV, CMV, rubella, toxoplasma, listeria, malaria.

- Ascending maternal infection following prolonged rupture of membranes (PROM). This results in chorioamnionitis.
- Perinatal infection acquired during birth via the hematogenous or genital route. Infections are HIV, HZV, HBV and chlamydia.
- Perinatal infection transmitted via breastfeeding.

Parturition is a risk factor to the neonate due to contamination with maternal blood and genital tract secretions. Risk is high when there is prolonged or PROM.

Q. What are the special reasons for increased risk of congenital perinatal infections?

Ans.
- At birth infant's immune system remains immature.
- Transfer of maternal antibodies [immunoglobulin G (IgG)], protects the infant through transplacental passage.
- This process is less effective in the premature infant.
- Moreover, infection acquired by the mother close to the time of delivery, puts the infant at increased risk of severe disease. This is due to lack of time for the mother to develop protective antibody IgG.

73. Congenital HIV Infection and AIDS

Q. What are different modes of MTCT for human immunodeficiency virus (HIV)?
Ans.
- Overall mother to child transmission (MTCT) is 25–40%.
- Only 1.5–2% transplacental.
- Vast majority acquire infection during late pregnancy, parturition and breastfeeding (30–40%).

Q. How much is the risk of MTCT for HIV when correct interventions are done?
Ans. With appropriate interventions [highly active antiretroviral therapy (HAART), elective cesarean delivery and absence of breastfeeding], transmission rates can be reduced to less than 1%.

Q. What are the risk factor for increased rate of MTCT?
Ans.
- Father with high viral load
- Mother with AIDS
- Previous baby with HIV infection
- First born twin
- Preterm delivery
- Low maternal $CD4^+$ count
- Chorioamnionitis
- Premature rupture of membranes (PROM)
- Breastfeeding.

Q. What are the common presentations of the child born with HIV?
Ans. The child presents with the features of impaired cellular immune defense.
Common features are:
- Recurrent bacterial infections, meningitis, pneumonia
- Persistent oral candidiasis that fails to respond with standard therapy
- Recurrent viral infections (e.g. herpes simplex, CMV)
- Unusual infections, e.g. *Mycobacterium avium, Pneumocystis jirovecii*
- Hepatomegaly, splenomegaly, cardiomyopathy.

Q. What are the different diagnostic tests for HIV in a child born to an HIV-positive mother?
Ans.
- An enzyme-linked immunosorbent assay (ELISA) is unreliable for the first 18 months due to transmission of maternal antibodies.

- Polymerase chain reaction (PCR) of viral DNA is to be done at day(s) 0, 2 and 6 weeks and again at 3 months time.

Second-line confirmatory tests are:	Additional tests:
- HIV, RNA, PCR	Serology for:
- CD4 count	- HBV, HCV
- HLA B5701	- CMV, VDRL
	- Mantoux test

Q. What are stages of pediatric HIV (CDC-1994)?
Ans. Stages are:
- **Category N**—asymptomatic
- **Category A**—mildly symptomatic, e.g. lymphadenopathy, hepatomegaly, splenomegaly, recurrent respiratory tract infections.
- **Category B**—moderately symptomatic. These include meningitis, pneumonia, chronic diarrhea, nephropathy, oropharyngeal thrush > 2 months.
- **Category C**—severely symptomatic with an AIDS-defining illness.

Q. What are the different management issues to prevent MTCT?
Ans. Mother is helped to make an informed choice as regard breastfeeding versus bottle feeding. Breastfeeding doubles the risk of MTCT. WHO recommends exclusive breastfeeding in the developing countries for the first 6 months. Exclusive replacement feeding is done only when **AFASS** (A = Affordable, F = Feasible, A = Accessible, S = Sustainable and S = Safe) criteria is fulfilled.

Q. Describe the management of neonates born to HIV-infected mothers.
Ans.
- Antiretroviral (ARV) therapy to be started within 4 hours of birth.[1]
- Most neonates are treated with zidovudine monotherapy but neonates with higher risk are treated with highly active antiretroviral therapy (HAART). However, single dose nevirapine have been shown to be effective.[2]
- Prophylaxis against pneumocystis pneumonia (PCP) (cotrimoxazole) is to be given.
- Children with confirmed HIV seroconversion should be treated at specialist pediatric infectious disease center.

WHO and National guideline (2011) for the feeding of HIV-infected infants is exclusive breastfeeding for at least first 6 months. Exclusive replacement feeding may be done on mother's choice or when she fulfills the criteria of AFASS.

Q. When should HAART to be started?
Ans. HAART can reduce the risk of opportunistic infection significantly. HARRT is to be started in a case where the risk of progression of the disease is more based on CD4 counts and viral load. Serial measurements of these values and clinical assessments are the most useful indicator.[3]

Q. What is the immunization protocol for such infants?
Ans.
- Routine immunization schedule to be followed.

- Live immunizations (except MMR) are to be avoided.
- Children with AIDS have poor immune response.

Q. What is the prognosis of the children born with HIV infection?

Ans.
- Perinatal infection promotes accelerated disease progression compared to adults.
- Approximately 25% of children develop AIDS in the first year of life.
- Mortality is > 50% by 2 years of age.

References

1. Panel on Antiretroviral Therapy and Medical Management of HIV-Infected Children. (2016). Guidelines for the Use of Antiretroviral Agents in Pediatric HIV Infection. [online] Available from http://aidsinfo.nih.gov/contentfiles/lvguidelines/pediatricguidelines.pdf. [Accessed June, 2016]
2. Volmink J, Siegfried NL, van der Merwe L, et al. Antiretrovirals for reducing the risk of MTCT of HIV infection (review). Cochrahe database Syst Rev. 2007;(1):CD003510.
3. Siegfried N, van der Merwe L, Brocklehurst P, et al. Antiretrovirals for reducing the risk of mother-to-child transmission of HIV infection. Cochrane Database Syste Rev. 2011;(7):CD003510.

74 Varicella Zoster Virus (Chickenpox) Infection

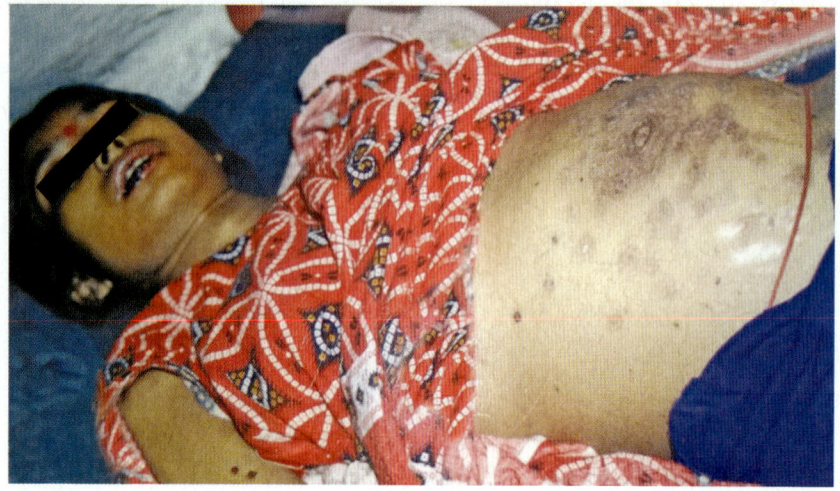

Fig. 74.1: Mrs C, 27-year-old woman, at 33 weeks of pregnancy, admitted with Varicella Zoster Virus infection in pregnancy. Different stages of rash formations are seen. Centripetal macular rash is seen. The rash has spread to the extremities and the face. Skin excoriation and scabbed lesions are also seen

- Chickenpox is a DNA virus of Herpesviridae family.
- It is highly infectious.
- In 90% of cases, it occurs before adolescence.

Q. What are the high-risk factors for VZV infection?
Ans. The infection may be severe in pregnancy to affect both the mother and fetus.
High-risk factors are:
- Immunosuppression
- Older age
- Steroid use
- Malignancy.

Q. What is the clinical presentation of the case?
Ans. Viral entry through upper respiratory tract → incubation period 10–14 days → fever (3–4 days: 38–39°C) → appearance of crops of vesicles (3–5 days) → site-head, neck, trunk (macule, papule vesicle and pustule) → crusts formation → scar formation (usually not long-lasting) (Fig. 74.1).

Q. What are the management issues for a pregnant or breastfeeding woman when infected with VZV?

Ans.
- Supportive—adequate diet and fluid intake.
- Symptomatic treatment—analgesics and antipyretics (paracetamol).
- Antiviral therapy: Acyclovir is to be started if the woman presents within 24 hours or has severe chickenpox or if they are at risk of complications.
- With the onset of complications (pneumonia, encephalitis) women needs to be hospitalized.
- Women going to preterm labor increases the risk of neonatal chickenpox.

Oral acyclovir is started 800 mg for 5 times a day for 5–7 days.

Q. What are the risk of chickenpox infection in pregnancy?

Ans.
- **Infection in pregnancy < 20 weeks:** Congenital varicella syndrome—about < 2%.
- **Infection > 20 weeks:** Neonatal chickenpox, preterm labor. This is more so if the mother infected within 7 days of birth.
- **Neonatal chickenpox** is also a problem when the rash appears within 2 days after delivery.

Neonatal chickenpox is mainly due to transplacental transfer of virus but no antibody. In such a situation there is no time for IgG to develop as the onset of infection and delivery is very short.

Q. What are the complications of neonatal chickenpox?

Ans.
- Severe pneumonia
- Fulminant hepatitis
- Risk of neonatal death up to 30%.

Q. How neonatal chickenpox should be treated?

Ans. Treatment is done with immunoglobulin and acyclovir therapy.

Q. What are the maternal complications of VZV infections?

Ans.
- Viral pneumonia may be life-threatening. Secondary bacterial infections—streptococcal infection to cause necrotizing fasciitis and toxic shock syndrome.
- Chest pain.
- Encephalitis—may need ICU admission.
- Myelitis.

Q. What is congenital varicella syndrome?

Ans. It is observed in < 2% of cases when infection occurs at < 20 weeks of gestation.

FGR	Cataracts
Microcephaly	Microphthalmia
Cortical atrophy	Chorioretinitis
Limb hypoplasia	Skin scarring

Q. How VZV infection could be prevented?

Ans.
- Mass chickenpox vaccination (to children 1–12 years age)
- 2 doses of vaccine 4–8 weeks apart—98% protection in children.

75. Rubella in Pregnancy

Rubella infection though common in many parts of the world is an uncommon infection in UK. This is mainly due to widely accepted vaccination program and antenatal screening. It is a self-limiting viral infection.

Q. What is the major concern with rubella infection in pregnancy?
Ans. Maternal infection in early pregnancy results in congenital rubella syndrome (CRS).

Q. How the mother presents when infected with rubella?
Ans. About 20–50% of rubella infections are subclinical.
- There may be macular rash, posterior auricular lymphadenopathy, arthralgia, low-grade fever and malaise.
- It is a self-limiting illness.

Q. How the fetus is affected?
Ans. Risk of fetus depends upon the period of gestation.

Gestational age (weeks)	Risk of damage (%)
8–10	90
11–16	10–20
> 16	Rare

Q. At what period of gestation the risks of fetal damages are high?
Ans. Damages involve multiple organs. Risks of damage are high (90%) when infection occurs in the first 8–10 weeks of pregnancy. Thereafter risk of fetal damage is reduced to 10–20% in the first 11–16 weeks. Fetal damage is rare after 16 weeks of pregnancy.

Q. What are the different types of damages in the neonate that may occur?
Ans.

Transient damages	Developmental damages	Permanent damages
IUGR, thrombotic thrombocytopenic purpura (blueberry skin), hemolytic anemia, hepatosplenomegaly, jaundice, meningoencephalitis, neurological damages and radiolucent bone disease.	Sensorineural deafness (80%), mental retardation, IDDM (20%) diarrhea, pneumonitis and high mortality.	Congenital heart disease, pulmonary artery stenosis, PDA, eye defects including cataracts, pigmentary retinopathy (salt and pepper), microphthalmia, severe myopia and microcephaly.

Q. How could rubella be distinguished from other viral infections?
Ans. *Differential diagnosis:* Rubella is indistinguishable from infections like parvovirus B_{19} and other viruses like TORCH (toxoplasmosis, other rubella, cytomegalovirus, herpes simplex) group.

Q. How is the infection to be investigated?
Ans. *In the mother*
- Rubella-specific IgM (saliva)
- Rise in IgM titer over 2 weeks
- Rubella-specific IgM—indicates primary infection.

In the baby
- Presence of IgM antibodies—suggests infection acquired after birth
- Persistence of rubella IgM (which is usually cleared by 6 months)
- Polymerase chain reaction (PCR) is a sensitive test for rubella.

Q. Discuss the management issues for rubella infection:
Ans.
- Termination of pregnancy is offered when the mother is positive for IgM antibodies in the first 16 weeks of pregnancy.
- Special educational support for the children with mental, hearing and visual defects.
- Cochlear implants.
- Cardiac surgery.

Q. Discuss the different preventive measures for rubella infection:
Ans.
- Immunization of adolescents and women of childbearing age to prevent CRS.
- Checking rubella antibody status in antenatal care (ANC) is too late for the current pregnancy. It should ideally be done during preconception counseling.
- Human immunoglobulin IV is not protective.

76 Cytomegalovirus Infection in Pregnancy

Cytomegalovirus (CMV) infection is usually asymptomatic (50–80%). Mode of infection is via body fluids, e.g. blood transfusion, sexual intercourse or by tissue donation.

Q. What are the complications of CMV infection?
Ans. Complications of primary CMV infection in an immune competent, individual are uncommon. But when the individual is immunocompromised almost every organ of the body is affected. Combined infection with CMV and human immunodeficiency virus (HIV) is very serious.

Complications are:
- Guillain-Barré syndrome
- Myocarditis
- Pneumonia
- Neuropathy
- Meningoencephalitis
- Thrombocytopenia
- Uveitis
- Pulmonary hemorrhage.
- Pericarditis
- Hepatitis
- Retinitis

Q. How does congenital CMV infection occur?
Ans. CMV is a common congenital acquired infection in infants.
- Transplacental infection is common for primary infection.
- CMV is present in both cervical secretion and breast milk.
- Children infected *in utero* may manifest late.

Q. What are the risks of damage with congenital CMV disease?
Ans.
- **A neurological damage:** Sensorineural hearing loss, neurodevelopmental delay (mental and motor) microcephaly.
- **Cytomegalic inclusion disease:** Jaundice, splenomegaly, thrombocytopenia, fetal growth restriction (FGR).
- **CMV secretion** is common in children with congenital infection. Infected child may act as a reservoir of infection for other children.

Q. What are the risks of organ transplantation and CMV infection?
Ans.
- It is associated with increased morbidity and mortality.
  - All organ donor and recipients should be screened for CMV prior to any organ transplantation.
  - Seronegative recipients who received a solid organ transplant from a seropositive donor should be offered valacyclovir as a prophylaxis against primary infection.

Q. How to confirm the diagnosis of CMV infection?

Ans.
- CMV antibodies—IgM and IgG. There is four-fold increase in IgG levels.
- **Polymerase chain reaction (PCR)**—has been used to detect CMV in blood and tissues. It is a very sensitive test.
- **Biopsy**—detection of intranuclear inclusion is the hallmark of CMV infection.
- **Others**—chest X-ray/computed tomography (CT) for lung infiltrates.

Q. Discuss the management issues of congenital CMV infection?

Ans. Ganciclovir (IV) or valganciclovir orally for 14 days is to be given.
- Ganciclovir is more active but more toxic than acyclovir.
- Foscarnet is used as a second-line agent and is more toxic.
- Cidofovir is given for acquired immune deficiency syndrome (AIDS) patients.

Duration of therapy and efficiency of treatment is assessed by monitoring the viral load using PCR tests.

77. Viral Hepatitis in Pregnancy

Hepatitis B virus (DNA virus) is the most common cause of viral hepatitis. Worldwide 350 million people are chronically infected with hepatitis B virus (HBV) infection (WHO). Currently, there is a decline in HBV infection due to routine HBV vaccination. Other viral hepatitis are due to hepatitis C virus (HCV) and hepatitis D virus (HDV) infection.

Q. How the woman with HBV infection in pregnancy presents?
Ans. Infection may be in the subclinical state or may present with flue-like illness.
- There may be fever, malaise or jaundice.
- Occasionally causes fulminant hepatic necrosis.

Q. How the patient with chronic HBV infection presents?
Ans.
- Often these patients are healthy carriers. Few may present with fatigue, anorexia, nausea, right upper quadrant pain.
- Nearly 25% of adults who become chronically infected during childhood later die from hepatocelluar carcinoma or cirrhosis of liver.

Q. When a patient is defined to suffer from chronic HBV infection? What determines the progression of the disease?
Ans. Persistence of HBV surface antigen (HBSAg) in the serum of an individual for a period of 6 months or longer, is defined as chromic infection.
The risk of progression is related to the level of active viral replication in the liver as well as the immune status of the individual.
More than 90% of neonates whose mothers are hepatitis HBe antigen-positive, suffer from chronic hepatitis B infection.

Q. What are the different routes of transmission of HBV infection?
Ans.
- ***Sexual***—through vaginal or anal intercourse.
- ***Blood to blood contact***—sharing of needles, needle stick injury.
- ***Transfusion related***—infection is rare in the UK.
- ***Perinatal transmission*** from mother to child transmission (MTCT).

Q. What are the investigations to be performed for a woman with HBV infection?
Ans.
- Investigations for HBV:
  - Hepatitis B surface antigen (HBsAg)
  - Hepatitis Be antigen (HBeAg)

- Anti-HBe antibody
- Anti-HBs antibody
- Anti-HB core antibody
- Quantitative hepatitis B virus DNA
- Hepatitis B virus genotype (for those considered for interferon)
- Hepatitis delta virus (HDV) serology.
- General investigations:
  - Full blood count (FBC)
  - Serum AST and ALT levels
  - Serum bilirubin
  - Coagulation parameters.
- Investigations for HCV and HIV
- Others
  - Liver biopsy.

Q. What are the implications of the different serological markers?
Ans.
- HBsAg is detected during the first 3–5 weeks of infection (mean time: 30 days).
- Persistence of HBsAg for > 6 months indicates chronic carrier status which is observed in 5–10% of infections.
- HBsAg positive women having HBeAg detected in the serum, are highly infectious.
- Woman HBsAg-positive and HBeAg-negative are (anti-HBe antibody-positive) are of lower infectivity.
- Antibodies to HBcAg (anti-HBc antibody) imply past infection.
- Antibodies to HBsAg (anti-HB antibodies) alone indicates vaccination.
- Dane particles are HBV virions
- DNA polymerase when present indicates viral replication.
- Women with acute HBV infection have raised levels of IgM to HBcAg whereas women with chronic infection have positive HBsAg and negative IgM to HBcAg.

Q. When to stop antiviral therapy?
Ans. When a patient positive for HBeAg becomes negative for HBeAg or positive for anti-HBe antibody and there is sustained suppression of HBV-DNA after treatment withdrawal, can be considered for stopping therapy.

Q. What is the risk of viral transmission (mother to infant) during pregnancy?
Ans. Vertical transmission (mother to infant) occurs in 90% of pregnancies when the mother is HBeAg-positive. However, it is only 10% when the mother is HBeAg negative.

Q. How the infant born to an infected mother should be treated?
Ans. All infants should receive a complete course vaccine. HBIG should be given within 24 hours of birth. Baby should also be given HBV active immunization simultaneously (at a different site). This reduces vertical transmission by 90%.

Q. Who are risk group that they need screening and primary vaccination?
Ans. Hepatitis B testing should be considered in the following high-risk (asymptomatic) patients: (a) Sex workers, (b) IV drug users, (c) HIV positive patients, (d) Men who have sex with men, (e) Needle stick victims, (f) Sexual assault victims and (g) Sexual partner of positive patients.

Q. What are the complications of chronic HBV infection?
Ans.
- Chronic hepatitis
- Relapse
- Cholestasis
- Cirrhosis
- Hepatocellular carcinoma
- Concurrent infection with HCV, leading to fulminant hepatitis.

Q. Who are the patients that they need to be treated for chronic HBV infection?
Ans.
- Patients who have hepatic necrosis, fibrosis due to inflammation.
- Patients with high serum HBV-DNA.
- Patients with cirrhosis of liver irrespective of HBV-DNA titer.
- HBV-DNA quantification showing rising titer.

Q. How to treat a patient who is with chronic HBV infection?
Ans. Use of interferon and oral antiviral nucleoside/nucleotide analog have improved the outcome.
- Lamivudine, entecavir, adefovir, tenofovir are the potent antiviral drugs. These drugs suppress HBV replication.
- Pegylated interferon (weekly injection) gives an effective response in about 30% of patients. It is not commonly used due to its side effects.

However, it is not yet certain which drug works best.

Q. How the efficacy of antiviral therapy is assessed?
Ans. Antiviral efficacy is judged by the:
- Degree of HBV-DNA suppression
- Rates of HBVe antigen loss
- Improvement in liver histology.

Q. How to treat a patient who is viral resistant or who has HBV infection along with HIV infection?
Ans. Patient resistant to single antiviral agent may need combination of drugs.
Patients infected with combined HBV and HIV have higher risk of chronicity, decreased rates of seroconversion to become negative and increased viral multiplication rates. These are probably due to impairment of immune defense.

Q. Make an outline of the management issues of HBV infection.
Ans. **General:**
- Patients are advised against unprotected sexual intercourse. They should avoid oro and orogenital contact.
- Vaccination against HBV infection.
- Infected patients should not donate blood.

Treatment of infection with HBV infection: Treatment of acute infection is mainly supportive. Consultation with a hepatologist is ideal.

The goal of treatment:
- To prevent progression to cirrhosis
- To reduce the risk of complications (hepatic failure)
- To prevent the spread of the disease.

Q. How do you treat a woman with chronic infection?
Ans. Currently, there is improvement in the management of HBV infection. The different management options are:
- Use of interferon
- Lamivudine, entecavir, adefovir or tenofovir can be used. These drugs suppress HBV replication.

Q. How to prevent HBV infection?
Ans.
- Active immunization with recombinant HBV vaccine as an universal protocol to all or for the high-risk groups.
- Passive immunization with specific hepatitis B immunoglobulin to nonimmune contacts after high-risk exposure.

Q. What is the route of transmission for HCV?
Ans.
- Parenteral route: Intravenous drug use, blood transfusion
- Hemodialysis
- Sexual contact
- Needle stick injuries, sharing toothbrushes, tattooing
- Perinatal transmission (mother to infant).

Q. What is the long-term effect of chronic HCV infection?
Ans.
- Cirrhosis of liver (20–30%)
- Hepatocellular carcinoma
- Liver failure.

Q. How a patient with HCV chronic infection be treated?
Ans. Peginterferon (alfa-2a) weekly injection and daily oral ribavirin is effective (NICE-2010).
- Boceprevir and telaprevir are effective as they prevent viral replication particularly with genotype 1 chronic hepatitis C.
- Treatment is contraindicated in women who are pregnant or breastfeeding.
- No vaccine is currently available for HCV.
- About 50–80% of HCV infected patients become chronic carriers.

78. Listeriosis in Pregnancy

Listeria is gram-positive nonsporing rods. *Listeria monocytogenes* is the major pathogen. Others are *Listeria ivanovii* and *Listeria seeligeri*.

Q. What are the routes of transmission of the infection?

Ans. *Listeria monocytogenes* is common in wild and domesticated animals and also in soil and water.

Important modes of transmission are:
- Food borne (raw foods, refrigerated food—soft cheese, uncooked meats, smoked food).
- Direct contact with infected animals (during lambing, calving).
- *In utero* transfer from mother to fetus (transplacental).

Q. How does the woman commonly present?

Ans.
- Influenza like illness—myalgia, sore throat, cough, fever.
- Severe infection may cause—septicemia, meningoencephalitis.
- Infection in a pregnant woman may cause—miscarriage, intrauterine fetal death (IUFD), stillbirth, neonatal death (transplacental infection).
- Infants when infected present with—poor feeding, jaundice, respiratory distress syndrome (RDS), pneumonia, meningitis and even death.

Q. What investigations are done for the diagnosis?

Ans.
- Culture for amniotic fluid, blood and urine are done.
- Serological tests are not reliable.
- Chest X-ray, magnetic resonance imaging (MRI) for central nervous system (CNS) disease, electrocardiography (transesophageal) is informative for the diagnosis of endocarditis.

Q. What management is done for the infection?

Ans. Amoxicillin and ampicillin are used to treat infection in a pregnant woman. Severe infection (septicemia) needs to be treated with these drugs parenterally. Erythromycin is used when the woman is found allergic to penicillin group of drugs. Immunocompromised patients need longer courses of therapy.

Q. What are the long-term complications of listeriosis in an infected infant?

Ans.
- Neurological damage
- Delayed development.

Q. *How could the long-term complications of listeriosis in an infected infant be prevented?*
Ans.
- Pregnant woman should avoid contact with wild/domestic animals.
- She should avoid contaminated food, refrigerated food, soft cheese, cold salads and smoked sea food.
- Food should always be adequately cooked or reheated.

79 Toxoplasmosis in Pregnancy

Toxoplasmosis is due to *Toxoplasma gondii*. It is an intracellular parasite (protozoan). Its main host is the cat.

Q. What are the routes of transmission for toxoplasmosis?
Ans.
- Ingestion or handling of oocytes from cat feces through contaminated water, food or soil.
- Eating or handling of undercooked or raw meat which is infected (mainly pork and lamb).
- Mother to fetal transmission—when primary infection is acquired during pregnancy.
- Organ transplantation—in the context of a seropositive (*T. gondii*) donor and a seronegative recipient.

Q. What is the overall prevalence of infection with T. gondii?
Ans. There is wide variation of seroprevalence in pregnant women worldwide.
- In UK (London region), seroprevalence in pregnant women was 5.5–12.7%.
- In France, seropositivity is about 90%.
- In Japan, it is 12.5%.
- In Netherlands, it is about 60%.

Q. How the women present when infected with T. gondii during pregnancy?
Ans. Commonly this infection presents in four main types.
1. **Acquired infection in immunocompetent subjects:** (a) Asymptomatic in most cases. (b) About 10% presents with lymphadenopathy (occipital or cervical), rarely myocarditis, pneumonitis or myositis.
2. **Ocular toxoplasmosis:** (a) Chorioretinitis, (b) Reduced visual activity, (c) Anterior uveitis, endophthalmitis.
3. **Congenital infection in immunocompetent patients**.
   - Mother may present with malaise, lymphadenopathy.
   - **Fetal consequences:** Fetal risks are severe in early pregnancy. Risk of maternal and fetal transmission increases as pregnancy progresses but consequences are less severe. Overall fetal complications are:
     - Miscarriage, fetal abnormalities
     - Complications may develop later in life

- Hydrocephalus, microcephaly, chorioretinitis, epilepsy, anemia, thrombocytopenia and development delay
- **The classical triads of congenital infection are**—chorioretinitis, intracranial calcifications and hydrocephalus.

4. **Immunocompromised subjects**

Q. What are the consequences of infection in immunocompromised patients?

Ans. It may be life-threatening at times:
- Encephalitis
- Focal neurological deficits
- Cerebellar signs
- Neuropsychiatric features
- Others—chorioretinitis, pneumonitis, multiorgan involvement with respiratory failure.

Q. What are investigations to be done for the diagnosis?

Ans.
- **Serology**
  - IgG antibodies appear within 1–2 weeks of infection and persist for life.
  - Tests of the avidity of IgG can help to distinguish recent from previous infection.
  - IgM appears in the first week of infection, increases rapidly and thereafter declines.
  - IgM and IgA levels are useful for neonatal infection.
- **PCR amplification** can detect *T. gondii* in blood, tissues, fluids (amniotic fluid). It indicates acute infection.
- **Imaging:** MRI/CT/fetal/neonatal ultrasonography to detect ventriculomegaly, CNS calcification, hepatosplenomegaly, ascites, pericardial or pleural effusion.

Q. Outline the management of a woman in pregnancy with toxoplasmosis.

Ans.
- Nonpregnant women and children (immunocompetent)
  - Treatment is not usually required unless the symptoms are severe or persistent.
  - The usual drug combination is pyrimethamine, sulfadiazine and folinic acid for 4–6 weeks.
- **Maternal and fetal infection:** Recent versus past infection is to be differentiated. Treatment is started immediately for acquired infection.
  - **Treatment outline is** spiramycin is started soon when there is acute maternal infection. It is continued till term.
  - **For fetal infection:** Pyrimethamine/sulfadiazine plus folinic acid (not folic acid) is started after 14–18 weeks of gestation. Woman is monitored for hematotoxicity. Spiramycin can reduce vertical transmission. It does not cross the placenta well. Pyrimethamine and sulfadiazine can treat the fetus, but pyrimethamine is teratogenic. It should not be used in the first trimester.
  - Termination of pregnancy may be an option.

Q. What are the important complications of toxoplasmosis?

Ans.
- **CNS:** Seizures, deafness, developmental delay.
- **Ocular:** Visual impairment, blindness (rarely).
- Pneumonitis, carditis, respiratory failure, shock.
- Multiorgan involvement.

Q. What is the prognosis of women with toxoplasmosis?
Ans.
- Women who are immunocompetent and are asymptomatic, it resolves spontaneously. Over-all prognosis of maternal infection is fairly good.
- The overall risk of vertical transmission from a seropositive mother is 26%.
- Among the infected children retinal lesions are common (33%).

Q. How toxoplasmosis could be prevented?
Ans. Hygiene measures are important for pregnant women.
- To wash hands before handling food
- To wash fruits, vegetables before eating
- To cook meat and chilled meals thoroughly
- To avoid cat feces.

Routine screening of pregnant woman for toxoplasmosis is not recommended (NICE). It is routinely done in France but not in UK or USA.

80. Group B Streptococci Infection in Pregnancy

Q. What is the prevalence of group B streptococci (GBS) in pregnancy?
Ans. Group B streptococci are found in 12–26% of pregnant women, especially in the urine.

Q. What is the risk of maternal infection with GBS?
Ans. It is associated with higher risk of preterm labor and delivery. Ascending infection following rupture of membranes, chorioamnionitis and ultimately neonatal infection is common. The risk of recurrence of GBS infection in subsequent pregnancy is 38%.

Q. What is the risk of neonatal disease and its consequences?
Ans. Risk of neonatal GBS is about 0.9/1,000 births. Neonatal sepsis is associated with mortality of 6%.

Q. How the infection with GBS in pregnancy could be prevented?
Ans. There is no uniform strategy in this regard, however:
- **Some centers** treat on the basis of risk factors [previous pregnancy, preterm labor, premature rupture of membranes (PROM) > 18 hours], and targeted screening and treatment
- **Other centers:** Combined method of routine screening (vaginal swab) and risk factors evaluation.

However, routine screening of all pregnant women for antenatal GBS carriage is not recommended [Royal College of Obstetricians and Gynaecologists (RCOG)].

Q. How a woman with antenatal GBS infection should be treated?
Ans. *Intrapartum antibiotic prophylaxis (IAP):* Benzylpenicillin or ampicillin high dose intravenous (IV) is given to women who have:
- Positive vaginal swab for GBS
- GBS bacteriuria
- Previous baby with GBS
- PROM > 37.

IAP is not needed for women going for elective cesarean delivery with intact membranes. Women with chorioamnionitis need broad-spectrum antibiotic therapy by IV route.

SECTION 10

MRCOG Examination

Section Outline

Ch. 81. Part I MRCOG Examination
Ch. 82. Part II MRCOG Examination

81
PART I
MRCOG Examination

The examination system for the assessment of a candidate is different all over the world. Unfortunately no form of examination system is found to be perfect as yet. The Royal College of Obstetricians and Gynaecologists (RCOG) has designed the system to evaluate two important areas. First, the theoretical part is to assess the candidate's factual knowledge and the ability of organizing his/her thoughts logically. Second, the oral part of the examination is to assess the candidate's clinical competence, communication skill and the ability to formulate management plans. Since 1970, the examination has been divided into two parts: a basic science Part I and a clinically oriented Part II. Membership examination regulations are constantly under review. Aspiring candidates are requested to get existing ones directly from the college: Examination Department, Royal College of Obstetricians and Gynaecologists, 27 Sussex Place, Regent's Park, London NW1 4RG, UK. Tel: Secretary or Call: +44 20 7772 6200.

PART I MRCOG SYLLABUS SUMMARY

The Part I MRCOG examination covers the basic and applied sciences relevant to the clinical practice of obstetrics and gynecology. These are summarized as modules of the curriculum. Part I MRCOG candidate is expected to have the knowledge with clear understanding and skills over the following areas of modules. This page summarizes the syllabus, explaining what the candidates need to know for the Part I MRCOG examination.

Modules 2, 4 and 19 are not examined by the Part I MRCOG examination.
- Module 1: Clinical skills
- Module 3: Information technology, clinical governance and research
- Module 5: Core surgical skills
- Module 6: Postoperative care
- Module 7: Surgical procedures
- Module 8: Antenatal care
- Module 9: Maternal medicine
- Module 10: Management of labor
- Module 11: Management of delivery
- Module 12: Postpartum problems (the puerperium)
- Module 13: Gynecological problems
- Module 14: Subfertility

- Module 15: Sexual and reproductive health
- Module 16: Early pregnancy care
- Module 17: Gynecological oncology
- Module 18: Urogynecology and pelvic floor problems

FORMAT FOR THE PART I MRCOG EXAMINATION

Number of Papers

The examination consists of two written papers, each lasting 2 hours and 30 minutes (5 hours examining time in total).

Each paper contains 100 SBA. Marks are distributed evenly between the papers (i.e. paper 1 counts for 50% of the total marks and paper 2 also counts for 50% of the total marks).

Single Best Answer Questions

Please see the model single best answer (SBA) questions for a better understanding of this question format.

Answering the Questions

The answersheets are numbered 1–100. Against each number there are 5 lozenges labeled A–E. Each question in the question booklet consists of:
- A lead-in statement, which tells you clearly what to do
- An options list, labeled A–E to match the answersheet.

Answer each question by boldly blacking out the letter that corresponds to the SBA in the options list. It may appear that there are several possible answers, but one must choose only the most likely one from the options list.

Marking: Incorrect answers are not penalized.

Division of marks: Each SBA counts for the same number of marks, and each paper contributes the same proportion of marks to the overall total.

The distribution of marks across the two papers by subject domain varies from sitting to sitting. A typical distribution is shown below.

Part I MRCOG examination will have SBA only. The examination will be of the same length and still consist of two papers. However, there will be 100 SBA in each paper.

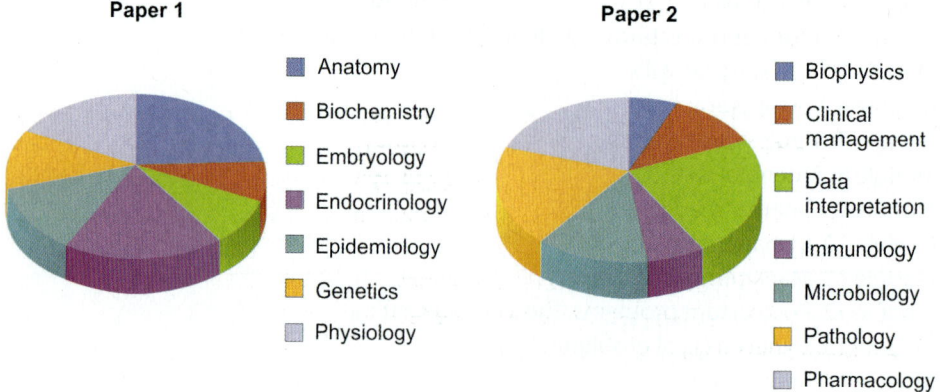

To contact college: For information, or have any questions, please email the Part I MRCOG Secretary or call +44 20 7772 6253.

MODEL SBA MRCOG PART I

Sample Single Best Answer

Part I MRCOG: Sample SBA

This page provides some example of SBA to help candidates preparing for the Part I MRCOG examination.

For each question, select the single most appropriate answer from the 5 options listed.

A 24-year-old woman has a miscarriage at 9 weeks of gestation. The next day she has a full blood count done and the results are tabulated below. Her blood pressure is 84/40 and pulse 95 beats per minute.

Any hospital					Laboratory medicine			
Hosp # 1010101M		Jane Doe			MR Noone			
Regd # 1010101M					U78			
25-AUG		Female			Gynecology ward			
Hb: 6.2 g/dL (12.0–15.0)		Plt: 264–10*9/L (150–400)			WBC: 8.53–10*9/L (4.00–10.0)			
RBC	10*12/L	2.29	(3.80–4.80)	Neut	10*9/L	8.24	(1.25–7.50)
HCT	1/1	0.29	(0.37–0.45)	Lymo	10*9/L	0.38	(1.00–4.00)
MCV	fl	84.5	(83.0–100)	Mono	10*9/L	0.88	(0.20–1.00)
MCH	pg	28.4	(27.0–0-32.0)	Eosi	10*9/L	0.10	(<0.51)
MCHC	g/dL	32.9	(31.5–34.5)	Baso	10*9/L	0.02	(<0.11)
Sample date 23-7-10								Reported 23-7-10
Our Ref: 1900073								
25000-1173								

Q.1 Which management option is most appropriate?
  a. Blood transfusion with 2 units of blood
  b. Colloid infusion
  c. Iron tablets 200 mg daily for 1 month
  d. Iron tablets 200–300 mg 2–3 daily for 2 months
  e. Parenteral iron infusion

Ans. a.

Q.2 A 24-year-old presents at 27 weeks into her second pregnancy feeling unwell, with backache, fever and rigors. She has a temperature of 39.5°C. Urinalysis shows leukocytes and protein +++. Her blood pressure is 80/50. Which action is most appropriate?
  a. Admit to ICU/HDU for intravenous antibiotics and supportive care
  b. Arrange ultrasound of renal tract
  c. Commence 7-day course of oral antibiotics
  d. Give intramuscular steroids to promote fetal lung maturity
  e. Make referral for physicians to review

Ans. a.

Q.3 Where in the body is angiotensin I converted to angiotensin II under the influence of angiontensin-converting enzyme?
a. Adrenal cortex
b. Blood vessel wall
c. Kidney
d. Liver
e. Lung

Ans. e.

Q.4 Which chromosome contains the gene that codes for the alpha globin chain (a constituent component of hemoglobin)?
a. Chromosome 5
b. Chromosome 11
c. Chromosome 16
d. Chromosome 18
e. Chromosome 21

Ans. c.

Q.5 Regarding cardiotocograph (CTG) analysis, what is the accepted normal range for variability?
a. 1–5 beats per minute
b. 1–15 beats per minute
c. 5–15 beats per minute
d. 10–20 beats per minute
e. > 15 beats per minute

Ans. c.

Q.6 A woman presents with a short history of vaginal spotting and cramping abdominal pain after 7 weeks of amenorrhea. A few days earlier she had a positive result on a home pregnancy test. The cervix is closed on examination. An ultrasound scan shows an intrauterine gestational sac. A fetal pole with cardiac activity is seen.
What is the most likely diagnosis?
a. Complete miscarriage
b. Incomplete miscarriage
c. Inevitable miscarriage
d. Septic miscarriage
e. Threatened miscarriage

Ans. e.

Q.7 In a trial where the null hypothesis is false (i.e. there is a real difference present) but a small trial does not find a statistically significant difference, what error is most likely to have occurred?
a. Confidence interval error
b. External validity error
c. P value error
d. Type I error
e. Type II error

Ans. e.

You receive the following result from a pregnant woman at 20 weeks who complained of vaginal discharge:

High vaginal swab
- *Neisseria gonorrhoeae* : Heavy growth
- Ceftriaxone-sensitive
- Penicillin-resistant
- Ciprofloxacin-sensitive
- Azithromycin-sensitive
- Tetracycline-sensitive

Q.8 What is the most appropriate course of action?
   a. Azithromycin 2 g PO single dose
   b. Ceftriaxone 500 mg IM plus 1 g oral azithromycin as single dose
   c. Ciprofloxacin 500 mg twice daily for 3 days
   d. Ciprofloxacin 500 mg twice daily and doxycycline 100 mg twice daily for 7 days
   e. Doxycycline 100 mg twice daily for 7 days

Ans. b.

Q.9 A 30-year-old woman with history of previous three recurrent miscarriages was investigated. Combined laparoscopy and hysteroscopy revealed bicornuate uterus. She was successful to have her fourth pregnancy and that continued to 35 weeks. Which obstetric phenomenon has an increased association with bicornuate uterus?
   a. Placental abruption
   b. Pre-eclampsia
   c. Placenta previa
   d. Breech presentation
   e. Fetal congenital malformations

Ans. d. Breech presentation. (*See* Dutta's Textbook of Gynecology, 7th Edition, p. 36)
Presence of bicornuate uterus is associated with increased risk of recurrent fetal loss, preterm labor and malpresentation (breech).

Q.10 Glucagon has the following effects:
   a. Decreases gluconeogenesis
   b. Decreases plasma glucose
   c. Increases glycogenolysis in the liver and skeletal muscles
   d. Reduces lipolysis
   e. Can be used for severe hypoglycemia of type-I diabetics

Ans. e.

Q.11 Substance(s) unable to bind to fetal hemoglobin:
   a. Carbon dioxide
   b. Nitrous oxide
   c. Carbon monoxide
   d. Oxygen
   e. 2,3-diphosphoglycerate

Ans. e. (*See* Dutta's Textbook of Obstetrics, 8th Edition, p. 47)

Q.12 Regarding oxytocin:
 a. It is an octapeptide
 b. Oxytocin agoinsts are helpful to manage preterm labor
 c. It is released from the adenohypophysis
 d. Administration can cause hyponatremia
 e. Bolus injections can cause hypertension

Ans. d. Oxytocin is a nonapeptide. Oxytocin antagonist, atosiban is used for preterm labor (tocolysis). Bolus administration causes hypotension.

Q.13 Concerning magnetic resonance imaging (MRI):
 a. MRI uses ionizing radiation
 b. In T_1-weighted images, water containing tissues appear white
 c. The international system unit used to measure magnetic field strength is tesla (T)
 d. In T_2-weighted images, bone appears bright
 e. Pregnancy is a contraindication

Ans. c. MRI uses magnetic field and not ionizing radiation. T_2-weighted images, bone and fat appear dark. (*See* Dutta's Textbook of Obstetrics, 8th Edition, p. 739).

Q.14 World Health Organization definition follows:
 a. Maternal mortality rate (MMR) is the number of maternal deaths, per 100,000 total births
 b. Perinatal mortality rate is the number of stillbirths or deaths in the first week of life per 1,000 livebirth
 c. Maternal death due to cardiac disease is a direct cause of maternal death
 d. Maternal death due to pre-eclamsia is an indirect cause of death
 e. Neonatal mortality rate is the number of such deaths in first 28 days per 1,000 livebirths

Ans. e.

Q.15 The posterior pituitary gland:
 a. Synthesizes oxytocin
 b. Releases vasopressin into the hypophyseal circulation
 c. Secretes prolactin
 d. Is known as adenohypophysis
 e. Both oxytocin and vasopressin are octapeptides

Ans. b.

Q.16 The nerve that traverse through the superficial inguinal ring:
 a. Nerve to the pectineus
 b. Genitofemoral nerve
 c. Ilioinguinal nerve
 d. Obturator nerve
 e. Femoral Nerve

Ans. c.

Q.17 About the diameters of the pelvis:
   a. True conjugate measures 10 cm
   b. Obstetric transverse diameter bisects the true conjugate
   c. Left oblique diameter ends at the left iliopubic eminence
   d. Anatomical transverse diameter may be shorter or equal to the obstetric transverse diameter
   e. The diagonal conjugate has no obstetric significance

Ans. b. Obstetric. (*See* Dutta's Textbook of Obstetrics, 8th Edition, p. 101).

Q.18 The following are the correlations of embryonic germ cell layers with the tissues differentiated:
   a. Ectoderm: Bones
   b. Ectoderm: Kidney
   c. Endoderm: Endocrine glands
   d. Mesoderm: Peripheral nervous system
   e. Mesoderm: Pituitary gland

Ans. c.

MOCK SBA MRCOG PART I: PAPER 2

Q.1 A woman attends the antenatal clinic at 16/40 after recently moving to the UK from China. Her booking bloods show her to be positive for HBsAg.
What is the risk of mother to baby transmission in this case, if no treatment is offered?
   a. 1%
   b. 5%
   c. 10%
   d. 50%
   e. 90%

Ans. e.

Q.2 Which drug is most effective in a severe case of Falciparum malaria?
   a. Artesunate
   b. Chloroquine
   c. Mefloquine
   d. Primaquine
   e. Proguanil

Ans. a.

Q.3 What is the risk of uterine rupture during vaginal birth after cesarean section?
   a. 0.1%
   b. 0.5%
   c. 1.5%
   d. 5%
   e. 10%

Ans. b.

Q.4 Which artery may be ligated in cases of massive postpartum hemorrhage where conservative measures have failed to stop the bleeding?
   a. Common iliac artery
   b. External iliac artery
   c. Inferior mesenteric artery
   d. Internal iliac artery
   e. Ovarian artery

Ans. d.

Q.5 Approximately how many pregnant woman per year in the UK are offered invasive prenatal testing [amniocentesis or chorionic villus sampling (CVS)]?
   a. 1,000
   b. 3,000
   c. 10,000
   d. 30,000
   e. 100,000

Ans. d.

Q.6 What percentage of complete hydatidiform moles arise as a consequence of duplication of a single sperm following fertilization of an 'empty' ovum?
   a. 5%
   b. 10%
   c. 30%
   d. 50%
   e. 75%

Ans. e.

Q.7 A pregnant woman who is HIV positive is taking antiretroviral therapy. Obstetrically she has an uncomplicated pregnancy and wishes to deliver vaginally.
At what viral load is it considered safe to deliver vaginally?
   a. 50 copies/mL
   b. 100 copies/mL
   c. 150 copies/mL
   d. 200 copies/mL
   e. 500 copies/mL

Ans. a.

Q.8 A woman with premature menopause has a dual-energy X-ray absorptiometry (DEXA) scan to assess her bone mineral density.
What t score is considered to be diagnostic of osteoporosis?
   a. +2.5
   b. +1.5+
   c. 0
   d. −1.5
   e. −2.5

Ans. e.

Q.9 A 24-year-old woman attends a genitourinary medicine clinic with vaginal discharge. Swabs are taken and she is found to be infected with Chlamydia.
Which antibiotic is an effective treatment for Chlamydia in a single dose?
   a. Azithromycin
   b. Doxycycline
   c. Erythromycin
   d. Tetracycline
   e. Vancomycin

Ans. a.

Q.10 What percentage of the UK antenatal population are seropositive for varicellazoster immunoglobulin G (IgG)?
   a. 10%
   b. 40%
   c. 70%
   d. 90%
   e. 100%

Ans. d.

Q.11 What percentage of twin pregnancies are monochorionic?
 a. 10%
 b. 25%
 c. 33%
 d. 50%
 e. 66%

Ans. c.

Q.12 A 68-year-old woman is referred to the gynecology clinic. A GP had arranged an ultrasound scan because the woman had some lower abdominal pain. This showed a 3.5 cm multilocular cyst in the right ovary but no other concerning features. A serum CA125 is requested, and this is found to be 50 u/mL.
The risk of malignancy index (RMI) for this woman is:
 a. 0
 b. 2
 c. 50
 d. 150
 e. 175

And. d.

Q.13 A 42-year-old woman has an ultrasound scan which shows a simple 5 cm cyst in her left ovary.
Which blood test is now required?
 a. α-fetoprotein
 b. CA125
 c. β-hCG
 d. Lactate dehydrogenase
 e. No blood test required

Ans. e.

Q.14 Which class of tocolytic drugs have the highest frequency of adverse effects?
 a. β-agonists
 b. Calcium-channel blockers
 c. Cyclo-oxygenase inhibitors
 d. Nitric oxide donors
 e. Oxytocin antagonists

Ans. a.

Q.15 Women with obstetric cholestasis often experience intense pruritus.
Which drug, that is commonly prescribed in obstetric cholestasis, effects the greatest improvement in pruritis?
 a. Chlorpheniramine
 b. Cholestyramine
 c. Dexamethasone
 d. S-adenosylmethionine
 e. Ursodeoxycholic acid

Ans. e.

Q.16 Patients with sickle-cell anemia have HbS rather than HbA. The formation of HbS is due to a mutation in which globin chain:
a. α
b. β
c. δ
d. γ
e. ε

Ans. b

Q.17 A 39-year-old woman presents to clinic with secondary amenorrhea. A pregnancy test is negative. Her BMI is 25 kg/m². She is otherwise fit and well. Blood tests are ordered with the following results:

Follicle-stimulating hormone (FSH): 73 IU/L
Luteinizing hormone (LH): 56 IU/L
Estradiol (E_2): <70 nmol/L
Anti-Mullerian hormone level (AMH): <1.2 U/L

What is the most likely diagnosis?
a. Asherman's syndrome
b. Imperforate hymen
c. Kallmann syndrome
d. Premature ovarian failure
e. Turner syndrome

Ans. d.

Q.18 You are called to the gynecology ward by a very concerned FY1 doctor. A 48-year-old woman who had a hysterectomy the day before has had a postoperative full blood count with the following result:
1. Hb: 7.2
2. Hematocrit: 23%
3. WBC: 9.6
4. Platelets: 278

The preoperative Hb was 12.3, so the FY1 doctor is very concerned. The patient is well with stable observations. The catheter bag is full.

What is the most likely diagnosis?
a. Excessive IV fluids
b. Hemolysis
c. Laboratory error
d. Normal results
e. Postoperative bleeding

Ans. a.

Q.19 An anxious 25-year-old woman who is 22/40 pregnant, is admitted with breathlessness and chest pain. Examination of her calves is normal. She has a ventilation/perfusion scan which is also normal.

Blood gases are taken with the following result:
1. PO_2: 13 kPa
2. PCO_2: 3.9 kPa
3. pH: 7.49
4. BE-2

What is the most likely diagnosis?
a. Metabolic acidosis due to gestational diabetes
b. Metabolic alkalosis due to indigestion medication
c. Normal blood gases
d. Respiratory acidosis due to asthma
e. Respiratory alkalosis due to hyperventilation

Ans. e.

Q.20 A woman attends the early pregnancy unit. It is 6 weeks since her last menstrual period and she had a positive pregnancy test 2 weeks ago.
She presents with a heavy per vaginam (PV) bleed.
An ultrasound scan is arranged with the following report:
Normal size uterus with endometrial thickness 5 mm. No evidence of a gestational sac. Both ovaries appear normal. No free fluid.

What is the most likely diagnosis?
a. Complete miscarriage
b. Ectopic pregnancy
c. Incomplete miscarriage
d. Heterotopic pregnancy
e. Missed miscarriage

Ans. a.

Q.21 An FY1 doctor evaluates the presence of glycosuria in the urine sample at booking for its ability to predict the development of gestational diabetes in women who have no history of diabetes.
100 women are assessed.

		Gestational diabetes	
		Develops	Does not develop
Glycosuria	Present	5	5
	Absent	45	45

What is the negative predictive value of glycosuria?
a. 5%
b. 10%
c. 45%
d. 50%
e. 90%

Ans. d.

Q.22 A 70-year-old preoperative patient who is taking lisinopril for hypertension, has an ECG performed.
What electrolyte disturbance is most likely to be present?
a. Hyponatremia
b. Hypernatremia
c. Hypokalemia
d. Hyperkalemia
e. Hypomagnesemia
Ans. a.

Q.23 An ST1 doctor in obstetrics is contracted urgently by a midwife. The midwife has recently seen a woman who is 36 weeks pregnant, who has intense itching, but is otherwise well, and blood tests were taken with the following results.
1. Albumin   30
2. Alkaline phosphatase   310
3. Alanine transaminase   28
4. Gamma-glutamyl transferase (GT)   9
5. Bile acids   3

The midwife is very concerned.

What do you advise?
a. Arrange an urgent review and ultrasound scan
b. Arrange a hepatitis screen
c. Arrange immediate delivery
d. Commence therapy with ursodeoxycholic acid
e. Reassure that everything is normal
Ans. e.

Q.24 An ST2 doctor decides to perform fetal blood sampling in labor due to a suspicious CTG. The results are as follows:
1. pH 7.28
2. BE –3

What is the correct management?
a. Repeat the sample immediately
b. Repeat the sample in 30 minutes if continue to be concerned about the CTG
c. Arrange category 1 cesarean section
d. Arrange category 2 cesarean section
e. Perform artificial rupture of membranes
Ans. b.

Q.25 A 30-year-old woman is referred to the gynecology clinic with menorrhagia, dysmenorrhea, dyspareunia and pelvic pain.
An ultrasound scan is arranged with the following report and image:
- Normal uterus and right ovary

- Within the left ovary there is a structure with a **ground glass appearance** measuring 25–30 mm
- Small amount of free fluid in the pouch of Douglas (POD).

What is this structure most likely to be?
a. Follicular cyst
b. Corpus luteum cyst
c. Dermoid cyst
d. Ovarian carcinoma
e. Endometrioma

Ans. e.

Q.26 A 23-year-old woman attends the genitourinary medicine (GUM) clinic with an offensive discharge. Triple swabs are taken and the endocervical swab yields the following result. Large numbers of Gram-negative diplococci identified.
Which organism is most likely to be causing the infection?
a. *N. gonorrhoeae*
b. *Chlamydia trachomatis*
c. *Trichomonas vaginalis*
d. *Candida albicans*
e. *Treponema pallidum*

Ans. a.

Q.27 A woman is seen in the early pregnancy unit. It is 7 weeks since her last menstrual period (LMP) and she has a positive pregnancy test. She has passed a small amount of brown discharge.
An ultrasound scan is arranged with the following results:
There is an intrauterine gestation sac which is collapsed without a fetal pole.
a. Normal early pregnancy <6/40 gestation
b. Missed miscarriage
c. Molar pregnancy
d. Ectopic pregnancy
e. Heterotopic pregnancy

Ans. b.

Q.28 Which physical principle does MRI use to form an image?
a. Stimulated emission of radiation
b. Acceleration of electrons
c. Vibration of a piezoelectric crystal
d. The alignment of protons in water
e. Conversion of low frequency current to high frequency current

Ans. d.

Q.29 Which two commonly performed tests of coagulation measure the extrinsic pathway of coagulation?
a. aPTT and prothrombin time
b. Prothombin time and INR

        c. aPTT and INR
        d. Platelet count and INR
        e. aPTT and bleeding time
Ans. b.

Q.30 Following a surgical evacuation of the uterus, you receive the following report: The sample contains hydropic villi with hyperplasia of villous trophoblast. No evidence of fetal parts.
What is the correct course of action?
   a. Arrange to re-evacuate the uterus
   b. Commence the COCP immediately
   c. Refer to a regional trophoblastic disease center
   d. Advise that is fine to try and conceive immediately
   e. Take no action

Ans. c.

Q.31 What is the mechanism of action of mifepristone?
   a. Selective estrogen receptor modulator
   b. Progesterone agonist
   c. Progesterone antagonist
   d. β2-agonist
   e. Cyclo-oxygenase inhibitor

Ans. c.

Q.32 What class of drug is tranexamic acid?
   a. Cyclo-oxygenase inhibitor
   b. Anti-fibrinolytic
   c. Progestagen
   d. Anti-androgen
   e. Estrogen

Ans. b.

Q.33 Immunoglobulin G consists of how many peptide chains:
   a. 2
   b. 3
   c. 4
   d. 5
   e. 6

Ans. c.

Q.34 A woman is referred to the antenatal clinic at 30/40 gestation; 2 weeks earlier she had developed a rash in her umbilicus which had now spread to cover her entire body, except her face. A few days earlier the rash had developed into large raised hot painful plaques, and these had now turned into tense blisters.
   a. Eczema
   b. Impetigo herpetiformis
   c. Pemphigoid gestationis
   d. Prurigo gestationis
   e. Pruritic folliculitis of pregnancy

Ans. c.

Q.35 What type of muscarinic receptors are found on the detrusor muscle?
   a. M1
   b. M2
   c. M3
   d. M4
   e. M5

Ans. c.

Q.36 Which complement protein is the most abundant, and whose cleavage results in activation of the lytic sequence?
   a. C1
   b. C2
   c. C3
   d. C4
   e. C5

Ans. c.

Q.37 Which cell type is the effector cell of the adaptive immune system?
   a. Basophil
   b. Eosinophil
   c. Lymphocyte
   d. Macrophage
   e. Monocyte

Ans. c.

Q.38 Which cell type is responsible for the majority of antibody production?
   a. B cells
   b. Cytotoxic T cells
   c. Helper T cells
   d. Macrophages
   e. Plasma cells

Ans. e.

Q.39 Ganciclovir is most effective against which species of herpes virus?
   a. Cytomegalovirus
   b. Epstein-Barr virus
   c. Herpes simplex virus 1
   d. Herpes simplex virus 2
   e. Varicella-zoster virus

Ans. e.

Q.40 Which subtypes of the human papillomavirus are responsible for the majority cases of genital warts?
   a. HPV 16
   b. HPV 18
   c. HPV 16, 18
   d. HPV 6, 11
   e. HPV 43, 53

Ans. d.

Q.41 What is the usual genetic origin and arrangement in a partial molar pregnancy?

Ploidy	Maternal genes	Paternal genes
a. Diploid	1 set	1 set
b. Diploid	2 sets	0 set
c. Diploid	0 set	2 sets
d. Triploid	1 set	2 sets
e. Triploid	2 sets	1 set

Ans. d.

Q.42 To which class of antiretroviral medication does the drug atazanavir belong?
   a. CCR5 antagonist/entry inhibitor
   b. Integrase inhibitor
   c. Non-nucleoside reverse transcriptase inhibitor
   d. Nucleoside reverse transcriptase inhibitor
   e. Protease inhibitor

Ans. e.

Q.43 The Jarisch-Herxheimer reaction may manifest as fever, rigors and hypotension. Typically, this reaction follows antibiotic treatment of which infection?
   a. Chlamydia
   b. Gonorrhea
   c. Molluscum contagiosum
   d. Syphilis
   e. *Trichomonas vaginalis*

Ans. d.

Q.44 An anxious patient had an intravenous bolus of midazolam prior to colposcopic treatment.
Following treatment she is excessively drowsy, with a low respiratory rate and hypotension.
Which drug would you administer?
   a. Adrenaline
   b. Buprenorphine
   c. Flumazenil
   d. Naloxone
   e. Pseudoephedrine

Ans. c.

Q.45 Acyclovir is an analog of which nucleoside?
   a. Adenosine
   b. Cytidine
   c. Guanosine
   d. 5-methyluridine
   e. Uridine

Ans. c.

Q.1 Which muscle is demonstrated in red in the diagram on right side?
a. Gluteus maximus
b. Gluteus minimus
c. Obturator internus
d. Vastus lateralis
e. Pyriformis
Ans. e.

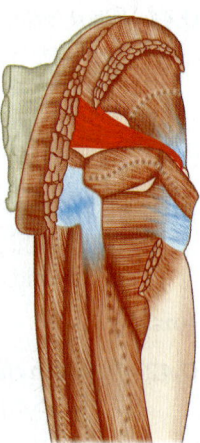

Q.2 Which anatomical structure can be used to distinguish between the body of the uterus and the cervix?
a. Broad ligament
b. Ovarian ligament
c. Round ligament
d. Sacrospinous ligament
e. Uterosacral ligament
Ans. e.

Q.3 At which vertebral level is the bifurcation of the aorta?
a. L1
b. L2
c. L3
d. L4
e. L5
Ans. d.

Q.4 Which structure makes a dimple in the skin of the buttock at S2?
a. Posterior inferior iliac spine
b. Posterior superior iliac spine
c. Sacrococcygeal ligament
d. Sacrospinous ligament
e. Supraspinal ligament
Ans. b.

Q.5 Which shape of pelvis most favors a normal vaginal delivery?
a. Android
b. Anthrapoid
c. Aysmmetrical
d. Gynecoid
e. Platypelloid
Ans. d.

Q.6 What is the value of the submentobregmatic diameter in a normal term infant?
a. 7.5 cm
b. 8.5 cm
c. 9.5 cm
d. 10.5 cm
e. 11 cm
Ans. c.

PART I MRCOG Examination

Q.7 The middle rectal artery is a branch of which artery?
   a. Anterior division of the internal iliac artery
   b. Posterior division mesenteric artery
   c. Inferior mesenteric artery
   d. Abdominal aorta
   e. Pudendal artery

Ans. a.

Q.8 Which muscle of the anterior abdominal wall has a free edge that forms the inguinal ligament?
   a. External oblique muscle
   b. Internal oblique muscle
   c. Transversus abdominis muscle
   d. Rectus abdominis muscle
   e. Pyramidalis

Ans. a.

Q.9 The facial nerve splits into several major branches in the parotid gland, into how many branches does it split?
   a. 2
   b. 3
   c. 4
   d. 5
   e. 6

Ans. d.

Q.10 When after birth does the anterior fontanel close completely?
   a. 6 weeks
   b. 6 months
   c. 1 year
   d. 18 months
   e. 2 years

Ans. d.

Q.11 What is the epithelial lining of the labia majora?
   a. Columnar
   b. Cuboidal
   c. Stratified squamous, keratinized
   d. Stratified squamous, non-keratinized
   e. Transitional

Ans. d.

Q.12 What is the root value of the obturator nerve?
   a. L1, 2, 3
   b. L2, 3, 4
   c. L3, 4, 5
   d. L4, 5, S1
   e. L5, S1, 2

Ans. b.

Q.13 In the mature placenta, how many cell layers are there between fetal blood and maternal blood?
   a. 1
   b. 2
   c. 3
   d. 4
   e. 5

Ans. e.

Q.14 At which receptor is ondansetron, an antagonist?
   a. $5\text{-}HT_{1a}$
   b. $5\text{-}HT_{1b}$
   c. $5\text{-}HT_{1c}$
   d. $5\text{-}HT_{2}$
   e. $5\text{-}HT_{3}$

Ans. e.

Q.15 Approximately how many times higher is the intratesticular concentration of testosterone compared to plasma?
   a. 10
   b. 30
   c. 100
   d. 300
   e. 1,000

Ans. e.

Q.16 At which gestation does plasma volume reach its maximal level?
   a. 12/40
   b. 16/40
   c. 24/40
   d. 38/40
   e. 32/40

Ans. e.

Q.17 What is the oxygen consumption of the fetus at term?
   a. 10 mL/min
   b. 20 mL/min
   c. 40 mL/min
   d. 80 mL/min
   e. 100 mL/min

Ans. b.

Q.18 Which neurotransmitter is antagonized by atropine?
   a. Acetylcholine
   b. Adrenaline
   c. Dopamine
   d. Noradrenaline
   e. Serotonin

Ans. a.

Q.19 What percentage of umbilical cords have a single umbilical artery?
- a. 0.1%
- b. 0.5%
- c. 1%
- d. 5%
- e. 10%

Ans. c.

Q.20 Which embryonic structure fail to fuse completely resulting in the development of bicornuate uterus?
- a. Metanephric duct
- b. Mesonephric duct
- c. Paramesonephric duct
- d. Promesonephric duct
- e. Vitelline duct

Ans. c.

Q.21 At which day, post-fertilization will a normal embryo have developed into the 49-cell stage?
- a. Day 0
- b. Day 1
- c. Day 2
- d. Day 4
- e. Day 8

Ans. d.

Q.22 What is the peak number of oocytes in the ovary in early fetal life?
- a. 100,000
- b. 500,000
- c. 1×10^6
- d. 3×10^6
- e. 7×10^6

Ans. c.

Q.23 At what gestational age would an experienced sonographer expect to see only a yolk sac on a transvaginal ultrasound scan in a normally developing pregnancy?
- a. 5/40
- b. 6/40
- c. 7/40
- d. 8/40
- e. 9/40

Ans. b.

Q.24 What is the most common cause of hyperthyroidism in reproductive age?
- a. Graves disease
- b. Thyroid follicular carcinoma
- c. Thyroiditis
- d. Toxic adenoma
- e. Toxic multinodular goiter

Ans. a.

Q.25 Which peptide of 31 amino acids is removed from proinsulin in the Golgi apparatus?
  a. A peptide
  b. B peptide
  c. C peptide
  d. D peptide
  e. E peptide
Ans. c.

Q.26 What is the main site of secretion of angiotensin-converting enzyme in the body?
  a. Adrenal
  b. Kidney
  c. Liver
  d. Lung
  e. Spleen
Ans. d.

Q.27 What is the embryological origin of the cells in the thyroid gland that produce calcitonin?
  a. Eustachian tube
  b. Foramen cecum
  c. Rathke's pouch
  d. Thyroglossal duct
  e. Ultimobranchial body
Ans. d.

Q.28 Which neurons in the hypothalamus are inhibited by leptin to give a feeling of satiety?
  a. α-melanocyte-stimulating hormone containing neurons
  b. GnRH containing neurons
  c. Neuropeptide Y containing neurons
  d. Somatostatin containing neurons
  e. VEGF containing neurons
Ans. c.

Q.29 Which enzyme converts pregnenolone to progesterone in the steroid synthesis pathway?
  a. 11 hydroxylase
  b. 17 hydroxylase
  c. 21 hydroxylase
  d. 3 hydroxysteroid dehydrogenase
  e. 5 reductase
Ans. d. (*See* Dutta's Textbook of Gynecology 7th Edition, p. 62).

Q.30 From where in the body is cholecystokinin secreted?
  a. Duodenal mucosa
  b. Gallbladder
  c. Liver
  d. Pancreas
  e. Spleen
Ans. a.

Q.31 Which protein binds 20% of estradiol in the plasma?
   a. Albumin
   b. Fibrinogen
   c. Lipoprotein
   d. Sex-hormone binding globulin
   e. Transferrin
Ans. a.

Q.32 Which enzyme is deficient in 95% of cases of congenital adrenal hyperplasia?
   a. 11 hydroxylase
   b. 17 hydroxylase
   c. 21 hydtoxylase
   d. 3 hydroxysteroid dehydrogenase
   e. 5 reductase
Ans. c.

Q.33 What is the half-life $(t_{1/2})$ of ethinyl estradiol?
   a. 3 hours
   b. 8 hours
   c. 15 hours
   d. 20 hours
   e. 36 hours
Ans. e.

Q.34 200 women with polycystic ovary syndrome but otherwise healthy are followed-up over a 10-year period. 100 women are taking metformin and 100 are taking placebo. After 10 years, the women are assessed for the development of type 2 diabetes.
In the metformin group, 20 women have type 2 diabetes
In the placebo group, 40 women have type 2 diabetes.
What is the relative risk of developing diabetes for women who take metformin?
   a. 0.1
   b. 0.2
   c. 0.4
   d. 0.5
   e. 1.0
Ans. d.

Q.35 16 patients have their diastolic blood pressure measured in an antenatal clinic. The mean diastolic:
BP is 70 mm Hg, with a standard deviation of 12 mm Hg.
What is the standard error of the mean in this population?
   a. 1.33
   b. 3
   c. 4
   d. 4.375
   e. 5.83
Ans. b.

Q.36 What type of data are the ABO blood group?
a. Discrete
b. Interval
c. Nominal
d. Ordinal
e. Ratio

Ans. c.

Q.37 What kind of error occurs when the null hypothesis is incorrectly rejected?
a. β error
b. γ error
c. δ error
d. Type I error
e. Type II error

Ans. d.

Q.38 What statistical test is used to compare the medians of two groups of nonparametric data?
a. Analysis of variance
b. Kruskal Wallis test
c. Mann Whitney U test
d. Sign test
e. Student's test

Ans. c.

Q.39 In statistical tests, what is an alternative name for the β level?
a. False-negative rate
b. False-positive rate
c. Negative predictive value
d. Power
e. True-negative rate

Ans. b.

Q.40 In a forest plot of a meta-analysis, the odds ratio of each contributing study is represented by a square. What is the size of the square proportional to?
a. Age of the study
b. Confidence interval of the study
c. Number in the study
d. Odds ratio of the study
e. Weighting used in the meta-analysis

Ans. e.

Q.41 Following an episode of hypoglycemia, glucagon is released. Which metabolic pathway is activated initially?
a. Gluconeogenesis in hepatocytes
b. Gluconeogenesis in cells of pancreas

c. Glycogenolysis in hepatocytes
   d. Glycogenolysis in cells of pancreas
   e. Lipolysis

Ans. c.

Q.42 Which compound is tested for in the Guthrie spot to screen for cystic fibrosis in the newborn?
   a. Chloride
   b. Free thyroxine
   c. Immunoreactive trypsinogen
   d. Medium-chain acyl-CoA dehydrogenase
   e. Phenylalanine

Ans. d.

Q.43 What is the correct order of potency of estrone, estradiol and estriol from strongest to weakest?
   a. Estradiol, estrone, estriol
   b. Estradiol, estriol, estrone
   c. Estriol, estrone, estradiol
   d. Estriol, estradiol, estrone
   e. Estrone, estradiol, estriol

Ans. b.

Q.44 What is the most prevalent cation in the intracellular fluid?
   a. Ca^{2+}
   b. Ca^{-}
   c. HCO_3
   d. K^+
   e. Na^+

Ans. d.

Q.45 Which vitamin facilitates the absorption of iron from the gut?
   a. Vitamin A
   b. Vitamin B_1
   c. Vitamin B_{12}
   d. Vitamin C
   e. Vitamin K

Ans. d.

82. PART II MRCOG Examination

The examination system for the assessment of a candidate is different all over the world. Unfortunately, no form of examination system is found to be perfect as yet. The Royal College of Obstetricians and Gynaecologists (RCOG) has designed the system to evaluate two important areas. First, the theoretical part to assess the candidate's factual knowledge and the ability of organizing his/her thoughts logically. Second, the oral part of the examination to assess the candidate's clinical competence, communication skill and the ability to formulate management plans. Since 1970, the examination has been divided into two parts: a basic science Part I and a clinically oriented Part II. Membership examination regulations are constantly under review. Aspiring candidates are requested to get existing ones directly from the college. Examination Department, Royal College of Obstetricians and Gynaecologists, 27 Sussex Place, Regent's Park, London NW1 4RG. Tel: Secretary or Call: +44 20 7772 6253.

PART II MRCOG SYLLABUS SUMMARY

The Part II MRCOG examination assesses the application of your knowledge in clinical scenarios. This page summarizes the syllabus, explaining what you will need to know for the Part II MRCOG examination.

Modules 4 and 19 are not examined by the Part II MRCOG.
- Module 1: Clinical skills
- Module 2: Teaching, appraisal and assessment
- Module 3: Information technology, clinical governance and research
- Module 5: Core surgical skills
- Module 6: Postoperative care
- Module 7: Surgical procedures
- Module 8: Antenatal care
- Module 9: Maternal medicine
- Module 10: Management of labor
- Module 11: Management of delivery
- Module 12: Postpartum problems (the puerperium)
- Module 13: Gynecological problems
- Module 14: Subfertility

- Module 15: Sexual and reproductive health
- Module 16: Early pregnancy care
- Module 17: Gynecological oncology
- Module 18: Urogynecology and pelvic floor problems

EXAMINATION

Theory Examination

Written: Paper 1: 50 SBAs and 50 EMQs
          Paper 2: 50 SBAs and 50 EMQs

Oral Examination

Candidates who pass the written examination must sit in the oral examination immediately following. The written mark does not contribute towards the oral score.

The Part II MRCOG oral examination consists of 12 stations. Ten of these stations will have an examiner present and two will be preparatory stations for the following one. **Each station is 15 minutes long, with 1 minute of that initial reading time**.

The format of questions may be as follows:

- You may be asked to describe an operation in detail, which may include preoperative and postoperative discussions.
- Your communication skills will be assessed by your interaction with a role-player depicting a particular scenario.
- Your history-taking skills may be assessed.
- You may be presented with a clinical problem and asked to explain it to a role-player.
- You may be faced with a number of clinical problems and have to set priorities what needs to be done and by whom.
- You may be asked to describe, demonstrate or assemble some surgical equipment or teaching skills using it.
- You may be asked to design an audit protocol.
- You may be asked to appraise critically an information leaflet.
  Each of the 10 active stations carry equal marks.

PART II MRCOG OBSTETRIC SBA

This page provides examples of obstetric single best answer questions for the Part II MRCOG examination. Answers and comments for each question can be found at the bottom of the page.
Practice SBA: Some examples of the SBA format are given below. Remember that for each question, you need to select the single most appropriate answer from the five options listed.

Q.1 A woman who is rhesus negative undergoes amniocentesis at 16 weeks. What dose of anti-D immunoglobulin should she receive immediately after the procedure?
  a. 250 IU
  b. 500 IU
  c. 1,000 IU

d. 1,500 IU
e. 2,000 IU

Ans. a.

Q.2 You have just examined a 28-year-old primigravida in spontaneous labor. Examination findings are 0/5 palpable per abdomen, cervix is 7 cm dilated, cephalic presentation-1 station, anterior fontanel palpable with orbital ridges and nasal bridge felt anteriorly. What is the presenting diameter of the fetus?
a. Mentovertical
b. Occipitofrontal
c. Submentobregmatic
d. Suboccipitobregmatic
e. Suboccipitofrontal

Ans. a. Brow presentation. Largest diameter 14 cm

Q.3 A 21-year-old woman, who is known to have beta thalassemia major, attends the clinic for preconception counseling.
What is the most relevant initial prepregnancy investigation to predict maternal complications of pregnancy?
a. Cardiac MRI
b. Chest X-ray
c. ECG
d. Echocardiogram
e. Pulmonary function tests

Ans. d.

Q.4 A 34-year-old woman attends for her booking in her third pregnancy. She had a cesarean section in her first pregnancy 4 years ago and has had a successful vaginal birth after cesarean section (VBAC) 2 years ago. She has a BMI of 26 kg/m².
What is the best predictor for a successful VBAC?
a. BMI of less than 30 kg/m²
b. Less than 35 years old
c. Previous vaginal birth
d. Short interpregnancy interval
e. Spontaneous onset of labor

Ans. c.

Q.5 You are asked to see a 21-year-old woman for preconceptual care. She was diagnosed with generalized tonic-clonic epilepsy 4 years ago. This is poorly controlled. She is currently on sodium valproate and levetiracetam.
What is the next step in her management?
a. Arrange an MRI
b. Arrange an EEG
c. Commence aspirin 75 mg
d. Commence folic acid 5 mg
e. Review medication

Ans. e. To consider the risks of antiepileptic drugs (AEDs) and use the lowest effective dose for each AED, avoiding polytherapy and commencing folic acid.

Q.6 A 28-year-old woman attends the mental health antenatal clinic at 12 weeks for a booking assessment. This is her first baby.
Which condition gives her the highest risk of puerperal psychosis?
a. Anorexia nervosa
b. Bipolar affective disorder (BPAD)
c. Moderate depression
d. Obsessive compulsive disorder
e. Recurrent anxiety

Ans. b. BPAD risk is up to 1 in 2–4 patients rest are not at increased risk of psychosis, i.e. 1–2 per 1,000.

Q.7 A woman has had a recent uncomplicated vaginal delivery but has developed a significant postpartum pyrexia and tachycardia. She is thought to be allergic to penicillin. You suspect puerperal sepsis and are keen to commence treatment prior to the investigations coming back.
What is the antibiotic regime of choice?
a. Cefuroxime
b. Clindamycin
c. Co-amoxiclav
d. Erythromycin
e. Metronidazole

Ans. a.

Q.8 In order to help plan the capacity required for providing future maternity services, you are asked to design a study to establish the incidence of vaginal birth following previous cesarean section. The study will require establishing the mode of delivery in women who have either had only vaginal delivery or have had a cesarean section in at least one previous pregnancy. You review the epidemiological study methods that may be appropriate for this type of study.
Which type of research study should you choose?
a. Case control
b. Cohort
c. Cross sectional
d. Ecological
e. Survey

Ans. b. The answer is cohort study. Cohort studies are longitudinal and follow subjects with or without exposure to a certain characteristic over time. The groups are then compared, e.g. for the development of a particular disease. Cohort studies can be used to measure incidence rates and relative risks.

Q.9 A woman has an instrumental delivery of a baby weighing 3,950 g in her first pregnancy. A Grade 3C tear of the anal sphincter is identified. An appropriate overlapping repair using 3/0 PDS is performed. Prior to discharge, she asks about the long-term risk of fecal or flatal incontinence.

What percentage risk would you advise?
a. 10%
b. 20%
c. 30%
d. 40%
e. 50%

Ans. d.

Q.10 The respiratory system undergoes immense changes in pregnancy in order to cope up with demands of the developing fetus and labor.
Which of the following parameters does not change?
a. Arterial pH
b. Functional residual capacity
c. PaO_2
d. Tidal volume
e. Vital capacity

Ans. e. (See Dutta Bedside Clinics and Viva-Voce, p. 102).

PART II MRCOG: GYNECOLOGY SBA

This page provides examples of gynecology SBA questions for the Part II MRCOG examination. Answers and comments for each question can be found at the bottom of the page.
Practice SBA: Some examples of the SBA format are given below. Remember that for each question, you need to select the single most appropriate answer from the five options listed.

Q.1 You have been asked to obtain consent from a 32-year-old woman with cyclical pelvic pain for a diagnostic laparoscopy under general anesthesia.
What would you advise her regarding the overall risk of a serious complication?
a. 1 in 50
b. 1 in 100
c. 1 in 250
d. 1 in 500
e. 1 in 1,000

Ans. d.

Q.2 A 28-year-old woman undergoes extensive laparoscopic surgery in the lithotomy position. She presents after 2 days with unresolved right-sided foot drop and paraesthesia over the calf and dorsum of the right foot.
Damage to which nerve is the most likely cause?
a. Common peroneal
b. Femoral
c. Ilioinguinal
d. Lateral cutaneous of the thigh
e. Obturator

Ans. a.

Q.3 A 19-year-old woman was seen in the gynecology clinic with a history of excessive growth of facial hair, she needs to wax every 2–3 weeks. Her menstrual periods last 7–8 days every 24–35 days. There is no change in her voice. Her BMI is 28 kg/m². Examination shows: Ferriman-Gallwey grade 2–3 hirsutism over chest and abdomen. A pelvic ultrasound showed no abnormality. Her day 2 hormone tests showed luteinizing hormone level 7.4 IU/L, follicle-stimulating hormone level 5.2 IU/L, serum testosterone level 2.3 nmol/L, SHBG 24 nmol/L.
What is the most likely diagnosis?
a. Adrenocorticotropic hormone (ACTH) tumor
b. Androgen-producing ovarian tumor
c. Cushing's syndrome
d. Idiopathic hirsutism
e. Polycystic ovary syndrome

Ans. d. Diagnostic criteria for PCOS in presence of at least two of the three following criteria: Polycystic ovaries [either 12 or more peripheral follicles or increased ovarian volume (greater than 10 cm³)], oligo or anovulation, clinical and/or biochemical signs of hyperandrogenism. Testosterone level will be raised in Cushing's syndrome, ACTH tumor and virilizing ovarian tumor.

Q.4 A 34-year-old woman complains of heavy periods. She is trying to get pregnant so you prescribe mefenamic acid for her, knowing it is very effective in reducing the blood flow.
What type of drug is this?
a. Cyclo-oxygenase inhibitor
b. Derivative of 17α-ethinyl testosterone
c. Gonadotropin-releasing hormone agonist
d. Plasminogen activator inhibitor
e. Synthetic steroid hormone

Ans. a.

Q.5 A 45-year-old woman with history of vulval itching and soreness for past 2 years attends the gynecology clinic. She is a smoker. She gives a history of using high-potency steroid ointment previously with no symptom relief. A biopsy in the clinic reports vulval intraepithelial neoplasia (VIN) 3. You counsel her for excision of the lesion.
What percentage of VIN ultimately have unrecognized invasion detected on excision?
a. 5%
b. 10%
c. 15%
d. 20%
e. 25%

Ans. d. Ref: RCOG Green Top Guideline No. 58, 2011

Q.6 A 55-year-old woman is due to come in for total abdominal hysterectomy and bilateral salpingo-oophorectomy for a large mucinous ovarian cyst. She takes sequential hormone replacement therapy (HRT) for menopausal symptoms.
You discuss with her the risk of venous thromboembolism. How long prior to surgery should she stop HRT?
a. 2 weeks
b. 3 weeks

    c. 4 weeks
    d. 5 weeks
    e. 6 weeks
Ans. c.

Q.7 A 22-year-old woman presents to the early pregnancy unit with mild left iliac fossa pain. Examination is normal. She has a positive urine pregnancy test. Her serum human chorionic gonadotropin (hCG) is 700 IU/L.
A transvaginal ultrasound scan reports:
'Bulky anteverted uterus with a 2 mm cystic area centrally located within the endometrial cavity. Both ovaries have normal ultrasonic appearances. There are no adnexal masses or free fluid in the pelvis.'
What is the most appropriate management?
    a. Diagnostic laparoscopy +/– proceed
    b. Methotrexate therapy
    c. Serum hCG (human chorionic gonadotropin) measurement in 48 hours
    d. Serum progesterone
    e. Ultrasound scan in 7 days
Ans. c. This is a pregnancy of unknown location (PUL). Ultrasound findings suggest a pseudosac. A true gestational sac would be eccentrically located and have a double decidual sac sign (two concentric rings surrounding an anechoic sac). The visualization of the yolk sac is the critical landmark of the gestational sac. Performing serial serum hCG measurements is the next most appropriate step to guide further management.

Q.8 A 70-year-old woman had noticed that her voice has deepened and she has increasing hair on her face over the last 3 years. Serum testosterone is elevated at 7.2 nmol/L and DHEAS (dehydroepiandrosterone) and urinary 17 ketosteroids are normal.
Which of the following is the most likely diagnosis?
    a. Adrenal carcinoma
    b. Congenital adrenal hyperplasia
    c. Ovarian hyperthecosis
    d. Polycystic ovary syndrome
    e. Sertoli-Leydig cell tumor
Ans. c.

Q.9 A 45-year-old woman underwent total abdominal hysterectomy for heavy menstrual bleeding. She has received treatment for cervical intraepithelial neoplasia (CIN) 3 and is on annual smears. Hysterectomy specimen has reported no CIN.
What would be the management plan?
    a. Continue annual smears
    b. Human papillomavirus testing
    c. No follow-up
    d. Vault smear in 6 months
    e. Vault smear in 12 months
Ans. d.

Q.10 A 30-year-old woman presents to the infertility clinic with primary infertility and dysmenorrhea and is found on ultrasound to have a 6-cm endometrioma in the left ovary.
What is the most appropriate initial management?
  a. Gonadotropin-releasing hormone agonist for 6 months
  b. *In vitro* fertilization
  c. Intrauterine insemination
  d. Laparoscopic drainage of the endometrioma
  e. Laparoscopic excision of the endometrioma

Ans. e.

SECTION 11

MRCOG (EMQs)

Section Outline

Ch. 83. Extended Matching Questions (EMQs)

83

Extended Matching Questions (EMQs)

EXTENDED MATCHING QUESTIONS (EMQs)

Royal College of Obstetricians and Gynaecologists (RCOG) has introduced the Extended Matching Questions (EMQs) as a part of written assessment. EMQs have considerable advantages over the Multiple Choice Questions (MCQs). EMQs need application of knowledge in a clinical scenario. MCQs only test the memory with simple factual recall without any clinical context.

The models of EMQs given in the book are to help the medical students for their preparation. The standards of the few EMQs given in the book are made easy so as to remove any fear of practice. Few models of EMQs are given from RCOG for exact standard. It is expected that many universities in UK and examination board in India and overseas are going to adopt this EMQs, replacing the older format of theory assessment. EMQs appear to assess the candidate much reliably compared to other methods of written assessment formats.

The answersheet is numbered 1–20 and against each number there are twenty lozenges labeled from A to T. Each question in the question booklet will consist of an option list (with same type of letter to reflect the answersheet). A lead-in statement (which tells the candidate clearly what to do) is there and then a list of one to five questions (each numbered, again to match the answersheet). Candidate is expected to judge each particular question and to answer by boldly blackening out the letter that corresponds the single best answer in the option list. In the examination, the option list may provide 10–14 answer options. The option lists will nearly always be in alphabetical or numerical order for ease of reference.

The candidate is expected to select the single answer that fits best. There may be several possible answers but only the most likely one from the option list must be chosen.

The model of a complete answersheet is shown with the EMQs section dealt below:

Marking: Incorrect answers are not penalized. Each correct EMQs answer will be scored three marks. Candidate is encouraged to fill one lozenge for each of the 20 answers. Marking of two or more boxes for one question, no mark is awarded. Any mistake must be erased clearly and completely.

Time management: It goes with the candidate's own decision. But college recommends spending about 24 minutes on the EMQs and 96 minutes on the MCQs would be a reasonable approach.

Examples of the EMQs Format

EMQs Sample 1. Theme: Neuroendocrinology in relation to reproduction

Options: A. Follicle stimulating hormone (FSH)
B. Gonadotropin releasing hormone (GnRH)

C. Calcitonin
D. Insulin
E. Luteinizing hormone (LH)
F. Oxytocin
G. Cortisol
H. Parathyroid hormone
I. Prolactin
J. Thyroxine
K. Growth hormone

Instructions: For each action described below, choose the single most likely causative hormone from the above option list. Each option can be used once, more than once or not at all.

Q.1 Causes hyperglycemia through lipolysis and opposing the effects of insulin.

Q.2 Function is essential for growth and development of central nervous system (CNS) and skeletal system.

Q.3 Induces aromatization in granulosa cells to convert androgens to estrogen.

Q.4 Continued stimulation may cause gonadotropic cells down regulation.

Q.5 Lowers plasma calcium concentration by reducing bone resorption.

Q.6 Inhibits glycogenolysis, increases glycolysis and promotes glycogenesis.

Q.7 Stimulates deposition of cartilage at the ends of bones.

Q.8 Initiates milk let-down reflex.

Q.9 Sustained and peak level augments ovulation.

Q.10 Enhances urinary excretion of calcium.

The answersheet area will look like this and correct responses are to be put as shown below:

1 [A] [B] [C] [D] [E] [F] [■] [H] [I] [J] [K] [L] [M] [N] [O] [P] [Q] [R] [S] [T]
2 [A] [B] [C] [D] [E] [F] [G] [H] [I] [■] [K] [L] [M] [N] [O] [P] [Q] [R] [S] [T]
3 [■] [B] [C] [D] [E] [F] [G] [H] [I] [J] [K] [L] [M] [N] [O] [P] [Q] [R] [S] [T]
4 [A] [■] [C] [D] [E] [F] [G] [H] [I] [J] [K] [L] [M] [N] [O] [P] [Q] [R] [S] [T]
5 [A] [B] [■] [D] [E] [F] [G] [H] [I] [J] [K] [L] [M] [N] [O] [P] [Q] [R] [S] [T]
6 [A] [B] [C] [■] [E] [F] [G] [H] [I] [J] [K] [L] [M] [N] [O] [P] [Q] [R] [S] [T]
7 [A] [B] [C] [D] [E] [F] [G] [H] [I] [J] [■] [L] [M] [N] [O] [P] [Q] [R] [S] [T]
8 [A] [B] [C] [D] [E] [■] [G] [H] [I] [J] [K] [L] [M] [N] [O] [P] [Q] [R] [S] [T]
9 [A] [B] [C] [D] [■] [F] [G] [H] [I] [J] [K] [L] [M] [N] [O] [P] [Q] [R] [S] [T]
10 [A] [B] [C] [D] [E] [F] [G] [■] [I] [J] [K] [L] [M] [N] [O] [P] [Q] [R] [S] [T]

EMQs Sample 2. Theme: Problems in early pregnancy

Options:
A. Threatened miscarriage
B. Incomplete miscarriage
C. Missed miscarriage
D. Ectopic pregnancy
E. Complete miscarriage
F. Molar pregnancy
G. Recurrent miscarriage

    H. Corpus luteal hemorrhage
    I. Fibroid with pregnancy
    J. Appendicitis

Instructions: For each of the case presentation below, select the most likely diagnosis from the options given above. Each option may be used once, more than once or not at all.

Q.11 Mrs AC, 22-year-old G2P0 with previous termination of pregnancy by medical methods at 8 week of gestation is seen due to her complaints of lower abdominal pain and vaginal bleeding. She reports her pregnancy status of 7 weeks according to her last menstrual period (LMP). Urine pregnancy test was positive but ultrasonography (TVS) failed to visualize any intrauterine gestational sac.

Q.12 A 23-year-old lady in her third pregnancy attends for routine antenatal clinic visit at 16 weeks of gestation. Her symptoms of nausea, vomiting, urinary frequency have subsided. She has no vaginal bleeding. On examination, she is normotensive. Abdominal palpation revealed that her uterus was not palpable above the symphysis pubis.

Q.13 Mrs CJ, 31-year-old G2P1 referred by her midwife at 14 weeks of gestation due to an episode of vaginal bleeding and pain in abdomen. Clinical examination revealed, she is hemodynamically stable. Her uterus is palpable above the symphysis pubis. Fetal heart sound (FHS) is audible with a handheld Doppler machine.

Q.14 Mrs LR, 29-year-old P2 is 15 weeks pregnant by her LMP. Her cycles were regular. She has been referred by her midwife due to excessive vomiting in the pregnancy. She noticed recurrent episodes of vaginal spotting. Her blood pressure measured 140/94 mm Hg. She was waiting for her dating ultrasound scan. On clinical examination, her uterus was found 20 weeks size.

Q.15 A 27-year-old G3P1 is admitted at 10 weeks of gestation with the problem of vaginal bleeding for last 4 days. She noticed increased bleeding with the passage of a big fleshy mass along with severe cramping pain of abdomen. Thereafter, she is relieved of her pain and the bleeding has resolved completely. On pelvic examination, the uterus is of normal size and the cervical os is found closed.

Ans. 11 = D, 12 = C, 13 = A, 14 = F, 15 = E. (*See* Dutta's Textbook of Obstetrics, 8th Edition, Chapter 16 under respective heads).

EMQs Sample 3. Theme: Pelvic Blood Vessels and Collateral Circulation

Options: A. Common iliac artery
    B. External iliac artery
    C. Anterior division of internal iliac artery
    D. Main trunk of internal iliac artery
    E. Middle rectal artery
    F. Uterine artery
    G. Ovarian artery
    H. Inferior epigastric artery
    I. Inferior gluteal artery
    J. Superior rectal artery
    K. Superior vesicle artery
    L. Inferior rectal artery
    M. Internal pudendal artery

Mrs AR, 27-year-old multiparous lady suffers from atonic postpartum hemorrhage, following forceps delivery. Decision was made to go for bilateral ligation of iliac arteries as the bleeding continued in spite of all medical measures. Regarding establishment of collateral circulation, the following points were discussed.

Instructions: For each question presented below choose the single most appropriate option from the list above. Each option may be used once, more than once or not at all.

Q.16 Which iliac vessels are to be ligated?

Q.17 Which other vessel anastomoses with superior rectal artery?

Q.18 Which vessel does inferior epigastric arise from?

Q.19 Which other vessel anastomoses with the uterine artery?

Q.20 Which vessel runs above and anterior to the ureter?

Q.21 Which vessel does internal pudendal artery arise from?

Q.22 Which vessel does inferior rectal artery arise from?

Ans. 16 = C, 17 = E, 18 = B, 19 = G, 20 = F, 21 = C, 22 = M.

EMQs Sample 4. Theme: Physiology of menstruation.

Options: A. Follicle stimulating hormone (FSH)
B. Luteinizing hormone (LH)
C. Estradiol (E2)
D. Progesterone (PGN)
E. Sex hormone binding globulin (SHBG)
F. Estriol (E3)
G. Gonadotropin releasing hormone (GnRH)
H. Androstenedione
I. Inhibin
J. Dehydroepiandrosterone

Instructions: For each of the following case presentation below, select the hormone most likely to be responsible in the options above. Each option may be used once, more than once or not at all.

Q.23 A 7-year-old girl presents with isosexual precocious puberty. She started menstruation also. Details of investigations revealed accelerated bone maturation. Endocrine assay revealed the case as the constitutional variety.

Q.24 A 22-year-old woman is being investigated for her inability to conceive. She is instructed to maintain the basal body temperature (BBT). The chart showed a rise of core body temperature by 1°F. (See Dutta's Textbook of Gynecology, 7th Edition, p. 193).

Q.25 A 29-year-old woman is being treated for primary infertility. She had regular menstrual cycle. She had been instructed to perform urine test using a kit at home on daily basis for 5 consecutive days in each cycle, depending on her cycle length. (See Dutta's Textbook of Gynecology, 7th Edition, p. 193).

Q.26 A 40-year-old woman with irregular cycles seeks investigations for her inability to conceive. Her doctor feels to perform a blood test to see her ability to conceive as regard the functional status of the ovary. (See FSH in Dutta's Textbook of Gynecology, 7th Edition, p. 200, 436).

Q.27 A 28-year-old woman attends the infertility clinic after 3 years of her marriage. Speculum examination was done for cervical smear. At the same time cervical mucus was taken for fern test, which showed characteristic fern-tree appearance. (See Dutta's Textbook of Gynecology, 7th Edition, p. 93).

Ans. 23 = G, 24 = D, 25 = B, 26 = A, 27 = C.

EMQs Sample 5. Theme: Infections during pregnancy
Options:

	Maternal diseases	Type	Risk of transplacental infection
A.	Malaria	Bacterium	Yes
B.	Malaria	Protozoan	Yes
C.	Malaria	Protozoan	No
D.	Malaria	Virus	Yes
E.	Syphilis	Bacteria	Yes
F.	Syphilis	Protozoan	No
G.	Syphilis	Spirochete	Yes
H.	Syphilis	Spirochete	No
I.	Tuberculosis	Bacterium	No
J.	Tuberculosis	Parasite	Yes
K.	Tuberculosis	Protozoa	No
L.	Tuberculosis	Bacterium	Yes
M.	Varicella	Fungus	Yes
N.	Varicella	Rickettsia	Yes
O.	Varicella	Virus	Yes
P.	Ancylostoma	Bacteria	Yes
Q.	Ancylostoma	Protozoa	No
R.	Ancylostoma	Rickettsia	No

Instructions: The options above are the different maternal infections in pregnancy. The microorganisms and the risk of transplacental spread are mentioned. Select the single correct profile for each of the microorganisms in the items below. Each option may be used once, more than once or not at all.

Q.28 *Plasmodium vivax.*

Q.29 *Treponema pallidum.*

Q.30 *Mycobacterium tuberculosis.*

Ans. 28 = B, 29 = G, 30 = L.

Options for Questions 31–32:
A. Amniotic fluid embolism
B. Cardiomyopathy
C. Chest infection
D. Cerebrovascular accident (CVA)
E. Endocarditis
F. Hemorrhage
G. HELLP syndrome
H. Myocardial infarction

I. Placental abruption
J. Placenta previa
K. Pulmonary embolism
L. Pulmonary hypertension
M. Sepsis
N. Substance misuse
O. Thromboembolism

Instructions: For each case described below, choose the single most likely cause of maternal death from the above list of options. Each option may be used once, more than once, or not at all.

Q.31 A previously healthy 18-year-old primigravida presents at 36 weeks, feeling unwell and tired. Her brother died unexpectedly aged 19 years. Her chest radiograph showed an enlarged heart. While being admitted, she developed increasing shortness of breath and died despite intensive resuscitation.

Q.32 A 30-year-old woman, 28 weeks of gestation in her sixth pregnancy presents to A and E with breathlessness and displays severe anxiety. She had complained of left-sided pelvic pain for a week. While being assessed, she collapsed and it was not possible to resuscitate her.

Ans. 31 = B, 32 = O.

Options for Questions 33–34:
A. Administer varicella zoster immune globulin (VZIG) as soon as possible to mother
B. Administer VZIG to mother if maternal serology –ve
C. Administer VZIG to neonate
D. Advise avoid contact with other pregnant women and neonates
E. Detailed ultrasound examination
F. Give intravenous acyclovir
G. Immediate cesarean section and transfer baby to the neonatal unit
H. Induction of labor
I. Reassurance
J. Separate mother and baby after delivery
K. Serum for VZV IgM antibodies
L. Treat with oral acyclovir

Instructions: For each scenario described below, choose the single most appropriate management from the above list of options. Each option may be used once, more than once, or not at all.

Q.33 A 26-year-old Para 1 + 0 at 38 weeks of gestation contacts her GP immediately after hearing that a child in her son's nursery has developed chickenpox. She has no memory of having the disease herself.

Q.34 Mrs Jones is seen in the antenatal clinic at 40 weeks. She has cough and smokes 20 cigarettes per day. She has a rash and feels generally unwell. Her sister's child has developed chickenpox. They spend a weekend together two weeks ago. She does not think she has ever had chickenpox. Serological investigation shows that she is susceptible to Varicella zoster.

Ans. 33 = B, 34 = L.

Extended Matching Questions (EMQs)

The answersheet area will look like this and correct responses are to be put as shown below:

31 [A] [■] [C] [D] [E] [F] [G] [H] [I] [J] [K] [L] [M] [N] [O]
32 [A] [B] [C] [D] [E] [F] [G] [H] [I] [J] [K] [L] [M] [N] [■]
33 [A] [■] [C] [D] [E] [F] [G] [H] [I] [J] [K] [L] [M] [N] [O]
34 [A] [B] [C] [D] [E] [F] [G] [H] [I] [J] [K] [■] [M] [N] [O]

Options for Questions 35–36:
- A. Atrophic vulvovaginitis
- B. Benign mucous membrane pemphigoid
- C. Paget's disease
- D. Contact dermatitis
- E. Eczema
- F. Herpes simplex infection
- G. HIV infection
- H. Human papillomavirus infection
- I. Lichen planus
- J. Lichen sclerosus
- K. Lichen simplex chronicus
- L. Psoriasis
- M. Vulval intraepithelial neoplasia
- N. Vulvodynia

Instructions: For each clinical scenario below, choose the single most likely diagnosis from the list above. Each diagnosis may be used once, more than once, or not at all.

Q.35 A 23-year-old woman presents with a two-year history of vulval, perineal and perianal irritation. The vulva is red, excoriated and there are areas of white, thickened skin. Application of 3% acetic acid shows areas of mosaic and coarse punctuation.

Q.36 A 68-year-old woman presents with vulval irritation, soreness and dysuria. On examination, the vulvar skin looks white. Vulvar biopsy revealed hyperkeratosis and thinning of the epithelium. There is hyalinization and chronic inflammatory cell infiltrate in the subepithelial zone.

Ans. 35 = M, 36 = J.

Options for Questions 37–39:
- A. Antihypertensive treatment
- B. Calculate the mean arterial blood pressure
- C. Carry out visual field assessment
- D. Immediate dose of 10 mL 10% calcium gluconate intravenously
- E. Insert central venous pressure line
- F. Intravenous magnesium sulfate
- G. Measure serum aspartate transaminase immediately
- H. Measure serum magnesium
- I. Monitor patellar reflex every 15 minutes
- J. Provide a fluid challenge with colloids
- K. Provide intravenous Hartmann's solution at the rate of 85 mL per hour
- L. Transfer to intensive treatment unit
- M. Transfer to the postnatal ward

Instructions: For each patient described below, choose the single most appropriate initial treatment option from the list. Each option may be used once, more than once, or not at all.

Q.37 A 20-year-old primigravida had a normal delivery of a live infant 12 hours previously. She has developed severe gestational proteinuric hypertension, her clotting is normal, serum albumin is 43 g/dL, there is no ankle clonus and her blood pressure is 160/100 mm Hg. She has been given one liter of Hartmann's solution intravenously since her delivery and has been anuric. The central venous pressure is +10 mm Hg, serum sodium 132 mmol/L, serum potassium 7.1 mmol/L and serum urea 22 mmol/L.

Q.38 A 20-year-old primigravida delivered a live infant 24 hours previously. She has developed severe gestational proteinuric hypertension. Treatment with intravenous magnesium was required. Her fluid balance is satisfactory and serum urea, electrolytes and clotting profile are all normal. Her respiratory rate falls to 6 per minute and she is drowsy but arousable.

Q.39 A 20-year-old primigravida is 30 weeks pregnant and has been transferred to the delivery suite with severe gestational proteinuric hypertension. She complained of severe frontal headache, but has no other symptoms. She has a normal respiratory rate and her urine output has been satisfactory. Her blood pressure is 140/100 mm Hg. There are five beats of bilateral ankle clonus.

Ans. 37 = L, 38 = H, 39 = F.

Options for Questions 40–42:

    A. Damage to bladder/ureter
    B. Damage to bowel
    C. Failure rate 1 in 200
    D. Failure to gain entry into abdominal cavity
    E. Failure to identify disease
    F. Failure to visualize uterine cavity
    G. Hemorrhage requiring blood transfusion
    H. Hemorrhage requiring return to theater
    I. Laparotomy
    J. Pain
    K. Premature menopause
    L. Removal of ovaries
    M. Urinary retention
    N. Uterine perforation
    O. Vaginal bleeding

Instructions: For each of the case histories described below, choose the single most relevant complication that you must discuss with the patient when taking consent prior to surgery from the above list of options. Each option may be used once, more than once or not at all.

Q.40 A 52-year-old woman with frequent heavy periods is listed for diagnostic hysteroscopy. She has had two children both delivered by cesarean section. She is hypertensive and her body mass index (BMI) is 26 kg/m².

Q.41 A 56-year-old woman is scheduled for laparotomy and possible bilateral salpingo-oophorectomy for an ovarian mass. She had a total abdominal hysterectomy at the age of forty for fibroids and is in discomfort with an ovarian mass which measures 15 cm in diameter on ultrasound examination.

Q.42 A 48-year-old nulliparous woman is scheduled for vaginal hysterectomy because of menorrhagia. Her uterus is enlarged equivalent to 14 weeks' gestation.

Ans. 40 = N, 41 = A, 42 = G.

Options for Questions 43–47:

    A. Wide local excision and biopsy
    B. Radical hysterectomy
    C. Wide local ablation
    D. Total abdominal hysterectomy with bilateral salpingo-oophorectomy
    E. Radical vulvectomy with bilateral inguinofemoral lymphadenectomy
    F. Debulking (cytoreductive) surgery
    G. Chemotherapy
    H. Trachelectomy
    I. Radiotherapy
    J. Concurrent chemoradiation

Instructions: For each of the clinical case presentation given below, select the most appropriate treatment from the list of options. Each option may be used once, more than once or not at all.

Q.43 Mrs AR, 32-year-old parous woman presents with moderate dyskaryotic smear. Subsequent colposcopy revealed well-defined area of acetowhite epithelium at the transformation zone. Colposcopy-directed biopsy confirmed CIN III. (See Dutta's Textbook of Gynecology, 7th Edition, p. 259)

Q.44 Mrs A, 67-year-old lady presents with vulval sore and discharge. Clinical examination revealed a 3 × 4 cm ulcerated lesion on inspection. Inguinal lymph nodes were enlarged. Biopsy from the lesion confirmed squamous cell carcinoma of the vulva. (See Dutta's Textbook of Gynecology, 7th Edition, p. 277)

Q.45 A 48-year-old lady presents with an abdominal mass of 20 weeks size. Serum CA 125 was 1020 IU/mL. She underwent laparotomy where stage IIIa. Ovarian cancer was diagnosed. (See Dutta's Textbook of Gynecology, 7th Edition, p. 311)

Q.46 A 39-year-old multiparous woman presents with postcoital bleeding. On speculum examination, cervix appeared abnormal. Punch biopsy confirmed squamous cell carcinoma of the cervix. FIGO staging made the case stage IIIb. (See Dutta's Textbook of Gynecology, 7th Edition, p. 290)

Q.47 A 57-year-old nulliparous woman, known to be diabetic and hypertensive, presents with postmenopausal bleeding. Hysteroscopy and endometrial biopsy revealed well-differentiated adenocarcinoma of the endometrium. (See Dutta's Textbook of Gynecology, 7th Edition, p. 295)

Ans. 43 = A, 44 = E, 45 = F, 46 = J, 47 = D.

Options for Questions 48–52:

    A. Occipitoposterior position
    B. Secondary arrest
    C. Fetal scalp blood sampling
    D. Oral misoprostol

E. Face presentation
F. Instrumental delivery
G. Deep transverse arrest
H. Immediate cesarean delivery
I. Partographic monitoring and repeat vaginal examination in 3–4 hours
J. Rupture the membranes and add oxytocin

Instructions: For each of the clinical case presentation given below, select the most appropriate diagnosis/treatment from the list of options. Each option may be used once, more than once or not at all.

Q.48 A 22-year-old primigravida admitted in the labor ward at 37 weeks of gestation with regular painful uterine contractions. On examination, uterine contractions were adequate, Fetal heart rate (FHR) was satisfactory. Cervix was 70% effaced, 3 cm dilated and station 'O', membranes were absent, liquor clear.

Q.49 A 27-year-old P2G4 is admitted in labor at 36 weeks gestation. Clinical examination revealed uterine fundus is of 34 weeks size. Uterus is contracting regularly. On vaginal examination, cervix was 6 cm dilated and the membranes were intact. Presenting part was the shoulder. FHR was satisfactory.

Q.50 A 25-year-old primigravida admitted in labor following a term pregnancy. She had spontaneous rupture of membranes with clear liquor. Partographic analysis revealed cervicograph was on the right side of the alert line. Augmentation with oxytocin was done. She complained of severe backache throughout. The presenting part (Head) remained one-fifth above the brim. On vaginal examination, the posterior fontanelle was felt near the left sacroiliac joint.

Q.51 A 32-year-old G1P0 with gestational diabetes mellitus was admitted in established labor at 39 weeks of gestation. Uterine contractions were 3–4 per 10 minutes and were lasting for 40 seconds. Cervix was 6 cm dilated, membranes were absent, with station '0'. Repeat examination after an interval of 4 hours the findings were the same despite adequate contractions.

Q.52 A 26-year-old, G1P0 at 38 weeks of gestation with hypertension was admitted in the labor ward for induction of labor. During labor examination revealed adequate uterine contractions. Cervix was 7 cm dilated and the head was below '+2' station, membranes were absent and liquor was clear. After a period of two hours cervix was fully dilated and station was same as before. CTG revealed recurrent late deceleration with a base line FHR 160 bpm.

Ans. 48 = I, 49 = H, 50 = A, 51 = B, 52 = F.

SECTION 12

In Whose Footsteps We Follow

Section Outline

Ch. 84. History in Obstetrics and Gynecology

84 History in Obstetrics and Gynecology

HISTORY IN OBSTETRICS AND GYNECOLOGY

List of eminent personalities with their contributions in Obstetrics and Gynecology has been presented in this section. Sometimes questions are asked by the examiner in relation to such personalities with their contributions. Failure to answer such question is not going to fail the candidate, but certainly this improves the impression of the candidate if he or she could answer it.

Apgar, Virginia (1909–1974): Anesthetist working in America. She introduced 'Apgar Score' for assessment of cardiopulmonary and neurological status of the newborn at birth. This was described in 1953. Virginia Apgar's newborn score is used almost universally. She was apparently a fast walker, fast talker and a fast driver. She started flying lessons when she was 59 years old. Apgar was a popular musician and played cello and violin. Virginia Apgar died in her sleep on 7th August 1974.

Asherman, Joseph (Born–1889): Gynecologist from Tel Aviv. Intrauterine adhesion (synechiae) associated with amenorrhea is recognized by his name Asherman's syndrome (*See* Dutta's Textbook of Gynecology, 7th Edition, p. 378). He was not the first to report the syndrome that bears his name. In fact, Asherman did not describe endometrial destruction and adhesions as the cause of amenorrhea. He described the amenorrhea to sclerosis of the internal os. Asherman was elected the first President of the Israeli Society of Obstetrics and Gynecology in 1972.

Ayre, James Ernest (1910–1974): He is recognized by his contribution of a special spatula for collecting cervical smear 'Ayre's spatula' (*See* Dutta's Textbook of Gynecology, 7th Edition, p. 517). He was the director of Papanicolaou Cancer Research Institute, Miami, Florida.

Bartholin, Caspar (1655–1738): He was the professor of anatomy, medicine and physics at the University of Copenhagen. He described Bartholin's gland (greater vestibular glands) in 1677. (*See* Dutta's Textbook of Gynecology, 7th Edition, p. 2).

Bonney, William Francis Victor (1872–1953): Gynecologist at the Middlesex Hospital, the Chelsea Hospital for women and the Postgraduate Medical School, London. His contributions to Gynecology are manifold. He is mostly remembered for his conservative surgery for fibroids (myomectomy). Unfortunately, before he pioneered myomectomy, his wife had subtotal hysterectomy for fibroid uterus. His significant contributions are:
- ***Bonney's hood myomectomy:*** Myomectomy using anterior hood type incision to prevent adhesions. (*See* Dutta's Textbook of Gynecology, 7th Edition, p. 229 and Bedside Clinics and Viva-Voce, p. 494).

- **Bonney's myomectomy clamps:** Special clamps used to compress the uterine arteries at the base of the broad ligament during myomectomy operation (*See* Dutta's Textbook of Gynecology, 7th Edition, p. 527, Fig. 38.22).
- **Bonney's myomectomy screw (*See Dutta's Textbook of Gynecology, 7th Edition, p. 526, Fig. 38.21*):** Special type of screw used to fix a big myoma after incising the capsule. Traction is maintained when the myoma is enucleated out of its bed (myomectomy).
- **Bonney's test:** Elevation of bladder neck during vaginal examination. It was used as a diagnostic test for stress urinary incontinence and its success for repair surgery. Currently this test is not practised.
- **Bonney's gynecological surgery:** Textbook of Operative Gynecology, first edition was in 1911.

Cloquet, Jules Germain (1790–1883): Professor of Anatomy and Surgery in Paris. He was the president of the French Academy of Medicine. He described the lymph gland of Cloquet (1817), which is the uppermost deep femoral node situated in the femoral canal. (*See* Dutta's Textbook of Gynecology, 7th Edition, p. 24, 275, 501).

Couvelaire, Alexandre (1873–1948) Paris Obstetrician: He described Couvelaire uterus (uteroplacental apoplexy) in 1911 (*See* Dutta's Textbook of Obstetrics, 8th Edition, p. 296).

Donald Ian (1910–1987): Professor of Obstetrics and Gynecology at Queen Mother's Hospital, Glasgow. He introduced the use of ultrasound, 'Sonar' in medicine. He was the author of the book, 'Practical Obstetric Problems'. Ian served in Royal Air Force as a Medical Officer from 1942–46. From the experience of the two World Wars, he thought of the echo sounding system that was used for antisubmarine detection. He worked with **Tom Brown**, a brilliant young engineer to produce the first contact compound sector scanner described in the Lancet in 1958.

Donald was an enthusiastic, ambitious and a revered man. His book, **Practical Obstetric Problems**, reflects his vast experience and the entertaining type of writing. He underwent cardiac surgery for rheumatic heart disease on three occasions. Besides all his medical carrier, Donald was an accomplished sailor, pianist and artist. He suffered repeated heart failures and died on 19 June 1987. Throughout the world, these days, ultrasound is in use in every hospital in almost every department—a great discovery by a great man.

Douglas, James (1675–1742): Anatomist and 'male midwife' working in London. He was the physician to Queen Caroline, the wife of George II. He is remembered by his descriptions:
- **Pouch of Douglas:** Rectovaginal pouch (*See* Dutta's Textbook of Gynecology, 7th Edition, p. 16).
- **Semicircular fold of Douglas:** Lower arcuate margin of the posterior rectus sheath, situated below the level of umbilicus.

Fallopio, Gabriele (1523–1563): He was the Professor of Surgery, Anatomy and Botany at the University of Padua, Italy. He described the fallopian tubes (Oviducts) in 1561.

de Graaf, Regnier (1641–1673): He was born in Holland and worked as an Anatomist and Physician in France. He described graafian follicle (mature ovarian follicle) in 1672 (*See* Dutta's Textbook of Gynecology, 7th Edition, p. 68).

Green-Armytage, Vivian Bartley (1882–1961): MB, worked as the captain in Indian Medical Service. He was the resident surgeon at Eden Hospital, Calcutta (1912). Later, he became the Professor of Obstetrics in the same department. He also worked in West London Hospital. He devised the forceps, 'Green Armytage forceps' for holding the uterine incision margins and the angles during cesarean section (*See* Dutta's Textbook of Obstetrics, 8th Edition, p. 756, Fig. 42.28).

Krukenberg, Friedrich (1871–1946): Pathologist and Professor of Ophthalmology, Halle. He described Krukenberg tumor in 1896 (*See* Dutta's Textbook of Gynecology, 7th Edition, p. 318).

Leventhal, Michael (1901–1971): American Obstetrician and Gynecologist. He along with **Stein, Irving** from Chicago, described **Stein-Leventhal syndrome (polycystic ovarian disease)** in 1935 (*See* Dutta's Textbook of Gynecology, 7th Edition, p. 378).

Meigs, Joseph (1892–1963): Professor of Gynecology at Harvard University. He described Meigs' syndrome in 1937 (*See* Dutta's Textbook of Gynecology, 7th Edition, p. 241).

Mitra, Subodh (1896–1961): Gynecological Cancer Surgeon and Vice-Chancellor, University of Calcutta, India. He is remembered for his new technique of operation, 'radical vaginal hysterectomy with bilateral extraperitoneal lymphadenectomy'. This operation is popularly known as 'Mitra's operation for cancer of the cervix'. (*See* Dutta's Textbook of Gynecology, 7th Edition, p. 286).

Purandare, BN (1911–1990): Gynecologist from Mumbai, India, is recognized by his abdominal cervicopexy operation for cases with nulliparous prolapse (Prolapse without a cystocele) (*See* Dutta's Textbook of Gynecology, 7th Edition, p. 182).

Shirodkar, VN (1899–1971): Gynecologist from Grant Medical College, Mumbai, India. He introduced 'Shirodkar's Stitch' cervical encirclage operation in 1955, for cases with cervical incompetence and recurrent midtrimester abortion (*See* Dutta's Textbook of Obstetrics, 8th Edition, p. 200). He was the President of the Federation of Obstetric and Gynecological Societies of India. He received the Honorary Fellowship of the Royal College of Obstetricians and Gynecologists (RCOG), London. He was a good golf and tennis player.

Sims, James Marion (1813–1883): An American Gynecologist and is recognized by his pioneering work on vesicovaginal fistula repair. Some of his many other contributions are: **Sims' Speculum, Sims' position and Sims' wire** (*See* Dutta's Textbook of Gynecology, 7th Edition, p. 84, 347, 518). Sims bought a malleable pewter spoon and fashioned it into a retractor for the posterior vaginal wall. This was the forerunner of **Sims' Speculum** (*See* Dutta's Textbook of Gynecology, 7th Edition, p. 518, Fig. 38.2). Sims made many contributions to surgery and Gynecology. He studied infertility in relation to survival of spermatozoa in the cervical and vaginal secretions—the forerunner of the **Sims Huhner postcoital test**. In 1876, he was elected the President of American Medical Association and in 1880 became the President of the American Gynecological Society.

Sims published an account of his surgical technique in 1852 using **silverwire as suture material** for repair of vesicovaginal fistula (VVF). Sims' relentless pursuit of surgical cure of VVF was recognized almost a century later by **John Chassor Moir**, a subsequent master of surgery of VVF. He died of coronary thrombosis on 13 November 1883. A bronze statue of James Marion Sims stands in Central Park, New York.

Turner, Henry (1892–1970): Professor of Medicine, Oklahoma University, USA. He described Turner's syndrome, (Ovarian dysgenesis 45XO) (*See* Dutta's Textbook of Gynecology, 7th Edition, p. 363). He became the doyen of clinical endocrinology in United States. He diagnosed his own lung cancer as inoperable. He worked until his death on 4th August, 1970.

Wertheim, Ernst (1864–1920): Gynecologist from Vienna. He described **Wertheim's operation (Radical hysterectomy)** in 1900 (*See* Dutta's Textbook of Gynecology, 7th Edition, p. 286, 501). He worked as assistant to Friedrich Schauta. Later on, he became the Professor of Gynecology.

Wertheim was an excellent sportsman particularly in skiing and skating. He died of influenza at 56 years of age.

Wolff, Kaspar (1733–1794): Professor of Anatomy and Physiology at St. Petersburg. He described Wolffian duct (mesonephric duct) in 1759 (*See* Dutta's Textbook of Gynecology, 7th Edition, p. 28).

Steptoe, Patrick Christopher (1913–1988), Edwards, Robert Geoffrey (Born 1925): Patrick Steptoe was a consultant Obstetrician and Gynecologist in the district hospital Oldham, Lancashire, England. World's first test tube baby, Louise Joy Brown was born in July 25, 1978. This was the culmination of 10 years collaborative research between **Patrick Steptoe** and **Robert Edwards** the two men residing 250 km apart. Bob Edwards was the geneticist and embryologist working at Cambridge. They faced criticism about the ethics. They worked against the hardship of fund and repeated failures to achieve implantation. Patrick Steptoe was a talented musician. After the retirement from the National Health Service (NHS), he worked at Bourn Hall to train others. He died on March 21, 1988 from prostate cancer. **Bob Edwards** was born in Yorkshire, England. He received PhD in animal genetics in Edinburgh. He conducted further research on induction of ovulation and IVF in animals. This knowledge, in fact, led Edwards to meet Steptoe as his clinical partner. In 1968, Edwards approached Steptoe at Royal Society of Medicine, London, where Steptoe presented his work on gynecological laparoscopy. Bob Edwards was appointed the Scientific Director of the Bourn Hall Clinic in 1980.

The revolution in reproductive medicine made by Steptoe and Edwards came following the years of tenacious endeavor with limited resources and in the face of opposition (*See* Dutta's Textbook of Gynecology, 7th Edition, p. 204).

Friedrich, Schauta (1849–1919) Radical vaginal hysterectomy: Schauta popularized the vaginal radical hysterectomy to reduce the operative mortality of abdominal procedure (*See* Dutta's Textbook of Gynecology, 7th Edition, p. 286). Schauta's technique was later modified by Alfred Amreich (1885–1972) to remove more pelvic connective tissues. This procedure is often known as **Schauta-Amreich operation**. He was head of the department in University of Vienna in 1891. Later on Schauta had disagreement with his assistant, Wertheim, who left him in 1897.

Chamberlen, Peter (1601–1683) Obstetric forceps: The modern obstetric forceps is the modification of original forceps designed by Chamberlen. Much had been written about the Chamberlen family (*See* Dutta's Textbook of Obstetrics, 8th Edition, p. 651, 754). William Chamberlen was a Huguenot Surgeon in Paris. He fled to England in 1569 due to religious persecution. He had two sons, Peter (elder) and Peter (younger). The son of Peter (younger) was also named Peter (1601–1683). He was known as Dr Peter as he received medical degrees from Padua, Oxford and Cambridge. Forceps were kept secret within the family for about a century. Four pairs of Chamberlen forceps are now on display at the RCOG, London.

Palmer, Raoul (1905–1985): Raoul Palmer used his technique of laparoscopy in gynecology in 1943. Besides laparoscopy, he was also a noted surgeon for his skills in tubal and vaginal surgery, 'Palmer's Point' in laparoscopic surgery goes by his name (*See* Dutta's Textbook of Gynecology, 7th Edition, p. 503, 508). He assisted Vivian Green-Armytage, while in Paris, in vaginal hysterectomy operation.

Pinard, Adolphe (1844–1934): Pinard was a great clinical teacher in Obstetrics during his time. He was the first to promote antenatal care and to establish the value of logical and systematic approach for abdominal palpation in pregnancy. His contributions in Obstetrics for the management of pregnancy and labor are many. Obstetric maneuvers—the external cephalic version, bringing down the extended leg in frank breech presentation, go by his name (Pinard's maneuvers). He is also remembered for the Pinard fetal stethoscope (*See* Dutta's Textbook of Obstetrics, 8th Edition, p. 757).

Pomeroy, Ralph Hayward (1867–1925): Ralph Pomery developed the simple procedure of tubal ligation which goes by his name 'Pomeroy tubal ligation'. It was not Ralph himself but two of his colleagues Dr Eliot Bishop and WF Nelms, presented his technique at the New York State Medical Society on June 1929, 4 years after his death. This method is accepted as a simple, safe and effective method all over world.

Spencer Wells, Thomas: History: Sir Spencer Wells Thomas (1818–1897) was a surgeon at the Samaritan Free Hospital for Women and Children, London (UK). He devised the clamp to place across the ovarian pedicles. He established himself as the most prolific ovariotomist of his era. In 1884, he was elected the President of Royal College of Surgeons (*See* Dutta's Textbook of Gynecology, 7th Edition, p. 530).

Index

Page numbers followed by f refer to figure, and t refer to table, respectively.

A

Abortion
  causes of 159
  midtrimester recurrent 49
  missed 49
  unsafe 454f
Abruptio placentae 10, 52
Abruption, placental 214, 227, 258, 287, 420
Acanthosis nigricans 323f
Acardius amorphus 248
Acidosis 506
  metabolic 503
Acquired immunodeficiency syndrome (AIDS) 212, 527
Adenine 442
Adenocarcinoma 135f
  serous 463
Adenomyosis 113, 114, 155, 348, 492
  treatment of 114
Adrenal disease 371
Adrenal disorders 116
Adrenal hyperplasia,
  cause of 171
  congenital 117f, 198, 571
Adrenogenital syndrome 117, 117f, 198
  congenital 176
Adult respiratory distress syndrome 258
Air embolism 444
Airway 277
Ambiguous genitalia 209
Amenorrhea 158, 552
  postpill 81
  primary 115, 116, 158, 165, 175
  secondary 118, 158, 169, 559
ACOG 293
American Society for Reproductive Medicine 393t
Amino acids 570
  placental transfer of 78
Amniocentesis 68, 75, 556, 575
Amnioinfusion 87, 511
  advantages of 512
Amniotic fluid 72, 79, 103
  embolism 451, 452
Analgesia, epidural 81
Anaphylaxis 458
Androgen 184
  insensitivity syndrome 117
  role of 397
Anemia 96, 280, 407, 407t
  aplastic 407
  classification of 407t, 408t
  deficiency of 407
  hemolytic 407, 532
  megaloblastic 82
  microcytic hypochromic 87, 408
  pre-existing 489
  pregnancy 407
  treatment of 410
  types of 409
Anesthesia 269
  general 578
Angiotensin
  converting enzyme 261, 552
  secretion of 570
  infusion test 6
  receptor-blocking drugs 261
Anorectal dysfunction 291
Anovulation 107
Antibiotic 225, 283
  prophylaxis, intrapartum 545
Anticoagulation therapy 426
Anticonvulsants 484
Antihypertensive drug 258, 260
  selection of 261
Antimuscarinic drugs 320
Antioxidant food supplement 384
Antiphospholipid antibody 302
  syndrome 299-301, 432
Antiretroviral therapy 557
Antithrombin deficiency 432
Antithyroid drugs 419, 420t
Antiviral therapy 537
Anuria 260

Aorta, bifurcation of 566
Aortic lymphadenectomy 146
Aortic root dissection 453
Aortocaval compression 458
Apheresis 442
Apoptosis 132
Appendicitis 56
Arrhythmias 456
    cardiac 426, 453
Arterial ligation, bilateral 34
Arteriovenous pseudoaneurysm formation 28
Artery
    pulmonary 453
    stenosis, pulmonary 532
    umbilical 50, 95, 569
Asherman's syndrome 192, 198
Aspiration pneumonitis 269
Assisted reproductive technology 121, 249, 389
    methods of 125
Assisted vaginal breech delivery 100
Asthenospermia 386
Atelectasis 456
Atenolol 261
Atosiban 227
Atresia 362
    cervical 185
Atrophic vaginitis 200
Atropine 568
Augmentation cystoplasty 321
Australian Carbohydrate Intolerance Study 231
Autoimmune hyperthyroidism 419
Autosomal chromosomal syndrome 215
Azithromycin 553
Azoospermia 384
    classification 384
    obstructive 386
    post-testicular 385
    pretesticular 384

B

Bacterial vaginosis 195, 301
Bacteriuria, asymptomatic 90
Banana sign 44*f*
Bandl's ring 56
Bariatric surgery 469-471
Barrier method 428
Bartholin's gland 186
Basal antral follicle count 381
Bicornuate uterus 553
    development of 569

Biguanides 234
Biopsy 351
    endometrial 593
    testicular 171
Biparietal diameter 77
Birth asphyxia 430
Blastocyst transfer 392
Blastomere size 393
Blood
    coagulation disorders 52
    components 441
        type of 441
    pressure 451
    tests 559
    transfusion 290, 416, 444
        arrangement of 268
    values 48, 280
Blueberry skin 532
Body
    mass index 592
    stalk anomaly 251
Bone mineral density 485, 557
Bonney's gynecological surgery 598
Bonney's myomectomy
    clamps 598
    screw 598
Bonney's test 598
Bony pelvis 97, 102
Botulinum toxin, injection of 321
Brace suture 26
Bradycardia 221
    fetal 17, 74
Brain metastasis 335
Breast 219, 280
    milk 241
Breastfeeding 37, 517-520
    higher rates of 290
Breech
    delivery 86
    presentation 43, 90
Broad-spectrum antibiotics 281, 484
Bromocriptine 173, 177
    therapy 177
Bronchopulmonary dysplasia 225
Burch colposuspension 204

C

Call-Exner bodies 214, 215
Cancer
    antigen 347
    cervical 171, 193, 476

cervix, management of 133*f*
testicular 333
vulval 166
Carcinoma 172
    cervix 131, 131*f*, 132-134, 141, 141*f*, 142, 146, 157, 163, 164, 183
        pathogenesis of 132
        treatment of 164
        type of 131
    endometrial 135, 136, 136*f*, 144, 149, 150, 154, 166, 194, 339*f*, 340, 466, 478, 479, 492
    fallopian tube 175
Cardiac failure, congestive 420
Cardiotocography 15, 16*f*, 18, 247, 509
    antenatal 86
Cardiovascular disease 262, 325, 333
Cataracts 531, 532
Ceftriaxone 553
Cell death 132
Cephalopelvic disproportion 14
Cerebellar signs 543
Cerebellum, abnormal 250
Cerebral palsy 225
Cerebrospinal fluid 43
Cervical
    cerclage 310, 312, 313
        operation, type of 311
    dilatation 20, 22
    ectopy 492
    fibroid 130
    incompetence 79, 302, 311
    insufficiency 310
    intraepithelial neoplasia 157, 166, 580
    stroma 341
    weakness 301
Cervix
    adenocarcinoma of 168
    carcinoma 82
    microinvasive carcinoma of 157
    squamous cell carcinoma of 141, 593
Cesarean
    delivery 36, 237*f*, 238, 246, 283*f*, 289, 291, 292, 429
    hysterectomy 81, 99
    on request 267
    perimortem 276
    section 267, 268*t*, 269, 290*t*, 457
Chemotherapy, prophylactic 49
Chest compression 277
Chickenpox 63, 67, 69, 590
    infection 530, 531
    neonatal 531

Chlamydia 525
Chocolate cyst 381
Cholelithiasis 414
Cholestasis
    intrahepatic 89
    obstetric 445
Chorioamnionitis 178, 227, 280
Choriocarcinoma 172, 206, 210, 334*f*, 335*f*
Chorionic villus sampling 99, 215, 216, 253, 556
Chorioretinitis 531
Choroid plexus cyst 250, 252
Chromosomal pattern, abnormal 116
Ciprofloxacin 553
Circulation, collateral 218*f*
Cloaca 179
Clomiphene citrate 159, 199
Clonus 260
Clostridial infection 282
Club feet 252
Coagulation profile, abnormal 283
Colposcopy 166
Confusion 260
Congenital infection 525*t*, 542, 543
    type of 525
Console 356
Contraception 62, 428, 480
    emergency 93
    method of 53, 62, 93, 213, 328
Convulsions 258
Coombs' test 55
Conservation, fertility 437
Cord
    compression 506
    umbilical 72, 242*f*, 252, 569
Corpus luteal insufficiency 156
Corpus luteum 154
    formation of 371
Cortical atrophy 531
Corticosteroid 422
    antenatal 225, 226
Couvelaire uterus, management of 52
Craniopharyngioma 196
Cryopreservation, method of 394
Cryptomenorrhea 115
    causes of 116
Cyanosis, acute 286
Cycloxygenase inhibitors 227
Cystadenoma, serous 217
Cystic fibrosis 573
    transmembrane regulator gene 385
Cystic hygroma 44, 214, 250, 252

Cystitis, interstitial 204
Cytology 202
Cytomegalovirus 525
   infection 53, 534
      congenital 535

D

Danazol 112, 496
   therapy 182
Darifenacin 320
Deep dyspareunia 110
   causes of 178
Deep vein thrombosis 80
Defibrillation 277
Dehydroepiandrosterone 373, 580
Detrusor muscle 564
Dextrose 442
Diabetes 17, 56, 280, 571
   mellitus 282, 301
      gestational 53, 88, 230, 233, 235, 238, 239, 325, 594
   severity of 446
Diabetic nephropathy 446
Diabetic retinopathy 446
Diaphragmatic hernia 251
Diarrhea 453, 532
Diastolic flow velocity waveform 506*f*
Diathermy 330, 332
Dichorionic placenta 243
Dichorionic twin 247, 522
   pregnancy 245
Diphtheria 518, 520
Distal tubal
   block 377
   intraepithelial carcinoma 463
Docking 355
Dominant follicle
   emergence of 362
   growth of 365
   selection of 371
Donor
   insemination 386
   oocyte 394
Doppler flow velocimetry 85
Douglas, semicircular fold of 598
Down's syndrome 94, 215
Drug therapy 321
Duodenal atresia 214, 251, 252
Dysfunctional uterine bleeding 158
Dysgerminoma 170, 217

Dysmenorrhea 561, 581
   intractable 113*f*
   primary 208
Dyspareunia 561
   causes of 119

E

Eclampsia 6, 76, 258, 259, 287, 420, 450, 458
Ectopic pregnancy 7, 7*f*, 79, 206, 287, 307, 331, 344, 345
Ectopy 177
Edema
   cerebral 455
   pulmonary 258, 260, 284, 288
Edwards' syndrome 251*f*
Electrocardiography 509
Elevated liver enzymes 263
Embolectomy 457
Embryo cryopreservation 394
Embryo transfer 122, 389
   number of 393*t*
   procedure 394
Embryonic urogenital structures 191
Encephalitis 543
Encephalopathy syndrome 5
Endocarditis, infective 453
Endometrial
   ablation methods 316
   cancer 149, 478
      surgical staging of 151
   carcinoma
      management of 341
      types of 135
   hyperplasia, types of 144
Endometrioma 129
Endometriosis 110, 111, 129, 182, 207, 497
   complication of 111
   pelvic 110-112, 177, 376, 497
   sites of 110
   treatment of 217
Endometrium
   adenocarcinoma of 135, 593
   carcinoma of 135, 339
   transcervical resection of 200, 316*f*
Epididymal sperm aspiration 386
Epilepsy 65, 450
Episiotomy 64
Epithelial ovarian cancer 140, 217
Epithelium and organ, type of 201
Erb's palsy 86
Erythropoiesis, fetal 72

Escherichia coli 525
Esophageal atresia 214
Estrogen 151
    dominant follicular microenvironment 365
Estrogenic stimulation 150

F

Facial
    clefts 250
    hair, growth of 579
    nerve splits 567
Falciparum malaria 556
Fallopian tube 186, 212, 329*f*
    cancer 492
Female genital organs
    cancer of 206
    development of 184
Femoral
    artery catheterization 488*f*
    triangle 208
    vein 457
Fertility 197, 470
    conservation 473
Fetal
    abnormalities 250
    anomalies 506
    biophysical profile 439
    bradycardia, causes of 17
    chromosomal abnormalities 301, 302, 521
    circulation 87, 102
    congenital malformations 40
    consequences 542
    death 248
    distress, management of 85
    ECG 509
    growth restriction 258, 415
    heart rate abnormalities, causes of 221
    heart rate, variability 505
        acceleration 507
        sinusoidal pattern 507
    hypoxia, grades of 503
    infection 543
    loss, recurrent 304
    malformations 246, 436
    monitoring 67
        intrapartum 503
    movements 15*f*
    physiology 84
    reduction 249
    sleep 506
    spine anterior or posterior 435
    squamous cells 453
    termination 249
    testis 176
    thyroid dysfunction 422
Fetoplacental circulation 503
Fetus
    oxygen consumption of 568
    papyraceus 38
    ultrasonography of 44*f*
Fever 453
Fibroid 195, 492
    red degeneration of 54
    uterus 315*f*
        multiple 148
FIGO grading system 339
Fimbrioplasty, laparoscopic 125*f*
Fistula 291
Fitz-Hugh-Curtis syndrome 167
Folic acid
    deficiency 63
    prepregnancy 42
    supplementation of 42
Follicle stimulating hormone 197, 363, 366
Follicular
    androgens, role of 398
    atresia 361
    growth 361, 362, 364, 390
        monitoring of 121
    luteinization, premature 390
    maturation 362
Folliculogenesis 361, 398
Forceps delivery 64
    types of 102
Fresh frozen plasma 441, 443
Friction rub 456
Frozen embryo transfer 394
Furosemide therapy, hazards of 76

G

Galactorrhea 157, 371
Gamete intrafallopian transfer 181, 389
Ganciclovir 564
Gastrointestinal tract 276
Gastroschisis 214
Genital
    malignancy 173
    organs 167
        development of 187, 209, 210
    sepsis 453*t*
    tract, developmental defect of 116

tuberculosis 155, 160, 177, 182, 190, 301
warts 564
Genitalia
  external 180, 187
  internal 116
Genuine stress incontinence 192, 204
Germ cell 46
  migration 361
  tumor 212, 217
    malignant 217
Gestational diabetes, development of 560
Gestrinone 496
Gland
  adrenal 170
  endometrial 180
Glomerular filtration rate 90
Glucagon 553
Glucocorticoids, antenatal administration of 225
Glucose tolerance test 73, 239
Glycosuria 560
Golgi apparatus 570
Gonadotropin 169, 197, 375
  releasing hormone 198
    analog 316
    use of 388
  stimulation 388, 391, 396
  therapy 120
Gonads, development of 170, 209
Gonorrhea 525
Granulosa cells 154, 197
  luteinization of 365
  proliferation of 364
  tumor 165, 210
Graves' disease 418, 419
Gravid uterus 272*f*

H

Harmonic scalpel 353
Headache 260
Heart
  block, fetal 506
  disease 53, 82, 425
    congenital 74, 453, 532
    organic 53
    rheumatic 453
  rate 451
    fetal 505, 594
HELLP syndrome 3, 4, 50, 79, 260, 263-265, 287
  classification of 263
  management of 264
  maternal complications of 264

Hematocolpos 123
Hematoma formation 457
Hematometra 187
Hematosalpinx, causes of 168
Hemoglobin, fetal 100, 101, 553
Hemoglobinopathy 411
Hemolysis 263
Hemopoiesis 67
Hemorrhage 27, 427
  atonic postpartum 588
  cerebral 5
  cerebrovascular 258
  intraventricular 225
  life-threatening 457
  obstetric 99
  postpartum 29, 58, 73, 238, 287, 289, 487, 556
  retroplacental 214
Hemotherapy 265
Heparin
  therapy 305
  unfractionated 240, 305, 433
Hepatitis
  A 518, 520
  B surface antigen 536
  B virus infection 539
    chronic 536, 538
    transmission of 536
  viruses 525
Herpes
  genitalis 181
    infection 190
  virus 564
High grade serous ovarian cancers 464, 464*t*
History, Obstetrics and Gynecology 597
Hobnail cells 215
Hormonal hypothesis 463
Hormone replacement therapy 144, 203, 579
  postmenopausal 203
Human
  chorionic gonadotropin 47, 98, 347, 580
  growth hormone, role of 398
  immunodeficiency virus (HIV) 58, 65, 103, 525, 527
    infection 83, 527
    treatment of 60
  papillomavirus 564
    testing 132
    vaccines 519
  placental lactogen 78, 347
  semen volume contribution 205
  seminal fluid 191

Hybrid 348
Hydatidiform mole 49, 60, 126, 126*f*, 334, 335, 557
Hydramnios 50
Hydration, maternal 511
Hydrocephalus 5, 43, 251
Hydropic villi 563
Hydrops, fetal 214, 252
Hydrosalpinx 122
Hyperandrogenemia 109
Hyperandrogenism 107, 109
Hyperbilirubinemia 283
Hyperemesis gravidarum 48, 89
Hypergonadotropic hypogonadism 116, 371, 372
Hyperhomocysteinemia 304
Hyperinsulinemia 109, 178, 301
Hyperplasia 171, 348
    adrenal 174
    endometrial 150, 492
Hyperprolactinemia 371
Hypertension 51, 261, 262, 594
    diastolic 259
    gestational 51
    maternal 17
    pulmonary 414
    systolic 259
Hypertensive crisis 261
Hypertensive disorders 287
Hyperthyroid state, control of 421
Hyperthyroidism 205, 371, 419, 569
    causes of 418, 419
    complications of 420*t*
    fetal 422
    gestational 419
    management of 420
    neonatal 422
Hypogastric artery 34*f*
    bilateral ligation of 218
    close origin, ligation of 34*f*
    ligation 30, 31
        rationale of 31
Hypoglycemia 430, 572
Hypogonadotropic hypogonadism 116, 371
Hypotension 283, 456, 565
Hypothalamic pituitary
    dysfunction 371, 373
    failure 371
Hypothermia 284, 444, 450
Hypothyroidism 371, 423, 423*f*
    complications of 424
    management of 423
    primary 423
Hypovolemia 450
Hypoxia 450, 453, 503, 504, 506, 510
Hysterectomy 144, 146, 148, 157, 163, 200, 273, 289, 291, 317, 318
    abdominal 163, 341, 579, 580, 592
    advantages of 49
    indications of 317, 479
    laparoscopic 466
    peripartum 290
    radical 141, 163, 599
    route of 317
    type of 132
Hysterosalpingogram 124*f*
Hysteroscopic myomectomy 316*f*
Hysteroscopy 162, 315, 494
    advantages of 494

I

Idiopathic thrombocytopenic purpura 492
Iliac artery
    bilateral ligation of 588
    internal 186, 187
    ligation, internal 33
        steps 33
Immunization 517
In vitro fertilization 389
    embryo transfer 121
    insemination 392
Infections, perinatal 525
Infertility 120, 124, 156, 385
    anovulatory 120*f*
    causes of 111
    duration of 381
    female 156, 370
    male 196, 383, 384, 386
    unexplained 368, 379, 386
Influenza 518, 520
    virus 525
Inguinal
    canal 208
    ligament 567
    lymph nodes 593
Inherited cancers 152
Injectable contraceptive steroids 93
Internal iliac artery
    bilateral ligation of 92, 217
    ligation 31, 32, 33*f*, 92, 163
        indications of 31
Interventional radiology 487
Intracytoplasmic sperm injection 386, 389
    procedure 386*f*
    intralipid 457

Intrauterine
  contraceptive devices 213, 428, 480
  fetal death 258
  gestation sac 562
  growth restriction 17, 227, 246, 250
  insemination 385, 389
    indications of 121
Invasive carcinoma cervix 132, 182
  development of 161
Iron
  absorption 408, 409
  deficiency 74
    anemia 52, 408
Ischemic heart disease 238
Isosexual precocious puberty, causes of 181
Isoxsuprine therapy 74

J

Japanese encephalitis 518
Jarisch-Herxheimer reaction 565
Jaundice 286, 532
Joel-Cohen incision 269
  advantages of 270

K

Kallmann's syndrome 197
Klinefelter's syndrome 385
Kroener technique 329
Krukenberg tumor 156

L

Labetalol 261
Labia majora 208, 567
Labia minora 208
Labor
  active management of 81
  augmentation of 22
  management of 20, 22
  nonprogress of 13
  normal 48
  preterm 90, 304, 415, 420
  progress of 94
  second stage of 95, 98
  slow progress of 13
  third stage of 99
Lactation 62, 85, 92
  failure 238
Laparoscopy 183, 378

Laser energy 353
Leg ulcers 414
Leiomyoma 348
  subclassification of 348
Lemon sign 44*f*
Leptin 372
Leukemia 492
Levator ani 186
Levonorgestrel intrauterine system 66, 93, 314
Leydig cells 384
Ligation, techniques of 32
Limb hypoplasia 531
Listeria monocytogenes 525
Listeriosis 76, 540
Live vaccines 518
Liver
  disease 495
  functions of 220
  tenderness 260
Low grade serous ovarian cancers 464, 464*t*
Lugol's iodine solution 422
Lung 280
  disease, chronic 225
  fetal 101
  maturation, fetal 96, 431
Lupus anticoagulant 68
Luteal phase
  defect 199, 381
  pregnancy 330, 331
Lutein cyst 155, 175
Luteinized unruptured follicle syndrome 380
Luteinizing hormone 197, 363, 366
  releasing hormone 366
Lymph node 163
  dissection 140
  pelvic 157, 467
Lymphadenectomy, para-aortic 340, 341
Lymphadenectomy, pelvic 141

M

Macrosomia 238
Madlener technique 329
Magpie trial 260
Magnetic Resonance Imaging 4, 455
Management
  NRFS 511
Malaria 79, 525
Male contraception, permanent method of 486
Malignancy index 138, 558
Mass, abdominal 593

Massive proteinuria 260
Maternal
   age, advanced 301
   blood pressure 22
   death 258
      causes of 259
   immunoglobulins 419
   medical complications 435
   morbidity 285, 291
   near miss 285
   request 289
   serum alpha fetoprotein 78, 255
Mayer-Rokitansky-Kuster-Hauser syndrome 116
McCune-Albright syndrome 209
McDonald's operation 311
Measles 525
Meconium 512
   stained amniotic fluid 17
Mefenamic acid 579
Meigs syndrome 217
Membranes
   preterm rupture of 74
   prolonged rupture of 280
Meningoencephalitis 532
Menopausal symptoms 168
Menopause 144, 169, 203
Menorrhagia 113*f*, 561, 593
   cause of 157
Menstrual abnormality 107
Menstrual bleeding 189
   heavy 314, 315, 315*f*, 580
Menstrual cycle 154, 316, 361, 364
   normal 196, 207, 209
Menstrual period 560
Menstruation 371
   cessation of 118
Mental retardation 532
Mesosalpinx 180
Metabolic disorders 116
Metaplastic epithelium 132
Metformin 234, 325, 374
   dose schedule of 325
   therapy 167, 324, 325
Methicillin-resistant *Staphylococcus aureus* 281
Methimazole 420
Methotrexate 308, 346
Methyldopa 261
Methylenetetrahydrofolate reductase 432
Micrognathia 250
Microphthalmia 531, 532
Midtrimester fetal loss, recurrent 310

Mifepristone 201
Miscarriage 238, 299, 300, 415, 420, 499
   first trimester 48
   midtrimester 49
   recurrent 96, 299-301, 305, 306, 325
Mitral valve replacement 425*f*
Molar pregnancy 49
Monochorionic monoamniotic twin
   pregnancy 249
Monochorionic twin 243, 245, 247, 522
   pregnancy 242, 244, 246
      placenta of 242*f*
Monosomy 250
Monozygosity 50
Monozygotic twin 50
   pregnancy 83
   type of 50
Mortality index 288
Mucus debris 376
Müllerian duct 160, 213
Multilocular cyst 558
Multiple pregnancy, management of 38
Muscles 282
Mycobacterium tuberculosis 589
Myocardial infarction 453
Myomas
   enucleation of 352*f*
   interstitial 379
   submucosal 379
Myomectomy 173, 317, 318
   laparoscopic 352*f*, 353
Myometrial invasion 150
   depth of 340
Myopia 532

N

Nasal bone 252
Natural killer cells 302
Nausea 587
Neck lipoma 251
Necrotizing enterocolitis 225
Necrotizing fasciitis 281, 282, 283*f*
Neisseria gonorrhoeae 553
Neoadjuvant chemotherapy 140
Neonatal
   chickenpox, complications of 531
   death 238
   infections 525
   intensive care unit 290
Nephritis, chronic 82

Neural tube defect 40, 41, 214, 250, 252, 304
Newborn care 96
Nifedipine 227, 228
Nitroglycerine 227
Nitroprusside 261
No scalpel vasectomy 331, 332*f*
Nonhysterectomy surgery 316
Nonimmune hydrops fetalis, causes of 76
Nonnucleoside reverse transcriptase inhibitors 484
Nonovulatory cycle 366
Non-reassuring fetal status, management of 511
Nonsteroidal antiinflammatory drugs 316
Nonstress test 15, 15*f*
   abnormal 18*f*
Norethisterone 316
Nuchal translucency 243, 251, 253, 255
Nucleoside reverse transcriptase inhibitors 484

O

Obesity 109, 237, 238, 282, 371, 432, 435, 469, 470
   classification of 238
   complications of 469
   management of 470
   maternal 522
   prevalence of 238
Obstetric shock, causes of 450, 451*f*
Obstructed labor, management of 58
Obturator nerve, root value of 567
Ocular toxoplasmosis 542
Oligoasthenoteratozoospermia syndrome 188
Oligohydramnios 214, 244, 250
Oligospermia 386
Oliguria 260, 286
Omphalocele 214
Oocytes
   cryopreservation 394, 474
   meiosis, complication of 365
   primary 361
Oophorectomy 148, 317, 318
   bilateral 148
Oral
   biguanide 374
   contraceptive, combined 80, 316, 482
   progestogen 318
Organ transplantation 534
Osteomyelitis 415
Osteoporosis 144, 199, 220, 305, 557
   postmenopausal 202
Ovarian
   cancer 138, 140, 148, 179, 189, 152, 463, 474, 475
      management of 140

   carcinoma
      pathogenesis of 463
      type of 463
   cycle, physiology of 371
   cyst 380, 579
   drilling 326
      laparoscopic 162, 170, 213
   dysfunction 111, 497
   electrodiathermy 326
   factors 118
   failure, premature 199, 371
   follicular 205
   fossa 184
   hyperstimulation syndrome 122
   insufficiency 373
      premature 372
   ligament 201
   malignancy 473
      algorithm 138
      primary 169
   mass 592
   pregnancy 69
   reserve 372
   stimulation 380, 388, 391, 498
   structures 186
   tissue cryopreservation 474
   transposition 474, 476
   tumor 172, 202, 217
      malignant 473
      occurrence of 217
Ovary 173, 211
   carcinoma of 138
   development of 187
   epithelial tumors of 217
   feminizing tumors of 214
   follicular cysts of 155
   hormone producing tumors of 214
   neoplasms of 194
   virilizing tumors of 213
Ovulation 159, 193, 209, 361, 365, 371
   causes of 172
   endocrine control of 361, 363
   failure of 366
   induction of 109, 120, 199
   physiology of 361
Ovulatory disorders 120, 370, 371
   classification of 371
   management of 371
Ovulatory dysfunction 370
Oxygen deficiency 503
Oxytocin 85, 98, 425, 554
   infusion 60, 511

P

Paget's disease 176, 192
Pain 260, 578
    abdominal 552, 558, 587
    epigastric 260
    pelvic 110, 119, 291, 561
    testicular 333
Painful crisis, acute 417
Palpation 406
Papilledema 260
Paralytic ileus 284
Paraovarian cyst 160
Partial mole, triploid chromosomal pattern of 128*f*
Parvovirus 525
    B19 infection 251
Paternal age, advanced 301
Pelvic
    endometriosis, treatment of 111
    floor muscle exercise 320
    infection 201, 492
    inflammatory disease, acute 189
    ureter, female 186
Pelvis 91
    diameters of 555
    normal 48
    ultrasonography of 108*f*
Percutaneous epididymal sperm aspiration 386
Perinatal
    death, cause of 65
    infections, congenital 525, 526
Peritoneal adenocarcinoma, primary 181
Persistent
    anticardiolipin antibodies 432
    ectopic pregnancy 309
    lupus anticoagulant 432
    trophoblasts 309
Pertussis 518
Phimotic ostium 125
Phosphate 442
Pictorial blood loss chart 314
Pituitary gland, posterior 554
Pituitary tumor 371
Placenta accreta 67, 161, 291
    management of 274
Placenta previa 10, 11, 51, 271, 273, 287, 290
    accreta 271, 273
        management of 272, 273
Placenta, hemangiomas of 214
Plasma 441
    bilirubin 283

Plasmodium vivax 589
Platelet count 260, 283
Pleuritic chest pain 456
Pneumonia 430
Pneumonitis 532
Pneumoperitoneum 183, 185
Poliomyelitis 518
Polycystic
    kidney disease 214
    ovarian
        disease 599
        syndrome 107, 167, 169, 195, 301, 323-325, 371, 492, 521
Polyhydramnios 244, 250
Polyp 348
Polysaccharide 518
Pomeroy's method 161, 329*f*
Postcoital bleeding 593
Posterior reversible encephalopathy syndrome 4*f*
Postmaturity syndrome 80
Postmenopausal bleeding 135, 149, 593
    causes of 119, 144
Post-tubal sterilization syndrome 331
Pouch of Douglas 598
Pre-eclampsia 3, 6, 75, 227, 238, 258, 260, 287, 415, 420, 454, 455
    severe 258, 261
Pregnancy 68, 75, 76, 79, 82, 88, 103, 237, 492
    abdominal 68
    associated plasma protein 255, 347
    first trimester of 68, 84
    loss 216
    medical termination of 72, 80
    multiple 38, 214, 228, 522
    normal 90, 98
    termination of 259, 499
    test 562
    unknown location 343
Premature ovarian
    failure, causes of 158
    insufficiency, causes of 372
Premenstrual syndrome 199
Prenatal genetic screening tests 255*t*
Preterm labor, prevention of 226, 228
Primordial follicles, development of 362
Procidentia, urinary symptoms of 164
Progesterone 62, 102, 344
    secretion of 365
Progestin
    only contraception 485
    therapy 479

Prolactinomas 196
Propylthiouracil 420
Prostaglandins 60
Prostate cancer 333
Prosthetic heart valves, type of 426
Protein C deficiency 432
Proton pump inhibitors 269
Proximal tubal block 376
Psammoma bodies 215
Pseudohermaphroditism, male 198
Pseudoprecocious, causes of 184
Puberty 175, 184, 361
   delayed 220
   precocious 172, 197, 588
   pseudoprecocious 183
Pubic hair distribution, male pattern of 323*f*
Pudendal nerve 185, 219
Puerperal foot drop 59
Puerperal psychosis 577
Puerperal pyrexia 37, 279
Puerperal sepsis 279, 280, 283, 577
   management of 281*t*
   pathogenesis of 280
   treatment of 279
Pulse rates 456
Pyelectasis 252
Pyometra 174
Pyosalpinx 124
Pyrexia, postpartum 577

Q

Quad screen 253, 254
Quintero system of classification 245

R

Rabies 518, 520
Radiation therapy 282, 341
Radical vaginal trachelectomy, laparoscopic
   assisted 146
Radiolucent bone disease 532
Radiotherapy, advantages of 131
Rectovaginal fistula 162
Rectus muscle 268
   suturing 268
Rectus sheath 268
Reinke's crystal 215
Renal agenesis 214
Renal dysfunction 414, 495
Renal papillary necrosis 415
Reproductive organs, male 384

Reserve
   ovarian 372
Respiratory distress syndrome 225, 430
Resuscitation
   cardiopulmonary 277
   neonatal 85
Retinal disease 414
Retinopathy 225, 446
   pigmentary 532
Retraction ring 56
Rhesus-antigen 55
Robertsonian translocation 302
Robotic assisted laparoscopic hysterectomy 466
Robotic surgery 355, 466
   advantages of 356
   complications of 357
   disadvantages of 357
Robotic technology 355
Rocker bottom feet 250, 252
Roll over test 6
Rosiglitazone 374
Round ligament 185, 211
Routine nodal dissection 467
Rubella 525, 532
   infection 70, 532, 533
      maternal 216
   syndrome, congenital 216
Rupture uterus, surgical treatment of 59
Ruptured tubal ectopic pregnancy, management
   of 103
Rutledge's classification 132

S

Sacral nerve stimulation 321
Sacrococcygeal teratoma 214
Sacrosciatic notch 70
Saline infusion sonography 315, 491
Salpingectomy, prophylactic 463
Salpingitis 167
   tuberculous 155, 376
Salpingo-oophorectomy 463
   bilateral 341, 579, 592
Sarcoma botryoides 194
Scar
   endometriosis 113
   rupture 290
Schauta-Amreich operation 600
Schiller-Duval body 215

Sclerosis, tuberous 258*f*
Seizures 450
Semen analysis 384
Sensorineural deafness 532
Sepsis 288, 453
    resuscitation bundle 454
SERMs 183
Sertoli cells 384
Serum AFP 214
Serum anti-Müllerian hormone 373
Severe pre-eclampsia, complications of 258
Sex cord stromal tumors 175
Sexual dysfunction, male 367
SHBG 196
Sheehan's syndrome 167
Shirodkar's operation 311
Shock 101, 221, 286, 288
    index 29
    hemorrhagic 450
    non hemorrhagic 450, 458, 459
    obstetric 450
Shoulder dystocia 58, 88, 231
Sickle cell
    anemia 53, 559
    disease 74, 414
    hemoglobinopathy 417
    trait 415
Signet ring cells 215
Sims' Huhner postcoital test 599
Sims' position 599
Sims' speculum 599
Sims' wire 599
Sinusoidal patterns 15, 19, 507, 508
Skin 280
    incision 268, 270
    rash 453
    scarring 531
    suture 268
Sling procedures, complications of 162
Sodium
    citrate 442
    valproate 576
Soft tissue 280
Solifenacin 320
Spasmodic dysmenorrhea, primary 169
Sperm
    aspiration, testicular 386
    extraction, testicular 386
    recovery, methods of 386
    transfer 389
Spermatogenesis 205

Spiegelberg's criteria 69
Squamocolumnar junction 132
Stein-Leventhal syndrome 174, 599
Sterilization 161, 376, 428
    electrocoagulation, laparoscopic 213
    female 193, 327, 328, 329*f*
    laparoscopic method of 330
    male 327, 328
    method of 331
    transcervical 486
    voluntary 332
Steroid therapy 265
Stillbirth 238
Stress urinary incontinence 203, 319, 321
Stroke 286
Struma ovarii 215
Subcapsular liver hematoma 258, 260
Subcutaneous tissue, closure of 270
Sulfonylureas 233
Superficial inguinal glands 185
Surgery over radiotherapy, advantages of 133
Surgical site infection
    classification of 489
    prevention of 490
Surrogacy 400
    full 400
    gestational 400, 401
    host 400
    IVF 400
    natural 400
    partial 400
Symphysiotomy 64
Symphysis pubis 587
Syphilis 525
Systemic lupus erythematosus 95, 432

T

Tachycardia 17, 221, 456, 506, 577
    fetal 17
Tachypnea 456
    transient 430
Tamoxifen 494
Tamponade 450
Tension-free vaginal tape 162
Tension pneumothorax 450
Teratospermia 386
Testicular feminization syndrome 117*f*, 161, 166
Testing, perinatal 521
Testis, function of 190
Tetanus 518, 520
Tetracycline 553

Thalassemia 82
    treatment of 53
Thanato dysplasia 251
Theca cell tumor 175
Theca lutein cyst 157
Thiazolidinediones 234, 374
Third generation robotic system 357
Thrombocytopenia 75, 263, 283, 288, 305, 492
Thromboembolism 238, 289, 450
Thrombophilia 89, 300, 304
    acquired 432
Thrombophilic syndrome 374
Thromboprophylaxis 270, 432, 456
Thrombosis, microvascular 282
Thrombotic thrombocytopenic purpura 532
Thyroid
    disease 422
    disorders 116
    dysfunction 301, 371, 418, 492, 495
        neonatal 422
        postpartum 424
    function 206, 221, 418
        tests 418f
    gland 570
Thyroid hormones 220
Thyroiditis
    chronic 418
    postpartum 423
Thyrotoxicosis 83, 172, 420
    gestational 419
Tocolysis, rational use of 226
Tocolytic drugs 228, 511
Tolterodine 320
Tonic-clonic epilepsy 576
Toxic shock syndrome 206
Toxoplasma 525
Toxoplasmosis 542-544
    complications of 543
Trachelectomy, radical 147
Tranexamic acid 316, 317, 496, 563
Transabdominal infraumbilical route 32
Transvaginal sonography 347, 491
Treponema pallidum 589
Trisomy 215, 250
    21, screening of 256
Trophoblast 453
    cells 97
    membranes 305
Trophoblastic disease, gestational 50, 205, 334

Tubal
    block 376
    dysfunction 111, 497
    ectopic pregnancy 8f, 9, 211, 307, 308
    endometriosis 376
    occlusion
        method of 330
        timing of 330
    patency tests 376
    polyps 376
    reconstructive surgery, contraindications
        of 179
    sterilization 213, 328, 330, 377
        failure of 330
        laparoscopic method of 330
        procedure 170
        reversal of 170
    surgery 376, 377
        advantages of 377
        disadvantages of 377
Tubectomy 428
Tuberculosis 82, 116
Tubo-ovarian mass 492
Tumor
    adrenal 171
    endometrial 136f
    grades of 340
    marker 138
    necrosis factor 347
    size 340
Turner's syndrome 116, 178, 201, 209
Twin
    placenta of 71
    pregnancy 51, 61, 246, 337f, 558
Twin-to-twin transfusion syndrome 38, 243-245
    management of 242
Typhoid 518, 520

U

Uchida technique 329
Ultrasonography 90, 126f, 249, 347
Ultrasound 315
    Doppler study 247
Umbilical artery
    doppler evaluation of 506f
    flow velocimetry of 87
Umbilical cord clamping, timing of 96
Unruptured tubal ectopic pregnancy 49, 91, 309

Ureter
  accidental injury of 161
  pelvic 184
Urethral competence, tests of 321
Urge urinary incontinence 204, 319
Urinary
  bladder 219
  diversion 321
  fistula 203
  frequency 587
  incontinence 204, 289, 319
    management of 321
  tract 280
    infections 415
Urodynamic stress incontinence 162, 164, 176
Urogenital sinus 180
Uterine
  anomalies 305
  arteriovenous malformations 27
    causes of 492
  artery 141*f*, 211
    Doppler velocimetry of 6*f*
    embolization 28, 190, 487, 488*f*
    flow velocity waveform of 6*f*
    ligation 30, 30*f*
  bleeding, abnormal 152, 331, 348, 491
  compression sutures 30
  contractions 21
  devascularization 30
  fibroids 169
    treatment of 190
  fundus 594
  incision 268
    extension of 270
  malformations, congenital 301
  sarcoma 203, 492
  synechiae 171, 379
  vascular malformations 27
Utero-ovarian vessels 30*f*
  ligation 30
Uterus 350*f*
  congenital malformation of 174
  primary carcinoma body of 166
  rupture of 287, 289, 290
  sarcoma of 173

V

Vagina 212
  agenesis of 159
  carcinoma of 206
  clear cell carcinoma of 166
  complete absence of 115*f*
  development of 203
Vaginal
  agenesis, congenital 159
  birth 36, 99, 292
  bleeding 587
  breech delivery 292
  delivery 68, 87, 246, 566, 577
    traumatic 280
  discharge 453
  hysterectomy 466, 593
    laparoscopic assisted 466
  route misoprostol 499
  spotting 552, 587
  swab 553
  trachelectomy 477
    radical 476
Vaginitis 196
Valves, type of 426
Varicella 520
  syndrome, congenital 531
  zoster virus 525
    infection 530
Vas occlusion, methods of 332
Vasa previa 11, 271, 274
Vascular endothelial growth factor 347
Vasectomy 327, 331, 333, 428, 486
  failure of 333
  methods of 331
  operation 64
  over tubectomy, advantages of 486
Ventouse 78
Vesicovaginal fistula 174
  combined 162
Villi, deeper penetration of 47
Villus sampling, chronic 255
Viral
  hepatitis 536
  infections 191, 533
  transmission 537
Vomiting 75, 260, 453, 587
von-Willebrand disease 492
Vulva 187
  squamous cell carcinoma of 593
Vulval pain, causes of 202
Vulvar intraepithelial neoplasia 211
Vulvodynia 207

W

Weight gain, excessive 371
Weight loss, excessive 371
Wertheim's operation 599
Wolffian duct 180
Wound infections 238
Wurm's operation 311

Y

Y chromosome, microdeletions of 385
Yellow fever 518

Z

Zygote intrafallopian transfer 389